Pediatric Hand Therapy

Pediatric Hand Therapy

Edited by

JOSHUA M. ABZUG, MD
Associate Professor
Departments of Orthopedics and Pediatrics
University of Maryland School of Medicine

Director
University of Maryland Brachial Plexus Practice
Director of Pediatric Orthopedics
University of Maryland Medical Center
Deputy Surgeon-in-Chief
University of Maryland Children's Hospital
Baltimore, MD, United States

SCOTT H. KOZIN, MD
Clinical Professor
Orthopaedic Surgery
Lewis Katz School of Medicine at Temple University
Philadelphia, PA, United States

Clinical Professor
Orthopaedic Surgery
Sidney Kimmel Medical College at Thomas Jefferson University
Philadelphia, PA, United States

Chief of Staff
Shriners Hospital for Children
Philadelphia, PA, United States

REBECCA NEIDUSKI, PHD, OTR/L, CHT
Dean of the School of Health Sciences
School of Health Sciences
Elon University
North Carolina
United States

ELSEVIER

Publisher: Cathleen Sether
Acquisition Editor: Kayla Wolfe
Editorial Project Manager: Sandra Harron
Production Project Manager: Sreejith Viswanathan
Cover Designer: Alan Studholme

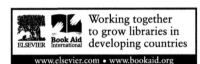

Working together
to grow libraries in
developing countries

www.elsevier.com • www.bookaid.org

List of Contributors

Joshua M. Abzug, MD
Associate Professor
Departments of Orthopedics and Pediatrics
University of Maryland School of Medicine
Director
University of Maryland Brachial Plexus Practice
Director of Pediatric Orthopedics
University of Maryland Medical Center
Deputy Surgeon-in-Chief
University of Maryland Children's Hospital
Baltimore, MD, United States

Allison Allgier, OTD, OTR/L
Cincinnati Children's Hospital
Cincinnati, OH, United States
Clinical Program Manager
Occupational and Physical Therapy
Cincinnati Children's
Cincinnati, OH, United States

Sarah Ashworth, OTR/L, BS
Occupational Therapist
Rehabilitation Services
Shriners Hospital for Children
Philadelphia, PA, United States

Jamie Berggren, OTR/L, BS
Division of Pediatric Rehabilitation Medicine
Occupational Therapist
Children's Hospital Los Angeles
Los Angeles, CA, United States

Matthew B. Burn, MD
Hand Fellow
Hand & Upper Limb Fellowship
Stanford University
Redwood City, CA, United States

Alexandria L. Case, BSE
Research Coordinator
Department of Orthopedics
University of Maryland School of Medicine
Baltimore, MD, United States
Department of Orthopaedics
University of Maryland
Baltimore, MD, United States

Jennifer M. Chan, OTR/L, CHT
Hand Therapist
Rehabilitation Therapy
Lucile Packard Children's Hospital
Palo Alto, CA, United States

Roger Cornwall, MD
Cincinnati Children's Hospital
Cincinnati, OH, United States
Professor
Orthopaedic Surgery and Developmental Biology
Cincinnati Children's Hospital
Cincinnati, OH, United States

Jenny M. Dorich, MBA, OTR/L, CHT
Occupational Therapist III
Adjunct Faculty
Cincinnati Children's Hospital Medical Center
Univeristy of Cincinnati College of Health Sciences
Cincinnati, OH, United States

Reeti R. Douglas, OTD, OTR/L
Texas Scottish Rite Hospital for Children
Dallas, TX, United States

Kelly Anne Ferry, MOTR/L
Rick Gardner FRCS (Trauma & Orthopaedics)
CURE Ethiopia Children's Hospital
Addis Ababa, Ethiopia

Theodore J. Ganley, MD
Director of Sports Medicine at the Children's Hospital
    of Philadelphia
Professor of Orthopaedic Surgery at the University of
    Pennsylvania
Associate Professor of Orthopaedic Surgery
Director of Sports Medicine
Division of Orthopaedic Surgery
Children's Hospital of Philadelphia
Philadelphia, PA, United States

Richard Gardner, FRCS
CURE Ethiopia Children's Hospital
Addis Ababa, Ethiopia

Ritu Goel, MS, OTR/L
Occupational Therapist
Department of Orthopaedics
University of Maryland School of Medicine
Baltimore, MD, United States

Donald Goldsmith, MD
Professor
Pediatrics
Drexel University College of Medicine
Philadelphia, PA, United States

Director
Section of Rheumatology
St Christopher's Hospital for Children
Philadelphia, PA, United States

Namrata Grampurohit, PhD, OTR/L
Assistant Professor
Department of Occupational Therapy
Jefferson College of Rehabilitation Sciences
Thomas Jefferson University
Philadelphia, PA, United States

Elliot Greenberg, PT, DPT, PhD
Board Certified Specialist in Orthopaedic Physical
    Therapy
Sports Medicine & Performance Center
The Children's Hospital of Philadelphia Care Network,
    Pediatric & Adolescent Specialty Care
Bucks County
Clinical Specialist / Research Scientist
Sports Medicine Physical Therapy
Philadelphia, PA, United States

Christine A. Ho, MD
Staff Orthopaedist
Dept of Orthopaedics
Texas Scottish Rite Hospital for Children
Dallas, TX, United States

Division Director
Department of Pediatric Orthopaedics
Children's Health Dallas
Dallas, TX, United States

Associate Professor
Department of Orthopaedics
University of Texas Southwestern Medical School
Dallas, TX, United States

Danielle A. Hogarth, BS
Department of Orthopaedics
University of Maryland
Baltimore, MD, United States

Research Coordinator
Orthopaedics
University of Maryland School of Medicine
Batlimore, MD, United States

Deborah Humpl, OTR/L
Children's Hospital of Philadelphia
Department of Occupational Therapy
Philadelphia, PA, United States

Clinical Specialist Outpatient Occupational Therapy
Occupational Therapy Department
Children's Hospital of Philadelphia
Philadelphia, PA, United States

Gina Kim, MA, OTR/L
Division of Pediatric Rehabilitation Medicine
Occupational Therapist
Children's Hospital Los Angeles
Los Angeles, CA, United States

Scott H. Kozin, MD
Clinical Professor
Orthopaedic Surgery
Lewis Katz School of Medicine at Temple University
Philadelphia, PA, United States

Clinical Professor
Orthopaedic Surgery
Sidney Kimmel Medical College at Thomas Jefferson
    University
Philadelphia, PA, United States

Chief of Staff
Shriners Hospital for Children
Philadelphia, PA, United States

Ryan Krochak, MD
Orthopaedic Sports Medicine Fellow at the University
  of Pennsylvania
Orthopedic Surgeon
Orthopedic Sports Medicine
Orlin & Cohen Orthopedics/Northwell Health
Long Island, NY, United States

Amy L. Ladd, MD
Elsbach-Richards Professor of Surgery
Orthopaedic Surgery
Stanford University School of Medicine
Stanford, CA, United States

Amy Lake, OTR, CHT
Occupational Therapy
Texas Scottish Rite Hospital for Children
Dallas, TX, United States

Carolyn M. Levis, MD, MSc, FRCSC
Division of Plastic Surgery
McMaster University
St. Joseph's Healthcare Hamilton
Hamilton, ON, Canada

Kevin J. Little, MD
Director
Pediatric Hand and Upper Extremity Center
Fellowship Director
Mary S. Stern Hand Surgery Fellowship
Associate Professor of Orthopaedic Surgery
Cincinnati Children's Hospital Medical Center
University of Cincinnati School of Medicine
Cincinnati, OH, United States

Director, Hand and Upper Extremity Surgery
Division of Pediatric Orthopaedics
Cincinnati Children's Hospital Medical Center
Cincinnati, OH, United States

Erin Meisel, MD
Assistant Professor of Orthopaedic Surgery
Children's Hospital Los Angeles
University of Southern California
Los Angeles, CA, United States

Michelle Hsia, MS, OTR/L
Outpatient Supervisor
Occupational Therapy
The Children's Hospital of Philadelphia
Philadelphia, PA, United States

M.J. Mulcahey, PhD, OTR/L, FASIA
Professor of Occupational Therapy
Director, Center for Outcomes and Measurement
Jefferson College of Rehabilitation Sciences
Thomas Jefferson University
Philadelphia, PA, United States

Rebecca Neiduski, PhD, OTR/L, CHT
Dean of the School of Health Sciences
Professor of Health Sciences
School of Health Sciences
Elon University
Elon, NC, United States

Scott Oishi, MD
Director of Hand Service
Orthopaedics
Texas Scottish Rite Hospital for Children
Dallas, TX, United States

Heta Parikh, OTR/L, MPH
Occupational Therapist
Department of Orthopedics
University of Maryland School of Medicine
Baltimore, MD, United States

Meagan Pehnke, MS, OTR/L, CHT, CLT
Senior Occupational Therapist
Occupational Therapy
The Children's Hospital of Philadelphia
Philadelphia, PA, United States

Nicholas Pulos, MD
Texas Scottish Rite Hospital for Children
Pediatric Upper Extremity Fellow
Dallas, TX, United States

Lydia D. Rawlins, MEd, OTR/L
Children's Hospital of Philadelphia
Department of Occupational Therapy
Philadelphia, PA, United States

Roberta Ciocco, MS, OT
Senior Occupational Therapist
Out patient Occupational Therapy
Children's Hospital of Philadelphia
Philadelphia, PA, United States

Daniel W. Safford, PT, DPT
Board Certified Orthopaedic Specialist
Certified Strength & Conditioning Specialist
Penn Therapy and Fitness at Arcadia University
Good Shepherd Penn Partners
Research Physical Therapist
Physical Therapy Department
Arcadia University
Glenside, PA, United States

Sandra Schmieg, MS, OTR/L, CHT
Senior Occupational Therapist
Occupational Therapy
The Children's Hospital of Philadelphia
Philadelphia, PA, United States

Apurva S. Shah, MD, MBA
Assistant Professor of Orthopaedic Surgery
Division of Orthopaedic Surgery
The Children's Hospital of Philadelphia
Department of Orthopaedic Surgery, Perelman School
    of Medicine at the University of Pennsylvania
Philadelphia, PA, United States

Francisco Soldado, MD, PhD
Pediatric Hand
Nerve and Microsurgery Institute
Barcelona, Spain

Milan Stevanovic, MD
Physician
Professor of Orthopaedic Surgery
Department of Orthopaedic Surgery
Division of Orthopedic Surgery
Keck School of Medicine of USC
Los Angeles, CA, United States

Tami Konieczny, MS, BS
Supervisor Occupational Therapy
Occupational Therapy
Children's Hospital of Philadelphia
Philadelphia, PA, United States

Kathleen Tate, MS, OTR/L
Children's Hospital of Philadelphia
Department of Occupational Therapy
Philadelphia, PA, United States

Daniel Waltho, MD
Resident
Plastic Surgery
McMaster University
Hamilton, ON, Canada

Heather Weesner, OT
Occupational Therapist
University of Maryland Rehabilitation
    and Orthopedic Institute
Baltimore, MD, United States

Aviva Wolff, EdD, OT, CHT
Clinician Investigator
Rehabilitation
Hospital for Special Surgery
New York, NY, United States

Cheryl Zalieckas, OTR/L, MBA
Department of Orthopaedics
University of Maryland
Baltimore, MD, United States

Dan A. Zlotolow, MD
Hand and Upper Extremity Surgeon
Shriners Hospitals for Children Philadelphia and
    Greenville
The Hospital for Special Surgery
The Philadelphia Hand to Shoulder Center
Professor of Orthopaedics
The Sidney Kimmel Medical College of Thomas
    Jefferson University
Philadelphia, PA, United States

Attending Physician
Shriners Hospital for Children
Philadelphia, PA, United States

Acknowledgments—Pediatric Hand Therapy

This book is dedicated to all healthcare providers who care for the child's upper limb. Specifically, the goal of this book was to provide a resource for the occupational therapist who cares for children's upper limbs. Several of the conditions and injuries are somewhat rare to see for most providers and therefore, we have tried to make a quick, easy to read resource for these providers and people interested in caring for the child's upper extremity. The work performed to bring this book to completion would not have been possible without the collaboration and efforts of all of the authors of the various chapters as well as my coeditors. I must also thank my parents for their continued support and encouragement. Most importantly, I want to thank my wife, Laura, and our three boys, Noah, Benjamin, and Zachary, for always loving and supporting me. Although I know the time necessary to do projects like this takes away some of our time together, you always continue to support me, understand the work that I am doing, and most importantly love me——and for that I thank you.

Joshua M. Abzug, MD

Hand surgery and hand therapy are synergistic. The results of hand surgery require preoperative and postoperative communication between the surgeon and the therapist. Our therapists provide invaluable preoperative input into the families and their children regarding expected outcomes, cooperation, and compliance. Our therapist provides critical postoperative care. This care requires communication as the therapist must understand the procedure performed and the status of any repaired structures, such as a nerve or tendon. A stout repair can be managed with early mobilization. In contrast, a weaker repair must be treated with gentle mobilization. At Shriners Hospitals for Children-Philadelphia, hand surgeon and hand therapist work in tandem. We work as a team to provide state-of-the-art surgery and optimum therapy to maximize our children's outcome. Complex procedures mandate a skilled and talented therapist. We require our families to travel back to Philadelphia to begin their rehabilitation process. This prerequisite avoids miscommunication and initiates the rehabilitation process with a therapy team accustomed to the surgical procedure. Our therapists are familiar with the potential trials and tribulations in the early therapy period. Addressing these problems can avoid a suboptimal outcome, which is disappointing to the family, therapist, and surgeon. Over the last 25 years at Shriners Hospitals for Children, I have had the privilege to work with many gifted therapists. They have enhanced our patient's outcomes and made me a better surgeon. I want to thank each and every one of them for all their knowledge, for all their expertise, and for all their service to the children at Shriners Hospitals for Children.

Scott H. Kozin, MD

The key to achieving excellent outcomes in upper extremity rehabilitation is relationships. The relationship between hand surgeon and hand therapist creates the foundation on which communication, shared values, trust, and collaboration are built. The relationship between therapists in the subspecialty of pediatric hand provides a network of colleagues and problem solvers who share resources and opportunities. The relationships among healthcare providers, children, caregivers, and families enable our youngest clients to embrace possibility and participation through surgery, therapy, and adaptation. This text was built on invaluable relationships between therapist and surgeons, and we hope it adds an impactful resource to your pediatric hand therapy practice.

Rebecca Neiduski, PhD, OTR/L, CHT

Preface

Caring for the child's upper extremity is challenging due to the rarity of various injuries and/or conditions as well as the child's inability to cooperate and understand instructions. Despite these obstacles, occupational therapy is a critical component of caring for the child's upper limb. Whether the therapist is helping a child with a congenital limb difference learn how to perform activities of daily living or rehabilitating a child following a traumatic injury, the occupational therapist is maximizing the function of the child. Despite this critical role, few resources exist to aid the occupational therapist in caring for the child's upper limb. The purpose of this book is to provide a comprehensive, easy to read and use reference for the healthcare provider who is caring for pediatric and adolescent upper extremities. The book details the formation and functional development of the child's upper limb. Subsequently, the necessary details and key points of the examination are discussed along with details of various outcome measures. In addition, splinting and taping techniques as well as prosthetic use are emphasized. The remainder of the book is organized into various sections to permit the reader easy access to specific diagnoses. Although the book provides a concise, yet thorough discussion regarding these topics, we envision that the treater will keep the book at "arm's length" as a resource for caring for children with an upper extremity condition. Many of the chapters provide protocols to use during rehabilitation as well as specific splints that are necessary to improve function or during the postoperative course. The goal of this book is to provide the reader with the knowledge to perform a thorough examination, establish an accurate diagnosis, refer for timely treatment, and perform specific rehabilitation including therapy and splinting to maximize the child's outcome.

Contents

CHAPTER 1

Embryology and Intrauterine Diagnosis

FRANCISCO SOLDADO, MD PHD • SCOTT H. KOZIN, MD

INTRODUCTION

Someone's first-ever sip of coffee is often an unpleasant experience that renders them pondering how they could ever learn to like such a foul-flavored drink. Similarly, many health professionals' first exposure to embryology, and the basic science that is so integral to it, is often a bitter experience. However, over time, dedicated professionals learn how interesting the field is and how essential the knowledge gleamed is pertinent to patient care. This fundamental principle is particularly true for those who choose to enter a field that evaluates and treats newborns with congenital defects.

Congenital anomalies affect somewhere between 1% and 3% of newborns. Among these infants, roughly 1 in 10 has one or more abnormalities that affect their upper extremities.[1,2] In prevalence, upper-extremity anomalies rank second only to congenital heart defects among malformations present at birth.[3] Most limb anomalies manifest spontaneously or are inherited, with congenital anomalies secondary to teratogens decidedly rare.[4,5]

For those clinicians that evaluate newborns with hand anomalies as patients, or counsel parents who have already born such a child, a basic understanding of embryogenesis, limb formation, and genetics is utterly essential. Also crucial is understanding how these anomalies may relate to more systemic conditions, as these healthcare providers often are required to counsel parents about the potential effect on future pregnancies and what intervention can and should be done. Understanding genetic criteria and their associated anomalies affords such healthcare providers the capacity to make appropriate recommendations to families and/or referral to clinical geneticist and/or genetic counseling.

The requirements are not the same with all upper-limb congenital anomalies. For example, transverse deficiencies are usually sporadic and carry no appreciable hereditary risk. As such, subsequent pregnancies require no more monitoring than standard care,[1] and there is no need to refer this family to a clinical geneticist. However, concerns about the risks of teratogen exposure elevate when multiple limbs are affected and deficient. This clinical finding suggests some widespread insult to all the developing limb buds and potential teratogen or bleeding abnormality.

Conversely, many other upper-limb anomalies (e.g., radial deficiency) are associated with concomitant, systemic defects (Fig. 1.1).[6] At the same time during embryogenesis when upper-limb anomalies are in their formative stage, other organ systems are developing at the same time. These organ systems can be affected and require evaluation. It is essential that the clinician recognizes those anomalies that typically occur in isolation versus those anomalies that are associated with concomitant anomalies; many of these anomalies may initially be unapparent with dire consequences. This principle is especially crucial when the concomitant anomalies of other organ systems are of greater clinical importance than the limb anomalies. Hand surgeons assessing such patients must focus on the infant's general health before addressing hand malformations.

Some congenital hand anomalies are linked to other musculoskeletal problems, such as ulnar deficiency.[7] Some anomalies can even be associated with more than one musculoskeletal disorder. For example, central deficiency may be linked to the triad of ectrodactyly ectodermal dysplasia and facial clefts (the so-called EEC syndrome) or lower-limb hemimelia (in which

Pediatric Hand Therapy. https://doi.org/10.1016/B978-0-323-53091-0.00001-4

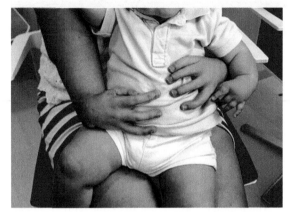

FIG. 1.1 Nine-month-old boy with an inherited radial deficiency associated with Holt–Oram syndrome. Mother and child's heart anomalies were surgically treated.

either the tibia or fibula is absent or inadequately formed) (Fig. 1.2).

HOW LIMBS DEVELOP IN UTERO
Embryogenesis
After an egg is fertilized, the first stage of growth is called embryogenesis. During this period of time, a sequence of events occurs that will determine the number of limbs, their location, and their orientation.[8] In addition, during this time, between the fourth and eighth week of gestation, most upper-extremity congenital anomalies occur. The sequence of events that determines upper-limb development is as follows:

- Day 26 after fertilization: The limb buds initially become visible. The embryo is only about the size of a single grain of rice, roughly 4 mm in length.[9,10]
- Days 27–47: Over the next 3 weeks, limb buds develop rapidly, but the fingers and toes are not yet identifiable. Even at the end of this period of time, the entire embryo is still only about the size of a lima bean, roughly 20 mm in length.
- Days 48–53: Over the next five or so days, the fingers and toes separate, so that hands and feet become clearly recognizable.
- Day 56: By the end of the eighth week after fertilization, all the essential limb structures are present. Embryogenesis is complete and the next stage of development, the fetal period, has begun.

Fetal Period
Upon the completion of embryogenesis, the fetal period begins. During this stage of development existing structures differentiate, mature, and grow.[3–13] In the limbs, part of the differentiation and maturation process involves the creation of articulations. Joints form as chondrogen condenses into dense plates between limb structures that will ossify to become bones.[14] Joint cavitation develops the articulation further, though each joint's development ultimately requires fetal movement to ensure the joint surface is modeled into its final prenatal form.

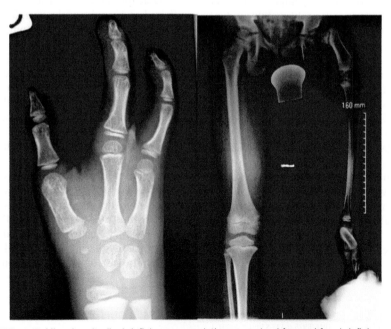

FIG. 1.2 Ulnar longitudinal deficiency associating a proximal femoral focal deficiency.

At a cellular level, limb buds are an outgrowth of mesoderm into overlying ectoderm. Cells from two mesodermal sources—lateral plate mesoderm and somatic mesoderm. These cell lines migrate from their origins into the limb bud.[3,14] The lateral plate cells eventually become bone, cartilage, and tendon. The somatic cells form muscles, nerves, and vascular elements. Blastemas are clusters of cells that all are destined to differentiate into the same type of tissue. In the fetus's developing limbs, muscular and chondrogenic blastema, derived from lateral plate mesoderm differentiate into muscles and bones, respectively.[15] The level of oxygen tension appears to play a part in this differentiation process. Chondrogenic blastema is located more centrally within the limb bud where oxygen tension is relatively low. Muscular blastema is more peripheral in location where oxygen tension is greater. Both muscles and the cartilaginous structures that ultimately will ossify to become bones develop sequentially, starting proximal and progressing in a distal direction.

Joints form between the ends of adjacent blastemas, a joint capsule surrounding the interzone and the intervening blastemas cavitating within the interzone's center to create the articular space. Joint fluid is produced within this space, while cartilage caps the two ends of each bone. Joints ossify and fuse, resulting in synostosis, when the process mentioned earlier fails. Two joints commonly effected by are the proximal radioulnar and ulnohumeral joints (Fig. 1.3). Another component of fetal development that is required for the formation of a functional mobile joint is movement. When fetuses fail to move adequately, as in arthrogryposis, joint spaces become infiltrated by fibrous tissue resulting in contracted and immobile joints (Fig. 1.4).

Signaling Centers

Three growth signaling centers—the apical ectodermal ridge (AER), the zone of polarizing activity (ZPA) and the Wnt (Wingless type)—central to limb patterning align the three spatial axes of limb development. The axes are labeled proximodistal, anteroposterior, and dorsoventral, respectively (Table 1.1).[14–17] As demonstrated later, our understanding of embryogenesis has been advanced by ingenious experiments performed by embryologists. In these experiments, animal models with limb patterning have been manipulated to permit the dissection and alteration of crucial signaling centers that effect limb development and orientation.[12,13,18]

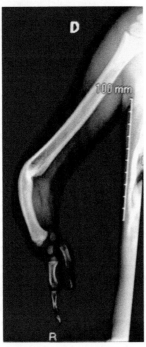

FIG. 1.3 Ulnohumeral fusion or synostosis associated with ulnar longitudinal deficiency.

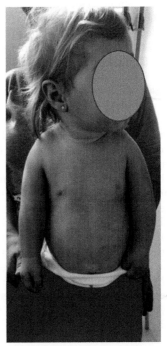

FIG. 1.4 Eleven-month-old girl with arthrogryposis involving predominantly the shoulder girdles. Absence of elbow creases revealing intrauterine poor motion.

TABLE 1.1
Spatial Axes of Limb Development, their Signaling Centers and Malformation Associated.

Signaling Center	Signaling molecule	Limb Axis	Malformation
Apical ectodermal ridge	Fibroblast growth factors	Proximal to distal	Transverse deficiency
Zone of polarizing activity	Sonic hedgehog protein	Radioulnar	Mirror hand
Wnt pathway	Transcription factor, Lmx-1	Ventral and dorsal	Abnormal nail and pulp arrangement Nail-patella syndrome

Proximodistal limb development

Limbs develop in a proximal to distal direction, from shoulder → arm → forearm → hand. The proximodistal signaling center, called the apical ectodermal ridge (AER), is a thickened layer of ectoderm that condenses over each limb bud[14] and secretes proteins that create this effect.[19,20] Experimental models have been developed to mimic proximodistal limb development. They include removing the AER, which results in limb truncation. Conversely, ectopic implantation of the AER induces the formation of additional limbs.[10,12,14] Interestingly, however, removing the AER can be overridden by administering certain fibroblast growth factors that are released by the AER. Moreover, mice deficient in these fibroblast growth factors exhibit complete transverse limb defects.[21,22]

Given these results, transverse deficiencies are now attributed to deficits in the AER or certain signaling molecules, such as fibroblast growth factors, that it produces (Fig. 1.5).

Anteroposterior limb development

In animal models, both transplantation of the anteroposterior (i.e., radioulnar or preaxial–postaxial) signaling center, called the zone of polarizing activity (ZPA), and transplanting the sonic hedgehog protein that the ZPA secretes have been demonstrated to cause mirror duplication of the ulnar aspect of the limb.[23] Mutant mice with sonic hedgehog protein in their anterior limb bud develop polydactyly.[24] Also in models, triphalangeal thumbs (thumbs with three phalanges, instead of the usual two) have been found to arise secondary to point mutations that generate ectopic sonic hedgehog compound at the anterior margin of the limb bud.[25] In humans, therefore, both mirror hand and certain forms of polydactyly are now attributed to deficits in the ZPA or sonic hedgehog protein (Fig. 1.6).[3,18]

Dorsoventral limb development

The mechanism behind the development of the dorsum of the finger with its fingernail and the volar surface

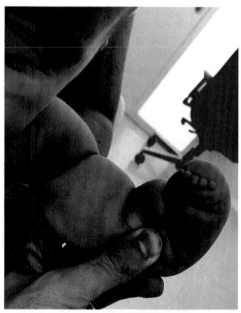

FIG. 1.5 Adactylous form of symbrachydactyly a manifestation of transverse deficiencies. "Nubbins" are the vestiges of digits and are the hallmark of symbrachydactyly. The nubbins are comprised of the remaining ectodermal structures of the distal finger (the pulp, nail fold, and nail).

with its abundant pulp tissue are differentiated and developed is not well understood.[11] The pathway responsible for this differentiation produces one transcription factor, Lmx-1, that induces the mesoderm to adopt dorsal characteristics.[26] In the ventral ectoderm, the Wnt pathway is blocked by a product of a gene called engrailed-1 (En-1). Mice lacking the anteroposterior Wnt signaling pathway, which resides in dorsal ectoderm and secretes Lmx-1, exhibit ventralization of the dorsal surface of their limbs, such that they manifest palmar pads on both sides of their hand: front and back.[27] Conversely, mice lacking the engrailed-1 protein exhibit dorsalization of their limbs' volar surfaces

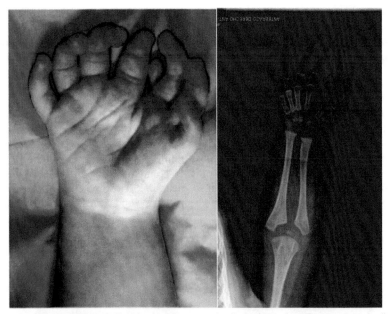

FIG. 1.6 Mirror hand attributed to abnormal anteroposterior limb patterning. The result is duplication of the ulnar field but absence of the radial field.

(so-called bidorsal limbs).[28] Alterations in this latter pathway are relatively rare. Loss of Lmx-1 is associated with a condition called *nail-patella syndrome*, in which affected individuals have small, poorly developed nails and kneecaps. Affected individuals also have musculo-skeletal defects in other areas of the body including their elbows, hips, and chest.[29] Other children may present with anomalies that include extraneous nail or abnormal pulp development, both linked to an altered Wnt signaling pathway.[30] In humans, dorsal dimelia with the nails may present on the palmar surface of fingers, is explained by alterations in the Wnt signaling pathway or Lmx-1 (Fig. 1.7).[23]

Programmed Cell Death

Programmed cell death (PCD) is another essential component of proper limb development. PCD is an active process that is genetically controlled. PCD eliminates un-wanted cells during embryogenesis.[23] Apoptotic cells undergo a degenerative process, associated with DNA fragmentation, and eventually are engulfed by phago-cytes. A clear example of this is the separation of fingers and toes during days 48–53 of gestation. Before day 48, all human digits are webbed. Over the next 5-day period of gestation, interdigital necrosis occurs with extraneous, web-like tissue between fingers and toes undergoing PCD. Failure of interdigital PCD results in syndactyly.[31]

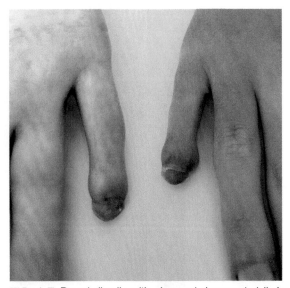

FIG. 1.7 Dorsal dimelia with abnormal dorsoventral limb patterning can cause duplication of the dorsal field resulting in the presence of a nail both in the dorsal and volar sides of the finger.

Widely recognized for their role in chondrogenesis and osteogenesis, bone morphogenetic proteins (BMPs) also trigger apoptotic pathways in interdigital mesenchyme to separate the fingers.[23] Antagonists to

BMP are capable of blocking BMP signaling and preventing this process of apoptosis and interdigital necrosis. An obvious animal example of this are bats, mammals whose limbs are webbed, and whose BMP has been shown to be blocked during limb embryogenesis.[32] Similarly, altered signaling of fibroblast growth factors can negate BMP-mediated apoptosis and result in syndactyly, which occurs in individuals with Apert syndrome (Fig. 1.8).

Genes and Molecular Abnormalities and www.omim.org

Research on gene misexpression and altered anatomical and functional development has enhanced general understanding about how limbs develop in utero.[3,18] This research has included intense work focusing on genotype–phenotype correlations that may have substantial clinical implications.

Online Mendelian Inheritance in Man (OMIM, www.omim.org) is a reliable and comprehensive, online compendium of human genes and genetic phenotypes that is updated daily and freely available to help clinicians, investigators, and other interested parties understand the vast evolving field of genetics and countless number of different phenotypes.

Numerous congenital deformities have a known genetic link. However, most possess variable inheritance patterns and breadths of expression. Healthcare

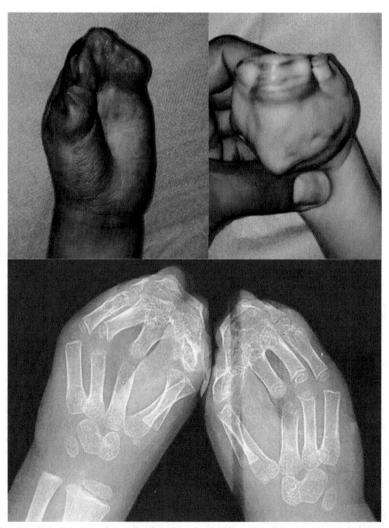

FIG. 1.8 Syndactyly in Apert syndrome is related to altered signaling of fibroblast growth factors resulting in abnormal BMP-mediated apoptosis.

providers who evaluate patients with hand deformities must have basic knowledge about congenital differences that are familial and potentially inherited versus those differences that are not inheritable. This understanding will justifiably recommend to families whether or not they should undergo evaluation by a clinical geneticist. Parents also require appropriate counseling pertaining to the spectrum of phenotypic expressions that can occur with a particular mutation. One misconception that frequently affects parents with a mild phenotype of a congenital disorder is that the extent and severity of their own disorder is a "worst-case scenario" for their child. This misperception can lead such parents to purse with pregnancy and birth, naïve to the possibility that their offspring may have a phenotypically much worse form of their difference. Their severely affected offspring renders those parents devastated, ill prepared, and engulfed with feelings of guilt. Appropriate genetic counseling referral can mitigate the misconception of variable phenotype with similar genotype.

Mutations that encode signaling proteins, receptor molecules, and transcription factors can alter normal limb arrangement, resulting in anomalies that range from almost imperceptible to complete limb absence. The number of molecularly identifiable congenital anomalies that practicing hand surgeons are seeing is steadily increasing. Other anomalies, though less well defined at a molecular level, have been mapped to specific chromosomal segments.[3] Table 1.2 lists examples of genes that encode transcription factors and exert some crucial level of control over upper-limb formation (Figs. 1.9 and 1.10).[33–36]

Intrauterine Diagnostics and Treating Upper-Limb Anomalies

Diagnosing congenital anomalies in utero can lead to parental counseling by a geneticist and/or by a surgeon who specializes in the anomaly identified and its treatment. In utero diagnosis may guide parental decisions on difficult personal and ethical questions, such as should gestation be terminated? In addition, in-utero procedures reevolving and may be considered based upon the certainty of diagnosis.[37] In addition, in utero diagnosis permits investigations to screen for associated anomalies, via further imaging studies or other procedures such as amniocentesis and chorionic villus sampling for fetal karyotyping and genetic analysis.[38]

To date, ultrasound remains the primary modality for fetal evaluations and/or monitor fetal development. Ultrasound also guides prenatal care and identifies fetal abnormalities (Fig. 1.11A).[39,40] Ultrasound-based prenatal diagnosis has improved substantially over the last several decades because of technological advances, improved image resolution, increased standardization of prenatal ultrasound protocols, and enhanced training of diagnosticians.[37] Prenatal ultrasound has the potential to identify isolated musculoskeletal abnormalities, including a broad range of hand and upper-limb condition including transverse and longitudinal deficiencies, syndactyly, polydactyly, clinodactyly, and clasped thumbs (Fig. 1.12).[40]

Both the American College of Radiology and American Institute of Ultrasound in Medicine recommend routine second-trimester screening with transabdominal ultrasound, between 18 and 22 weeks of

TABLE 1.2
Consequence of Mutation of Some Genes Encoding Transcription Factors Crucial for Limb Formation.

Gen	Syndrome	Limb anomaly	Inheritance
Hox	Synpolydactyly	Synpolydactyly (Fig. 1.9)	A.D.
	Hand-foot-genital syndrome	Short great toes and hipoplastic thumbs	
	Leri-Weill dyschondrosteosis	Madelung's deformity	
T-Box	Holt-Oram Sd (Tbx-5)	Radial deficiency	A.D.
	Ulnar-mamary Sd (Tbx-3)	Ulnar digits hipoplasia	
Cartilage-derived morphogenetic protein	Grebe chondrodysplasia	Brachidactily	A.R.
	Hunter-Thompson chondrodysplasia	Brachidactily (Fig. 1.10)	

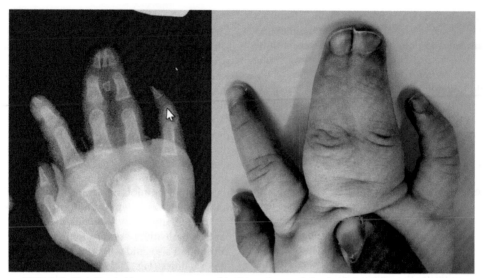

FIG. 1.9 Mutation in Hox genes can result in this autosomal dominant familial synpolydactyly.

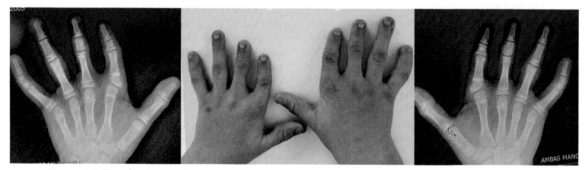

FIG. 1.10 This familial brachydactyly may be explained by an underlying mutation in cartilage-derived morphogenetic protein gen.

gestation, to confirm the fetuses gestational age, evaluate their intrauterine development, and screen for congenital anomalies. Current recommendations only require that the ultrasonographer document that all four extremities are present, although enhanced ultrasound imaging will likely change this basic recommendation. Currently, even with level-2 ("targeted") ultrasound studies, further detailed assessment of the extremities is "encouraged," but formalized standards are nonexistent.[41] In fact, despite improvements in ultrasound technology and techniques, its sensitivity detecting upper-limb anomalies remains low.[42]

At one tertiary level hospital, the postnatally confirmed sensitivity of prenatal ultrasound detecting upper-extremity anomalies was approximately 40%.[42]

This sensitivity was lower when the anomalies were limited to the upper extremities (25% vs. 55%). Sensitivity for upper-limb anomalies was highest for conditions affecting the entire upper extremity (85%) and lowest for those affecting the digits alone (10%). Fetuses with limb-reduction defects, radial longitudinal deficiency, phocomelia, arthrogryposis, abnormal hand positioning, and cleft hand were more likely to be accurately diagnosed, because they were more likely to have an associated anomaly.

Several strategies can be utilized to enhance the sensitivity and accuracy of ultrasound imaging. One such technique is transvaginal ultrasound, which allows better visualization of the fetus and limbs.[40] In some high-risk groups, early risk assessment with ultrasound is performed between 11 and 14 weeks of gestation.

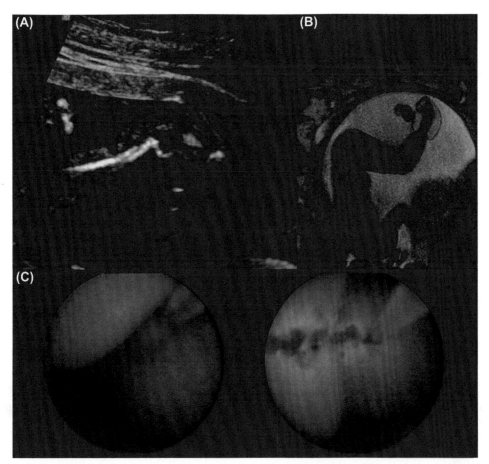

FIG. 1.11 Ultrasound showing severe leg constriction with markedly distal edema and risk of intrauterine amputation **(A)** Prenatal MRI confirming the ultrasound findings **(B)** Fetoscopic image of the leg constriction and longitudinal release with a Yag-Laser fiber **(C)**.

Within this time period and by employing transvaginal techniques, initial limb development can be assessed. Three-dimensional (3-D) ultrasound also improves the modality's diagnostic potential, allowing for the identification and characterization of more-complex anatomical structures. Authorities have advocated adopting 3D ultrasound as the imaging modality of choice for analyzing fetal limbs, particularly their hands (Fig. 1.13).[43]

The hand is best visualized by ultrasound during the late part of the first and early part of the second trimester. At this time, the fingers are large enough to be visualized and characteristically extended and abducted, facilitating the examiner's ability to discern anatomical alterations. Later in gestation, the hands often position in a clasped fist-like appearance obscuring hand anomalies. Additionally, the relative decrease in intrauterine space and amniotic fluid in later gestation limits fetal motion and the likelihood that the fetus will move into a position more suitable for detailed ultrasound assessment.

Magnetic resonance imaging (MRI) has particular advantages for evaluating neural axis, thoracic, and head or neck abnormalities, relative to the conventional ultrasound, because imaging the fetus with MRI is less dependent upon the presence of normal amniotic fluid volume, fetal position, and maternal body habitus.[44] However, due to artifacts caused by moving extremities, the accuracy of MRI in evaluating the hand and remaining upper limb remains to be determined (Fig. 1.11B).

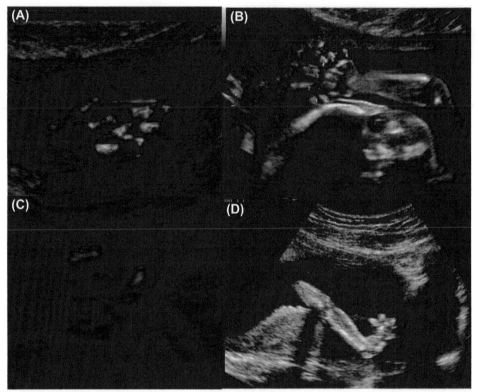

FIG. 1.12 A variety of congenital differences diagnosed by ultrasound at 21 weeks of gestational age: **(A)** complex syndactyly, **(B)** postaxial polydactyly, **(C)** ulnar deficiency with oligosyndactyly, and **(D)** radial clubhand with absent radius.

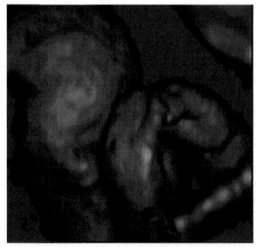

FIG. 1.13 27 weeks 3D ultrasound showing an Apert's hand.

PRENATAL TREATMENT

Fetal surgery is an emerging and established procedure. Intrauterine surgery was initially restricted to the treatment of life-threatening anomalies, given risks to both the mother and fetus (e.g., diaphragmatic hernia, twin–twin transfusion syndrome, giant teratomas, etc.).[45] As the prerequisite of anesthesia (maternal and fetal) and technology (fetal endoscopy) have improved, the risks have been reduced and the indications for intrauterine surgery have been extended to include nonlethal orthopedic conditions, including myelomeningocele and amniotic band syndrome.[46]

Currently, the only upper-limb indication for fetoscopic examination and treatment is the risk of limb amputation by an extremity amniotic band (Fig. 1.11C). The progressive strangulation of a limb by an intrauterine amniotic band leads to gradual worsening of the deformity and ultimate amputation. Prenatal band release arrests the progression of strangulation and allows the fetal tissue's natural healing capacity to potentially restore the affected limb's normal morphology and function (Fig. 1.11C).[36] Fetal wound repair also occurs without scar formation, which yields the potential application to treating other congenital upper limb deformities (e.g., syndactyly). As future advances in technology and anesthesia decrease maternal—fetal risks further, the indications for prenatal interventions to correct congenital anomalies will likely expand.

REFERENCES

1. Kozin SH. *Embryology of the Upper Extremity*. In: *Green's Operative Hand Surgeryc*. 6th ed. Philadelphia: Churchill Livingstone; 2011.
2. Parker SE, Mai CT, Canfield MA, et al. Updated National Birth Prevalence estimates for selected birth defects in the United States, 2004—2006. *Birth Defects Res A Clin Mol Teratol*. 2010;88:1008.
3. Bamshad M, Watkins WS, Dixon ME, et al. Reconstructing the history of human limb development: lessons from birth defects. *Pediatr Res*. 1999;45:291.
4. Taussig HB. A study of the German outbreak of phocomelia the thalidomide syndrome. *J Am Med Assoc*. 1962;180:1106.
5. Temtamy SA, McKusick VA. The genetics of hand malformations. *Birth Defects Orig Artic Ser*. 1978;14(1).
6. Lourie GM, Lins RE. Radial longitudinal deficiency. A review and update. *Hand Clin*. 1998;14:85.
7. Schmidt CC, Neufeld SK. Ulnar ray deficiency. *Hand Clin*. 1998;14(65).
8. O'Rahilly R, Gardner E. The timing and sequence of events in the development of the limbs in the human embryo. *Anat Embryol*. 1975;148(1).
9. Uthoff HK. *The Embryology of the Human Locomotor System*. Berlin: Springer-Verlag; 1990.
10. Zaleske DJ. Development of the upper limb. *Hand Clin*. 1985;1(383).
11. Moore KL. *The Developing Human: Clinically Oriented Embryology*. Philadelphia: W.B. Saunders; 1988.
12. Riddle RD, Tabin C. How limbs develop. *Sci Am*. 1999;280(74).
13. Shubin N, Tabin C, Carroll S. Fossils, genes and the evolution of animal limbs. *Nature*. 1997;388:639.
14. Daluiski A, Yi SE, Lyons KM. The molecular control of upper extremity development: implications for congenital hand anomalies. *J Hand Surg Am*. 2001;26(8).
15. Al-Qattan MM, Yang Y, Kozin SH. Embryology of the upper limb. *J Hand Surg Am*. 2009;34:1340.
16. Laufer F, Nelson CE, Johnson RL, et al. Sonic hedgehog and Fgf-4 act through a signaling cascade and feedback loop to integrate growth and patterning of the developing limb bud. *Cell*. 1994;79:993.
17. Niswander L, Jeffrey S, Martin GR, et al. A positive feedback loop coordinates growth and patterning in the vertebrate limb. *Nature*. 1994;371:609.
18. Riddle RD, Johnson RL, Laufer E, et al. Sonic hedgehog mediates the polarizing activity of the ZPA. *Cell*. 1993;75:1401.
19. Mariani FV, Ahn CP, Martin GR. Genetic evidence that FGFs have an instructive role in limb proximal-distal patterning. *Nature*. 2008;453:401.
20. Niswander L, Martin GR. FGF-4 expression during gastrulation, myogenesis, limb and tooth development in the mouse. *Development*. 1992;114:755.
21. Fallon JF, Lopez A, Ros MA, et al. FGF-2: apical ectodermal ridge growth signal for chick limb development. *Science*. 1994;264:104.
22. Niswander L, Tickle C, Vogel A, et al. FGF-4 replaces the apical ectodermal ridge and directs outgrowth and patterning of the limb. *Cell*. 1993;75:579.
23. Chen Y, Zhao X. Shaping limbs by apoptosis. *J Exp Zool*. 1998;282:691.
24. Masayu H, Sagai T, Wakana S, et al. A duplicated zone of polarizing activity in polydactylous mouse mutants. *Genes Dev*. 1995;9:1645.
25. Lettice LA, Hill AE, Devenney PS, et al. Point mutations in a distant sonic hedgehog cis-regulator generate a variable regulatory output responsible for preaxial polydactyly. *Hum Mol Genet*. 2008;17:978.
26. Riddle RD, Ensini M, Nelson C, et al. Induction of the LIM homeobox gene Lmx1 by WNT7a establishes dorsoventral pattern in the vertebrate limb. *Cell*. 1995;83:631.
27. Parr BA, McMahon AP. Dorsalizing signal Wnt-7a required for normal polarity of D-V and A-P axes of mouse limb. *Nature*. 1995;374:350.
28. Loomis CA, Harris E, Michaud J, et al. The mouse Engrailed-1 gene and ventral limb patterning. *Nature*. 1996;382:360.
29. Dreyer SD, Zhou G, Baldini A, et al. Mutations in LMX1B cause abnormal skeletal patterning and renal dysplasia in nail patella syndrome. *Nat Genet*. 1998;19(47).
30. Al-Qattan MM. Classification of dorsal and ventral dimelia in humans. *J Hand Surg Eur*. 2013;38:928.
31. Zakeri Z, Quaglino D, Ahuja HS. Apoptotic cell death in the mouse limb and its suppression in the hammertoe mutant. *Dev Biol*. 1994;165:294.
32. Oberg KC, Feenstra JM, Manske PR, et al. Developmental biology and classification of congenital anomalies of the hand and upper extremity. *J Hand Surg Am*. 2010;35:2077.
33. Basson CT, Bachinsky DR, Lin RC, et al. Mutations in human TBX5 cause limb and cardiac malformation in Holt-Oram syndrome. *Nat Genet*. 1997;15(30).
34. Goodman FR, Bacchelli C, Brady AF, et al. Novel HOXA13 mutations and the phenotypic spectrum of hand-foot-genital syndrome. *Am J Hum Genet*. 2000;67:197.
35. Polinkovsky A, Robin NH, Thomas JT, et al. Mutations in CDMP1 cause autosomal dominant brachydactyly type C. *Nat Genet*. 1997;17:18.

36. Ross JL, Scott Jr C, Marttila P, et al. Phenotypes associated with SHOX deficiency. *J Clin Endocrinol Metab.* 2001;86:5674.

37. American College of Obstetricans and Gynecologists. ACOG practice bulletin No. 101: ultrasonography in pregnancy. *Obstet GyneCol.* 2009;113(2 Pt 1):451e461.

38. Drummond CL, Gomes DM, Senat MV, Audibert F, Dorion A, Ville Y. Fetal karyotyping after 28 weeks of gestation for late ultrasound findings in a low risk population. *Prenat Diagn.* 2003;23:1068–1072.

39. Chitty LS, Hunt GH, Moore J, Lobb MO. Effectiveness of routine ultrasonography in detecting fetal structural abnormalities in a low risk 40 population. *BMJ.* 1991;303:1165–1169.

40. Bronshtein M, Keret D, Deutsch M, Liberson A, Bar Chava I. Transvaginal sonographic detection of skeletal anomalies in the first and early second trimesters. *Prenat Diagn.* 1993;13:597–601.

41. Wientroub S, Keret D, Bronshtein M. Prenatal sonographic diagnosis of musculoskeletal disorders. *J Pediatr Orthop.* 1999;19:1–4.

42. Piper SL, Dicke JM, Wall LB, Shen TS, Goldfarb CA. Prenatal detection of upper limb differences with obstetric ultrasound. *J Hand Surg Am.* 2015;40(7):1310–1317.

43. Kos M, Hafner T, Funduk-Kurjak B, Bozek T, Kuriak A. Limb deformities and three-dimensional ultrasound. *J Perinat Med.* 2002;30:40–4424.

44. Breysem L, Bosmans H, Dymarkowski S, et al. The value of fast MR imaging as an adjunct to ultrasound in prenatal diagnosis. *Eur Radiol.* 2003;13:1538–1548.

45. Cortes RA, Farmer DL. Recent advances in fetal surgery. *Semin Perinatol.* 2004;28(3):199Y211.

46. Soldado F, Aguirre M, Peiró JL, et al. Fetoscopic release of extremity amniotic bands with risk of amputation. *J Pediatr Orthop.* 2009;29(3):290–293. https://doi.org/10.1097/BPO.0b013e31819c405f.

CHAPTER 2

Hand Function: Typical Development

AVIVA WOLFF, EDD, OT, CHT

INTRODUCTION

Hand motor skill development begins early in utero with spontaneous movements and is fully completed during adolescence with the mastery of fine motor skills and coordination. During the first few years of a child's life, the hand motor skills undergo rapid and remarkable developmental change to allow for exploration and use of objects.[1-3] Early spontaneous movements give way to nonspecific, generalized movements. The infant uses the generalized movements to explore the surrounding area and gather information from the environment. These critical sensory experiences are fundamental to the development of voluntary controlled hand movements.[1,4,5] Nonspecific movements further evolve into exploratory movements that begin with rudimentary grasp patterns and develop into precise movements that allow for dexterous manipulation of objects. The skills required for functional hand use encompass multiple discreet sequential components: recognition of an object, accurate reach for the object, proper hand orientation, proper calibration of aperture (hand opening) as it approaches the object, proper calibration of forces to grasp the object, and finally, grasp and manipulation of the object with one or both hands for the intended use.[6] Timing and coordination for each of these subskills develop throughout early childhood, as the reach-to-grasp movements develop from an immature feedback mechanism to a mature feedforward, anticipatory approach.[6-8] In late childhood and early adolescence, these skills continue to develop for maximum control of speed, accuracy, and coordination.[6,7] Fig. 2.1 represents a timeline of key components of hand motor skill development from the prenatal period through adolescence.

The development of hand skills integral for hand use and function emerges from a complex interaction of multiple systems and maturation of the central nervous system that is further influenced by many contributing factors such as postural control, cognitive and perceptual abilities, vision, sensory experiences, and interaction with the environment.[9,10] The developmental process parallels the typical sequential progression of neuromotor maturation yet varies in timing of onset among children. Typical patterns of hand skill development emerge at specific stages and age ranges with a wide variation in individual development that corresponds to maturation of the central nervous system.[6,9] Influences of the environment and sensory experience on development of hand skills are believed to be largely responsible for this variation.[9-12] Visual, tactile, and proprioceptive sensory experiences play an important role in the development of hand function. Sensory and visual stimulation provide essential feedback for ongoing development of skills and can be manipulated by caregivers and clinicians to enrich the environment and promote and encourage development in typically and atypically developing children.

The purpose of this chapter is to provide clinicians with an understanding of how hand skills develop from basic crude movements to precise patterns that enable skilled manipulation of objects for functional use. This chapter will review the motor development of the range of skills necessary for functional use of the hand for each of these skills: the reach-to-grasp movement, object release, object manipulation, and bimanual coordination. The first section describes the characteristics of spontaneous movements, the second section covers the development of unimanual skills and function, and the third section describes the development of bimanual hand skills and function. Each section explicates the specific characteristics and skills that emerge and mature throughout the developmental continuum and the important factors that influence and shape development. The components and characteristics of key hand motor skills with the corresponding developmental age ranges are listed in Table 2.1.

SPONTANEOUS MOVEMENTS

The earliest movements exhibited by infants are nonspecific, nonpurposeful, and seemingly random. These

Pediatric Hand Therapy. https://doi.org/10.1016/B978-0-323-53091-0.00002-6

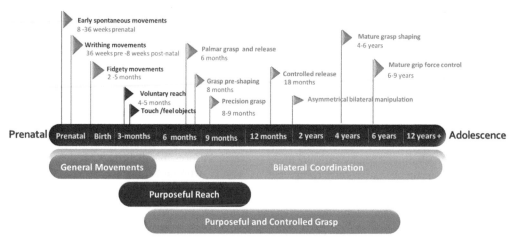

FIG. 2.1 Timeline of key components of hand motor skill development.

movements, called as generalized movements, are not isolated to the upper extremity and occur in all four limbs. They are described as spontaneous movements because they are not elicited by any cause.[13] In the upper limb, general movements have been identified as early as 8 weeks of gestation and continue through early infancy until purposeful and directed reach emerges by approximately 16 weeks.[4,14] Early fetal preterm general movements show large variability until 36–38 weeks of gestation. These movements are replaced by writhing movements that are observed between 36 weeks of gestation to 2 months postterm. Writhing movements are proximal, and characterized by a slow-to-moderate speed and small-to-moderate amplitude.[15] Fidgety movements appear next between 2 and 5 months old, and are more distal, have smaller amplitude, lower speed, and varied acceleration.[15] General movements of the arms are thought to be precursors to reaching and grasping movement and are described in the literature as prereaching behavior[16] because they allow infants to explore their own bodies and surrounding surfaces to gather information critical for future development of reach and grasp.[1,17] Absent, abnormal, and erratic spontaneous movements (especially fidgety movements between 2 and 5 months) are highly predictive of risk for later neurologic dysfunction and conversely, normal movements are predictive of normal development.[14,18,19] When impairment is suspected, the environment can be manipulated by caregivers and clinicians to provide opportunities for enriched sensory experiences to allow for early intervention and further stimulate development.

The general movement assessment is the most commonly used early screening tool to assess abnormal motor activity and identify infants at risk for developmental disorders.[14,15,18–20] It is the most reliable clinical assessment currently available and considered highly predictive for cerebral palsy.[21] Motion capture techniques also provide the opportunity to detect, assess, and track hand and arm movements in infants over the course of development. These techniques are not as well developed but are becoming more available and feasible for use. An extensive review of the advantages and disadvantages of various movement recognition technology (video cameras, 3D motion capture, and direct sensing) in assessing spontaneous general movements was recently published by Marcroft et al.[22] Regardless of the method used, early detection of infants at risk allows for early intervention with a focus on encouraging and facilitating motor control of the hand and arm by providing opportunities that encourage increased use.

UNIMANUAL FUNCTION
Unimanual Reaching
Voluntary, goal-directed, functional movements begin to emerge by 3 months old and replace spontaneous movements. These changes are associated with changes in neuromotor developmental processes and a shift from subcortical to cortical processing.[23,24]

The reach movement observed in early infancy broadly encompasses two types of reach: reaching toward an object, a precursor for a reach-to-grasp movement, and reaching toward the self that is described as bringing the hand to the face (usually mouth and eye). Both movements have a directed arm movement in common. The movements differ in the sensory

TABLE 2.1
Components of Upper Limb Movements

Category	Movement	Developmental Age Range	Characteristics/Examples
Spontaneous movements	Generalized movements	8–36 weeks prenatal	Spontaneous, large variability, reach to mouth
	Writhing movements	36 weeks prenatal –8 weeks postnatal	Proximal, slow-to-moderate speed, small-to-moderate amplitude
	Fidgety movements	2–4 months postnatal	Distal, smaller amplitude, low speed, varied acceleration
Reach	Spontaneous reach	Birth to 2 months	Gross, symmetrical, swipe for objects, predominantly bilateral
	Voluntary unilateral reach	4–5 months	Irregular trajectory, variable movement patterns
	Voluntary bilateral reach	4 months	Attempted bilateral movements
	Mature reach	1–2 years	Straighter, smoother movement path, consistent trajectory
Grasp	Reflexive	1–4 months	Grasp objects placed in hand, nonpurposeful
	Instinctive/Squeeze	5 months	Touching, feeling, raking, beginning anticipatory grasp
	Ulnar palmar grasp	6 months	Four finger grasp, no thumb
	Radial palmar grasp (superior palmar grasp)	7 months	Radial fingers and thumb press object into palm
	Scissors grasp	9 months	Small objects picked up with thumb and lateral border of finger
	Inferior pincer	10 months	Objects held between pads of thumb and fingertip
	Superior pincer	12 months	Objects held between tips of thumb and fingertip
	Deft and precise grasp	15 months	Adjustments for weight and size, varies grip
	Dexterity and manipulation	18 months	Increased control for speed and precision, manipulates utensils
Release	Reflexive	1–4 months	Response to tactile stimulation of extensors
	Accidental release	5 months	Object falls out of hand
	Forced withdrawal	6 months	Pulling
	Release to table or surface	7 months	Variable, and clumsy
	Intentional dropping	10–11 months	Throwing/dropping food
	Precision release	12 months	Graded release, stacking blocks
	Controlled release	18 months–2 years	Accurate, precise release, puzzle pieces
Manipulation	Premanipulation	1–4 months	Object exploration, fingering, raking, shaking objects
	Transfer objects	4–6 months	Transfer from hand to hand, banging, wave and rotate objects
	Finger differentiation	9–10 months	Able to isolate finger movements, pointing
	In-hand manipulation	1–2 years	Move items from palm to fingers

determination of the target. The reach-to-self target is determined by proprioceptive input, whereas the reach-to-object target is determined by visual input.[5,25] The earliest observation of reaching to a target has been documented prenatally at 22 weeks of gestation in the context of reaching toward the mouth.[5]

Reach to grasp
Reach

The phases of a mature reach-to-grasp movement include reach, grasp, transport, and object release. The reach component refers to the movement of the arm toward a target and occurs in parallel with the hand opening and shaping in preparation to grasp the object. Although these movements occur simultaneously in mature reaching, each component develops sequentially during infancy with voluntary goal-directed reaching preceding grasp formation.[26] Successful reaching toward a target requires integration of visual and proprioceptive information. A mature reach is characterized by a smooth trajectory with a consistently continuous straight path to the target, although the speed and trajectory of reach vary depending on the size and location of the target and the intended action. The velocity of a mature reach has a defined acceleration and deceleration phase as the arm approaches the target and concludes with a grasp phase as the hand prepares to grasp the object. These distinct phases are indicative of motor planning and reflect the ability for anticipatory control[27] (Fig. 2.2).

In infants, goal-directed reaching that is characterized as anticipatory and visually guided emerges by the age of 4 months.[4] Before this, infants may attempt to occasionally swipe at objects within their visual field with occasional success. Over time with repeated exposure and experience, hand and arm movements become more purposeful and directed toward a target. However, this early reach is characterized by an irregular trajectory that lacks smoothness and consistency and is highly variable. During early reaching, infants must learn to coordinate the movements of the shoulder, arm, and hand. They begin by using the shoulder and torso to move the hand to the target, while keeping the elbow stiff in an attempt to control the degrees of freedom.[28] Movement trajectories of reach begin to stabilize at the age of 1 year with straighter movement paths, and stereotypical patterns by the age of 2−3 years.[29,30]

Grasp

Successful manipulation of objects is achieved through a combination of several discreet components of hand motor skills: controlled grasp and release, the ability to transfer an object from one hand to another, and individuation of the fingers. Mature grasp is characterized by an anticipatory mechanism that evolves during the reach movement with the hand simultaneously opening and shaping to match the approximate size and shape of the object. The timing of hand opening and closing is critical for smooth and coordinated grasp. Closing the hand too early or too late results in unsuccessful or awkward grasp. During mature grasp, the hand opening (aperture) reaches the maximum opening at about 75% of the reach movement and begins to close as it nears the object.[27,31]

In infants, purposeful grasp is preceded by spontaneous opening and closing of the fingers. These nonpurposeful "pregrasp" hand movements have been called as "vacuous hand babbling."[32] Reflexive grasp exists in infancy from birth to 4 months and is observed as infants curl their fingers around an object in response to stimulation of the palm. Purposeful grasp control develops between 4 and 6 months through exposure to tactile and verbal stimulation.[33] During this time, infants begin to integrate visual information to prepare the hand in anticipation of grasping an object. The combination of tactile and visual stimulation is critical for the development of the ability to grasp, orient, and adjust the hand to objects for purposeful grasp.[9] Grasp patterns emerge over time

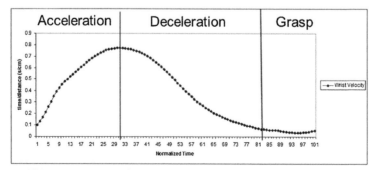

FIG. 2.2 Wrist velocity curve of mature reach-to-grasp movement over the course of time.

from experience and interaction with a variety of object shapes and sizes. At 5 months, a child will touch and feel an object. Voluntary grasp develops through these experiences and is at first accidental. Subsequently, a range of grasp patterns develop through stimulation and exposure to various objects and toys. The characteristics and development of the repertoire of grasp patterns is discussed and detailed later. The earliest anticipatory grasp ability is seen in 5–6 month olds as they open the hand in preparation for grasp and start to close the hand before making contact with the object.

Preshaping the hand to match the object size begins to develop by 8 months old and continues over the next year.[26] Young children, up to age 6, overshoot when reaching for objects and open their hands wider than necessary (Fig. 2.3). Older children demonstrate accurate grip formation to the size and shape of the object with normalization of hand shaping occurring by age 6–8.[34,35] The ability to adjust and orient the grip orientation to the object begins to develop at 6 months and continues to become more accurate up to the age of 15 months.[16,26] Calibration of force control is another critical component of precision grasp that allows for objects to be held without being dropped or crushed. The amount of force generated during grasp is dependent on the size, friction, weight, and texture of the object.[8,36–38] The ability to anticipate force control develops gradually beginning in the second year. Before that, infants control force development via a feedback mechanism. Fingertip force control continues to develop throughout early childhood and reaches adult levels by age 6–9.[39]

Grasp patterns

Mature grasp encompasses a larger repertoire of patterns utilized for the performance of an infinite number of everyday tasks. The specific grasp pattern employed for

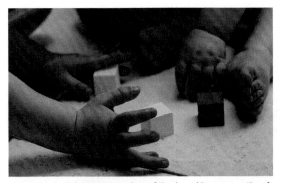

FIG. 2.3 Anticipatory opening of the hand in preparation for grasp. Note: the hand is opening wider than necessary to grasp the cube. (Photo credit: Naomi Polatsek)

a given task is determined by the size and shape of the object, location, and intended use.[9] Grasp patterns have been classified historically into either power or precision grips.[39] In a power grip, the finger and thumb are directed to the palm and the force is directed at the object. Types of power grip include cylindrical grasp (holding a cup or glass), spherical grasp (holding a round object), and a hook grasp (carrying a bag with handles). In precision grasp, the object is held between the thumb and fingers to allow for manipulation of the object relative to the hand and the force is transmitted between the thumb and fingers. Types of precision grasp include tip-to-tip pinch (picking up a marble), pad-to-pad pinch (squeezing a clothespin), three-point pinch or three-jaw chuck (picking up a cube), and lateral pinch (pulling a zipper).[39]

In infants, early spontaneous grasp movement is governed by reflexes from birth to 4 months. The development of purposeful grasp follows a consistent trajectory that begins with a raking and scratching movement of the fingers in 4–5 month olds.[9,40] This is important for tactile stimulation. At first, the fingers flex and extend simultaneously and by 5–6 months most infants exhibit individual finger differentiation and isolated finger movements, most notably the ability to extend the index finger for pointing.[41] These behaviors are largely automatic with the occasional "accidental" grasp. Early grasp at this age (5 months) is instinctive and resembles a squeezing motion. Voluntary grasp begins at age 6 months and has been studied for the last century. Although the development of grasp patterns has traditionally been described in a sequential manner, there is recent evidence to suggest that the emergence of grasp patterns may be more dependent on the object and the requirements of the task.[42,43] The common grasp pattern development described historically is detailed later, and begins with the emergence of a palmar grasp of the four fingers without the thumb that is often more ulnar-based (Fig. 2.4).[9,39,40]

Palmar grasp is succeeded by a radial grasp (also known as a superior palmar grasp) at 7 months. The infant uses the radial fingers and thumb to press the object into the palm when using this pattern (Fig. 2.5A). This allows for easy access to the mouth when the forearm is supinated (Fig. 2.5B). Infants frequently mouth objects during this phase as a method of exploring and learning object properties. In this position objects can also be easily transferred from one hand to the other.

At 8–9 months, precision grasp begins to emerge, and most infants can grasp an object with the distal aspects of the fingers without use of the palm. For small objects, a scissors grasp is used between the thumb and

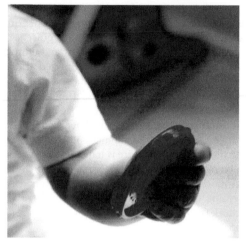

FIG. 2.4 Palmar grasp—object is grasped with four fingers against the palm without the thumb. (Photo credit: Naomi Polatsek)

lateral border of the index with the hand stabilized on a surface (Fig. 2.6). This is an important developmental step toward being able to manipulate and use objects.

At 10 months, small objects can be held with the distal fingertip pads. This grip allows for greater control for release and is called as inferior pincer grasp or forefinger grasp (Fig. 2.7A). The superior pincer grasp, tip-to-tip pinch, emerges at 12 months and allows for greater accuracy and stabilization (Fig. 2.7B).

At this stage, the child is also able to begin adjusting for size and weight of the object. By 15 months, the infant becomes more adept at using a variety of grasps

with increased precision. The ability to manipulate objects with increased dexterity continues over the next few months and by 18 months, there is an increase in dexterity and manipulation of tools and utensils such as using a spoon for self-feeding.[9,39,40]

Object release

Object release emerges following the development of early grasp patterns. Similar to grasp, object release is first observed in infants as reflexive behavior in response to stimulation of primitive reflexes. Brushing the back of the hand elicits a spontaneous extension of the fingers.[44] Purposeful release is seen at 5—6 months, at first inconsistently and accidentally. By 6 months, release of objects is consistent and purposeful and mostly observed when bringing an object to the mouth. Initially, there is a forced withdrawal as the child uses one hand to pull the object out of the other hand. By 7 months, the child is able to release objects on to a surface (table), and object release occurs consistently during bilateral transfer of objects. Sophisticated release in the context of play is seen by 10—11 months.[9] This is the time that children revel in this newfound ability and create a game out of dropping items and food from their high chair.[9] Graded hand opening for precision release such as stacking blocks is achieved by 12 months. At first, the child will press hard while releasing, and lack the ability to precisely and gently release the object. Controlled release continues to develop between ages 1 and 2 for more complex tasks that require precise release of small objects with greater accuracy (placing puzzle pieces, small items in jar). Timing and controlling release continues to be

(A)

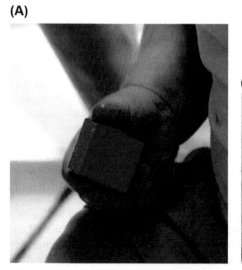

(B)

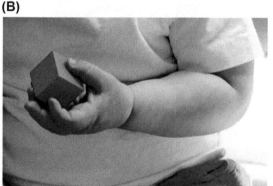

FIG. 2.5 **(A)** Radial grasp—object is grasped by radial fingers and thumb and pressed into palm, **(B)** Forearm is supinated to allow easy access to the mouth. (Photo credit: Naomi Polatsek)

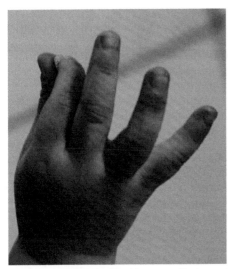

FIG. 2.6 Scissors grasp—object is grasped between thumb and lateral border of the index with the hand stabilized on a surface. (Photo credit: Naomi Polatsek)

difficult for 2–3 year olds, who often exhibit difficulty with delicate tasks.[45] This skill continues to develop by age 5–6 for improved accuracy, speed, and dexterity.[9]

Manipulation

Efficient manipulation of objects requires a combination of skills and the ability to differentiate movement between the fingers, calibrate grip force, regulate precise release, and control timing and speed. Dexterous manipulation of objects is a skill that develops from infancy through adolescence.

Premanipulation behavior is observed in early infancy, even before voluntary grasp and reach is developed. In early infancy (1–4) months, arm movements are used for object exploration. When an object is placed in the hand of a 1–2-month-old child, the child will twist the wrist to move the object when it is within the visual field (rotation).[46,47] A child will also use movements of the arm to deliberately change the location of the object (translation), or to shake the object (vibration). An increase in fingering and raking behavior is observed at age 4 months.[48] Object exploration continues to develop at 5–6 months with the ability to transfer objects. By 6 months, infants are able to rotate, wave, and bang objects as well as transfer from one hand to the other. With the ability to differentiate finger movements and control release at age 9–10 months, manipulation skills further develop allowing for poking, prodding, and picking up small objects.

In-hand manipulation skills begin to develop at the age of 1 year. The term was first described by Exner

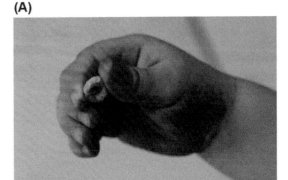

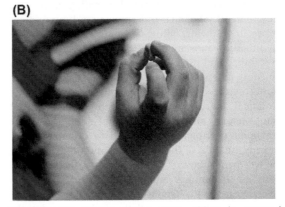

FIG. 2.7 **(A)** Inferior pincer grasp—object is grasped between pads of thumb and index finger. **(B)** Superior pincer grasp—object is grasped between tips of thumb and finger. (Photo credit: Naomi Polatsek)

(1992) who described in hand manipulation as the adjustment of objects by movements of the fingers so that the objects are placed in a more appropriate position to accomplish the task.[49] Exner defines several subcomponents of this skill:

1. The ability to move an object from the palm to the fingers (translation) as in moving a coin to the fingers from a fistful of change.
2. The ability to rotate an object in the pads of the finger as in loosening a screw.
3. Using the thumb to move an object in a linear direction on the finger (shift) as in rolling a pencil.

Finger to palm translation and simple rotation occur by 2 years old, and complex rotation movements such as manipulating a pencil for writing use continues to develop until age 7.[49] Between ages 3 and 7 years old, children master more complex manipulation skills such as fastening buttons and manipulating writing and eating utensils. The ability to perform these skills with precision is directly related to the concurrently developing ability to properly calibrate grip forces.[8] Finger movements continue to become more accurate in older children (ages 6–12) with demonstrated improvements in reaction times and speed.[34,50] By age 12, fine motor coordination and accuracy approximate adult behavior.[34]

BIMANUAL FUNCTION

Bimanual Reach to Grasp

Most daily tasks require some level of bimanual function where demands are required of both hands. This adds a level of complexity on both a functional and neural control level for regulation of timing and coordination between the two hands. Depending on the task requirements, bimanual movements can be symmetrical as in throwing, lifting, pushing, and pulling, or asymmetrical movements where either one hand acts to stabilize and the other manipulates, or both hands function independently in a differentiated role as in typing on a keyboard or playing a musical instrument.[51] Bimanual function is controlled by interactions of many neural structures, and the development of bimanual coordination is related to the maturation and myelination of the corpus callosum that connects the two hemispheres.[52] In early infancy, these connections are incomplete and continue to develop over several years. As the nervous system develops, the intermanual control improves with the ability to regulate the timing and spatial coordination of both hands for complex tasks.[52] Additionally, bimanual tasks require mature postural and trunk control to allow for both hands to function independently.

Bimanual Reaching

Bilateral asymmetric and symmetric arm movements are present from early infancy, first as spontaneous general movements. Although most spontaneous arm movements appear to be simultaneous and symmetrical, alternating arm movements are also typically present from birth to 2 months when elicited by reflexes and tactile input. Voluntary bimanual reach first emerges at 2 months as gross symmetrical movements of both hands reaching for objects, although swiping movements tend to be predominantly unilateral.[9] Symmetrical bilateral reaching continues to evolve and predominate by 4 months as trunk stability increases. There is also an increased drive toward symmetrical movements to midline. By 5 months, the bilateral approach for reach to grasp becomes more consistent as both hands move toward the object simultaneously. At this age, in spite of the bilateral reach, the grasp remains unilateral.[1,6,9]

Bimanual Grasp

Bilateral fingering precedes bilateral grasp and is evident in 4–5 month olds. Between the ages of 6–8 months, objects are approached most frequently with both hands. During this stage, both simultaneous and sequential bilateral reach-to-grasp patterns emerge[9,53] (Fig. 2.8).

At 7 months, infants appear to use both a unilateral and bilateral approach depending on the size and position of the object, and the amount of external support provided. They tend to use a bilateral approach to grasp large objects and a unilateral approach for small objects. In an unsupported environment, they may utilize a unilateral strategy while using the other arm for stabilization. By 8–11 months, improved motor and postural control allows for increased discriminatory ability of unimanual and bimanual strategies as they are now unconstrained by factors that predispose a specific strategy.[12,54] However, a return to a predominant bilateral reach-to-grasp strategy emerges when postural stability is challenged as seen with early walking.[55]

Bimanual Manipulation

Transfer from hand to hand is evident as early as 4–6 months and becomes more consistent and fluid by 7–8 months once the infant masters radial grasp.[56] This is the age when infants will begin to play with two objects simultaneously by banging them together, waving them in the air, or banging on a surface[57] (Fig. 2.9).

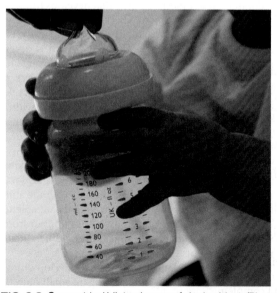

FIG. 2.8 Symmetrical bilateral grasp of single object. (Photo credit: Naomi Polatsek)

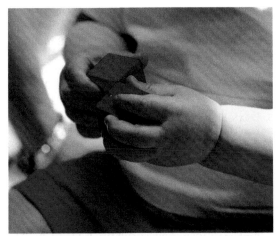

FIG. 2.9 Symmetrical bilateral grasp of two independent objects. (Photo credit: Naomi Polatsek)

The repertoire of symmetrical bimanual skills continues to expand to include bimanual squeezing, pulling apart, and pushing together. Toys with multiple parts encourage these activities and can be used in therapy sessions to provoke responses.[54] Asymmetrical skills develop simultaneously to allow for exploratory behavior with one hand, while the other hand is grasping the object. By 9 months, the child has acquired a larger repertoire of bimanual skills and is able to position an object with one hand while manipulating it with the other.[58] At this time, the ability to rotate and reposition objects begins to develop with the recent acquisition of grip orientation ability. Between 9 and 12 months, coordination improves and greater independence between the two hands emerges allowing for rotation of toys with both hands. From 1 to 2 years old, the infant continues to develop greater control over bimanual skills and mastery of more difficult tasks such as symmetrical bimanual drumming. Asymmetrical independent use of each hand, such as removing objects from inside another or stringing small beads, is also observed in children between the ages of 1–2.[9,46,54] Between the ages of 2–4, children begin to master more difficult tasks that require simultaneous efficient use of independent movements in both hands such as buttoning, zippering, and opening a snack bag or candy wrapper.[9,46,54] More complex bimanual coordination skills continue to develop along with the development of cognitive and perceptual skills throughout early childhood and adolescence, allowing for complex two-handed tool use such as cutting food, or sequenced and complementary movements of both hands such as using scissors for cutting. The speed, efficiency, timing, and accuracy continue to improve with less variability throughout early adolescence where skills approximate those of adults.

CONCLUSION

Assessment and treatment of pediatric hand conditions require intimate knowledge of the stages of typical development of hand motor skills from infancy to adolescence. An understanding of age appropriate function also allows for early detection of impaired hand motor control and delayed skill development. Early identification of infants at risk affords early intervention so that children are stimulated in sensory rich environments that encourage the emergence of hand function skills. Familiarity with age appropriate skills and function enable the clinician to select the appropriate assessment tools and develop suitable treatment strategies. Proper toy selection during each phase is critical to stimulate and encourage developmentally appropriate skills.

ACKNOWLEDGMENTS
Photo credits: Naomi Polatsek

REFERENCES

1. Lobo MA, Galloway JC, Heathcock JC. Characterization and intervention for upper extremity exploration & reaching behaviors in infancy. *J Hand Ther*. 2015;28(2):114–124. https://doi.org/10.1016/j.jht.2014.12.003. quiz 125.
2. Lobo MA, Harbourne RT, Dusing SC, McCoy SW. Grounding early intervention: physical therapy cannot just be about motor skills anymore. *Phys Ther*. 2013;93(1):94–103. https://doi.org/10.2522/ptj.20120158.
3. Thelen E, Schöner G, Scheier C, Smith LB. The dynamics of embodiment: a field theory of infant perseverative reaching. *Behav Brain Sci*. 2001;24(1):1–34. discussion 34-86.
4. Berthier NE, Keen R. Development of reaching in infancy. *Exp Brain Res*. 2006;169(4):507–518. https://doi.org/10.1007/s00221-005-0169-9.
5. Zoia S, Blason L, D'Ottavio G, et al. Evidence of early development of action planning in the human foetus: a kinematic study. *Exp Brain Res*. 2007;176(2):217–226. https://doi.org/10.1007/s00221-006-0607-3.
6. Charles J. Typical and atypical development of the upper limb in children. In: Eliasson A-C, Burtner PA, eds. *Improving Hand Function in Children with Cerebral Palsy:Theory, Evidence and Intervention*. London: Mac Keith Press; 2008.
7. Shumway-Cook A, Woollacott MH. Reach, grasp, and manipulation: changes across the life span. In: *Motor Control: Translating Research into Clinical Practice*. Third. Philadelphia: Lippincott; 2007.
8. Forssberg H, Eliasson AC, Kinoshita H, Johansson RS, Westling G. Development of human precision grip. I: basic coordination of force. *Exp Brain Res*. 1991;85(2):451–457.

9. Case-Smith J. Hand skill development in the context of infant's play: birth to 2 years. In: Henderson A, Pehoski C, eds. *Hand Function in the Child: Foundations for Remediation*. Second. St. Louis: Mosby; 2006:117–143.

10. Thelen E. Motor development: a new synthesis. *Am Psychol*. 1995;50(2):79–95.

11. Thelen E, Corbetta D, Spencer JP. Development of reaching during the first year: role of movement speed. *J Exp Psychol Hum Percept Perform*. 1996;22(5):1059–1076.

12. Corbetta D, Thelen E. The developmental origins of bimanual coordination: a dynamic perspective. *J Exp Psychol Hum Percept Perform*. 1996;22(2):502–522.

13. Ferrari F, Prechtl HF, Cioni G, et al. Posture, spontaneous movements, and behavioural state organisation in infants affected by brain malformations. *Early Hum Dev*. 1997; 50(1):87–113.

14. Einspieler C, Prechtl HFR. Prechtl's assessment of general movements: a diagnostic tool for the functional assessment of the young nervous system. *Ment Retard Dev Disabil Res Rev*. 2005;11(1):61–67. https://doi.org/10.1002/mrdd.20051.

15. Prechtl HF, Einspieler C, Cioni G, Bos AF, Ferrari F, Sontheimer D. An early marker for neurological deficits after perinatal brain lesions. *Lancet Lond Engl*. 1997; 349(9062):1361–1363. https://doi.org/10.1016/S0140-6736(96)10182-3.

16. von Hofsten C, Fazel-Zandy S. Development of visually guided hand orientation in reaching. *J Exp Child Psychol*. 1984;38(2):208–219.

17. Lobo MA, Galloway JC. Assessment and stability of early learning abilities in preterm and full-term infants across the first two years of life. *Res Dev Disabil*. 2013;34(5): 1721–1730. https://doi.org/10.1016/j.ridd.2013.02.010.

18. Prechtl HF. State of the art of a new functional assessment of the young nervous system. An early predictor of cerebral palsy. *Early Hum Dev*. 1997;50(1):1–11.

19. Einspieler C, Peharz R, Marschik PB. Fidgety movements - tiny in appearance, but huge in impact. *J Pediatr*. 2016; 92(3 Suppl 1):S64–S70. https://doi.org/10.1016/j.jped.2015.12.003.

20. Kwong AKL, Fitzgerald TL, Doyle LW, Cheong JLY, Spittle AJ. Predictive validity of spontaneous early infant movement for later cerebral palsy: a systematic review. *Dev Med Child Neurol*. 2018;60(5):480–489. https://doi.org/10.1111/dmcn.13697.

21. Bosanquet M, Copeland L, Ware R, Boyd R. A systematic review of tests to predict cerebral palsy in young children. *Dev Med Child Neurol*. 2013;55(5):418–426. https://doi.org/10.1111/dmcn.12140.

22. Marcroft C, Khan A, Embleton ND, Trenell M, Plötz T. Movement recognition technology as a method of assessing spontaneous general movements in high risk infants. *Front Neurol*. 2014;5:284. https://doi.org/10.3389/fneur.2014.00284.

23. Hitzert MM, van Geert PLC, Hunnius S, Van Braeckel KNJA, Bos AF, Geuze RH. Associations between developmental trajectories of movement variety and visual attention in fullterm and preterm infants during the first six months postterm. *Early Hum Dev*. 2015;91(1):89–96. https://doi.org/10.1016/j.earlhumdev.2014.12.006.

24. Ouss L, Le Normand M-T, Bailly K, et al. Developmental trajectories of hand movements in typical infants and those at risk of developmental disorders: an observational study of kinematics during the first year of life. *Front Psychol*. 2018;9:83. https://doi.org/10.3389/fpsyg.2018.00083.

25. Zoia S, Blason L, D'Ottavio G, Biancotto M, Bulgheroni M, Castiello U. The development of upper limb movements: from fetal to post-natal life. *PLoS One*. 2013;8(12): e80876. https://doi.org/10.1371/journal.pone.0080876.

26. von Hofsten C, Rönnqvist L. Preparation for grasping an object: a developmental study. *J Exp Psychol Hum Percept Perform*. 1988;14(4):610–621.

27. Jeannerod M. The timing of natural prehension movements. *J Mot Behav*. 1984;16(3):235–254.

28. Berthier NE, Clifton RK, McCall DD, Robin DJ. Proximo-distal structure of early reaching in human infants. *Exp Brain Res*. 1999;127(3):259–269.

29. Konczak J, Dichgans J. The development toward stereotypic arm kinematics during reaching in the first 3 years of life. *Exp Brain Res*. 1997;117(2):346–354.

30. von Hofsten C. Structuring of early reaching movements: a longitudinal study. *J Mot Behav*. 1991;23(4):280–292. https://doi.org/10.1080/00222895.1991.9942039.

31. Jakobson LS, Goodale MA. Factors affecting higher-order movement planning: a kinematic analysis of human prehension. *Exp Brain Res*. 1991;86(1):199–208.

32. Wallace PS, Whishaw IQ. Independent digit movements and precision grip patterns in 1-5-month-old human infants: hand-babbling, including vacuous then self-directed hand and digit movements, precedes targeted reaching. *Neuropsychologia*. 2003;41(14):1912–1918.

33. Bruner JS, Koslowski B. Visually preadapted constituents of manipulatory action. *Perception*. 1972;1(1):3–14. https://doi.org/10.1068/p010003.

34. Kuhtz-Buschbeck JP, Stolze H, Boczek-Funcke A, Jöhnk K, Heinrichs H, Illert M. Kinematic analysis of prehension movements in children. *Behav Brain Res*. 1998;93(1–2): 131–141.

35. Wolff AL, Raghavan P, Kaminski T, Hillstrom HJ, Gordon AM. Differentiation of hand posture to object shape in children with unilateral spastic cerebral palsy. *Res Dev Disabil*. 2015;45–46:422–430. https://doi.org/10.1016/j.ridd.2015.07.002.

36. Gordon AM, Forssberg H, Johansson RS, Westling G. The integration of haptically acquired size information in the programming of precision grip. *Exp Brain Res*. 1991; 83(3):483–488.

37. Forssberg H, Kinoshita H, Eliasson AC, Johansson RS, Westling G, Gordon AM. Development of human precision grip. II. Anticipatory control of isometric forces targeted for object's weight. *Exp Brain Res*. 1992;90(2): 393–398.

38. Eliasson AC, Gordon AM, Forssberg H. Tactile control of isometric fingertip forces during grasping in children with cerebral palsy. *Dev Med Child Neurol*. 1995;37(1):72–84.

39. Napier JR. The prehensile movements of the human hand. *J Bone Joint Surg Br.* 1956;38-B(4):902–913.

40. Halverston H. A further study of Grasping. *J Gen Psychol.* 1932;7:34–63.

41. Nagy E, Compagne H, Orvos H, et al. Index finger movement imitation by human neonates: motivation, learning, and left-hand preference. *Pediatr Res.* 2005; 58(4):749–753. https://doi.org/10.1203/01.PDR.000018 0570.28111.D9.

42. Duff S. Functional development. In: Abzug J, Kozin SH, Zlotolow DA, eds. *The Pediatric Upper Extremity.* Vol. 1. Philadelphia: Springer; 2015.

43. Lantz C, Melén K, Forssberg H. Early infant grasping involves radial fingers. *Dev Med Child Neurol.* 1996;38(8): 668–674.

44. Twitchell T. Reflex mechanisms and the development of prehension. In: Conolly K, ed. *Mechanisms of Motor Skill Development.* London: Academic Press; 1970.

45. Gesell A, Halverston H, Thompson H, et al. *The First Five Years of Life.* New York: Harper and Brothers; 1940.

46. Pehoski C. Object manipulation in infants and children. In: Henderson A, Pehoski C, eds. *Hand Function in the Child: Foundations for Remediation.* Second. Mosby; 2006: 143–163.

47. Karniol R. The role of manual manipulative stages in the infant's acquisition of perceived control over objects. *Dev Rev.* 1989;9:205–233.

48. Rochat P. Object manipulation and exploration in 2 to 5 month-old infants. *Dev Psychol.* 1989;25:871–884.

49. Exner CE. The zone of proximal development in in-hand manipulation skills of nondysfunctional 3- and 4-year-old children. *Am J Occup Ther.* 1990;44(10): 884–891.

50. Garvey MA, Ziemann U, Bartko JJ, Denckla MB, Barker CA, Wassermann EM. Cortical correlates of neuromotor development in healthy children. *Clin Neurophysiol.* 2003; 114(9):1662–1670.

51. Swinnen SP, Wenderoth N. Two hands, one brain: cognitive neuroscience of bimanual skill. *Trends Cognit Sci.* 2004;8(1):18–25.

52. Fagard J, Hardy-Léger I, Kervella C, Marks A. Changes in interhemispheric transfer rate and the development of bimanual coordination during childhood. *J Exp Child Psychol.* 2001;80(1):1–22. https://doi.org/10.1006/jecp .2000.2623.

53. Castner B. The development of fine prehension in infancy. *Genet Psychol Monogr.* 1932;12:105–193.

54. Greaves S, Imms C, Krumlinde-Sundholm L, Dodd K, Eliasson A-C. Bimanual behaviours in children aged 8–18 months: a literature review to select toys that elicit the use of two hands. *Res Dev Disabil.* 2012;33(1): 240–250. https://doi.org/10.1016/j.ridd.2011.09.012.

55. Corbetta D, Bojczyk KE. Infants return to two-handed reaching when they are learning to walk. *J Mot Behav.* 2002;34(1):83–95. https://doi.org/10.1080/002228902 09601933.

56. Pierce D, Munier V, Myers CT. Informing early intervention through an occupational science description of infant-toddler interactions with home space. *Am J Occup Ther.* 2009;63(3):273–287.

57. McCall RB. Exploratory manipulation and play in the human infant. *Monogr Soc Res Child Dev.* 1974;39(2):1–88.

58. Kimmerle M, Ferre CL, Kotwica KA, Michel GF. Development of role-differentiated bimanual manipulation during the infant's first year. *Dev Psychobiol.* 2010;52(2):168–180. https://doi.org/10.1002/dev.20428.

CHAPTER 3

Physical Examination of the Pediatric Upper Extremity

SARAH ASHWORTH, OTR/L, BS

Physical examination of the upper extremity in the pediatric client includes the same components pertinent to the adult population. However, methods of assessment must be tailored to the developmental level of the patient. Infants and young children have limited attention spans, less ability to follow directions, and are often uncooperative with unfamiliar adults. Patience, age-appropriate language, and a ready supply of toys and props will lead to a more successful evaluation. Evaluations performed on the floor, at a child-sized table, or from a trusted caregiver's lap can build rapport and improve participation. When working with children, including the family is imperative. Caregivers often provide history; explain what the child can do and actually does on a daily basis; and are important to supporting carryover at home. Videos or photographs of participation in daily activities in the child's environment provide valuable information that may be difficult to elicit in the clinic.

Children will often try to "get the right answer" on the examination, especially when they know what the clinician is assessing. For example, a 6-year-old child with a history of pollicization may demonstrate consistent incorporation of her thumb when handed various objects by the therapist. However, in the waiting room, she demonstrates interdigital scissoring pinch for small objects. Her mother reports that she uses her thumb for cups and balls, but prefers scissor pinch for small items. A combination of formal assessment, observation, and family interview provides a more accurate picture of the child's true function.

RANGE OF MOTION

A precise assessment of range of motion is essential to identify limitations and tracking progress with intervention. Active range of motion (AROM) and passive range

of motion (PROM) measurements can be challenging with infants and young children due to pain, fearfulness, limited attention span, and small hand size. Children may be afraid when they see an unfamiliar tool. When possible, handing the goniometer to the child to "measure" a parent or clinician often helps to reduce fear. At times, the goniometer will not be tolerated and the therapist is required to use his or her "ocular goniometer" to assess motion. Beginning with AROM measurements can help to build trust before handling, however if the child has difficulty following instructions starting with PROM can model the desired movement. For children having difficulty tolerating the assessment, prioritizing the most important measures and completing others later is a necessary strategy.[1]

With young children, it is often challenging to take accurate goniometric measurements of active motion. Small hand size can make measuring active and passive digital movement difficult.[2,3] Alternative play-based measurements may be necessary. For example, composite flexion may be quantified by measuring the diameter of the smallest marker the child can grasp. Alternative measures should be objective and repeatable to track progress over time. Limited attention spans or ability to follow directions can lead to difficulty maintaining maximum effort at end range. Having the goniometer in position to measure quickly and engaging a parent to elicit the desired motion can assist the process. Games, such as Simon Says, can also help engage and build rapport with younger clients.[4] Patients who have sustained a traumatic injury may have their effort limited by pain or fear of pain. Beginning with moving unaffected adjacent joints may reduce guarding postures. A functional task may produce more movement than instructions to move in a particular plane.

Pediatric Hand Therapy. https://doi.org/10.1016/B978-0-323-53091-0.00003-8

The concept of scaffolding should be utilized to elicit challenging motions.[5,6] This refers to beginning in the range where the child experiences success and gradually building the challenge, rather than starting in a range that is out of reach. For example, a toddler with a brachial plexus injury with limited shoulder abduction may not even attempt to reach for a sticker held overhead. By presenting the sticker at chest height, the child experiences success. From here, the stimulus can be gradually raised higher until the AROM limit is achieved (Fig. 3.1).

PROM assessment is often difficult for clients who have pain or have had negative experiences with stretching over time. Other children may have limited tolerance for handling or being still for the assessment. Distractions such as music or videos may help the child relax for the exam. Patience and time may be necessary to slowly move the affected joint and avoid eliciting muscle guarding and discomfort. Any stretches that are anticipated to cause discomfort should be saved for the end of the examination. One example is passive shoulder external rotation for children with brachial plexus palsy and suspected internal rotation contracture. Initiating the evaluation with this stretch in an infant or toddler may cause them to shut down, negating any additional assessment of arm function.

Children with range of motion deficits, especially congenital conditions, will develop adaptations to function within their abilities. Careful observation of these

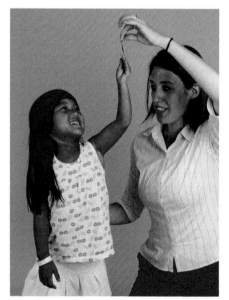

FIG. 3.1 Slowly raising the sticker to provide the "just right" challenge to elicit overhead reach. (Courtesy Shriners Hospital for Children, Philadelphia.)

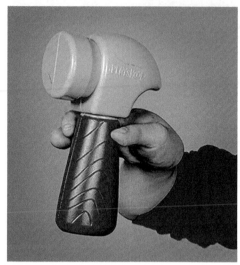

FIG. 3.2 A child with a congenital hand difference grasps a toy, which was selected by the clinician to be an appropriate width and weight for success in play. (Courtesy Shriners Hospital for Children, Philadelphia.)

compensatory strategies will highlight areas that require further assessment. Excessive wrist flexion can be observed during midline function in children with brachial plexus birth palsy who demonstrate limitations in internal rotation limitation. Wrist flexion is also used as a compensatory strategy for self-feeding in a child lacking elbow flexion after an elbow injury. Patients with arthrogryposis multiplex congenita (AMC) often develop several compensatory patterns to overcome limitations (Fig. 3.2). For clients with chronic conditions that create limited potential for improvement in range of motion, these patterns are encouraged. However, in conditions where further recovery is expected, these movement patterns are discouraged to eliminate ongoing and unnecessary compensatory movement patterns.

STRENGTH

Strength assessment in pediatric clients can be challenging for many of the reasons noted in the previous section. Manual muscle testing (MMT) can be utilized in older children and adolescents. Beginning with larger joints, clear instructions and comparison to the unaffected side, when possible, will allow the clinician to assess if a child is able to participate in the exam. For patients with limited attention spans, focus on the key muscles to test to elicit maximum effort.[1] Making strength testing a game can help to increase participation. In addition to MMT, dynamometry for grip and pinch strength has established norms for children as young as 6 years old.[7]

Upper extremity strength in infants and toddlers should be assessed through observation of function.[2,3] This can be objectively measured by presenting toys with different sizes and monitoring how long the child can maintain grasp or lift the toy. Movement is compared in antigravity and gravity-eliminated planes. As the child moves through developmental positions, such as quadruped or pulling to stand, assess for symmetrical weight bearing and inclusion of the affected side. The Active Movement Scale was developed for measuring strength in infants with obstetrical brachial plexus palsy.[8] Although reliability studies focus on this population, this scale can be used clinically for infants with other diagnoses to obtain an objective comparison of strength changes.

Compensatory movements may conceal weaknesses and require careful scrutiny. A teenage patient with absent triceps from a C6 spinal cord injury may appear to have 2/5 MMT strength via shoulder external rotation and supination. However, palpation, blocking external rotation, and any attempt at antigravity movement will reveal that the triceps is not functioning. Extensor digitorum communis and the long finger flexors (flexor digitorum profundus and superficialis) can act upon the wrist in the presence of weak wrist extension or flexion, respectively (Fig. 3.3). Proximal momentum can be utilized to augment shoulder or elbow flexion. In the absence of active elbow flexors, children may utilize the Steindler effect. This occurs when forearm pronation and wrist and finger flexion are paired with momentum to initiate elbow flexion. The child is able to hold the elbow in flexion by contracting the flexor/pronator muscles that originate proximal to the elbow.[9] When in doubt, having the child reproduce the movement slowly can often elucidate what is powering the motion.

It is also important to consider the effect of concomitant weakness on distal and proximal control. For children with trunk weakness, proximal support from adaptive seating or alternative positions might be necessary to fully assess strength in the upper extremity. In the example of the teen with C5 spinal cord injury, when asked to perform shoulder abduction, they may initially demonstrate very limited motion against gravity. Raising the arm above shoulder height may cause loss of sitting balance and passive elbow flexion causing the hand to fall into the client's face. Providing appropriate support at the trunk and maintaining elbow extension will allow for a more accurate assessment of shoulder function. Creative variations from standard testing positions may be necessary to fully assess a child's strength.

SENSIBILITY TESTING

Sensibility assessment requires concentration, focus, and participation of a patient. Different from most other aspects of upper extremity evaluation, occluding vision is necessary for accuracy. Many of the tests require tedious test procedures with multiple stimuli applied in each area of the hand. These aspects make formal sensation testing challenging with the pediatric population.[1]

As with the other areas of evaluation, clinical observation is valuable with regards to sensibility testing. Observing how the child spontaneously incorporates the affected area into play is critical information. Provide bimanual toys such as hook and loop, food, pop beads, and stickers to peel from backing paper. Bypassing digits or avoiding use of the hand is indicative of decreased sensibility. Observe for motor changes such as claw posturing or altered thumb movement patterns indicating underlying nerve injury. Sympathetic dysfunction should raise suspicion for loss of sensibility in peripheral nerve injuries, as the sympathetic fibers are more resistant to damage from traumatic injury.[10] Observations or parent reports of sympathetic dysfunction may include skin color and temperature changes (cold or bluish area, redness in the bath or summer heat); excessive or absent sweat; and trophic changes such as smooth, shiny, or excessively dry skin, tapered appearance of digits, and nail and hair abnormalities[11] (Fig. 3.4). Signs of self-mutilation from biting can be present in young children with suspicion of abnormal sensation (Fig. 3.5). In the clinic, this can appear to begin with nerve regeneration, possibly as a way to dampen neurogenic discomfort. Children often lack the vocabulary to verbalize pain or sensory changes. Some may describe feeling "ants crawling" or "electric shocks," others may react with nonverbal gestures. For example, patients may react with leg twitching when light touch stimuli or stroking is applied to a hypersensitive hand.

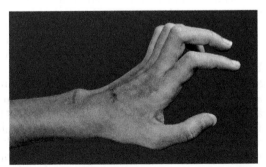

FIG. 3.3 12-year old child utilizing extensor digitorum communis to aid weak wrist extensors. (Courtesy Shriners Hospital for Children, Philadelphia.)

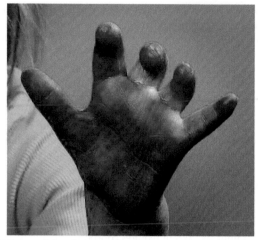

FIG. 3.4 A hand presenting with trophic changes following nerve injury. (Courtesy Shriners Hospital for Children, Philadelphia.)

Threshold and functional sensibility tests can be incorporated in the pediatric population. Avoid words that may elicit a fearful response before application. Substituting "warm" for "hot" and "pointy" for "sharp" can improve participation. Allowing the child to see and feel the stimulus in an unaffected area before testing gives them better understanding of the exam and what to expect. The Semmes Weinstein Monofilament Test may be utilized with older children and adolescents. The entire exam includes 20 monofilaments and can document small changes; however, the evaluation is lengthy

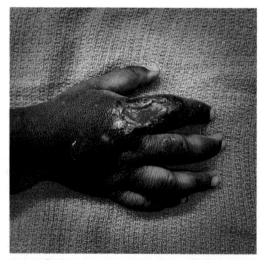

FIG. 3.5 Digit injury secondary to self-mutilating behaviors in a 4-year-old girl following nerve injury. (Courtesy Shriners Hospital for Children, Philadelphia.)

to complete. The Weinstein Enhanced Sensory Test (WEST) can be utilized with children as young as 6 years old and only includes five monofilaments that are connected to one handle. This allows for quickly switching between monofilaments for more efficiency with testing. In normal pediatric upper limbs, it has moderate to excellent test—retest reliability.[12,13]

Functional sensibility assessments include static and moving two-point discrimination, Moberg Pickup Test, and stereognosis testing. Two-point discrimination is commonly utilized following nerve repair to track recovery. In addition, it can be used in children with cervical spinal cord injuries to assist in determining if sensibility will allow for spontaneous hand function without visually observing the hand during manipulation.[14] Static two-point discrimination has been found to be reliable in children as young as 6 years old.[15,16] The Moberg Pickup Test presents the child with a set of objects to pick up with each hand, with and without vision.[17] In addition to observing hand function relying on sensibility, this test allows the clinician to observe in hand manipulation skills and which parts of the hand are incorporated. Stereognosis testing involves presenting familiar objects to the patient with vision occluded for the child to identify with sensation only. Pictures of the objects can be incorporated when testing younger children. This test can allow the clinician to observe manipulation patterns and can be presented as a fun game.

The Wrinkle Test can be administered to assess vasomotor function. The test is relatively simple to use and only requires tolerance of water play. This assessment includes submerging the hand in warm water, 40°C for 20—30 min as described by O'Riain.[18] After soaking, the hand is observed for even wrinkling throughout the nerve distributions. Affected areas will remain smooth while intact skin will appear wrinkled. Incorporating toys for water play encourages bimanual submersion, which can be helpful for comparison.[1] This test is most useful to indicate complete peripheral nerve lacerations. Patients with nerve compression injuries will often maintain sympathetic function.[19]

DEXTERITY

Dexterity is simply defined as using the hands to manipulate objects. The developmental context of acquiring grasp, pinch, release, and in-hand manipulation skills is further discussed in Chapter 2. These movement patterns are multifactorial. Assessment of dexterity requires mindfulness of hand development and the impact of strength, range of motion, muscle tone, and sensation on typical hand function.

Assessment of dexterity can be particularly difficult in children under 3 years old. Developmental motor assessments with fine motor subscales can be utilized to identify delays, such as the Peabody Developmental Motor Scales (PDMS-2).[20] Often, more specific hand function measures are desired. Ho describes a consistent developmental approach for young children.[3] She recommends preparing a consistent set of toys, carefully selected with objects of different shapes and sizes, to elicit a variety of grasp and manipulation patterns. When possible, the unaffected limb is assessed as the reference point to compare function. By utilizing the same set of objects, serial assessments can be utilized to track progress over time.[3] Safety must be considered when introducing small objects to assess pincer grasp. Consider utilizing individually appropriate edible props, such as cereals, to avoid choking hazards.

Many additional assessment tools have been found to be reliable for children. The Functional Dexterity Test (FDT), box and block test, and 9-hole peg test all have norms established from 3 years old through adulthood.[7,21–23] The FDT assesses in-hand manipulation skills. The test consists of a pegboard with 16 pegs that the client picks up, turns over, and replaces into the board. Performance is timed with penalties for dropped pieces.[21] The box and block test has clients pick up one inch blocks, lift over a divider, and drop into the other side of the box. Scoring is based on how many blocks are moved in 1 min. This assessment can be utilized with children with limited hand function; however, it requires proximal function to cross over the divider.[7,22] In addition to objective measures to assess progress over time, these tests provide observation of repeated hand movement patterns. Compensatory movements and other concerns should be noted with results.

Physical examination of the pediatric upper extremity can present unique challenges. This population is very rewarding to treat, as children often heal better and are more resilient than older patients. Caregivers are vital to provide an accurate picture of functional limitations and day-to-day symptoms. Approaching the assessment with patience, a playful attitude, and toys builds rapport to facilitate a successful evaluation.

REFERENCES

1. Ho ES. Evaluation of pediatric upper extremity peripheral nerve injuries. *J Hand Ther.* 2015;28:135–143.
2. Aaron DH. Pediatric hand therapy. In: Henderson A, Pehoski C, eds. *Hand Function in the Child: Foundations for Remediation.* 2nd ed. St Louis: Mosby Elsevier; 2006: 367–400.
3. Ho ES. Measuring hand function in the young child. *J Hand Ther.* 2010;23:323–328.
4. Ashworth S, Kozin SH. Brachial plexus palsy reconstruction tendon transfers, osteotomies, capsular release and arthrodesis. In: Skirven TM, Osterman AL, Fedorczyk JM, Amadio PC, eds. *Rehabilitation of the Hand and Upper Extremity.* 6th ed. Philadelphia: Elsevier; 2011:792–812.
5. Wood D, Bruner J, Ross G. The role of tutoring in problem solving. *J Child Psychol Psychiatry.* 1976;17:89–100.
6. Maybin J, Mercer N, Stierer B. "Scaffolding" learning in the classroom. In: Norman K, ed. *Thinking Voices: The Work of the National Oracy Project.* London: Hodder and Stoughton; 1992:186–195.
7. Mathiowetz V, Federman S, Wiemer D. Box and blocks test of manual dexterity: norms for 6–19 year olds. *Can J Occup Ther.* 1985;52:241–245.
8. Curtis C, Stephens D, Clarke HM, Andrews D. The Active Movement Scale: an evaluative tool for infants with obstetrical brachial plexus palsy. *J Hand Surg Am.* 2002;27(3): 470–478.
9. Al-Qattan MM. Elbow flexion reconstruction by Steindler flexorplasty in obstetric brachial plexus palsy. *J Hand Surg.* 2005;30B:424.
10. Tindall A, Dawood R, Povlsen B. Case of the month: the skin wrinkle test: a simple nerve injury test for paediatric and uncooperative patients. *Emerg Med J.* 2006;23: 883–886.
11. Duff S, Estilow T. Therapist's management of peripheral nerve injuries. In: Skirven TM, Osterman AL, Fedorczyk JM, Amadio PC, eds. *Rehabilitation of the Hand and Upper Extremity.* 6th ed. Philadelphia: Elsevier; 2011: 619–633.
12. Weinstein S. Fifty years of somatosensory research: from the Semmes-Weinstein monofilaments to the Weinstein enhanced sensory test. *J Hand Ther.* 1993;6(1):11–22.
13. Thibault A, Forget R, Lambert J. Evaluation of cutaneous and proprioceptive sensation in children: a reliability study. *Dev Med Child Neurol.* 1994;36(9):796–812.
14. McDowell CL, Moberg EA, House JH. The second international conference on surgical rehabilitation of the upper limb in tetraplegia (quadriplegia). *J Hand Surg.* 1986; 11(4):604–608.
15. Cope EB, Antony JH. Normal values for the two-point discrimination test. *Pediatr Neurol.* 1992;8:4.
16. Dua K, Lancaster TP, Abzug JM. Age-dependent reliability of Semmes-Weinstein and 2-point discrimination tests in children. *J Pediatr Orthop.* 2016. https://doi.org/10.1097/BPO.0000000000000892.
17. Moberg E. Objective methods for determining the functional value of sensibility in the hand. *J Bone Joint Surg Br.* 1958;40-B:454–476.
18. O'Riain S. New and simple test of nerve function in hand. *Br Med J.* 1973;3:615–616.
19. Phelps PE, Walker E. Comparison of the finger wrinkling test results to established sensory tests in peripheral nerve injury. *Am J Occup Ther.* 1977;31(9):565–572.

20. Exner CE. Development of hand skills. In: Case-Smith J, ed. *Occupational Therapy for Children*. 5th ed. Philadelphia: Elsevier; 2005:304−355.
21. Gorgola GR, Velleman PF, Shuai X, Morse AM, Lacy B, Aaron D. Hand dexterity in children: administration and normative values of the Functional Dexterity Test. *J Hand Ther*. 2013;38:2426−2431.
22. Jongbloed-Pereboom M, Nijhuis-van der Sanden MWG, Steenbergen B. Norm scores of the box and block test for children ages 3−10 years. *Am J Occup Ther*. 2013;67:312−318.
23. Wang Y, Bohannon RW, Kapellusch J, Garg A, Gershon RC. Dexterity as measured with the 9-hole peg test (9-HPT) across the age span. *J Hand Ther*. 2015;28:53−60.

CHAPTER 4

Outcome Measures

NAMRATA GRAMPUROHIT, PHD, OTR/L • M.J. MULCAHEY, PHD, OTR/L, FASIA

INTRODUCTION

Upper extremity capabilities of varied prehension, reach, object transport, and sensing can challenge the measurement of outcomes in therapy.[1] The growth and development in children along with differential opportunities for play and education can further impact functional upper extremity measurement. Multifaceted assessment by therapists of children with upper extremity impairments and limitations involves the use of standardized observation and assessment of impairment (manual muscle testing, sensation, lower motor neuron deficits, spasticity, etc.), performance-based measures, child-reported outcomes, and parent-reported outcomes. Therapy-related objectives for assessment include screening; diagnosing functional limitations to develop benchmark, reimbursement, evaluation, and goal setting; prioritization of treatment goals; monitoring change over time; building evidence to support treatment for individualized data-driven decision making; and comparing outcomes among treatments. This chapter is an update to a prior publication that provided a description of outcome measures and their psychometric properties.[2] This chapter provides an overview of different types of tests; details the psychometric properties of outcome instruments and their interpretation; updates the therapists on the literature on outcome instruments with particular focus on functional pediatric upper extremity instruments; and further discusses scoring and interpretation of traditional and modern item response theory (IRT)-based measures. Finally, the chapter provides resources for therapists to maintain ongoing competency in assessment of the pediatric upper extremity.

The scope of this chapter includes functional assessments of the upper extremity. The existing classification systems such as the Manual Ability Classification System for children with Cerebral Palsy (CP),[3] the Mallet Classification and Active Movement Scale for children with brachial plexus birth palsy (BPBP),[4] the International Standards for Neurological Classification of Spinal Cord Injury,[5] and Classification of the Upper Extremity in Tetraplegia for children with spinal cord injury (SCI)[6] will not be discussed in this chapter as they are not outcome measures, but classification systems. The scope of this chapter also excludes impairment-based measures for muscle strength, sensibility, joint range of motion, pain, and spasticity. Information on these methods can be found in other excellent resources.[2,7–11] Impairment-based methods have traditionally been used during therapy and do not suffice as functional endpoints for outcomes assessment in children. The scope of this chapter also excludes assessments using mobile health technology and activity trackers as the literature on these technology-based measures is in its early stages with no consensus; however, preliminary evidence can be found in some recent studies.[12,13] Of note, the terms tests, tools, scales, instruments, measures, and assessments will be used interchangeably in this chapter, as is the case in much of the literature.

TYPES OF OUTCOME INSTRUMENTS

The selection of outcome instruments is guided by determining if the scores need to be compared to a level of performance or criterion, or to the typical population. Thus, there are two types of instruments that differ in how scores are interpreted: criterion-referenced and norm-referenced tests. Criterion-referenced tests enable interpretation of test score in relation to a certain level of benchmark performance.[14,15] For example, Shriners Hospitals Upper Extremity Evaluation (SHUEE) is a criterion-referenced test where children with cerebral palsy are compared on predefined criteria for assessment of their performance. In contrast, norm-referenced tests can be interpreted in the individual's performance relative to performance of some known typical or normative group.[14] An example of commonly used norm-referenced tests is the developmental motor scales wherein scores are interpreted against "normal"

Pediatric Hand Therapy. https://doi.org/10.1016/B978-0-323-53091-0.00004-X

development. For norm-referenced instruments, the mean scores from the reference sample provide a standard and variability is used to determine how an individual performs relative to the reference sample.[15] Norm-referenced tests are usually used for diagnosing, while criterion-referenced tests are used to examine proficiency of performance along a continuum. An example of a criterion-referenced test continuum is the range from inability to do a task to ability to complete the task and is felt to be more useful for developing and evaluating rehabilitation outcomes.[15]

There are two types of assessments based on the use of scores: formative and summative assessments. An assessment that provides information to guide ongoing planning of treatment is called as a formative assessment. The criterion-referenced instruments provide the ability to examine ongoing performance and are used as formative assessments. In contrast, a summative assessment enables initial or discharge assessment of function and typically is a norm-referenced test.[16] The knowledge of the original purpose of the test as described by the test author can help identify the recommended use of the instrument as a formative or summative assessment. Therapists need to be aware of the author-intended use of the instrument and to avoid inaccurate representation of the scores.

The assessments can also be categorized as generic versus disease specific. Generic measures are used across diagnostic conditions but need to be validated for their use in the population of interest. The disease-specific measures are only used with certain diagnoses with their items customized for the symptoms, features, or functional implications of the diagnosis. For example, the Jebsen Test of Hand Function[17] and the Box and Block Test[18] are generic performance measures for the upper extremity that assess function and dexterity, respectively. Although these measures have been originally developed for adults, their measurement properties have been studied in children. In contrast, the Prosthetic Upper Extremity Functional Index (PUFI) and the Child Amputee Prosthetics Project-Functional Status Inventory (CAPP-FSI) are disease-specific instruments developed for children with limb deficiency. The selection between generic and disease-specific instruments is determined by the purpose of assessment. The generic measures enable comparison of outcomes across diagnostic conditions; whereas, the specialized therapy centers prefer to use disease-specific instruments as they typically work for most patients seen within the clinic. Disease-specific instruments have the advantage of highly relevant items and response scales to the diagnostic population and may also function

better at detecting change than a generic measure.[19] For example, the PUFI has items probing the usefulness of the prothesis for the activity and items that have response options that take into consideration the use of prosthetic hand actively and passively.[20]

The International Classification of Functioning, Disability, and Health (ICF) has also been used to categorize outcome instruments into body structure and function, activity, or participation level of measurement. Although measurement of performance in each of these domains is important for a comprehensive assessment of functioning, the currently available measures lack adequate coverage of all three domains, particularly those related to participation. Hao et al.[21] described the expert consensus on musculoskeletal pediatric upper extremity outcome instruments according to ICF domains. For the activity domain, the bilateral tasks were highly valued by experts along with the instruments Assisting Hand Assessment (AHA), Pediatric Evaluation of Disability Inventory (PEDI), SHUEE, and Jebsen Hand Function Test. For the participation domain, the Canadian Occupational Performance Measure (COPM), Pediatric Outcomes Data Collection Instrument (PODCI), and Disabilities of the Arm, Shoulder, and Hand (DASH) were highly valued by experts. Other sources have provided detailed ICF classification of outcome instruments for children with CP[22] and linking of individual outcome measures such as the PEDI.

There are different types of assessments based on the individual completing the items, that is, performance-based measures, parent/teacher/proxy-reported measures, and child-reported measures. Therapists typically use performance-based measures wherein the items are scored based on observed performance of the tasks for the test and used to be the data collection method preferred within the clinical setting. However, in the changing healthcare environment, to adhere to patient-centered clinical practice, there is also a need to collect patient-reported outcomes[23] and a battery of outcome measures may be needed to fully assess the client's functioning. Child-reported outcomes are equally important to collect within pediatric therapy practice and children as young as 3 years old could participate in reporting their experiences on appropriately designed measures.[24]

PSYCHOMETRIC PROPERTIES OF OUTCOME INSTRUMENTS

The measurement or psychometric properties of an instrument provide the therapist with evidence on the accuracy and appropriateness of the tool for the intended purpose. The properties should be considered during selection of the outcome measure particularly when decisions related to treatment and reimbursement are based on the scores. These properties include evidence of reliability, validity, and responsiveness. The definitions of these properties and their interpretation guidelines are provided in Table 4.1. Reliability evidence for a tool is the most basic of the three measurement properties and needs to be examined carefully. Reliability evidence for total scores is usually determined using Intraclass Correlation Coefficient,[25] while those on individual items can be determined using kappa coefficients.[15] For using a measure repeatedly with a

TABLE 4.1
Description of Measurement Properties and Their Interpretation.

Measurement Property	Definition	Interpretation Guidelines	References
RELIABILITY			
Test−retest Intrarater Interrater Alternate forms	Stability of scores free from measurement error across the specified condition (e.g., across time, within one rater, among different raters, and varied forms)	Intraclass correlation coefficient for total scores 0.7 and 0.9 are recommended for outcome instruments Higher than 0.9 are preferred	Andresen (2000)[139], Fitzpatirck et al.,[38] Portney and Watkins [141], Portney and Watkins,[15] Streiner and Norman[25]
Internal consistency	The degree of **interrelatedness** among items in a measure	Cronbach's α >0.9 strong effect 0.70−0.80 moderate effect <0.70 weak effect	Portney and Watkins [141], Portney and Watkins[15]
Measurement error	The **systematic or random error** not related to a change in function	Scores/points	Portney and Watkins[141]
RESPONSIVENESS			
Effect size	The degree to which the score on an instrument is capable of **detecting change** in function. Responsiveness can be determined in a longitudinal study	Cohen's d <0.2 weak effect 0.2−0.5 moderate effect 0.5−0.8 strong effect	Andresen (2000)[139]
Minimal detectable change	The degree to which the score on an instrument is capable of **detecting important changes** in function beyond measurement error	Scores/points greater than measurement error	Guyatt et al.[33]
Minimal clinically important difference	The degree to which the score on an instrument is capable of detecting **clinically important** changes in function. Also called as minimal important difference, minimally important changes, clinically meaningful differences		
Floor effect	The degree to which the score on an instrument is not capable of detecting changes at the **lower end** of function	15%−20% of individuals achieved the lowest (floor) or highest (ceiling) score	Andresen (2000)[139]
Ceiling effect	The degree to which the score on an instrument is not capable of detecting changes at the **higher end** of function		

Continued

TABLE 4.1
Description of Measurement Properties and Their Interpretation.—cont'd

Measurement Property	Definition	Interpretation Guidelines	References
VALIDITY			
Validity	The degree to which the instrument measures what it is **supposed** to measure	There are multiple ways in which validity can be reported. The unified concept of validity considers all psychometric properties as contributing evidence of validity	Messick[26]
Face	The degree to which the instrument **appears** to measure what it intends to measure	Qualitative and content expert agreement	Portney and Watkins[141], Portney and Watkins[15]
Content	The degree to which the **items** in the instrument reflect the construct to be measured based on theory and expert opinion	Qualitative and content expert agreement	Portney and Watkins[141], Portney and Watkins[15]
Criterion—concurrent	Degree to which the scores on the instrument are related to scores on a **gold standard measure** of the same construct	Correlation coefficient r or ρ <0.30 weak 0.30–0.60 moderate >0.60 strong	Andresen (2000)[139], Portney and Watkins[141], Portney and Watkins[15]
Construct—convergent	The degree to which the scores on the instrument are related to scores on **another instrument** with the same construct		
Construct—divergent/discriminant	The degree to which the scores on the instrument are not related to scores on another instrument with a **different** construct		
Factorial	The degree to which the items on the instrument represent **factors** within the construct	Confirmatory factor analysis indicating how much variance in scores is explained by the factors. Measures can have one or more dimensions	Andreson (2000)[139], Mokkink et al.[31]
Known groups	The degree to which the scores on the instrument are able to **differentiate** or discriminate between known groups	Statistically significant difference between groups	Andresen (2000)[138]
Cross-cultural	The degree to which the scores on the instrument are able to measure the same construct in a new cultural cohort	Cultural adaptation, front and back translation, and adaptation of the measure with establishment of relevant measurement properties	Andresen (2000)[138]

patient, strong evidence of test–retest and intrarater reliability is desired. When there are multiple therapists involved in the assessment of a patient, a measure with strong evidence of interrater reliability estimates is preferred. When using different formats of the same instrument, alternate forms reliability should be examined for the evidence it provides to justify the use of differing formats. Internal consistency is a form of reliability assessed using Cronbach's α coefficient for each dimension and is usually the most commonly reported evidence for reliability of a tool.[15] However, internal consistency alone is not sufficient evidence of reliability.

The evidence for construct validity encompasses all measurement properties.[26] Face and content validity evidence is the most basic form of validity.[27] Content validity evidence for patient-rated outcomes is gathered during the development and field-testing of the items with experts and users in an iterative cognitive testing methodology.[28–30] The evidence for construct validity can be evaluated using hypothesis testing with a correlation coefficient for convergence with scores from instruments measuring similar constructs and divergence with scores from instruments measuring dissimilar constructs. The evidence for construct validity can also be informed by inferential tests for group differences of scores among known groups, such as those with and without upper extremity impairments. The evidence from exploratory or confirmatory factor analysis can further inform the validity evidence. The language adaptations for the patient-reported instrument should be accompanied with cultural adaptations, backward and forward translations, and measurement properties for the translated instrument. For the evidence of validity to be applicable for the diagnostic condition, measurement studies need to be conducted in the population of interest, the design needs to be intended for measuring psychometric properties, missing data should be reported accurately, and adequately powered for good quality.[31]

The responsiveness of the scores of a measure can help the therapist determine its use as an outcome measure for the clinic. There are multiple methods used to report responsiveness such as effect size, standard response mean, minimal detectable change (MDC), and minimal clinically important difference (MCID).[32,33] The MDC and MCID values should be greater than the measurement error values of the instrument. Floor and ceiling effects provide the therapist with information regarding the range of deficit for which the measure will not be useful.[32] The clinical utility of a measure, although not a measurement property, includes the appropriateness of the measure based on construct and psychometrics, acceptability, practicability, and accessibility.[34] Outcome measures that are lengthy, difficult to administer, or expensive and those lacking accommodations for disabilities lose clinical utility due to factors beyond those of psychometrics and therapists must consider these pragmatic aspects during selection of outcome measures.

The measurement properties discussed thus far and described in Table 4.1 provide description and interpretation guidelines using traditional measurement theory approach. The newer methods of item response theory employ modern statistical tools to analyze items calibrated on a continuum from low to high levels of the construct or trait. The properties of reliability and validity have different interpretation guidelines for studies using item response theory. For example, the National Institutes of Health Patient-Reported Outcomes Measurement Information System measures are developed using the modern measurement techniques.[35] More information on use of item response theory applications to patient-reported outcome measures can be found in other useful sources[36,37] (Table 4.1).

CONSIDERATIONS IN SELECTION OF OUTCOME INSTRUMENTS

Selection of instruments in the clinic can be a time-intensive task and a systematic approach can enhance efficiency. The UK Patient Reported Outcomes Measurement Group has set forth eight criteria for selection of instruments.[38] These include appropriateness of the instrument to the needs of the construct to be assessed; acceptability of the instrument to the patients; feasibility to easily administer and score the instrument; interpretability and precision of the scores of the instrument; reliability of the instrument's results; reproducibility and internal consistency; and responsiveness of the instrument to detect changes over time that matter to the patients. The Pediatric Section of the American Physical Therapy Association has enabled ease of access to this information for therapists and categorized by the ICF to facilitate the selection of measures. A systematic approach in the clinical setting can involve listing the characteristics of the population served by the clinic (e.g., age, diagnosis, and severity); thorough literature search on the instruments available for the population at impairment, activity and participation levels; examining the eight selection criteria; obtaining the instruments; and periodically reviewing the needs of the patient population to update the inventory. The outcomes used to track groups of patients at the clinic can also dictate the selection of instruments. These criteria can be applied within a program or department for systematic process of staff training using an educational framework for competence. The iterative process can involve conducting a pretraining needs assessment; establishing preliminary face validity of the measures; analyzing the needs of the learners such as time and learning preferences; assessing for initial competency; developing a posttraining competency assessment; developing training modules; delivering learning modules that involve problem-based, real-life learning opportunities; completing posttraining competency assessment; sharing results with learners; and discussion, evaluating the learning experience and updating the training and assessment based on feedback.

The guidelines for selection of instruments set forth by national organizations over the past decade are presented as core datasets or common data elements. The common data elements are essential or highly recommended elements of data for a particular diagnostic condition or for the general population as determined by scientific task forces convened to develop these guidelines. The outcome measures are only a subset of the common data elements that also include essential data to be reported during clinical trials such as height, weight, etc. Table 4.2 provides a description and link to the U.S. National Institute of Health, National Quality Forum, International Spinal Cord Injury Core Outcome Sets, Core Outcome Measures for Effectiveness Trials, American Physical Therapy Association's EDGE Task Force Recommendations, and the ICF Core Sets. Although the common data elements were developed for uniform data collection in research studies, their translation to clinical practice can lead to standardized measurement variables collected across various diagnoses to enable creation of larger data repositories. This work is currently being done within the specialized model systems in the United States, for example the Spinal Cord Injury Model System. The field of rehabilitation can greatly benefit from adoption of common data elements within clinical practice.

The advanced user of assessments in the clinic can go beyond the evidence of measurement properties and utility of the instrument to consider the consequences of testing.[26] The consequences of testing are not only experienced by the therapist, organization, and payers, but also by the child, parents, and other team members. The therapist must pay close attention to the undesired consequences of testing such as value judgements and social desirability. For example, the value assigned to a developmental test to determine the services needed for a child can place undesired burden on the tester

and the test-taker both and deter from unbiased performance from both entities. The high-stakes embodiment of the instruments may not match the original purpose of the test and can also affect the validity of the instrument's scores. The advanced user needs to consider the positive and negative impact of testing as contributing to the validity evidence of the instrument.

ADMINISTRATION, SCORING, AND INTERPRETATION

To get the child and parent engaged in the process of assessment, it is important to share the rationale, purpose, and interpretation of scores in an easy to understand language.[39] The consent for testing should be routinely obtained and participant's feedback on the process and results should be incorporated into future testing situations.[40] The structured and standardized administration of a measure includes acquiring the necessary training in setup, instructions to the patient, recording, scoring, and continued competency. Many of the upper extremity performance measures require extensive set up, standard workspaces for reaching and placing objects, and differing sizes and weights of objects. They are prone to observer bias introduced due to fatigue, lack of interest, or accumulation of compensatory movements.[41] For patient-reported outcome measures, the framing of questions can change the responses obtained. For example, task performance of children is indicated by asking if they "did" something and capacity is indicated by asking if they "can do" a task.[42] There was a difference of 18% detected between performance and capacity in children with physical disabilities.[43]

Instruments should be accompanied by instructional manuals that provide detailed information on set up, ideal testing conditions, administration, methods for calculating total and subscale scores, handling missing items, and interpretation of scores. Raw scores are obtained by manual calculations. Raw scores often need to be converted to standard scores, which allow for comparison across individuals and variables with different normal distributions. Calculating a standard score requires one to know the raw score, the mean score, and the standard deviation. For example, IQ scores are traditionally expressed with a mean of 100 and standard deviation of 15 (Fig. 4.1). A conversion to Z-score has a mean of 0 and standard deviation of 1. The Z-score is the distance from the mean in standard deviation units. A T-score on the other hand is a transformed score with a mean of 50 and standard deviation of 10. For example, Pediatric Evaluation of

TABLE 4.2
Outcome Measures for Functional Assessment of the Pediatric Upper Extremity.

Outcome Measure	Description	Number of Items	Supplier/Source	References
FUNCTIONAL PERFORMANCE MEASURES				
Assisting Hand Assessment (AHA)	Assesses the use of the assisting hand while performing bimanual play in usual environments; uses Rasch measurement model	22	http://www.ahanetwork.se/	Chang et al.,[58] Bialocerkowski et al.,[59] Krumlinde-Sundholm and Eliasson,[54] Gordon,[56] Hoare et al.,[63] Krumlinde-Sundholm et al.,[55] Holmefur et al.[57] Mini-AHA in CP: Greaves et al.[60]
Box and Block Test (BB)	Performance measure that requires picking up blocks and placing; norms available	1	Sammons Preston	Mathiowetz et al.,[18] Chen et al.,[48] Desrosiers et al.,[49] Lin et al.,[50] Platz et al.,[51] Jongbloed-Pereboom,[52] Mulcahey et al.,[118] Ekblom et al.[53]
Capabilities of the Upper Extremity Test (CUE-T)	Performance measure with unilateral and bilateral tasks scored on repetitive actions, progressive actions, and timed tasks	17	Dent et al.[140]	Dent et al.[140]
Graded Refined Assessment of Strength, Sensation, and Prehension (GRASSP)	Strength, dorsal and palmar sensation, prehension ability and prehension performance are assessed	25 items per hand	https://www.grassptest.com/	Mulcahey et al.[107]
Jebsen Test of Hand function	It requires manipulation of objects that reflect everyday tasks and one writing task; norms available	7	Sammons Preston	Bovend'Eerdt et al.,[142] Jebsen et al.,[17] Taylor et al.,[46] Noronha et al.,[143] Mulcahey et al.,[143] Aliu et al.,[145] Klingels et al.,[146] Netscher et al.,[147] Lee et al.,[68,69] Shingade et al.,[148] Hiller and Wade[149], Brandao et al.,[150] Staines et al.,[151]
Melbourne Assessment of Unilateral Upper Limb function (MUUL)	Assesses unilateral upper extremity quality of movement in children with neurological impairments	14	https://www.rch.org.au/melbourneassessment/how-to-order/	Randall et al.,[61,62]; Spiritos et al.,[152] Klingels et al.[66]
Quality of Upper Extremity skills Test (QUEST)	Criterion-referenced measurement tool, developed to evaluate upper extremity quality of movement in children with CP	36	https://www.canchild.ca/en/shop/19-quality-of-upper-extremity-skills-test-quest	Klingels et al.,[66] DeMatteo et al.,[153,154]

Continued

TABLE 4.2

Outcome Measures for Functional Assessment of the Pediatric Upper Extremity.—cont'd

Outcome Measure	Description	Number of Items	Supplier/Source	References
Shriners Hospitals Upper Extremity Evaluation (SHUEE)	Video-based tool for the assessment of upper extremity function in children with hemiplegic cerebral palsy	Tone, range of motion, and 16 manual function tasks	http://shrinerschildrens.org/shuee-test-scoring-and-interpretation/	Klingels et al.,[66] Sakzewski et al.,[70] Bard et al.,[64] Randall et al.,[62] Klingels et al.,[67] Lee et al.,[68,69] Thorley et al.,[71,72] Davidson et al.,[65] Gilmore et al.[47]
CHILD AND PARENT-REPORTED OUTCOME MEASURES				
ABILHAND-Kids	Manual ability in children; uses Rasch measurement model	21	http://www.rehab-scales.org/abilhand-kids-downloads.html	Arnould et al.,[89] Penta et al.,[155] Vandervelde et al.,[156] Aarts et al.,[157] Klingels et al.,[146] Sgandurra et al.,[158] Foy et al.,[90] Spaargaren et al.,[91] Buffart et al.,[92] Kumar and Phillips[93]
Activities Scale for Kids (ASK)	Assesses physical function with a capability and performance version	30	http://www.activitiesscaleforkids.com/	Young et al.,[159] Plint et al.[160]
Canadian Occupational Performance Measure (COPM)	Semistructured interviews for parents and children to identify performance activities that are perceived as important by the parent, child, and/or society	5	http://www.thecopm.ca/	Law et al.,[95] Cup et al.,[161] Eyssen et al.,[162] Cusick et al.,[163,164] Carswell et al.,[165] McColl et al.,[166] Mulcahey et al.,[118] Davis et al.,[167] Pollock et al.,[168] Brandao et al.[150]
Cerebral Palsy profile of Health and function (CP-PRO)				
Child Health Questionnaire (CHQ)	Assesses health related quality of life	50 or 28	https://www.healthactchq.com/survey/chq	Landgraf et al.[85]
Child Amputee Prosthetics project-Functional Status Inventory (CAPP-FSI)	Assesses functional status in children with limb deficiency including preschool children and toddlers	40	Pruitt et al.[169]	Pruitt et al.[169,170]
Children's Hand-use Experience Questionnaire (CHEQ)	Assesses the experience of children and adolescents in using the affected hand in activities where usually two hands are needed. New version uses Rasch model	29 Mini-CHEQ for ages 3–8 years: 21	http://www.cheq.se/	Sköld et al.[171]

TABLE 4.2
Outcome Measures for Functional Assessment of the Pediatric Upper Extremity.—cont'd

Outcome Measure	Description	Number of Items	Supplier/Source	References
Disabilities of the Arm, Shoulder and Hand (DASH) and QuickDASH	Physical function and symptoms in patients with several musculoskeletal disorders of the upper limb	30; QuickDASH: 11	http://www.dash.iwh.on.ca/	Quatman Yates et al.[88]
Goal Attainment Scaling	Evaluates performance on each goal using specified possible outcomes, and evaluates the extent of goal attainment	Variable	https://www.kcl.ac.uk/nursing/departments/cicelysaunders/attachments/Tools-GAS-Practical-Guide.pdf	Bovend'Eeerdt et al.,[96] Kiresuk et al.,[172] Mailloux et al.,[173] Ten Berge et al.,[174] Wesdock et al.,[175] Lowe et al.,[176] Steenbeek et al.,[177] Bovend'Eerdt et al.[178]
Motor Activity Log: Pediatric and Infant	Structured interview to examine how often and how well a child uses his/her involved upper extremity in their natural environment outside the therapy setting	22	https://www.uab.edu/citherapy/images/pdf_files/CIT_PMAL_Manual.pdf	Uswatte et al.,[179] Wallen et al.[180]
Pediatric Evaluation of Disability Inventory (PEDI)	Functional skills, level of independence, and modifications required for functional activities are assessed	197	https://www.pearsonclinical.com/childhood/products/100000505/pediatric-evaluation-of-disability-inventory-pedi.html	Haley et al.[86]
Pediatric Outcomes Data Collection Instrument (PODCI)	Upper extremity function as well as physical function, activity and sports, mobility, pain, happiness, and satisfaction with treatment	86	https://www.aaos.org/research/outcomes/Pediatric.pdf	Daltroy et al.,[181] Hunsakar,[182] Amor et al.,[183] Kunkel et al.,[184] Matsumoto et al.,[185] Lee et al. (2010), Nath et al.,[186] Dedini et al.,[187] Huffman et al.[188]
Pediatric Measure of Participation (PMoP)	Assesses the child's self-participation relative to how much the child's friends participate	51 self-participation 53 friends-participation	Mulcahey et al.[114,118]	Mulcahey et al.[114,118], Mulcahey et al. (2016)
Pediatric Quality of Life Inventory (PedsQL)	Assesses quality of life in children with chronic illnesses	23	https://www.pedsql.org/	Varni et al.[84]
Piers-Harris Children's self-concept scale	Assesses behavior, intellectual and school status, physical appearance and attributes, anxiety, popularity, happiness, satisfaction	80	https://www.mhs.com/MHS-Assessment?prodname=piersharris2	Piers et al.[189]

Continued

TABLE 4.2
Outcome Measures for Functional Assessment of the Pediatric Upper Extremity.—cont'd

Outcome Measure	Description	Number of Items	Supplier/Source	References
Prosthetic Upper Extremity Functional Index (PUFI)	Evaluates the extent to which a child actually uses a prosthetic limb for daily activities, the comparative ease of task performance with and without the prosthesis, and its perceived usefulness	38	Wright et al.[20]	Buffart et al.,[190] van Dijk-Koot et al.,[191] Wright et al.[20,94]
COMPUTER ADAPTIVE TESTS AND SHORT FORMS				
Pediatric Evaluation of Disability Inventory Computer Adaptive Test (PEDI-CAT)	Assesses self-care mobility and social function in children across different diagnoses	Variable from 197 item pool	https://www.pedicat.com/	Haley et al.,[101,103] Coster et al.,[99] Allen et al.,[98] Dumas et al.,[100] Mulcahey et al.[102]
CP PRO	Parent-reported assessment of physical	Can be limited to 5,	University of Utah	Grampurohit et al.[109]

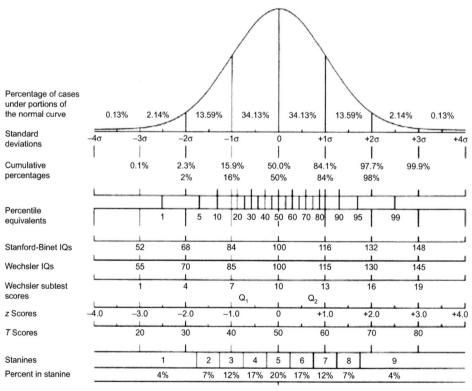

FIG. 4.1 Description of the Wechsler scale IQ scores and their relationship to the various types of standard scores and the normal curve.

Disability Inventory's standard score is a T-score.[42] A high T-score needs to be interpreted based on the desirability of the skill assessed. A high T-score for an undesirable trait is worse performance. For example, in the Children's Depression Inventory,[44] a higher T-score would indicate more depression. In contrast, the PROMIS Upper Extremity Item Bank developed using Item Response Theory methods is scored on a T-score metric where higher scores indicate better function.[45]

For norm-referenced tests, percentile scores are indicative of how the child ranked relative to the normative sample. A percentile rank of 95 indicates that a child scored at or above 95% of the students in the normative sample. Age equivalencies, on the other hand, provide an equivalent age based on the performance of the child on the measure. The interpretation of the equivalent age provided on such measures should be interpreted in light of the other scaled or standard scores. The scaled score is the performance on a subtest that assesses a particular skill. It is combined with other scaled scores to form standard scores. A standard error of measurement is provided based on the normative sample, and two standard errors on either side of the score provide the confidence interval. Thus, the confidence interval is the hypothetical range of scores predicted if a child were given the test multiple times. Criterion-referenced test scores are interpreted with a cut-score or percent correct; however, standard and scaled scores may also be used. Interpretation for criterion-referenced test scores is based on how much of the skill the child can perform and is beneficial for children with moderate-to-severe disability where comparisons with normative sample do not serve the intended purpose of testing.

FUNCTIONAL PERFORMANCE MEASURES

The functional performance measures involve demonstration of functional arm and hand tasks that are rated by observation of quality, completion, assistance, or speed of performance. These measures require standard setup, administration, scoring, and interpretation guidelines typically provided in a manual. Table 4.2 lists some of the available functional performance measures that can be used with children with pediatric upper extremity disorders, and other sources listed in Table 4.3 can provide a detailed listing of the psychometric properties of these measures. Therapists should note that many of these performance measures were field-tested with adults. The Jebsen Test of Hand Function is a norm-referenced, timed test of hand function that was originally established for adults[17] and subsequently field-tested in children.[46] It requires

manipulation of everyday objects and one writing task. Although it has been used with children with varying diagnoses, sound psychometric studies in samples of pediatric populations with upper extremity impairments are lacking.[47] The Box and Block Test[18] is another generic performance measure that evaluates unilateral hand function as assessed by the number of blocks acquired, carried, and released in 1 min. Although most psychometric studies have been conducted with adults with neurologic and orthopedic impairments,[48-51] studies have also been done with children 3 years and older and with conditions such as brachial plexus birth palsy, limb deficiency.[52,53] The AHA is an upper extremity performance measure that measures assisting hand use during bimanual play in child's typical environment.[54] It has been studied for children with spastic hemiplegia, cerebral palsy, and other orthopedic conditions.[55-59] The Mini-AHA has been established for babies with CP between 8 and 18 months of age and further psychometric testing is needed.[60] The Melbourne Assessment of Unilateral Upper Limb Function (MUUL),[61,62] the Quality of Upper Extremity Skills Test (QUEST), and the SHUEE are performance measures for children with cerebral palsy that assess upper extremity function. The MUUL, QUEST, and SHUEE are impairment or body structure-level measures.[63] All three instruments have strong psychometric properties when used with children with CP, provide important information about upper limb function, and have been used in treatment effectiveness studies.[47,62,64-72] Based on a systematic review of psychometric studies,[47] for children with CP and upper limb involvement, the MUUL is recommended for assessment of unilateral performance and, when used with the AHA, is most effective at measuring change in unilateral and bimanual hand function over time or following treatment.

PATIENT-REPORTED OUTCOME INSTRUMENTS

The importance and use of patient-reported outcome instruments has received widespread attention in the past decade.[73,74] Agencies such as the US Food and Drug Administration[75] recommend studies include patient-reported outcomes. Child-reported outcomes are a growing area of work within pediatric instruments and studies have reported children as young as 3 and 6 years can report on their own health.[24,76] Proxy reporting by parents, guardians, or teachers can provide important but different perspectives when measuring similar outcomes.[77-80] Although only a few instruments are developed and validated for child report of

TABLE 4.3
Resources to Aid in the Selection of Outcome Instruments.

Resource	Website*	Details
DATABASES		
PROQUOLID	https://eprovide.mapi-trust.org/about/about-proqolid	A database of patient centered outcomes that assists selection of clinical outcome assessments based on recommended sources such as US food and Drug Administration, European Medicines Agency, and the research community
Rehab Measures Database	https://www.sralab.org/rehabilitation-measures	A database of over 400 existing measures in rehabilitation. The psychometric properties are provided within each instrument summary for the various populations
Spinal Cord Injury Research Evidence (SCIRE) Outcome Measures	https://scireproject.com/outcome-measures/	A database that provides information on common outcome measures used in spinal cord injury clinical practice. Also provides resources for selection of measures such as the Outcome Measures Toolkit with 33 tests
MEASUREMENT SYSTEMS		
CanChild	https://www.canchild.ca/	An accessible resource for children, families and healthcare providers regarding outcome measures and other aspects care for autism spectrum disorder, brain injury, concussion, cerebral palsy, developmental coordination disorder, down syndrome, fetal alcohol spectrum disorder, and spina bifida
Health Measures: A U.S. National Institute of Health (NIH) distribution center for Neuro-QoL, PROMIS, NIH Toolbox, and ASCQ-Me	http://www.healthmeasures.net	Quality of Life in Neurological Disorders (Neuro-QoL): A measurement system developed and validated for common neurological conditions to evaluate physical, mental, and social domains across the lifespan Patient-Reported Outcome Measures Information System (PROMIS): Self-reported and parent-reported measures developed and validated for global, physical, mental, and social health across the lifespan for general population and chronic conditions NIH Toolbox: Performance tests developed and validated for cognitive, motor, and sensory function. Self-reported measures developed and validated for emotional function across the lifespan ASCQ-Me: Self-reported measures developed for physical, mental, and social health in sickle cell disease
COMMON DATA ELEMENTS OR CORE SETS		
American Physical Therapy Association (APTA)	http://www.neuropt.org/professional-resources/neurology-section-outcome-measures-recommendations	Academy of Neurologic Physical Therapy EDGE Recommendations: Details of outcome measures for clinical practice, research and education are provided for many conditions including stroke, brain injury, and spinal cord injury
	https://pediatricapta.org/includes/fact-sheets/pdfs/13%20Assessment&screening%20tools.pdf	Pediatric APTA: List of outcome measures in pediatrics organized by International Classification of Functioning, Disability, and Health Framework

Core Outcome Measures in Effectiveness Trials (COMET)	http://www.comet-initiative.org/	Core Outcome Sets recommended by scientific panels for reporting outcomes within clinical trials
International Classification of Functioning, Disability, and Health (ICF) Framework	http://www.who.int/classifications/icf/en/	The ICF framework recommends coresets for various ICF domains that can be populated into a documentation form with a response scale that can be completed online to generate a functional profile
The International Spinal Cord Society (ISCOS) Core Data Sets	https://www.iscos.org.uk/international-sci-core-data-sets	International spinal cord injury datasets integrated with NINDS CDE resources
U.S. National Institute of Health (NIH) Common Data Elements	https://www.nlm.nih.gov/cde/	NIH repository of common data elements with outcome measures recommended by scientific advisory panels including those set up by the National Institute of Neurological Disorders and Stroke (NINDS) and National Cancer Institute (NCI)
U. S. National Quality forum (NQF)	http://www.qualityforum.org/Setting_Priorities/Improving_Healthcare_Quality.aspx	NQF invites authors to submit their measure for a thorough evaluation by their standing committee or to be guided by a measure incubator to be part of the portfolio of endorsed measures with a rigorous consensus development process

*This information is current as of March 20, 2019, and websites are subject to updates\changes.

the upper extremity, there is overwhelming consensus that child and parent outcomes should be obtained.[81−83] The patient-reported outcomes PODCI and Activities Scale for Kids include specific upper extremity items. The child-reported outcomes targeting global functioning are Pediatric Quality of Life Inventory (PedsQL),[84] the Child Health Questionnaire,[85] and the PEDI.[86] The most widely used upper extremity patient-reported outcome measure is the DASH, designed to measure physical function and symptoms in patients with musculoskeletal disorders of the upper limb. The QuickDASH is a shortened version of the DASH and, despite question about its dimensionality,[87] it has good reliability and internal consistency in older children.[88] There are other disease-specific patient-reported outcome instruments for children. The ABILHAND-Kids questionnaire is a 21-item measure of manual ability developed for and field-tested in children between 6 and 16 years old with CP[89] and has been used with children with arthrogryposis,[90] brachial plexus birth palsy,[91] limb deficiencies,[92] and muscular dystrophy.[93] The PUFI[20,94] and the CAPP-FSI are patient-reported outcome instruments developed for children with limb deficiency. The COPM[95] and Goal Attainment Scaling[96] are unique from other standardized patient-reported outcome instruments due to the individualized approach they use to establish goals. The COPM utilizes semistructured interviews through which parents and children identify performance activities that are perceived as important by the parent, child, and/or society (e.g., activities that a child is expected to perform). Performance is rated on a scale between 0 (cannot do) and 10 (can do very well) and the activities are used to establish goals for treatment. Goal Attainment Scaling (GAS) involves identification of patient-defined goals and weighted on importance or priority. The advantage of GAS is that goals can be established across the ICF domains.

COMPUTER ADAPTIVE TESTS AND SHORT FORMS

Modern measurement techniques and computer adaptive testing (CAT) are transforming the assessment approaches in healthcare globally.[97] The CAT format can reduce the number of items administered to an individual and select the items tailored to the individual's functional level with a simple artificial intelligence software platform. The scores can be compared across a standard metric even with a varied number of items for each patient. The CATs can be shortened to develop fixed-length short forms in the clinic. There are excellent resources for therapists to get familiar with CATs and short forms. The PEDI-CAT is an example of a commonly used CAT instrument[98−101] with evidence for validity in respiratory disease[100]; infantile, juvenile, and idiopathic scoliosis[102]; and mobility impairments.[103] The National Institutes of Health have developed patient-reported outcome measures as CATs and short forms for various domains with the Neuro-QoL and PROMIS initiatives. The domains relevant to therapists include physical functioning, global health,

TABLE 4.4
Summary of Notable Studies on Outcome Instruments for Children With Upper Extremity Impairments.

Study	Design	Instrument(s)	Population(s)	Salient Findings
Adkinson et al.[125]	Review	Multiple instruments including PUFI, DASH, Childhood Experience Questionnaire, and Pediatric Quality of Life Inventory	Children with congenital hand differences, 0—18 years	Only the child behavior checklist and the Piers-Harris Children's self-concept scale captured all ICF domains. The PUFI, the only patient-reported outcome validated for children with congenital longitudinal and transverse deficiency
Ardolino et al.[192]	Mixed Methods Psychometric Study	Pediatric Neuromuscular Recovery Scale, inclusive of three upper extremity items	Children 1—12 with SCI	Initial set of items including 3 that measure recovery of the upper limb
Aslam et al.[193]	Review	Multiple instruments including PODCI, AMPS, and Jebsen Hand function Test	Children 2—19 years	Mapping of 19 assessment tools by ICF domains indicated activities domain was well represented in all tools, highest number of domains were represented in musculoskeletal questionnaires and lowest in pegboard tests
Bell et al.[194]	Review	Multiple instruments including GRASSP, CUE-T, SCIM-III and Pediatric Neuromuscular Recovery Scale	Children with SCI	SCI clinical trial outcome instruments are being field-tested in pediatrics to establish psychometric properties
Bialocerkowski et al.[195]	Systematic review	Multiple instruments including AHA, Arm and Hand function Brachial Plexus Outcome Measure, PEDI, PODCI, MUUL	Children and adolescents with BPBP	PODCI, PEDI, and AHA have the strongest psychometric properties for BPBP Additional psychometric studies are needed for more robust measures
Bieber et al.[133]	Systematic review	Multiple instruments including the MABC-2, BOT-2, and SOS	Children with Developmental Coordination Disorder, 3—18 years	The fine-motor subdomain of the MABC, the BOT-2 and the Functional Strength Measurement, with adequate reliability and validity properties, might be useful for manual function capacity assessment. SOS and the Detailed Assessment of Speed of Handwriting could be adopted for handwriting assessment, respectively, from 6 to 9 years old
Buffart et al.[126]	Repeated measures, psychometric study	AHA, PUFI, ABILHAND	Children, age 4—12, with radial deficiency (RD), types I—IV	Each of the measures has good psychometric properties for children with RD types I—IV

			Unilateral and bilateral	AHA and PUFI have the strongest correlation with type of RD, hand grip, and global assessment of hand function No instrument is optimal
Burger et al.[127]	Cross-sectional, psychometric study	UNB, CAPP-FSIP, CAPP-FSI	Children with limb deficiency	No instrument is optimal
Chang et al.[58]	Systematic review	Multiple instruments including AHA, ABILHAND, PODCI	Children with BPBP	Serious void in validated instruments for population with BPBP Disparity in use of classification systems and instruments limiting ability to evaluate outcomes
Chien et al.[137]	Systematic review	Multiple instruments including SFA, Pediatric Activity Card sort, Pediatric ADL	Children 2–12 years	SFA-Participation section comprised 100% participation items. Child and Adolescent Scale of Participation and the Participation and Environment Measure for Children and Youth covered all domains
Chien et al.[138]	Systematic review	Multiple instruments related to hand use	Children 2–12 years	CHORES contained all items related to hand use. CAPE/PAC, SFA-Participation and CPQ revealed sufficient evidence of validity and reliability
Christakou and Laiou[128]	Critical review	PODCI and ASK	Children with orthopedic impairment	ASK has the stronger psychometric properties when compared to PODCI Further psychometric work is needed on both instruments
Dekkers et al.[7]	Systematic review	Multiple muscle strength instruments including Jamar Dynamometer and manual muscle strength (MMT) testing	Children with cerebral palsy	Jamar Dynamometer is recommended for grip strength, hand held dynamometer for other muscle groups. MMT can be used for limited wrist strength (less than grade 4) and total upper limb muscle strength
Dent et al.,[140]	Multicenter, repeated measures	Capabilities of the Upper Extremity Test	Children with SCI	Children 6 years old and older were able to complete the CUE-T, and strong test–retest reliability was demonstrated
Elvrum et al.[121]	Systematic review	Multiple instruments of hand function	Children with cerebral palsy	Strongest level of evidence for aspects of validity and reliability was found for the MUUL 2, and for the questionnaire ABILHAND-Kids

Continued

TABLE 4.4

Summary of Notable Studies on Outcome Instruments for Children With Upper Extremity Impairments.—cont'd

Study	Design	Instrument(s)	Population(s)	Salient Findings
Gerber et al.[134]	Systematic review	Multiple instruments	Children with central neuromotor disorders, 1–18 years	MUUL showed moderate positive evidence for interrater and a fair positive level of evidence for intrarater reliability. The Pediatric-MAL Revised revealed moderate positive evidence for test–retest reliability
Gilmore et al.[196]	Systematic review	Multiple instruments including MUUL, AHA, ABILHAND, QUEST, SHUEE	Children, age 5–16 years, hemiplegic cerebral palsy	The best performance measure with strong psychometric properties for bimanual function is AHA, unilateral function is MUUL, and capability and parent report is ABILHAND Multiple measures may be needed based on purpose of use
Grampurohit et al.[109]	Multicenter, repeated measures	Upper Extremity CP-PRO CAT, PODCI-UE, ABILHAND-Kids, and BB	Children, age 2–20 years,	Upper extremity CP-PRO CAT is significantly better in detecting change in function in the first 6 months postmusculoskeletal surgery for the upper extremity and comparable to other measures at 12 and 24 months
Harvey et al.[122]	Systematic review	Multiple instruments including PODCI, PEDI, ASK	Children with cerebral palsy	ASK and GMFM have the strongest psychometric properties for measuring activity limitation No one instrument addresses all aspects of the ICF; multiple instruments should be selected based on psychometric properties and purpose of measurement
Haywood et al.[136]	Systematic review	Multiple instruments	Children with Chronic Fatigue syndrome/Myalgic encephalomyelitis	With the exception of the generic SF-36, all measures had mostly limited evidence of measurement and/or practical properties
Haywood et al.[135]	Systematic review	Multiple patient-reported outcome instruments assessing severity of illness and outcomes of treatment	Children with chronic fatigue syndrome/myalgic encephalomyelitis	No instrument is optimal

Kleeper[131]	Critical review	CHA-Q, ASK, PODCI, JAFAS	Children with rheumatic disease	Each of the measures contains activities relevant to children across broad age range ASK is the only instrument that is child report and PODCI is the most comprehensive Using two or more measures is recommended to obtain the best understanding of child's functioning
Kingels et al. (2010)	Systematic review	Multiple instruments including QUEST, SHUEE, AHA, MUUL, PEDI, ABILHAND	Children, age 2–18 years, hemiplegic cerebral palsy	MUUL is recommended for capacity measure, AHA for performance measure, and ABILHAND for patient-reported outcome instrument
Lindner et al.[129]	Critical review	Multiple pediatric and adult instruments including PUFI, UBET, CAPP-FSI, CAPP-PSI	Children and adults using upper limb prostheses	Multiple instruments are needed to assess the constructs across the ICF Most pediatric instruments measure activity and participation domain of ICF Assessment with children requires measures that evaluate social interactions
Mazzone et al.[132]	Critical review	Multiple instruments including ABILHAND, self-reported Scale of Activity Limitation, Muscular Dystrophy Functional Rating Scale, Jebsen Test of Hand function, Upper Limb Functional Ability Test	Children with muscular dystrophy (MD)	Many of the instruments reviewed are psychometrically sound, although not with samples of children with MD None covers the full ability range of children with MD (ceiling and floor potential)
Mulcahey et al.[107]	Multicenter, repeated measures	GRASSP	Children with SCI	Lower age for GRASSP motor and sensory examinations is 6 years old. Lower age for GRASSP prehension examinations is 8 years old. When administered by trained raters, test retest reliability is string. Normative references for the prehension examinations would aid in the interpretation of GRASSP scores
Sakzewski et al.[70,a]	Systematic review	Multiple instruments including COPM, GAS	Children with CP	All instruments measure aspects of childhood participation, no one instrument covers all aspects of participation Responsiveness of all instruments is unknown

Continued

TABLE 4.4

Summary of Notable Studies on Outcome Instruments for Children With Upper Extremity Impairments.—cont'd

Study	Design	Instrument(s)	Population(s)	Salient Findings
Wagner and Davids[123]	Systematic review	Multiple instruments including AHA, BB, MUUL, QUEST, SHUEE, PEDI, PODCI, ASK, COPM, GAS	Children with CP	The understanding of psychometric properties will assist therapists with selecting the most useful instruments based on purpose of measurement
Wallen et al. (2014)	Systematic review	Multiple parent report measures.	Children with cerebral palsy	Children's Hand-use Experience Questionnaire holds most promise for guiding treatment planning. ABILHAND-Kids bimanual, good psychometrics and Pediatric Motor Activity Log unimanual only measure for 25 years old children
Wright[130]	Systematic review	Multiple instruments including AHA, PUFI, ABILHAND, CAPP-FSI, PODCI	Adult and pediatric prosthetic users	Comprehensive summary of instruments used with adults and children with limb deficiency
				Measures have varying degree of psychometric properties
				Further research is needed

Note: Shaded rows are articles included in the book The Pediatric Upper Extremity by Abzug et al. 2015.

ADL, Activities of Daily Living; *AHA*, Assisting Hand Assessment; *ASK*, Activities Scale for Kids; *BB*, Box and Block Test; *BOT*, Bruininks Oseretsky Test of Motor Proficiency; *BPBP*, Brachial Plexus Birth Palsy; *CAPP-FSI*, Child Amputee Prosthetics Project-Functional Status Inventory; *CAPP-FSIP*, Child Amputee Prosthetics Project-Functional Status Inventory for Preschool Children; *CAPP-PSI*; *C-HAQ*, Childhood Health Assessment Questionnaire; *CHORES*, Children Helping Out: Responsibilities, Expectations, and Supports; *CAPE/PAC*, Children's Assessment of Participation and Enjoyment/Preferences for Activities of Children; *CPQ*, Children Participation Questionnaire; *CP-PRO CAT*, Cerebral Palsy Profile of Health and Function Computer Adaptive Test; *COPM*, Canadian Occupational Performance Measure; *DASH*, Disabilities of the Arm Shoulder and Hand; *GAS*, Goal Attainment Scaling; *GMFM*, Gross Motor Function Measure; *ICF*, International Classification of Functioning Disability and Health; *JAFAS*, Juvenile Arthritis Functional Assessment Scale; *M-ABC*, Movement Assessment Battery for Children; *MAL*, Motor Activity Log; *MMT*, Manual Muscle Testing; *MUUL*, Melbourne Assessment of Unilateral Upper Limb Function; *PEDI*, Pediatric Evaluation of Disability Inventory; *PODCI*, Pediatric Outcomes Data Collection Instrument; *PUFI*, Prosthetic Upper Extremity Functional Index; *PRO*, Patient-Reported Outcomes; *QUEST*, Quality of Upper Extremity Skills Test; *SFA*, School Function Assessment; *SHUEE*, Shriners Hospital for Children Upper Extremity Evaluation; *SOS*, Systematic Detection of Writing Problems; *UBET*, Unilateral Below Elbow Test; *UE*, Upper Extremity; *UNB*, University of New Brunswick Test of Prosthetic Function.

[a] Studies that included outcome instruments not directly related to upper extremity but include COPM and GAS, two instruments/methods discussed in this chapter and have high relevance to evaluation of children with upper extremity impairments.

mental health, quality of life, and social participation. The instruments are not disease-specific and have been field-tested in diverse clinical samples. The PROMIS pediatric upper extremity instruments have been used for children with cerebral palsy, arthritis, asthma, attention deficit hyperactivity disorder, and congenital hand differences.[45,73,104–107] The measures have child and parent proxy versions with translations of the English measures available in Chinese-Simplified, Dutch, German, Korean, Spanish, Portuguese-Br, French, Italian, Japanese, Afrikaans, Swedish, Russian, and other ongoing translations. The PROMIS pediatric upper limb short form studied in children with cerebral palsy demonstrated acceptable internal consistency (Cronbach's α 0.85).[107] The CAT had a higher frequency of ceiling effects (29.5%) as compared to the short form (18.30%).[107] The PROMIS pediatric upper limb short form and CAT mean values were one standard deviation below the normal.[107] Lower mean values have also been reported in children with congenital hand differences particularly with comorbities and involvement of bilateral as compared to unilateral upper limb.[108]

Different from the PROMIS instruments, the Cerebral Palsy Profile (CP-PRO), the Pediatric Spinal Cord Injury Activity Measure (PEDI-SCI), and the Pediatric Measure of Participation (PMoP) are "disease-specific" IRT-based instruments that assess physical functioning in children with CP[109–113] and BPBP[114,115] and activity performance and participation in children with SCI.[116–118] The CP-PRO uses parent proxy reports and have been translated into Spanish. The PEDI-SCI AM and PMoP have been developed for both parent and child reports and have been linked to the adult SCI functional index (SCI-FI) CAT[119] developed by Jette and colleagues.[120] Among several strengths of the CP-PRO, PEDI-SCI AM and PMoP is that they have been administered to 2000 typically developing youth living in the United States, providing a basis for developing not only disease-specific trajectories of functioning but also a mechanism for normative comparison (Table 4.2).

RESOURCES TO MAINTAIN COMPETENCY

The resources that have emerged through many national and stakeholder organizations are primarily aimed at providing the most up-to-date information to healthcare providers regarding outcome measures. There is also detailed information on measurement properties to aid in the selection of outcome instruments. Some examples and websites are provided in Tables 4.2 and 4.3 and include Rehab Measures Database, Spinal Cord Injury Research Evidence Outcome Measures, PROQUOLID, and Common Data Elements or Core Sets. As summarized in Table 4.4, there are also notable critical and systematic reviews of outcome instruments for children with cerebral palsy,[7,47,67,70,121–124] BPBP,[58,59] limb deficiency,[125–130] rheumatic diseases,[131] muscular dystrophy,[132] developmental coordination disorder,[133] central neuromotor disorders,[134] chronic fatigue syndrome/myalgic encephalitis,[135,136] and participation-based outcomes for children.[137,138] Although these resources are not solely for pediatrics and not primarily related to the upper extremity, they are invaluable for the therapists. There have been concerted efforts to rate the quality of measurement studies included in systematic reviews and thereby raise the quality of original research. One example of such a multidisciplinary effort is the Consensus-based Standards for the Selection of Health Measurement Instruments that call for increased use of quality rating for measurement studies and stopping the use of poor measurement instruments.[31] The use of quality guidelines for measurement studies in future reviews can better serve the therapists with selection of outcome instruments (Tables 4.3 and 4.4).

SUMMARY

Several important contributions to the field have been made in the area of pediatric upper extremity measurement as the prior publication of this chapter.[2] Among these are widespread clinical adoption of patient-reported outcomes, commercial availability of computerized adaptive tests, application of modern measurement theory approaches, development of common data elements to aid in selection of instruments, and quality rating system for measurement studies. The advanced measurement practices have generated the need for therapists to be informed consumers and efficient users of outcome measures. Despite the wide range of outcome measures available for upper extremity function, there is reaming gap in the psychometric studies available to support their use. Therapists need to maintain their competency in selection, administration, and interpretation of outcome measures to meet the demands of the value-based healthcare systems.

REFERENCES

1. Jones LA, Lederman SJ. *Human Hand Function*. Oxford; New York: Oxford University Press; 2006.
2. Abzug JM, Kozin SH, Zlotolow DA. *The Pediatric Upper Extremity*. New York: Springer; 2015.
3. Eliasson AC, Krumlinde-Sundholm L, Rosblad B, Beckung E, Arner M, Rosenbaum P. The manual ability classification (MACS) for children with cerebral palsy: scale development and evidence of validity and reliability. *Dev Med Child Neurol*. 2006;48:549–554.
4. Bae DS, Waters PM, Zurakowski D. Reliability of three classification systems in measuring active motion in brachial plexus birth palsy. *J Bone Joint Surg Am*. 2003; 85:1733–1738.
5. Kirshblum SC, Waring W, Biering-Sorensen F, et al. Reference for the 2011 revision of the international standards for neurological classification of spinal cord injury. *J Spinal Cord Med*. 2011;34(6):547–554.
6. Mulcahey MJ, Weiss A. Upper extremity in tetraplegia. *Hand Clin*. 2008;24(2).
7. Dekkers KJ, Rameckers EA, Smeets RJ, Janssen-Potten YJ. Upper extremity strength measurement for children with cerebral palsy: a systematic review of available instruments. *Phys Ther*. 2014;94(5):609–622. https://doi.org/10.2522/ptj.20130166.
8. Gajdosik CG. Ability of very young children to produce reliable isometric force measurements. *Pediatr Phys Ther*. 2005;17(4):251–257.
9. Koman LA, Williams RM, Evans PJ, et al. Quantification of upper extremity function and range of motion in

children with cerebral palsy. *Dev Med Child Neurol.* 2008; 50(12):910–917.

10. Mulcahey MJ, Hutchison D, Kozin S. Assessment of the upper limb in tetraplegia. *J Rehabil Res Dev.* 2007;44(1): 91–102.

11. Van den Beld WA, Van der Sanden GA, Janssen AJ, Sengers RC, Verbeek AL, Gabreels FJ. Comparison of 3 instruments to measure muscle strength in children: a prospective study. *Eur J Paediatr Neurol.* 2011;15(6):512–518.

12. Evenson KR, Goto MM, Furberg RD. Systematic review of the validity and reliability of consumer-wearable activity trackers. *Int J Behav Nutr Phys Act.* 2015;18(12):159. https://doi.org/10.1186/s12966-015-0314-1.

13. Jabrayilov R, van Asselt ADI, Vermeulen KM, et al. A descriptive system for the Infant health-related Quality of life Instrument (IQI): measuring health with a mobile app. *PLoS One.* 2018;13(8):e0203276. https://doi.org/10.1371/journal.pone.0203276.

14. Hinderer SR, Hinderer KA. Principles and applications of measurement methods, chapter 6. In: DeLIsa JA, Gans BM, eds. *Rehabilitation Medicine: Principles and Practice.* Philadelphia: Lippincott-Raven; 1988: 109–136.

15. Portney LG, Watkins MP. *Foundations of Clinical Research: Application to Practice.* 3rd ed. Upper Saddle River: Pearson Prentice Hall; 2009.

16. Hinojosa J, Kramer P. *Evaluation in Occupational Therapy: Obtaining and Interpreting Data.* ISBN 10: 1569003564/ ISBN 13: 9781569003565. Bethesda, MD: AOTA Press; 2014.

17. Jebsen RH, Taylor N, Trieschmann RB, Trotter MJ, Howard LA. An objective and standardized test of hand function. *Arch Phys Med Rehabil.* 1969;50:311–319.

18. Mathiowetz V, Ferderman S, et al. Box and block test of manual dexterity: norms for 6–19 year olds. *Can J Occup Ther.* 1985;52(5):241–246.

19. Wiebe S, Guyatt G, Weaver B, Matijevic S, Sidwell C. Comparative responsiveness of generic and specific quality-of-life instruments. *J Clin Epidemiol.* 2003;56(1): 52–60.

20. Wright FV, Hubbard S, Jutai J, Naumann S. The prosthetic upper extremity functional index: development and reliability testing of a new functional status questionnaire for children who use upper extremity prostheses. *J Hand Ther.* 2001;14(2):91–104.

21. Hao Y, Bala K, McRae M, Carnahan H, Borschel GH, Ho ES. Establishing expert consensus on the evaluation of pediatric upper extremity function. *J Hand Ther.* 2015;28(2):151–156.

22. Schiariti V, Klassen AF, Cieza A, et al. Comparing contents of outcome measures in cerebral palsy using the International Classification of Functioning (ICF-CY): a systematic review. *Eur J Paediatr Neurol.* 2014;18(1): 1–12.

23. Weldring T, Smith S. Patient-reported outcomes (PROs) and patient-reported outcome measures (PROMs). *Health Serv Insights.* 2013;6:61–68.

24. Bevans KB, Riley AW, Moon JH, Forrest CB. Conceptual and methodological advances in child-reported outcomes measurement. *Expert Rev Pharmacoecon Outcomes Res.* 2010;10(4):385–396.

25. Streiner DL, Norman GR. *Health Measurement Scales: A Practical Guide to Their Development and Use.* 2nd ed. Oxford: Oxford University Press; 1995.

26. Messick S. Standards of validity and the validity of standards in performance asessment. *Educ Meas.* 1995;14:5–8. https://doi.org/10.1111/j.1745-3992.1995.tb00881.x.

27. Guyatt GH, Cook DJ. Health status, quality of life and the individual. *J Am Med Assoc.* 1994;272:630–631.

28. Dumas HM, Watson K, Fragala-Pinkham MA, et al. Using cognitive interviewing for test items to assess physical function in children with cerebral palsy. *Pediatr Phys Ther.* 2008;20(4):356–362.

29. Mulcahey MJ, Calhoun C, Riley A, Haley S. Children's reports of activity and participation after sustaining spinal cord injury: a cognitive interviewing study. *Dev Neurorehabil.* 2009;12(4):191–200.

30. Mulcahey MJ, Samdani A, Chafetz R, et al. Cognitive testing of the spinal appearance questionnaire with typically developing youth and youth with idiopathic scoliosis. *J Pediatr Orthop.* 2011;31(6):661–667.

31. Mokkink LB, Terwee C, Patrick, et al. COSMIN steering committee. *The COSMIN Checklist Manual;* 2012. Retrieved from: http://www.cosmin.nl/COSMIN.html.

32. Cook CE. Clinimetrics corner: the minimal clinically important change score (MCID): a necessary pretense. *J Man Manip Ther.* 2008;16(4):E82–E83.

33. Guyatt GH, Osoba D, Wu AW, Wyrwich KW, Norman GR. The Clinical Significance Meeting Group. Methods to explain the clinical significance of health status measures. *Mayo Clin Proc.* 2002;77:371–383.

34. Smart A. A multi-dimensional model of clinical utility. *Int J Qual Health Care.* 2006;18(5):377–382.

35. Fries JF, Bruce B, Cella D. The promise of PROMIS: using item response theory to improve assessment of patient-reported outcomes. *Clin Exp Rheumatol.* 2005;23(5 suppl 39):S53–S57.

36. Chakravarty EF, Bjorner JB, Fries JF. Improving patient-reported outcomes using item response theory and computerized adaptive testing. *J Rheumatol.* 2007;34(6): 1426–1431.

37. Chang CH, Reeve BB. Item response theory and its applications to patient-reported outcomes measurement. *Eval Health Prof.* 2005;28(3):264–282.

38. Fitzpatrick R, Davey C, Buxton MJ, Jones DR. Evaluating patient-based outcome measures for use in clinical trials. *Health Technol Assess.* 1998;2(14):1–74. i-iv.

39. Halle T, Zaslow M, Wessel J, Moodie S, Darling-Churchill K. *Understanding and Choosing Assessments and Developmental Screeners for Young Children: Profiles of Selected Measures.* Washington, DC: Office of Planning, Research, and Evaluation, Administration for Children and Families, U.S. Department of Health and Human Services; 2011.

40. Green LM, Friend AJ, Bardgett RJ, Darling JC. Including children and young people in assessments: a practical guide. *Arch Dis Child Educ Pract Ed.* 2017. https://doi.org/10.1136/archdischild-2017-313368. pii: edpract-2017-313368.

41. Girard JM, Cohn JF. A primer on observational measurement. *Assessment.* 2016;23(4):404–413. https://doi.org/10.1177/1073191116635807.

42. Knox V, Usen Y. Clinical review of the pediatric evaluation of disability inventory. *Br J Occup Ther.* 2000;63(1):29–32.

43. Young NL, Williams JI, Yoshida KK, Bombardier C, Wright JG. The context of measuring disability: does it matter whether capability or performance is measured? *J Clin Epidemiol.* 1996;49(10):1097–1101.

44. Kovacs M. The children's depression, inventory (CDI). *Psychopharmacol Bull.* 1985;21:995–998.

45. Waljee JF, Carlozzi N, Franzblau LE, Zhong L, Chung KC. Applying PROMIS to assess upper extremity function among children with congenital hand differences. *Plast Reconstr Surg.* 2015;136(2):200e–207e. http://doi.org/10.1097/PRS.0000000000001444.

46. Taylor N, Sand PL, Jebsen RH. Evaluation of hand function in children. *Arch Phys Med Rehabil.* 1973;54:129–135.

47. Gilmore R, Sakzewski L, Boyd R. Upper limb activity measures for 5- to 16-year old children with congenital hemiplegia: a systematic review. *Dev Med Child Neurol.* 2010;52:14–21.

48. Chen HM, Chen CC, Hsueh IP, Huang SL, Hsieh CL. Test retest reproducibility and smallest real difference of 5 hand function tests in patients with stroke. *Neurorehabilitation Neural Repair.* 2009;23(5):435–440.

49. Desrosiers J, Bravo G, Hebert R, Dutil E, Mercier L. Validation of the box and block test as a measure of elderly people: reliability, validity and norm studies. *Arch Phys Med Rehabil.* 1994;75(7):751–755.

50. Lin KC, Chuang LL, Wu CY, Hsieh YW, Chang WY. Responsiveness and validity of three dexterous function measures in stroke rehabilitation. *J Rehabil Res Dev.* 2010;47(6):563–571.

51. Platz T, Vuadens P, Eickof C, Arnold P, Van Kaick S, Heise K. REPAS, a summary rating scale for resistance to passive movement: item selection, reliability and validity. *Disabil Rehabil.* 2008;30(1):44–53.

52. Jongbloed-Pereboom M, Nijhuis-van der Sanden MW, Steenbergen B. Norm scores of the box and block test for children 3–10 years. *Am J Occup Ther.* 2013;67(3):312–318.

53. Ekblom AG, Dahlin L, Rosberg HE, Wiig M, Werner M, Arner M. Hand function in children with radial longitudinal deficiency. *BMC Muscoskelet Disord*; 2013. http://lup.lub.lu.se/record/3851474.

54. Krumlinde-Sundholm L, Eliasson AC. Development of the assisting hand assessment: a rasch built measure intended for children with unilateral upper limb impairments. *Scand J Occup Ther.* 2003;10:16–26.

55. Krumlinde-Sundholm L, Holmefur M, Kottorp A, Eliasson A. The assisting hand assessment: current evidence of validity, reliability and responsiveness to change. *Dev Med Child Neurol.* 2007;49:259–264.

56. Gordon AM. Measuring activity limitation in individuals with unilateral upper extremity impairments. *Dev Med Child Neurol.* 2007;49(4):245.

57. Holmefur M, Krumlinde-Sundholm L, Elisasson AC. Interrater reliability of the assisting hand assessment. *Am J Occup Ther.* 2007;61:79–84.

58. Chang KW, Justice D, Chung KC, Yang LJ. A systematic review of evaluation methods for neonatal brachial plexus palsy. *J Neurosurg Pediatr.* 2013. PMID 23931766.

59. Bialocerkowski A, O'Shea K, Pin TW. Psychometric properties of outcome measures for children and adolescents with brachial plexus birth palsy. *Dev Med Child Neurol.* 2013;55(12):1075–1088.

60. Greaves S, Imms C, Dodd K, Krumlinde-Sundholm L. Development of the mini-assisting hand assessment: evidence for content and internal scale validity. *Dev Med Child Neurol.* 2013;55(11):1030–1037.

61. Randall M, Johnson L, Reddihough D. *The Melbourne Assessment of Unilateral Upper Limb Function: Test Administration Manual.* Melbourne: Royal Children's Hospital; 1999.

62. Randall M, Imms C, Carey L. Establishing validity of a modified Melbourne assessment for children 2 to 4 years. *Am J Occup Ther.* 2008;63(4):373–383.

63. Hoare B, Imms C, Randall M, Carey L. Linking cerebral palsy upper limb measures to the international classification of functioning, disability and health. *J Rehabil Med.* 2001;43:987–996.

64. Bard R, Chaleat-Valayer E, Combey A, Bleu PE, Perretant I, Bernard JC. Upper limb assessment in children with cerebral palsy: translation and reliability of the French version for the Melbourne unilateral assessment (test de Melbourne). *Ann Phys Rehabil Med.* 2009;52(4):297–310.

65. Davidson JR, Peace LC, Wagner LC, Gidewell MA, Blackhurst DW, Robertson WM. Validation of the Shriners Hospitals for children upper extremity evaluation (SHUEE) for children with hemiplegia cerebral palsy. *J Bone Joint Surg Am.* 2006;88(2):326–333.

66. Klingels K, DeCock P, Desloovere K, et al. Comparison of the Melbourne assessment of unilateral upper limb function and the quality of upper extremity skills test in hemiplegia CP. *Dev Med Child Neurol.* 2008;50(12):904–919.

67. Klingels K, Jaspers E, Van de Winckel A, De Cook P, Molenaers G, Feys H. A systematic review of arm activity measures for children with hemiplegia cerebral palsy. *Clin Rehabil.* 2010;24:887–900.

68. Lee JS, Lee KB, Lee YR, et al. Botulinum toxin treatment on upper limb function in school age children with spastic cerebral palsy: one year follow up. *Ann Rehabil Med.* 2013;37(3):328–335.

69. Lee JA, You JH, Kiim DA, et al. Effects of functional movement strength training on strength, muscle size, kinematics and motor function in cerebral palsy: a 3-month follow up. *NeuroRehabilitation.* 2013;32(2):287–295.

70. Sakzewski L, Boyd R, Ziviani J. Clinimetric properties of participation measures for 5- to 13- year-old children with cerebral palsy: a systematic review. *Dev Med Child Neurol.* 2007;49(3):232–240.

71. Thorley M, Lannin N, Cusick A, Novak I, Boyd R. Construct validity of the quality of upper extremity skills test for children with cerebral palsy. *Dev Med Child Neurol.* 2012;54(11):1037–1043.

72. Thorley M, Lannin N, Cusick A, Novak I, Boyd R. Reliability validity of the quality of upper extremity skills test for children with cerebral palsy aged 2 to 12. *Phys Occup Ther Pediatr.* 2012;32(1):4–21.

73. Lai JS, Nowinski C, Victorson D, et al. Quality of life measures in children with neurological conditions: pediatric Neuro-QOL. *Neurorehabilitation Neural Repair.* 2012; 26(1):36–47.

74. Pencharz J, Young NL, Owen JL, Wirght JG. Comparison of three outcomes instruments in children. *J Pediatr Orthop.* 2001;21(4):425–432.

75. Food and Drug Administration (FDA). Guidance for industry on patient-reported outcome measures use in medical product development to support labeling claims. *Fed Regist.* 2009;74(235):65132–65133.

76. Riley A. Evidence that school-aged children can self-report on their health. *Ambul Pediatr.* 2004;4:21–26.

77. Eiser C, Morse R. Quality of life measures in chronic diseases of childhood. *Health Technol Assess.* 2001;5(4): 1–157.

78. Forrest C, Riley A, Vivier P, Gordon N, Starfield B. Predictors of children's health care use. The value of child versus parent perspective on health care needs. *Med Care.* 2004; 42:232–238.

79. Majnemer A, Sherell M, Law M, Poulin C, Rosenbaum P. Reliability in the ratings of quality of life between parents and their children of school age with cerebral palsy. *Qual Life Res.* 2008;17:1163–1171.

80. Sheffler LC, Hanley C, Bagley A, Molitor F, James MA. Comparison of self-reports and parent proxy-reports of function and quality of life of children with below-the-elbow deficiency. *J Bone Joint Surg Am.* 2009;91(12): 2852–2859.

81. Erhart M, Ellert U, Kurth BM, Ravens-Sieberer U. Measuring adolescent's HRQoL via self reports and parent proxy reports: an evaluation of the psychometric properties of both of the KINDL-R instrument. *Health Qual Life Outcomes.* 2009;7:77. https://doi.org/10.1186/1477-7525-7-77.

82. Tluczek A, Becker T, Grieve A, et al. Health-related quality of life in children and adolescents with cystic fibrosis: convergent validity with parent-reports and objective measures of pulmonary health. *J Dev Behav Pediatr.* 2013;34(4):252–261.

83. Varni JW, Burwinkle TM, Sherman SA, et al. Health-related quality of life of children and adolescents with cerebral palsy: hearing the voices of the children. *Dev Med Child Neurol.* 2005;47(9):592–597.

84. Varni J, Seid M, Rode CA. The PedsQL™: measurement model for the pediatric quality of life Inventory™. *Med Care.* 1999;37:126–139.

85. Landgraf JM, Abetzl L, Ware JE. *Child Health Questionnaire (CHQ): User's Manual.* Boston: The Health Institute NEMC; 1996.

86. Haley SM, Coster WJ, Ludlow LH, Haltiwanger JT, Andrellos PJ. *Pediatric Evaluation of Disability Inventory: Examiner's Manual.* New England Medical Center; 1992.

87. Gabel CP, Yelland M, Melloh M, Burkett B. A modified Quick DASH-9 provides a valid outcome instrument for upper limb function. *BMC Muscoskelet Disord.* 2009;10: 161. https://doi.org/10.1186/1471-2474-10-161.

88. Quatman-Yates CC, Gupta R, Paterno MV, Schih LC, Quateman CE, Ittenbach RF. Internal consistency and validity of the quick DASH instrument for upper extremity injuries in older children. *J Pediatr Orthop.* 2013;33(8): 838–842.

89. Arnould C, Penta M, Renders A, Thonnard JL. ABILHAND-Kids: a measure of manual ability in children with cerebral palsy. *Neurology.* 2004;63(6):1045–1052.

90. Foy CA, Miller J, Wheeler L, Ezaki M, Oishi SN. Long term outcome following carpal wedge osteotomy in the arthrogrypotic patient. *J Bone Joint Surg Am.* 2013;95(20).

91. Spaargaren E, Ahmed J, van Ouwerkerk WJ, de Groot V, Beckerman H. Aspects of activities and participation of 7–8 year-old children with an obstetric brachial plexus injury. *Eur J Paediatr Neurol.* 2011;15(4):345–352.

92. Buffart LM, Roebroeck ME, van Heijningen VG, Pesch-Batenburg JM, Stam HJ. Evaluation of arm and prosthetic functioning in children with congenital transverse reduction deficiency of the upper limb. *J Rehabil Med.* 2007; 39(5):379–386.

93. Kumar A, Phillips MF. Use of powered mobile arm supports by people with neuromuscular conditions. *J Rehabil Res Dev.* 2013;50(1):61–70.

94. Wright FV, Hubbard S, Naumann S, Jutai J. Evaluation of the validity of the prosthetic upper extremity functional index for children. *Arch Phys Med Rehabil.* 2003;84(4): 518–527.

95. Law M, Baptiste S, McColl M, Opzoomer A, Polatajko H, Pollack N. The Canadian occupational performance measure: an outcome measure for occupational therapy. *Can J Occup Ther.* 1990;57(2):82–87.

96. Bovend'Eeerdt TJ, Botell RE, Wade DT. Writing SMART rehabilitation goals and achieving goal attainment scaling: a practical guide. *Clin Rehabil.* 2009;23(4):352–361.

97. McHorney CA. Generic health measurement: past accomplishments and a measurement paradigm for the 21st century. *Ann Intern Med.* 1997;187(8 pt. 2):743–750.

98. Allen DD, Ni P, Haley SM. Efficiency and sensitivity of multidimensional computerized adaptive testing of pediatric physical functioning. *Disabil Rehabil.* 2008;30(6): 479–484.

99. Coster WJ, Haley SM, Dumas HM, Fragal-Pinkham MA. Assessing self-care and social functioning using a

computer adaptive testing version of the pediatric evaluation of disability inventory. *Arch Phys Med Rehabil.* 2008; 89(4):622–629.

100. Dumas H, Fragala-Pinkham M, Haley S, et al. Item bank development for a revised pediatric evaluation of disability inventory (PEDI). *Phys Occup Ther Pediatr.* 2010;30(3):168–184.

101. Haley SM, Ni P, Ludlow LH, Fragala-Pinkham MA. Measurement precision and efficiency of multidimensional computer adaptive testing of physical functioning using the pediatric evaluation of disability inventory. *Arch Phys Med Rehabil.* 2006;87(9):1223–1229.

102. Mulcahey MJ, Haley SM, Duffy T, Pengsheng N, Betz RR. Measuring physical functioning in children with spinal impairments with computerized adaptive testing. *J Pediatr Orthop.* 2008;28(3):330–335.

103. Haley SM, Raczek AE, Coster WJ, Dumas HM, Fragal-Pinkham MA. Assessing mobility in children using a computer adaptive testing version of the pediatric evaluation of disability inventory. *Arch Phys Med Rehabil.* 2005; 86(5):932–939.

104. DeWitt EM, Stucky BD, Thissen D, et al. Construction of the eight item patient reported outcomes measurement information system pediatric physical function scales: built using item response theory. *J Clin Epidemiol.* 2011; 64(7):794–804.

105. Gipson DS, Selewski D, Massengil S, et al. Gaining the PROMIS perspective from children with nephrotic syndrome: a Midwest pediatric nephrology consortium study. *Health Qual Life Outcomes.* 2013;11(3). http://www.hqlo.com/content/11/1/30.

106. Kratz AL, Salvin MD, Mulcahey MJ, Jette AM, Tulsky DS, Haley SM. An examination of the PROMIS pediatric instruments to assess mobility in children with cerebral palsy. *Qual Life Res.* 2013;22(10):2865–2876.

107. Mulcahey MJ, Slavin M, Ni P, et al. Examination of the PROMIS®: pediatric upper extremity measures in youth with cerebral palsy. *Br J Occup Ther.* 2018;81(7):393–401.

108. Bae DS, Canizares MF, Miller PE, Waters PM, Goldfarb CA. Functional impact of congenital hand differences: early results from the congenital upper limb differences (CoULD) registry. *J Hand Surg Am.* 2018;43(4):321–330. https://doi.org/10.1016/j.jhsa.2017.10.006.

109. Grampurohit N, Slavin M, Ni P, Kozin S, Jette A, Mulcahey MJ. Sensitivity of the cerebral palsy profile of health and function: upper extremity domain to change following musculoskeletal surgery. *J Hand Surg;* 2019. https://doi.org/10.1016/j.jhsa.2018.12.007.

110. Haley SM, Ni P, Dumas HM, et al. Measuring global physical health in children with cerebral palsy: illustration of a multidimensional bi-factor model and computerized adaptive testing. *Qual Life Res.* 2009;18(3): 359–370.

111. Haley SM, Chafetz RS, Tian F, et al. Validity and reliability of physical functioning computer adaptive tests for children with cerebral palsy. *J Pediatr Orthop.* 2010;30(1):71–75.

112. Tucker CA, Gorton G, Watson K, et al. Development of a parent report computer adaptive test to assess physical functioning in children with cerebral palsy I: lower extremity and mobility skills. *Dev Med Child Neurol.* 2009; 51(9):717–724.

113. Tucker C, Montpetit K, Bilodeau N, et al. Development of a parent reported computer adaptive test to assess physical functioning in children with cerebral palsy: upper extremity skills. *Dev Med Child Neurol.* 2009;51(9): 725–731.

114. Mulcahey MJ, Kozin S, Merenda L, et al. Evaluation of the box and blocks test, stereognosis and item banks of activity and upper extremity function in youths with brachial plexus birth palsy. *J Pediatr Orthop.* 2012; 32(suppl 2):S114–S122. https://doi.org/10.1097/BPO.0b013e3182595423.

115. Mulcahey MJ, Merenda L, Tian F, et al. Computer adaptive test approach to the assessment of children and youth with brachial plexus injuries. *Am J Occup Ther.* 2013;67(5):524–533.

116. Bent L, Mulcahey MJ, Kelly E, et al. Child- and parent-report computer-adaptive tests for assessing daily routines among youth with spinal cord injury. *Top Spinal Cord Inj Rehabil.* 2013;19(2):104–113.

117. Calhoun CL, Haley SM, Rile A, Vogel LC, McDonald CM, Mulcahey MJ. Development of items designed to evaluate activity performance and participation in children with spinal cord injury. *Int J Pediatr.* 2009:854905. https://doi.org/10.1155/2009/854904.

118. Mulcahey MJ, Calhoun C, Tian F, Ni P, Vogel L, Haley S. Evaluation of newly developed item banks for child reported outcomes of participation following spinal cord injury. *Spinal Cord.* 2012;50(12):915–919. https://doi.org/10.1038/sc.2012.80. Epub 2012 Aug 21.

119. Tian F, Ni P, Mulcahey MJ, et al. Tracking functional status across the spinal cord injury lifespan: linking pediatric and adult patient-reported outcome scores. *Arch Phys Med Rehabil.* 2014;95(11):2078–2085. https://doi.org/10.1016/j.apmr.2014.05.023. e15.

120. Jette AM, Tilsky DS, Ni P, et al. Development and initial evaluation of the spinal cord injury-functional index. *Arch Phys Med Rehabil.* 2012;93(10):1733–1750.

121. Elvrum AK, Saether R, Riphagen II, Vik T. Outcome measures evaluating hand function in children with bilateral cerebral palsy: a systematic review. *Dev Med Child Neurol.* 2016;58(7):662–671. https://doi.org/10.1111/dmcn.13119.

122. Harvey A, Robin J, Morris M, Graham HK, Baker R. A systematic review of measures of activity limitation for children with cerebral palsy. *Dev Med Child Neurol.* 2008;50:190–198.

123. Wagner LV, Davids JR. Assessment tools and classification systems used for the upper extremity in children with cerebral palsy. *Clin Orthop Relat Res.* 2012;470(5): 1257–1271.

124. Wallen M, Stewart K. Upper limb function in everyday life of children with cerebral palsy: description and review of parent report measures. *Disabil Rehabil.* 2015; 37(15):1353–1361. https://doi.org/10.3109/09638288.2014.963704.

125. Adkinson JM, Bickham RS, Chung KC, Waljee JF. *Clin Orthop Relat Res.* 2015;473:3549–3563. https://doi.org/10.1007/s11999-015-4505-5.

126. Buffart LM, Roebroeck ME, Janssen WG, Hoekstra A, Hovius SE, Stam HJ. Comparison in instruments to assess hand function in children with radius deficiencies. *J Hand Surg Am.* 2007;32(4):531–540.

127. Burger H, Brezovar D, Marincek C. Comparison of clinical test and questionnaires for the evaluation of upper prosthetic use in children. *Disabil Rehabil.* 2004;26(14–15):911–916.

128. Christakou A, Laiou A. Comparing the psychometric properties of the pediatric outcomes data collection instrument and the activities scale for kids. *J Child Health Care.* 2014;18(3):207–214. https://doi.org/10.1177/1367493513485651.

129. Lindner HY, Natterlund BS, Hermansson LM. Upper limb prosthetic outcome measures: review and content comparison based on international classification of functioning, disability and health. *Prosthet Orthot Int.* 2010;34(2):109–128.

130. Wright V. Prosthetic outcome measures for use with upper limb amputees: systematic review of the peer-reviewed literature, 1970–2009. *J Prosthet Orthot.* 2009;21(4):3–63.

131. Kleeper SE. Measures of pediatric function. *Arthritis Care Res.* 2011;63(s11):S371–S382.

132. Mazzone ES, Vasco G, Palermo C, et al. A critical review of functional assessment tools for upper limbs in Duchenne muscular dystrophy. *Dev Med Child Neurol.* 2012;54(10):879–885.

133. Bieber E, Smits-Engelsman BC, Sgandurra G, et al. Manual function outcome measures in children with developmental coordination disorder (DCD): systematic review. *Res Dev Disabil.* 2016;55:114–131. https://doi.org/10.1016/j.ridd.2016.03.009.

134. Gerber CN, Labruyère R, van Hedel HJ. Reliability and responsiveness of upper limb motor assessments for children with central neuromotor disorders: a systematic review. *Neurorehabilitation Neural Repair.* 2016;30(1):19–39. https://doi.org/10.1177/1545968315583723.

135. Haywood KL, Collin SM, Crawley E. Assessing severity of illness and outcomes of treatment in children with Chronic Fatigue Syndrome/Myalgic Encephalomyelitis (CFS/ME): a systematic review of patient-reported outcome measures (PROMs). *Child Care Health Dev.* 2014;40(6):806–824. https://doi.org/10.1111/cch.12135.

136. Haywood KL, Staniszewska S, Chapman S. Quality and acceptability of patient-reported outcome measures used in chronic fatigue syndrome/myalgic encephalomyelitis (CFS/ME): a systematic review. *Qual Life Res.* 2012;21(1):35–52. https://doi.org/10.1007/s11136-011-9921-8.

137. Chien CW, Rodger S, Copley J, Skorka K. Comparative content review of children's participation measures using the International Classification of Functioning, Disability and Health-Children and Youth. *Arch Phys Med Rehabil.* 2014;95(1):141–152. https://doi.org/10.1016/j.apmr.2013.06.027.

138. Chien CW, Rodger S, Copley J, McLaren C. Measures of participation outcomes related to hand use for 2- to 12-year-old children with disabilities: a systematic review. *Child Care Health Dev.* 2014;40(4):458–471. https://doi.org/10.1111/cch.12037.

139. Andresen EM. Criteria for assessing the tools of disability outcomes research. *Arch Phys Med Rehabil.* 2000;81(Suppl 2):S15–S20.

140. Dent K, Grampurohit N, Thielen C, Sadowsky C, Davidson L, Taylor H, Bultman J, Gaughan J, Marino R, Mulcahey MJ. Evaluation of the Capabilities of the Upper Extremity Test (CUE-T) in children with tetraplegia. *Topics in Spinal Cord Injury Rehabilitation.* 2018;24(3):239–251.

141. Portney LG, Watkins MP. *Foundations of clinical research: application to practice.* 3rd ed. Upper Saddle River: Pearson Prentice Hall; 2007.

142. Bovend'Eerdt TJ, Dawnes H, Johansen-Berg H, Wade DT. Evaluation of a modified Jebsen test of hand function and the University of Maryland Arm Questionnaire for Stroke. *Clin Rehabil.* 2004;18(2):194–202.

143. Noronha J, Bundy A, Groll J. The effect of positioning on the hand function of boys with cerebral palsy. *Am J Occup Ther.* 1989;43(8):507–512.

144. Mulcahey MJ, Smith BT, Betz RR, Weiss AA. The outcomes of surgical tendon transfers and occupational therapy in a child with a spinal cord injury. *Am J Occup Ther.* 1995;49(7):607–617.

145. Aliu O, Netscher DT, Staines KG, Thornby J, Armenta A. A 5-year evaluation of function after pollicization for congenital thumb aplasia using multiple outcome measures. *Plast Reconstr Surg.* 2008;122(1):198–205.

146. Klingels K, Feys H, Molenaers G, Verbeke G, Van Daele S, Hoskens J, Desloovere K, De Cock P. Randomized trial of modified constraint induced movement therapy with and without an intensive therapy program in children with unilateral cerebral palsy. *Neurorehabil Neural Repair.* 2013;27(9):799–807.

147. Netscher DT, Aliu O, Sandvall BK, Staines KG, Hamilton KL, Salazar-Reyes H, Thornby J. Functional outcomes of children with index pollicizations for thumb deficiency. *J Hand Surg Am.* 2013;38(2):250–257.

148. Shingade VU, Shingade RV, Ughade SN. Results of single-staged rotational osteotomy in a child with congenital proximal radioulnar synostosis: subjective and objective evaluation. *J Pediatr Orthop.* 2014;34(1):63–69.

149. Hiller LB, Wade CK. Upper extremity functional assessment scales in children Duchenne muscular dystrophy: a comparison. *Arch Phys Med Rehabil.* 1992;73(6):527–534.

150. Brandao MB, Ferre C, Kuo HC, Rameckers EA, Bleyenheuft Y, Hung YC, Friel K, Gordon AM. Comparison of structured skill and unstructured practice during intensive bimanual training in children with unilateral spastic cerebral palsy. *Neurorehabil Neural Repair.* 2014 Jun;28(5):452–461. https://doi.org/10.1177/1545968313516871.

151. Staines KG, Majzoub R, Thornby J, Netscher DT. Functional outcome for children with thumb aplasia

undergoing pollicization. *Plast Reconstr Surg.* 2005; 116(5):1314−1323.

152. Spirtos M, O'Mahony P, Malone J. Interrater reliability of the Melbourne Assessment of Unilateral Upper Limb Function for children with hemiplegic cerebral palsy. *Am J Occup Ther.* 2011 Jul-Aug;65(4):378−383.

153. DeMatteo C, Law M, Russell D, Pollock N, Rosenbaum P, Walters S. *Quality of Upper Extremity Skill Test. Ontario.* Neurodevelopmental Clinical Research Unit; 1992.

154. DeMatteo C, Law M, Russell D, Pollock N, Rosenbaum P, Walter S. The reliability and validity of the quality of upper extremity skills test. *Phys Occup Ther Pediatr.* 1993;13: 1−18.

155. Penta M, Thonnard JL, Tesio L. ABILHAND: a Rasch-built measure of manual ability. *Arch Phys Med Rehabil.* 1998; 79(9):1038−1042.

156. Vandervelde L, Van den Bergh PY, Penta M, Thonnard JL. Validation of the ABILHAND ques-tionnaire to measure manual ability in children and adults with neuromuscular disorders. *J Neurosurg Psychiatr.* 2012;81(5): 506−512.

157. Aarts PB, Jonqerius PH, Geerdink YA, van Limbeek J, Geurts A. Effectiveness of modified constraint induced movement therapy in children with unilateral spastic cerebral palsy: a randomized controlled trial. *Neurorehabil Neural Repair.* 2010;24(6):509−518.

158. Sgandurra G, Ferrari A, Cossu G, Guzzetta A, Fogassi L, Cioni G. Randomized trial of observation and execution of upper extremity actions versus action alone in children with unilateral cerebral palsy. *Neurorehabil Neural Repair.* 2013;27(9):808−815.

159. Young NL, Williams JI, Yoshida KK, Wirght JG. Measurement properties of the activities scale for kids. *J Clin Epidemiol.* 2000;53:12.

160. Plint AC, Gaboury I, Owen J, Young NL. Activities scale for kids: an analysis of normal. *J Pediatr Orthop.* 2003; 23:788−790.

161. Cup EH, Scholte op Reimer WJ, Thijssen MC, van Kuyk-Minis MA. Reliability and validity of the Canadian occupational performance measure in stroke patients. *Clin Rehabil.* 2003;17(4):402−409.

162. Eyssen IC, Steultjens MP, Oud TA, Bolt EM, Maasdam A, Dekker J. Responsiveness of the Canadian occupational performance measure. *J Rehabil Res Dev.* 2011;48(5): 517−528.

163. Cusick A, McIntrye S, Novak I, Lannin N, Lowe K. A comparison of goal attainment scaling and the Canadian occupational performance measure for pediatric rehabilitation research. *Pediatr Rehabil.* 2006;9(2):149−157.

164. Cusick A, Lannin NA, Lowe K. Adapting the Canadian occupational performance measure for use in a pediatric clinical trial. *Disabil Rehabil.* 2007;29(10):761−767.

165. Carswell A, McColl MA, Baptiste S, Law M, Polatajko H, Pollack N. *Can J Occup Ther.* 2004;71(4):210−222.

166. McColl MA, Law M, Baptiste S, Pollcock N, Carswell A, Polatajko HJ. Targeted applications of the Canadian occupational performance measure. *Can J Occup Ther.* 2005;72(5):298−300.

167. Davis SE, Mulcahey MJ, Smith BT, Betz RR. Outcome of functional electrical stimulation in the rehabilitation of a child with C5 tetraplegia. *JSCM.* 1999;22:107−113.

168. Pollock N, Sharma N, Christenson C, Law M, Gorter JW, Darrah J. Change in patient-identified goals in young children with cerebral palsy receiving a context-focused intervention: associations with child, goal and intervention factors. *Phys Occup Ther Pediatr.* 2013. PMID: 23713836.

169. Pruitt SD, Varni JW, Setoguchi Y. Functional status in children with limb deficiency: development and initial validation of an outcome measure. *Arch Phys Med Rehabil.* 1996 Dec;77(12):1233−1238.

170. Pruitt SD, Varni JW, Seid M, Setoguchi Y. Functional status in limb deficiency: development of an outcome measure for preschool children. *Arch Phys Med Rehabil.* 1998 Apr;79(4):405−411.

171. Sköld A, Hermansson LN, Krumlinde-Sundholm L, Eliasson AC. Development and evidence of validity for the children's hand-use experience questionnaire (CHEQ). *Dev Med Child Neurol.* 2011;53:436−442.

172. Kiresuk T, Smith A, Cardillo J. *Goal attainment scaling: applications, theory and measurement.* London: Erlbaum; 1994.

173. Mailloux Z, May-Benson TA, Summers CA, Miller LJ, Brett-Green B, Burke JP, Cohn ES, Koomer JA, Parham LD, Roley SS, Schaaf RC, Schoen SA. Goal attainment scaling as a measure of meaningful outcomes for children with sensory integration disorders. *AJOT.* 2007;61(2):254−259.

174. Ten Berge SR, Boonstra AM, Dijkstra PU, Hadders-Algra M, Haga N, Maathuis CG. A systematic evaluation of the effect of thumb opponens splints on hand function in children with unilateral cerebral palsy. *Clin Rehabil.* 2012;26(4):362−371.

175. Wesdock KA, Kott K, Sharps C. Pre and post surgical evaluation of hand function in hemiplegia cerebral palsy: exemplar cases. *J Hand Ther.* 2008;21(4):386−397.

176. Lowe K, Novak I, Cusick A. Repeat injection of botulinum toxin A is safe and effective for upper limb movement and function in children with cerebral palsy. *Dev Med Child Neurol.* 2007;49(11):823−829.

177. Steenbeek D, Ketelaar M, Galama K, Gorter JW. Goal attainment scaling in pediatric rehabilitation: a critical review of the literature. *Dev Med Child Neurol.* 2007;49(7): 550−556.

178. Bovend'Eeerdt TJ, Dawes H, Izadi H, Wade DT. Agreement between two different scoring procedures for goal attainment scaling is low. *J Rehabil Med.* 2011;43(1): 46−49.

179. Uswatte G, Taub E, Griffin A, et al. The pediatric motor activity log - revised: assessing real-world arm use in children with cerebral palsy. *Rehabil Psychol.* 2012;57: 149−158.

180. Wallen M, Bundy A, Pont K, Ziviani J. Psychometric properties of the Pediatric Motor Activity Log used for children with cerebral palsy. *Dev Med Child Neurol.* 2009;51: 200−208.

181. Daltroy LH, Liang MH, Fossel A, Golberg MJ. The POSNA pediatric musculoskeletal functional health questionnaire; report on reliability, validity and sensitivity to change. *J Pediatr Orthop*. 1998;18:561–571.

182. Hunsaker, American Academy of Orthopaedic Surgeons. *Pediatric Orthopaedic Society of North America, American Academy of Pediatrics, and Shriner's Hospitals*; 2005. www.aaos.org/research/outcomes/Pediatric.pdf.

183. Amor CJ, Spaeth MS, Chafey DH, Gogla GR. Use of the pediatric outcomes data collection Instrument to evaluate functional outcomes in arthrogryposis. *J Pediatr Orthop*. 2011;31(3):293–296.

184. Kunkel S, Eismann E, Cornwall R. Utility of the pediatric outcomes data collection instrument for assessing acute hand and wrist injuries in children. *J Pediatr Orthop*. 2011;31(7):767–772.

185. Matsumoto H, Vitale MG, Hyman JE, Roye DP. Can parents rate their children's quality of life? Perspectives of pediatric orthopedic outcomes. *J Pediatr Othop*. 2011;20(3):184–190.

186. Nath RK, Avila MB, Karicherla P, Somasundaram C. Assessment of triangle tilt surgery in children with obstetric brachial plexus injury using the pediatric outcomes data collection instrument. *Open Orthop J*. 2011;5:385–388.

187. Dedini R, Bagley A, Molitor F, James M. Comparison of pediatric outcomes data collection scores and range of motion before and after shoulder tendon transfers for children with brachial plexus birth palsy. *J Pediatr Orthop*. 2008;28(2):259–270.

188. Huffman GR, Bagley AM, James MA, Lerman JA, Rab G. Assessment of children with brachial plexus birth palsy using the pediatric outcomes data collection instrument. *J Pediatr Orthop*. 2005;25:400–404.

189. Piers EV, Herzberg DS. *Piers-Harris Children's Self Concept Scale-Second Edition manual*. Los Angeles, CA: Western Psychological Services; 2002.

190. Buffart LM, Roebroeck ME, Pesch-Batenburg JM, Janssen WG, Stam HJ. Assessment of arm/hand functioning in children with a congenital transverse or longitudinal reduction deficiency of the upper limb. *Disabil Rehabil*. 2006 Jan 30;28(2):85–95.

191. Van Dijk-Koot CA, Van DH, et al. Current experiences with the prosthetic upper extremity functional index in follow up of children with upper limb reduction deficiency. *J Prosthet Orthot*. 2009;21:110–114.

192. Ardolino EM, Mulcahey MJ, Trimble S, Argetsinger L, Bienkowski M, Mullen C, Behrman AL. Development and Initial Validation of the Pediatric Neuromuscular Recovery Scale. *Pediatr Phys Ther*. 2016;28:416–426.

193. Aslam R, van Bommel A, Southwood T, Hackett J, Jester A. An evaluation of pediatric hand and upper limb assessment tools within the framework of the World Health Organisation International Classification of Disability, Functioning, and Health. *Hand Therapy*. 2015;20(1):24–34.

194. Bell A, Guido T, Krisa L, Muhlenhaupt M, Mulcahey MJ. Measures and Outcome Instruments for Pediatric Spinal Cord Injury. *Current Physical Medicine and Rehabilitation*. 2016;4:200–207, 10.007/s40141-016-0126-5.

195. Bialocerkowski A, O'Shea K, Pin TW. Psychometric properties of outcome measures for children and adolescents with brachial plexus birth palsy. *Dev Med Child Neurol*. 2013;55(12):1075–1088.

196. Gilmore R, Sakzewski L, Boyd R. Upper limb activity measures for 5- to 16-year old children with congenital hemiplegia: a systematic review. *Dev Med Child Neurol*. 2010;52:14–21.

CHAPTER 5

Splinting, Taping, and Adaptation

DEBORAH HUMPL, OTR/L • KELLY ANNE FERRY, MOTR/L •
LYDIA D. RAWLINS, MED, OTR/L • KATHLEEN TATE, MS OTR/L

INTRODUCTION

Splinting, taping, and structural adaptations are common modalities in rehabilitating the injured or atypical hand. There are many options available for the pediatric therapist to adapt adult modalities for children; however, the materials, approach, and education may be very different in pediatrics. This chapter will highlight the uniqueness of pediatric splinting, taping, and adaptations, as well as techniques for successful design, fabrication, and carryover.

SPLINTING: MATERIALS AND TOOLS
Material Selection

Splinting is a modality that appears to have been used to support a body part as far back as 460 BC. Historically, materials were very rustic, using different wood shapes, sheet metals, belts, and eventually higher temperature plastics and foams. To this day, materials continue to evolve with a common goal of providing a splint that is lightweight, yet strong and functional enough to achieve the desired goal.[1] Splinting materials have many different properties that are designed to meet the very unique needs of varying diagnoses and clinical presentations.

Properties of Materials
Stretch and pliability of material

Splint sheets are flat and can bend very easily. The material only gains strength by molding contours into the splint. When the sheets are heated, resistance to stretch can range from minimal to highly resistant to stretch. Splint material that is minimally resistant to stretch uses gravity to mold and conform easily on a still and cooperative body part, requiring gentle handling to obtain the desired shape. In the adult hand clinic, Polyflex and Orfit varieties are used widely to achieve these parameters; however, children tend to have very busy hands that are constantly moving, pulling away with fear, or tightening with spasticity, not to mention hands of varying shapes and sizes. Therefore, materials that are more resistant to stretch are optimal. This allows the therapist to work at molding a busy and uncooperative hand without compromising the integrity of the splint. Materials such as Aquaplast and Prism are moderately resistive to stretch and have the ability to be wrapped and tacked along the arm when splinting without assistance[2] (see Fig. 5.1). EZ Form and Omega are more resistant to stretch that allows for more forgiveness when molding splints on busy little hands. Materials with higher resistance to stretch, such as Orthoplast and Synergy, tend to hold heat longer. More resilient materials also tend to hold heat longer and require the application of stockinette on a child's sensitive skin before the material is applied.

A small percentage of children with very cooperative hands may need a splint following a tendon repair or a fracture. This group may permit the therapist to use a lower resistant-to-stretch material such as Tailor Splint or Preferred, which will give a more intimate fit when molded; however, this case-by-case basis relies on the therapist's comfort with handling a material with minimal resistance to stretch.

Thickness and perforation

Splint material thicknesses range from 1/6″ to 3/16″. Thicker material will feel heavier on the arm, which can impact comfort on a child. The most versatile sheet

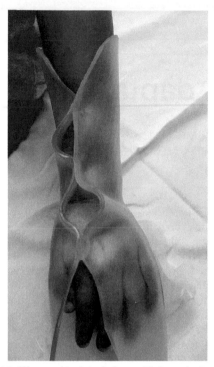

FIG. 5.1 Wrap and tack technique with Aquaplast or Prism secures material to the forearm so that the therapist can focus on molding the hand. (Courtesy Children's Hospital of Philadelphia.)

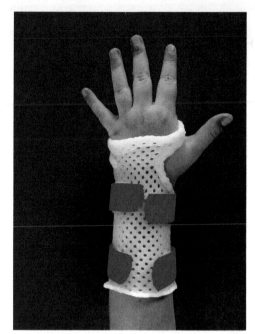

FIG. 5.2 Dorsal wrist cock up splint with perforated Aquaplast. (Courtesy Children's Hospital of Philadelphia.)

thicknesses for pediatrics are usually 1/16″ and 1/8″. Most clinics will stock 1/8″ material, as it is the most universal; however, 1/16″ and even 3/32″ materials are very useful for tiny hands, skinny body parts, and fractured fingers. Perforation in material provide aeration to the skin and will lighten the splint overall; however, cutting along the perforations may sometimes create a bumpy edge that is more challenging in creating a smooth finish (see Fig. 5.2).

Colors

A variety of colors for splint material can be attractive to a child's eye. The most child friendly colors are found in Aquaplast and Prism materials. Although a child's preference is very valid for aesthetics of the splint, it is more important that the therapist is comfortable handling the material. Splints can be made more child friendly by adding colorful straps, decorations, glitter paint, or even splint scrap enhancements.[2] See Figs. 5.3–5.5.

Other Materials

In lieu of prefabricated splints, making soft splints with materials, such as Neoprene and Fabrifoam, is

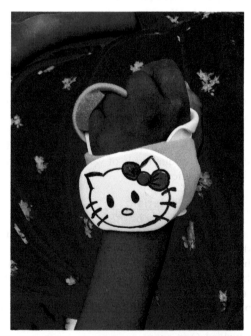

FIG. 5.3 Splint decorations made from scraps and permanent markers. (Courtesy Children's Hospital of Philadelphia.)

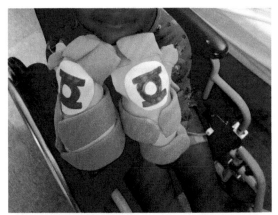

FIG. 5.4 Dorsal Hood splints with superhero designs. (Courtesy Children's Hospital of Philadelphia.)

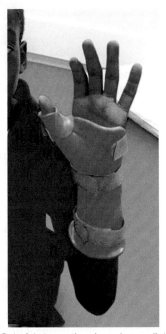

FIG. 5.5 Colorful long thumb spica splint. (Courtesy Children's Hospital of Philadelphia.)

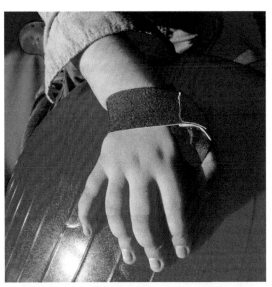

FIG. 5.6 Thumb abduction strap with Fabrifoam. (Courtesy Children's Hospital of Philadelphia.)

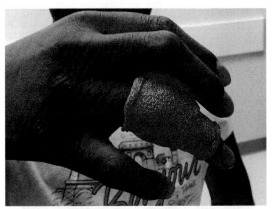

FIG. 5.7 Orficast semirigid material for serial splinting a proximal interphalangeal joint (PIP) flexion contracture. (Courtesy Children's Hospital of Philadelphia.)

advantageous as these materials are thinner, lighter, and able to be issued at the appointment versus ordering. These stretchy materials are great for simple thumb and supinator straps, as well as strapping on hard splints (see Fig. 5.6).

Orficast combines a soft webbing like material with imbedded Orfit splint material, to make an intimate semirigid splint (see Fig. 5.7). The therapist can also use Orficast to strengthen a soft splint, or even use it as an adhesive to attach Velcro onto a soft strap versus sewing Velcro (see Fig. 5.8). Delta Cast Conformable has also gained popularity for very lightweight circumferential splinting that can be cleaned in a washing machine (see Fig. 5.9).

Tools

In addition to a heat pan that can maintain a temperature of 160 °F, good tools are also essential for a well-made splint. A large, sharp, clean pair of sewing scissors should be designated solely for cutting splint material. This will allow for speed in cutting the hot material

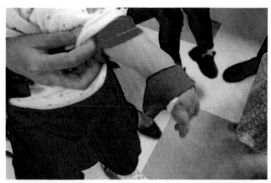

FIG. 5.8 Thumb abduction splint made with Fabrifoam (dark blue) and an Orficast web space support (light blue) to inhibit tone. (Courtesy Children's Hospital of Philadelphia.)

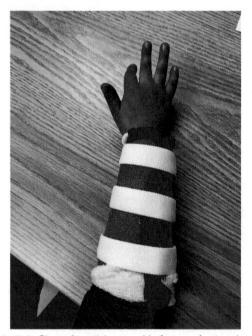

FIG. 5.9 Circumferential removable forearm fracture brace with Delta Cast Conformable. (Courtesy Children's Hospital of Philadelphia.)

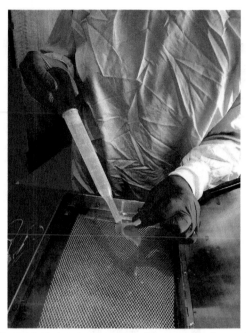

FIG. 5.10 Turkey baster with splint pan water is used for edge finishing small areas. (Courtesy Children's Hospital of Philadelphia.)

and promote smoother splint edges. The therapist also needs a pair of office scissors for cutting stockinette, Velcro, and foam. A spatula is needed to remove the heated material from the pan, and a sharp exacto knife is used to score and split the large splint sheets. Other tools that may be very helpful in pediatric splinting include small curved Mayo scissors for cutting thumb holes and curves of the splint and large curved scissors for cutting angles on the ends of the splints and elbow

joints. A turkey baster allows application of controlled heat onto a very small part of the splint, so the integrity is maintained with edge finishing (see Fig. 5.10). Although a heat gun's primary purpose is for edge finishing, the heat is very intense and can easily melt a very small splint. It is best to use the heat gun for heating Velcro to bond to the splint; as well as securing pieces on a splint, such as outriggers and universal cuff designs.

Patterns

Basic principles for making splint patterns are universal for adults and children. Paper towels make great templates for patterns, as they are more moldable than paper to test on the child before tracing it onto expensive splint material. Pattern making can be a challenge for the wiggly, fearful, or spastic hand, so the therapist needs to be as quick as possible without upsetting the child. When possible, patterns can be traced on an unaffected opposite extremity, and then flipped for use on the affected side.[2] Siblings or peers of similar size and age may also be called upon to have their hand traced. Adult patterns can be adapted for pediatrics by shrinking the patterns on a copy machine with card stock paper. The copies can then be laminated and wiped clean between patients.

SPLINTING: PSYCHOLOGICAL READINESS AND ENVIRONMENTAL PREPARATION

The pediatric patient requires special considerations when preparing for a splint fabrication visit. Certain amounts of compliance and participation are required of the patient and caregivers to create a custom splint that fits well and meets the criteria for the purpose of the splint. Efficient use of time is crucial for a successful session. Children generally lack the patience level of adults to sit and wait while material is heated or supplies are gathered; therefore, prepping the environment and the patient properly is essential. Creating a splint that is functional and extremely comfortable for the pediatric client takes 90% skillful preparation and 10% proper application.

Psychological Readiness

Psychological patient readiness is essential to the success of the splint fabrication visit. According to Meuthing et al., 2007, "The commonly accepted view of patients as passive recipients of health care is changing … The Accreditation Council for Graduate Medical Education has declared that residents must be able to provide family-centered patient care that is culturally effective, developmentally and age appropriate, compassionate, and effective as part of their core competencies."[3] Translating this ideology into everyday patient care takes a conscious effort. Although progress is being made in adult settings, these considerations are frequently undervalued and overlooked with regards to the pediatric client. Time constraints and lack of preparation time during busy days can lead a clinician to dismiss facilitating the child's mental acceptance of splint wear and readiness for the procedure ahead. In addition, it is common to observe dialogue being pursued with the caregiver versus the child in the medical setting. It is important to include the child when explaining the process. Carefully consider their level of cognition, sensory perception, and state of mind in the moment. A calm demeanor and kind and thoughtful eye contact can reduce anxieties in both the child and parent. Explain the process with language and terms the patient will understand. A statement such as "we are making a special glove to help your arm" is a helpful, child friendly, verbal approach. Taking the necessary time to prepare the child and caregiver's psychological readiness is instrumental to creating a product that best meet the patient's needs.

The therapist should try to consider the patient's entire day within context when approaching the patient. Did the child just spend 3 hours waiting to see the orthopedic surgeon before arriving for the occupational therapy visit? Is this the first time the child is seeing his or her stitches, wounds, or hardware upon cast removal? Was the commute long and stressful? Is the family anxious to get home to other siblings? Did the patient arrive late thus leaving limited time for the splint fabrication? Are there questions regarding the physician order that need to be clarified before splinting can begin? All of these factors and more can be part of a typical visit and could impact the outcome of the splint.

The patient's receptive and expressive language skills can widely vary. For the nonverbal patient, keen assessment skills are required to assess pain signs or notice discomfort. Although it is easy to dismiss the need to provide explanation to the nonverbal child, it should still be integrated into the visit with language at the child and caregiver's level of understanding.[4] For the child with neuromotor impairments and tone, consider using a quiet voice to reduce jerky movements and startle reflexes that may alter the molding process. Provide demonstrations on how to remain still using child friendly language, such as "still as a statue" and "quiet as a mouse." Even a sudden elevated pitch within a sentence or song from the caregiver during the molding process can startle the child and produce excessive muscle tone.

The medical setting and particularly the splinting process can be very intimidating. The sight of material being dropped in hot, steamy water can be enough to cause alarm. There are a number of good ways to allay the child's fears including allowing the child to play with a scrap material to make objects or jewelry, introducing the feeling and temperature to the unaffected side first, having the child along with a sibling to assist with making matching splints, fabricating a splint for a doll or stuffed animal, or even presenting premade samples of dolls or superheroes with splints[1,2] (see Fig. 5.11). Child life therapists can be utilized to help prepare the patient and provide distraction if necessary.

A child who is seen bedside in the hospital can have additional fears and anxiety. Good communication with the medical team can allow the therapist to find the best day or time for the patient, determine if the patient is medically stable enough for the splint, and communicate any other diagnostic tests that could impact patient comfort or timing. Nursing staff can also assist in making sure the patient has taken any prescribed pain medication at least 30 minutes before the splint is made.

Lastly, after all careful consideration of patient psychological readiness is complete, the ability to rapidly adapt to changing scenarios is a needed therapeutic skill

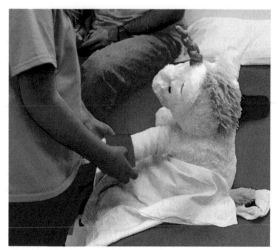

FIG. 5.11 Child splinting a stuffed animal to promote acceptance of own splint. (Courtesy Children's Hospital of Philadelphia.)

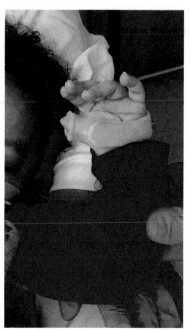

FIG. 5.12 Supine positioning with shoulder externally rotated for splint fabrication. (Courtesy Children's Hospital of Philadelphia.)

set. The therapist may begin with a very relaxed child, but loud noises, other children crying, or the need to go to the bathroom, may change the child's state quickly. The ability to remain flexible and make quick adjustments will lead to a more positive outcome.

Preparing the Environment

An organized and well-kept splint room leads to efficient and safe splint fabrication. Prepare the room with needed materials and have them ready before the client is brought into the treatment area. A binder stored in the splint room that includes a variety of splint patterns, along with a description of their use, is an extremely helpful resource. Safe and easy access to the tools and the patient are essential. Establish an organized work area before placing the splint material in the heat pan. Although in use, place tools in an area that are accessible to the therapist, yet out of reach of impulsive and curious children present. Sharp or potentially dangerous tools not in use should be stored in a locked drawer.

A child who is hospitalized, requiring bedside splint fabrication, poses unique challenges when obtaining environmental readiness. The team can work with therapists to make ready the environment by dimming lights or temporarily halting alarms. There are many obstacles at a patient's bedside such as tables, monitors, bed rails, and supply carts. All obstacles should be moved ahead of fabrication to allow for a clear path from the splint pan to the patient for molding. The patient should only be a few unobstructed steps from the splint pan and work station.

Proper positioning of the child can definitely help ease fabrication. Choose the patient's most desired and comfortable position that still allows good access to the arm. Placing the child supine on a mat or bed is often a preferred position as it fully supports the child and usually requires less handling from the therapist. In addition, it is easier to see the hand and arm surface being splinted, as the child's shoulder can be rotated safely for a better view (see Fig. 5.12). However, the best position can vary depending on your client. For example, if an infant arrives asleep in a car seat, take advantage of this supine positioning for splinting. A child may arrive in a tilt in space wheelchair with full head and trunk support. Sometimes simply tilting the chair back may be all that is necessary to reduce tone and achieve a semisupine position for better handling of the material. If a child has severe reflux, use of a beanbag chair or wedge can provide a fully supportive but upright position that can reduce reflux episodes and increase comfort.

Finally, there should be one last mental check before removing material from the splint pan to make sure that:

- The patient is positioned comfortably
- There is good access to the arm being splinted
- The arm is free of any items of clothing, jewelry, or identification bands

- Stockinette was applied to the arm
- Available helpers in the room have good direction and understanding of their role.
- The child is as mentally ready as possible

SPLINTING: FABRICATION PEARLS

Therapists with expert knowledge of splinting the pediatric patient often have a number of helpful hints or tricks they utilize to accomplish the task of creating a well-made splint. The following are highlights of some of the anecdotal methods frequently used when splinting the child.

- For the busy child, have a quick cooling method with paper towels dipped in cold water ready to apply to a warm splint material for faster set time once proper positioning is obtained.[2]
- Use the thenar eminence as a control point when splinting the hand by firmly supporting the child's thenar with the therapist's thenar when molding (see Fig. 5.13).
- Placement of 50/50 Elastomer putty in the hand pan can be very useful to prevent windswept fingers,

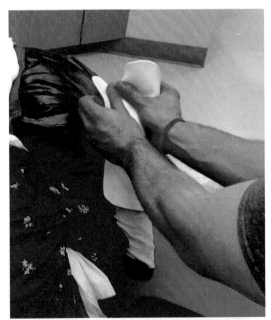

FIG. 5.13 To gain control with molding a splint on a busy hand, the therapist matches his thenar eminence to the teen's thenar to support the thumb, normalize tone, and prevent subluxation of the thumb metacarpophalangeal (MP) joint.

digits from crossing, and other deformities such as swan neck.[2]

- Consider comfort and function jointly. Monitor for signs of facial grimacing, white fingertips, or limb withdraw, which may indicate too much stretch has been elicited. A splint that provides maximal stretch to the elbow, wrist, thumb, and fingers is only effective if it can be worn comfortably by the patient. At times, allowing for slightly more finger flexion to obtain better wrist alignment is the best clinical decision.
- A 1-inch block may be useful for the child to pinch while making a thumb splint to optimize thumb position.
- If fabricating a splint with gloves donned for infection control purposes, applying lotion on the gloves will help prevent the gloves from sticking to the material.

Creative Splint Designs

As previously mentioned, pediatric splints can be adapted from adult patterns. There are many possibilities for creative splint design that can be used by the pediatric therapist.

The weight-bearing splint, typically used for patients with high tone, is used to properly achieve an upper extremity weight-bearing position. Use of a small dome, such as a smaller ball, is appropriate when molding the splint[5] (see Fig. 5.14). A cone splint can be a great option for serial wrist and finger splinting or as a secondary plan when molding the thumb becomes problematic[6] (see Fig. 5.15). A long arm extension splint that controls motion at three joints may be easier for a caregiver to manage than applying a separate elbow splint and forearm-based splint (see Fig. 5.16).

Traditional dynamic splints are not usually prescribed, as outriggers are very intricate and can be very dangerous if a child falls on or tries to play with them. There are some ways to use dynamic principles and functional splints for stretching. Dynamic elbow flexion splints with resistance band tension can help achieve end range elbow flexion, which is a challenge with prefabricated hinge splints in pediatrics[7] (see Fig. 5.17). Aquaplast tubes can be used to fabricate a dynamic wrist extension splint, and Fig. 5.8 splints can be used for swan necking or even as a thumb abduction splint (see Fig. 5.18). Finger cuffs and monofilaments can be added to a wrist splint for static progressive splinting (see Fig. 5.19). Soft materials can also be used for dynamic splints. As seen in Fig. 5.20, a dynamic elbow flexion/forearm supination splint is fabricated by sewing resistance cords into Fabrifoam bicep and

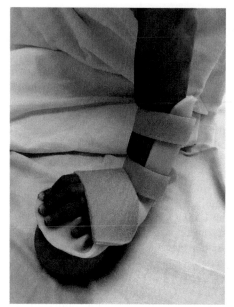

FIG. 5.14 Weight-bearing splint. (Courtesy Children's Hospital of Philadelphia.)

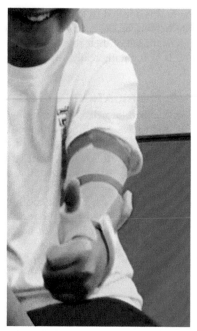

FIG. 5.16 Long arm extension splint. (Courtesy Children's Hospital of Philadelphia.)

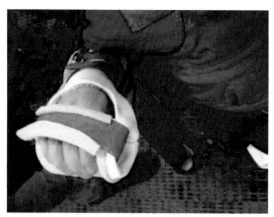

FIG. 5.15 Cone splint. (Courtesy Children's Hospital of Philadelphia.)

forearm cuffs. This allows the toddler with a C5-6 brachial plexus injury to overcome the typical waiter tip movement pattern and elicit activation of the triceps to help improve elbow flexion.

Strapping

There are many varieties of strapping and Velcro for splints. Although strap placement principles are usually

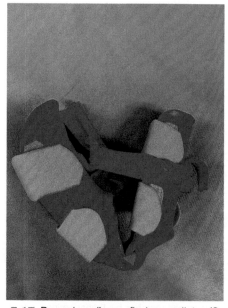

FIG. 5.17 Dynamic elbow flexion splint. (Courtesy Children's Hospital of Philadelphia.)

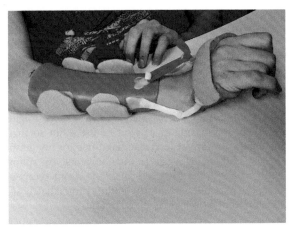

FIG. 5.18 A dynamic wrist extension splint with Aquatube hinges and resistance band tension. (Courtesy Children's Hospital of Philadelphia.)

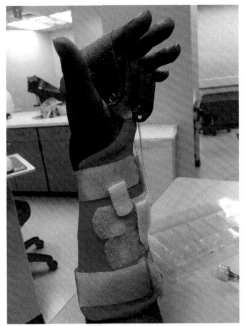

FIG. 5.19 Static progressive MP flexion splint for contracture management following a distal forearm tumor resection in a 9 year old.

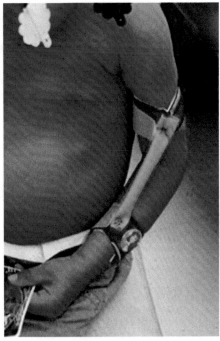

FIG. 5.20 Dynamic flexion/forearm supination assist splint made with Fabrifoam and resistance cords. (Courtesy Children's Hospital of Philadelphia.)

universal for pediatrics and adults, the child's ability to quickly remove a splint becomes a challenge for the caregiver and therapist. Over the years, many therapists have developed creative designs using shoelaces, diaper clips, and even zippers in the splints to prevent the child from removing it.[1,2,4] One quick trick is to cinch the middle of a piece of sticky back Velcro, which halts the leverage of one hand to remove the rest of the Velcro (see Fig. 5.21). The therapist can also try Polylock Velcro as it is also very hard for a child to remove.

For small hand splints with thumb holes, where there is not ample space for Velcro, the therapist can sew a strap through the thumb hole, to achieve better Velcro closure of the strap on the ulnar side (see Fig. 5.22). Foam may be added onto strapping to provide gentle compression and an extra soft surface on skin. In addition, thin strips of Terryfoam padding or moleskin can line the top of a resting hand splint so that the child does not incidentally scratch their face while sleeping.

Education

Education on use and care of the splint is a standard of care in pediatrics and adults. Skin checks and cleaning instructions are universal. It is important that the care principles and description of donning and doffing the splint are written clearly and reviewed with all of the caregivers who will be with the child while wearing it. Using a caregiver's cell phone to capture a donning and doffing video can help ensure splint adherence at home.

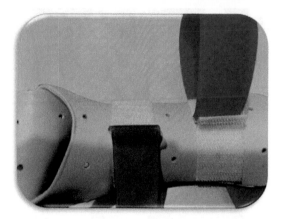

FIG. 5.21 Cinch the center of the Velcro strip so that the child cannot remove the splint. (Courtesy Cincinnati Children's Hospital.)

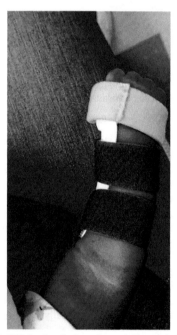

FIG. 5.22 Stitched soft strap through thumb hole of splint for better closure on ulnar side. (Courtesy Children's Hospital of Philadelphia.)

There is very inconsistent evidence to support wearing schedules for contracture prevention,[8] unless it is a specific protocol because of surgical intervention or a healing fracture.

For more chronic diagnostic groups, the authors educate caregivers on a 6–8 hour continual wear schedule in a resting hand splint to help decrease tone, prevent further deformity, and normalize hand arches. Ultimately, the therapist should discuss goals with the family to develop a wearing schedule that is realistic for their lifestyle.[8] Many children with neuromotor impairments may also wear lower extremity bracing at night that can really challenge the child's and caregiver's compliance with the ability to sleep with arms and legs fully immobilized. A suggested wearing pattern might be for alternating nights of wear of the splint so that the child can have at least one hand free for toy grasp or self-soothing. If sleep is truly impeded by splint wear, or the child feels self-conscious about wearing the splint in public, wearing the splint(s) immediately after school for 6 hours may be an option.

NICU CONSIDERATIONS

The neonatal intensive care unit (NICU) is a very complex and highly specialized hospital environment for premature or critically ill infants. The lifesaving technical equipment has been integral in saving lives. However, this often results in the infant having cognitive and musculoskeletal limitations, as well as long-term hearing, visual, and developmental issues.[9–11] Additionally, NICU babies often present with upper extremity dysfunction because of trauma to lower motor neurons during the intrauterine or perinatal period, fractures, dislocations, nerve injury, central nervous system damage, or prenatal exposure to drugs.[11]

Although upper extremity dysfunction in neonates is common, current research on evidence-based practice is limited to a specific diagnosis or case studies. There is considerable interest in the medical community to improve these infants overall neurodevelopmental outcomes; hence, therapists are seeing increased referrals for management of these patients.

Common upper extremity anomalies seen in the NICU include brachial plexus injuries, cortical thumb, radial club hands, and arthrogryposis. These will be described in detail in later chapters. Other causes of impairments may include infiltrates from IV's and contractures and tightness of the arm because of limited positioning in the NICU. Although early splinting can be paramount to improving upper extremity function, there is limited research available for the intensive care infant especially 6 months or younger. It should be noted that splinting before 28 weeks gestation is usually deferred due to the viability of infants before that age.

Environmental Considerations

The overall neurosocial behavioral state of the hospitalized neonate is generally diffuse. Their responses to handling often impact their autonomic status, therefore splinting needs to be provided in a manner that minimally impacts this status.[12] It is imperative for the therapist to coordinate the splint session with the medical team, particularly nursing, to ascertain the optimal time for splint fabrication. Use of sucrose or breast milk–dipped pacifiers, as the patient is medically able to accept, may also be helpful. Other nonpharmacological interventions to consider are swaddling the infant, offering bottle-feeding presplinting, offering splinting after a relaxing bath, and environmental adaptations such as soft music, dim lights, or overhead mobiles as distractions. The therapist may need to employ creativity in positioning the patient for comfort that may include splinting while the infant is in a crib, seated in a vibrating chair, or rocking in the caregiver's arms while the caregiver is seated or standing (see Fig. 5.23). If possible, it may also be beneficial to coordinate splinting with medical interventions that require sedation.

Materials

Splinting infants in the NICU is very unique, as it requires use of material that can be easily remolded due to the need for serial splinting to accommodate quick improvements with range and growth. Due to their sensitive skin and diminished fat pad, NICU infants are more at risk for skin breakdown, ulcers, and burns. Use of low temperature and lightweight thermoplastic material 1/16 to 1/8 of an inch in size such as Ezeform, Aquaplast, and Orfit are recommended. Splints may also be made out of soft fabric such as Softstrap, Fabrifoam, and Neoprene[12] (see Fig. 5.24). Elastomer can be used as another splint alternative or as finger and web spacers in the primary splint. Strapping size is ½ to 1 inch to accommodate to the small surface area of the splint.

Splint Types

The most common splints fabricated in the NICU include, but are not limited to the following:[13,14]

- Resting hand splint (Fig. 5.25)
- Thumb abduction splint (Fig. 5.26)
- Elbow extension splint (Fig. 5.27)
- Dorsal resting hand splint (Fig. 5.28)
- Radial and ulnar gutter splint

Skin Integrity/Risk for Factors

Skin integrity should be reviewed every hour for the first 4 hours (wearing tolerance schedule) as infants in the NICU are more at risk for fragile bones due to metabolic bone disease (MBD) and sensitive skin.[15,16] MBD occurs in up to 55% of babies born with a weight under

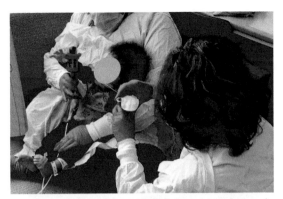

FIG. 5.23 Child fully supported by a caregiver using distraction with a toy on the right side while the splint is being fabricated on the left hand.

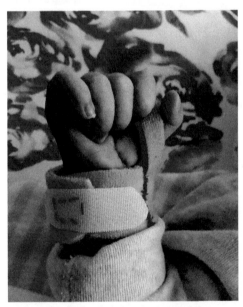

FIG. 5.24 Soft thumb strap splint.

1000 g and 23% of infants weighing <1500 g at birth.[10] It is especially prevalent in babies under 28 weeks of gestation. Careful and gentle handling should occur during splinting to prevent risk of fracture. The therapist should frequently check the splint material temperature on own their bare forearm, before, and during the molding process as the infant's skin will be very sensitive to warm material. This may place the infant at risk for burns. If an infant is teething or excessively mouthing hands, therapists should consider use of large splint over fabrication of a small splint to reduce chance of infant swallowing splint, use socks or gloves as covering over hands and splints, or hide splint under

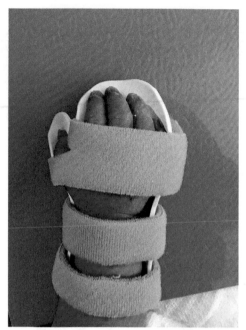

FIG. 5.25 Resting hand splint. (Courtesy Children's Hospital of Philadelphia.)

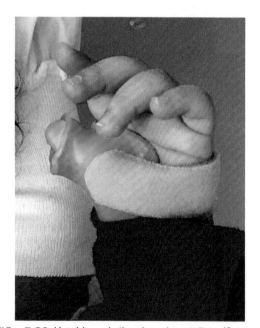

FIG. 5.26 Hand-based thumb spica splint. (Courtesy Children's Hospital of Philadelphia.)

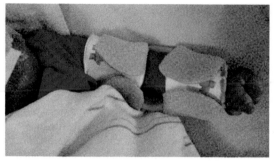

FIG. 5.27 1/16″ Ezeform Long arm extension splint with turtle decals made with Aquaplast. (Courtesy Children's Hospital of Philadelphia.)

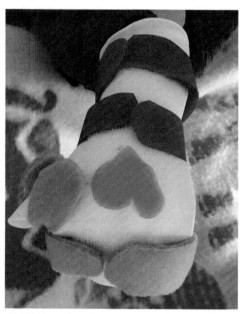

FIG. 5.28 Dorsal resting hand splint. (Courtesy Children's Hospital of Philadelphia.)

clothing. After the wearing tolerance schedule, the therapist should continue to perform frequent skin checks to reduce the opportunity for skin breakdown. Skin checks need to occur at minimum one time per shift; however, with every diaper change would be optimal.

Strapping

Strapping for the splint should be cut to cover a wide surface area of skin and edges should be rounded. This will reduce the chance for edema, circulation injuries, and skin irritations that can easily occur in fragile neonate skin. Colorful strapping and decals should be added to splints, as they provide accent to splints that reduce the chance of getting lost in the crib space. It is also as a creative way to normalize the infant experience, which is particularly meaningful to NICU parents (see Fig. 5.27).

Education

Education, whether it is for nurses, parents, or caregivers, is essential for proper follow through of the splint program. Instruction should include the purpose of splinting, donning and doffing of splints, wearing schedule, precautions, care of splint, and future plans. These areas may be captured succinctly in a bedside program (see Fig. 5.29).

Wearing Schedule

The wearing schedule will depend on the infant's needs and hand dysfunction. When a baby can accept a splint up to 4 hours, then the schedule can shift to overnight wear and a period of time during the day. As hand function increases, the time for wearing splints should be reduced. The therapist should reassess the wearing schedule every 2 weeks and change accordingly. In the hospital setting, the splint schedule and splints should be posted bedside for everyone to view. Small splints can be placed in a labeled plastic bag (see Fig. 5.30). This will aid in splint wear compliance and decrease chances of the splint being lost.

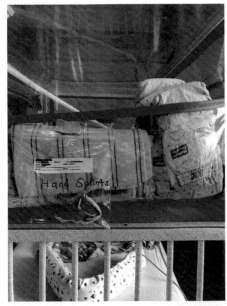

FIG. 5.29 Example of a simple bedside instruction and splint bag for easy storage and use. (Courtesy Children's Hospital of Philadelphia).

THERAPEUTIC TAPING

General Indications

Therapeutic taping is a technique in which elastic or inelastic tape is applied to one or more affected body parts using a specific technique to enhance function, support a limb, enhance posture and joint alignment, relax overused muscles, reduce edema, increase vascularity, and/or inhibit pain.[17] There are varying methods of taping practices that rely on specific properties for application. However, the most commonly recognized taping techniques for pediatric hand therapists are methods used with rigid and elastic tape.

Rigid taping provides firm support to a body part. It comprises a white skin barrier tape such as Hypafix or Anchor wrap that gets covered with a very strong, inelastic, sticky tape such as Rigid Strapping tape, Anchor tape, or Leukotape. When applied, tape is typically pulled in the direction of desired support. The California Tri-pull Taping method,[18] is primarily used to support a flaccid shoulder because of an acquired stroke in adults. However, this method has also been successful in children with acquired stroke and brachial plexus injuries, as well as supporting chronically weak shoulders in diagnoses such as high spinal cord injuries, spinal muscular atrophy, and transverse myelitis (see Fig. 5.31). Rigid tape is also valuable as a quick, temporary support to evaluate the need for a splint (see Fig. 5.32).

Use of therapeutic elastic taping (Kinesiotape or K Tape) in the pediatric population has gained popularity in recent history as an adjunctive therapy.[19] The properties of the tape give the client support without inhibiting dynamic movement, thus offering limitless possibilities for intervention. The therapist must first identify the primary goal for the use of K Tape and prioritize what body part to tape. Expert clinical observation of the patient is key to assessing the needs and selecting the correct application technique.

Strengths of Therapeutic Taping

Initial research analyzing short-term functional gain, particularly with children with cerebral palsy and brachial plexus injuries, show promise and therefore the use of the modality should not be discounted. Most studies to date measure functional change immediately after tape removal. There is strong initial evidence to support the use of K Tape for support and strengthening of the deltoid in patients with Erb's palsy.[20] The literature also shows immediate effects are observed with quality of movement and motor function in the child with cerebral palsy.[20] It may also be an essential benefit to encourage children to put to

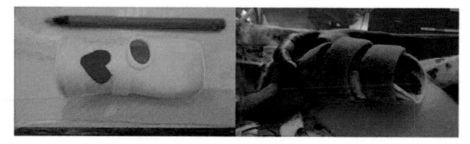

What: Modified Resting Hand Splint (Thumb should go through hole of splint. All other digits in hand portion of splint)

When: To be worn from 10:00 pm to 7:00 am

Why: To reduce tightness of Left Hand and Right Hand to maintain optimal ROM

Precautions: Please check capillary refill 1x per shift. Make sure splint straps are not too tight. Upon removal of splint, check for redness lasting greater than 30 minutes. Contact OT if this occurs. Keep away from heat of any kind or it will melt.

Care: Wash splint with cold soapy water and air day.

Plan: Splints should be reviewed by OT in one month to address progress of digit and wrist tightness. Pending that review, therapist will fabricate soft thumb abduction splint.

Please contact Jane Smith, Occupational Therapist, at 555-555-5555, if there are any questions Monday through Thursday.

FIG. 5.30 Typical NICU bedside splint program. (Courtesy Children's Hospital of Philadelphia.)

full use their few available motoric resources by influencing both cutaneous and sensorimotor receptors.[21,22]

Anecdotally, clinicians also find it useful as a "simulated test" before making a splint or ordering expensive, custom dynamic lycra garments for long-term functional use. It can also be extremely helpful for task analysis to gain better insight as to which muscle groups to relax or stimulate to obtain overall improved function. This information can be invaluable to the physical medicine and rehabilitation physician when selecting Botox injection dosage and placement. In addition, therapeutic tape applied after serial casting can be an effective intervention to encourage active movement through the full arc of the newly obtained range of motion and may replace the need for custom splints, especially those worn during the daytime.

Application: Test Patch and Frequency

After analyzing the patient's needs and establishing therapeutic goals surrounding tape application, a test patch should first be applied on the child's back close to the spine, as this area is very sensitive and out of sight

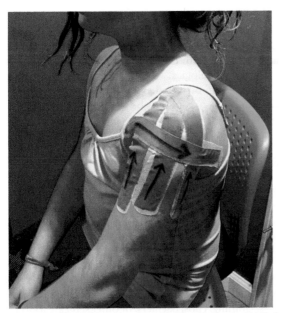

FIG. 5.31 Rigid Strapping tape for the California Tri-Pull Taping method supporting a hemi shoulder. Line of pull of tape is in the direction of humeral elevation and scapular retraction. (Courtesy Children's Hospital of Philadelphia.)

for the child to attempt to remove. The test patch should remain in place for at least 24–48 hours; however, it could take up to a week to determine if there is a potential irritation or allergy to the tape.[23]

Application: Tape Placement

As with splinting, setup and organization are key to successful tape application in pediatrics (see Figs. 5.33 and 5.34). The therapist should adopt similar environmental preparation and psychological readiness techniques and work quickly to obtain the proper pull and alignment of the tape without wrinkles, which can cause skin breakdown.

Tape application techniques are also similar in pediatrics and adults; however, tape widths may need to be narrowed to accommodate smaller arms, and children may enjoy the different colors and patterns of tape if available. However, tape removal can be anxiety and pain provoking, especially in cases where application is over body hair, the patient has underlying sensory issues, or the perception of pain is amplified. Educate the patient about the removal process and provide distraction. A heavy coating of citrus-based adhesive remover pads, olive oil, or thick unscented cream, applied generously over the whole taped area, at least 60 minutes before removing the tape, can begin to break down the adhesive to make removal easier.

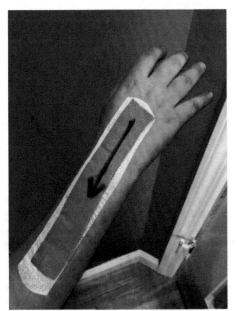

FIG. 5.32 Rigid taping used as temporary support for wrist extension. (Courtesy Children's Hospital of Philadelphia.)

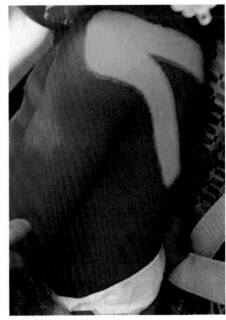

FIG. 5.33 K Tape facilitating shoulder external rotation.

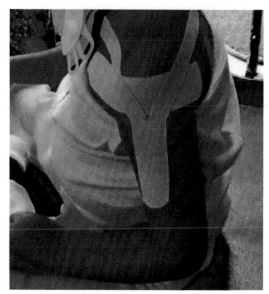

FIG. 5.34 K Tape supporting the humerus due to flaccidity.

Soaking the child in a tub with a lotion soap while removing the tape can also be effective. Best practice for tape removal is to provide a sensory distraction with quick rubbing and slowly removing the tape in the direction of hair growth. It is more beneficial to methodically work through a comfortable tape removal process versus quickly ripping off the tape. This will help the child and caregiver to gain acceptance, maintain trust with the modality, and prevent skin breakdown.

Education

Caregiver education is also key to success of the modality, especially in the outpatient setting where families are often asked to remove the tape after a certain period of time and report any significant functional gains or complications that may have occurred during tape wear. Help the caregiver understand the purpose and benefits the tape can provide, as well as the timeline and long-term plan for use. If the parent anticipates that removing the tape will be a struggle, then the parent can apply the remover at least 60 minutes before the scheduled visit, and the therapist can demonstrate tape removal during therapy.

It is important to teach the caregivers what movements to encourage from the child and give them concrete examples of age appropriate activities that will encourage specific actions. Offer examples of various positions in which the child can play, as well as ways to downgrade and upgrade the activity. Encourage capturing progress through video capture or photos to help plan optimal continuum of care with the tape in use.

ADAPTATIONS

The use of adaptations in the pediatric population can have tremendous implications on a child's success and function. With the ever changing and rapidly progressing technological world, adaptations for "making life easier" can be found everywhere, not just in medicine and will continue to be an area for therapists to be in the forefront of learning and application. One of the most unique skill sets of a pediatric therapist is the ability to modify adult adaptations to fit the pediatric population.

Adaptations can range from low technology to high technology. High technology adaptations are very complex and typically include mechanical, digital, or electronic components that require training and management in therapy sessions, such as power wheelchairs or myoelectric prosthetics.

Low technology adaptations are readily available, inexpensive, and do not require extensive training of complex mechanical parts. These may include adapting toys, clothing, cups, pacifiers, or other self-care tools for completion of activities of daily living (ADLs). In the clinic, most adaptations tend to happen organically when treating a patient through observation of skill or through goal setting with the patient or family. For example, a parent's goal may be for their child to brush their hair or hold a toy. The hand therapist can easily use splint material to mold custom handles onto almost any item for self-care or play. A parent may have been helping their child with ADLs, or setting up a play activity without the child's input in an attempt to achieve these goals in some capacity. The pediatric therapist can assess the skill level, environment, and tools needed to create adaptations that can help achieve actual involvement in the activity with a sense of independence for the child.

Examples of Pediatric Adaptations for the Upper Extremity
Custom-made adaptations

Scraps of splinting material allow the therapist to create many unique adaptations that fit specifically for a patient of any size. A low technology pencil grip can be made to assist a child with achieving a proper grasp while writing and help avoid positions of deformity (see Fig. 5.35). A width-adjustable shoe-tying trainer allows a child to slip their foot into it with or without a shoe to practice the shoe-tying sequence (see Fig. 5.36). Velcro hooks and loops can be added to a large number of items, most specifically self-care items, such as clothing and braces. These are used to allow a patient with limited range of motion and dexterity to

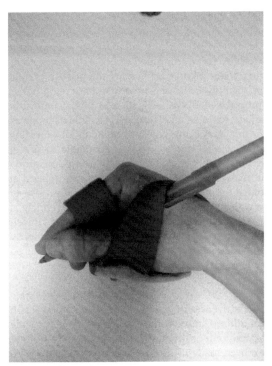

FIG. 5.35 Splint material is molded with three loops to encourage a three-jaw chuck pattern. (Courtesy Children's Hospital of Philadelphia.)

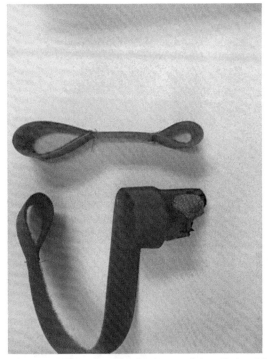

FIG. 5.37 A Velcro loop is added to a splint so that a child can achieve more independence with donning and doffing. (Courtesy Children's Hospital of Philadelphia.)

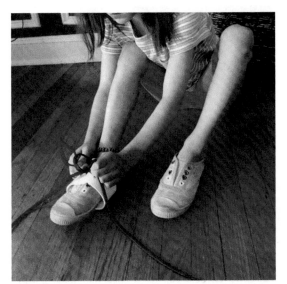

FIG. 5.36 A shoe-tying trainer made with splint material. (Courtesy Children's Hospital of Philadelphia.)

hook one digit into a Velcro-made loop to pull, adjust, tighten, or don an article of clothing or other material (see Fig. 5.37).

A face scratcher tool was developed so that a child could wipe sweat or adjust glasses by moving the head when the arms cannot reach the face (see Fig. 5.38). A sandwich holder was created for a child with upper limb deficiencies above the elbow to promote feeding independence (see Fig. 5.39). Although the parent may still need to set up the task, the experience of independence, even in the youngest child, can be a monumental reward.

Many adaptations are simply based on need of the current situation. There have been unique instances where therapists have received consults to fabricate protective splints for excessive self-chewing or nail biting that have caused infections, cellulitis, and subsequent treatment. By adding commercially available chewy tubes to a custom-made splint, a child can orally fixate on the tubes, and avoid the areas that were being protected with the splint (see Fig. 5.40).

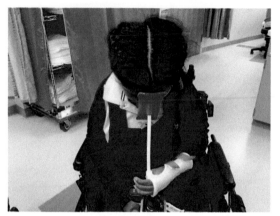

FIG. 5.38 A face scratcher tool for a teen with arthrogryposis. (Courtesy of Children's Hospital of Philadelphia.)

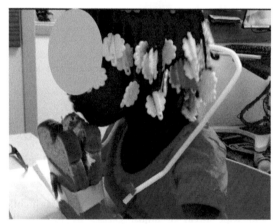

FIG. 5.39 A custom sandwich holder. (Courtesy of Children's Hospital of Philadelphia.)

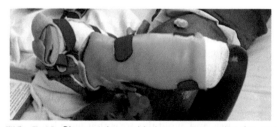

FIG. 5.40 Chewy tubes added to custom splint for oral fixation. (Courtesy of Children's Hospital of Philadelphia.)

Commercially available

The universal cuff is a simple and streamlined adaption designed to assist persons with decreased grip or dexterity to have more controlled use of ADL items, such as eating utensils When addressing the pediatric population, the universal cuff is used to hold developmentally appropriate items as well, such as toys, paintbrushes, markers, remotes, etc. The universal cuff has progressed over the years from large and bulky fabric and leather cuffs that were not hygienic or adaptable in size and did not work well with the pediatric population to multicolored, adaptable silicone that can be used and molded for individual use. The concept of silicone universal cuffs has been marketed and is now widely and commercially available, such as the EZ Hold Universal Cuffs. Occupational therapists have historically used splint material to create these types of cuffs as well (see Figs. 5.41 and 5.42).

Gravity-Reduced Weightlessness

The effectiveness of gravity-reduced weightlessness has been utilized since World War I to promote movement of paralyzed or dysfunctional limbs. Advancements have been made using simple and low technology options, such as pulleys, mobile arm support slings, and weight systems to newer exoskeletal systems that are portable and compact. The use of suspended resistance band springs is an example of a low technology option for gravity-reduced weightlessness. It is often used

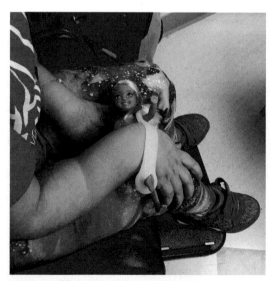

FIG. 5.41 EZ hold cuff for a child with weak grasp to engage in age appropriate doll play. (Courtesy of Children's Hospital of Philadelphia.)

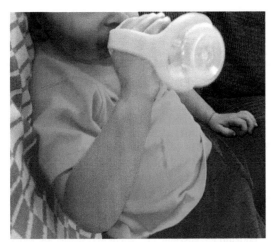

FIG. 5.42 Large EZ hold cuff to promote independence with bottle feeding. (Courtesy of Children's Hospital of Philadelphia.)

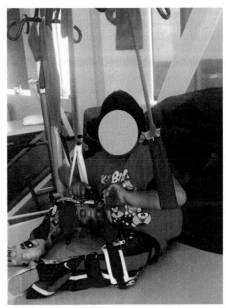

FIG. 5.43 Use of dynamic materials to suspend vertically to free arms for movement. (Courtesy Children's Hospital of Philadelphia.)

within pediatric acute care, rehabilitation, and outpatient settings, by hanging the bands from a hospital bed trapeze bar, Hoyer lift boom, ceiling mount swing hooks, an adjustable garment rack, or even an IV pole. This simple tool allows weightlessness to be achieved for exercise with active range of motion and affords easy adjustments with simple caregiver involvement, immediate gratification, and low cost (see Fig. 5.43). The WREX, or Wilmington Robotic Exoskeleton, is a lightweight exoskeleton that was created for individuals who experience chronic upper extremity weakness because of muscular dystrophy, spinal muscular atrophy, arthrogryposis, or high spinal cord injuries. It aims to mimic human movement patterns of the upper limb with elastic band-assisted elevation and can be attached to most wheelchairs or portable seating.[24] The WREX can promote independent self-feeding and self-grooming and can be used as a general assist for ADL. It can also be incorporated as an exercise modality in rehabilitation and recovery.

Tablet Adaptations

The use of iPads and tablets is now a norm in the pediatric population and creating adaptations for the use of these items will continue to grow and evolve. One area of need is the access of the iPad or tablet with users who have dexterity impairments or impaired muscle tone and are unable to isolate a single digit and not hit the screen with other digits. Items such as the Hand Glider were created to fix this problem and are an example of a universal adaptation that can be used with patients who have upper extremity impairments. There are also stylus

adaptations, such as the Faraday Stylus. This item was created to assist persons with decreased grip. The flexible body can be wrapped around the hand and wrist to allow manipulation of the stylus without actually gripping. Although these objects are commercially available, splint material can be used and manipulated to custom make and create these types of objects that fit directly to the patient.

CONCLUSION

Although pediatric modalities continue to be understudied, there are a wide variety of options to maximize positioning, comfort, and create potential functional gains with splinting, taping, and adaptations in the clinic. Possibilities for the pediatric therapist are endless with knowledge of tools, techniques, and supplies combined with a healthy dose of creativity.

REFERENCES

1. Fess EE, Gettle KS, Philips CA, Janson JR, et al. A history of splinting. Splinting the pediatric patient. In: *Hand and Upper Extremity Splinting: Principles and Methods.* 3rd ed. St. Louis: Mosby Incorporated; 2005. pp. 3–45 and 480-516.
2. Hogan L, Uditsky T. Pediatric splinting. In: Hogan L, Uditsky T, eds. *Pediatric Splinting; Selection, Fabrication, and Clinical Application of Upper Extremity Splints.* San Antonio: Therapy Skill Builders; 1998:32–78.

3. Meuthing SE, Kotagal UR, Schoettker PJ, Gonzalez-del Rey J, Dewitt TG. Family centered bedside rounds: a new approach to patient care and teaching. *Pediatrics*. 2007: 829−832.

4. Gabriel L, Duvall-Riley B. In: Coppard BA, Lohman H, eds. *Pediatric Splinting. Introduction to Splinting- A Clinical Reasoning and Problem Solving Approach*. 2nd ed. Philadelphia: Mosby; 2001:396−443.

5. Snook JH. Spasticity reduction splint. *Am J Occup Ther*. 1979;33(10):648−651.

6. Copley J, Kuipers K. *Management of Upper Limb Hypertonicity*. San Antonio: Therapy Skill Builders; 1999.

7. Altman E. Therapist's management of the stiff elbow. In: Skirven T, Osterman L, Fedorczyk J, Amadio P, eds. *Rehabilitation of the Hand and Upper Extremity*. 6th ed. Philadelphia: Mosby; 2011:1075−1088.

8. Jackman M, Noval I, Laninn N. Effectiveness of hand splints in children with cerebral palsy: a systematic review with meta-analysis. *Dev Med Child Neurol*. 2014;56:138−147.

9. March of Dimes. *2018 Premature Birth Report Card United States*. 2018.

10. Stensvold HJ, Klingenberg C, Stoen R, et al. Neonatal morbidity and 1-year survival of extremely preterm infants. *Pediatrics*. 2017:e20161821.

11. Su BH, Hsieh WS, Hsu CH, et al. Neonatal outcomes of extremely preterm infants from Taiwan: comparison with Canada, Japan, and the USA. *Pediatr Neonatol*. 2015; 56(1):46−52.

12. Anderson LJ, Anderson JM. Hand splinting for infants in the intensive care and special care nurseries. *Am J Occup Ther*. 1988;42(4):222−226.

13. Hunter JG. Neonatal intensive care unit. In: Case-Smith J, ed. *Occupational Therapy for Children*. Philadelphia: Mosby; 2011:649−677.

14. Currie DM, Mendiola A. Cortical thumb orthosis for children with spastic hemiplegic cerebral palsy. *Arch Phys Med Rehabil*. 1987;68(4):214−216.

15. Bozzetti V, Tagliabue P. Metabolic Bone Disease in preterm newborn: an update on nutritional issues. *Ital J Pediatr*. 2009;35(1):20.

16. Bishop N, Sprigg A, Dalton A. Unexplained fractures in infancy: looking for fragile bones. *Arch Dis Child*. 2007; 92(3):251−256.

17. Coopee RA. Elastic taping (Kinesio taping method). In: Skirven T, Osterman L, Fedorczyk J, Amadio P, eds. *Rehabilitation of the Hand and Upper Extremity*. 6th ed. Philadelphia: Mosby; 2011:1529−1538.

18. Chatterjee S, Hayner KA, Arumugam N, et al. The California Tri-Pull Method in the treatment of shoulder subluxation after stroke: a randomized clinical trial. *Natl J Med Sci*. 2016;8(4):175−182.

19. Guchan Z, Mutlu A. The effectiveness of taping on children with cerebral palsy: a systematic review. *Dev Med Child Neurol*. 2016:26−30.

20. ElKhatib RS, ElNegmy EH, Salem AH, Sherief AA. Kinesio arm taping as prophylaxis against the development of Erb's Engram. *J Adv Res*. 2012:485−491.

21. Shamsoddini A, Rasti ZK, Hollisaz MT, Sobhani V, Dalvand H, Bakhshandeh-Bali MK. The impact of Kinesio taping technique on children with cerebral palsy. *Iran J Neurol*. 2016:219−227.

22. Yasukawa A, Patel P, Sisung C. Pilot study: investigating the effects of Kinesiotaping in an acute pediatric rehabilitation setting. *Am J Occup Ther*. 2006;60(1):110−116.

23. Kase K, Martin P, Yasukawa A. *Kinesio Taping in Pediatrics. Orthopedic Physical Therapy & Rehabilitation Products*. 2006.

24. Haumont T, Rahman T, Sample W, et al. Wilmington robotic exoskeleton: a novel device to maintain arm improvement in muscle disease. *J Pediatr Orthoped*. 2011; 31:e44−e49.

CHAPTER 6

Pediatric Hand Therapy—Prosthetics and Training

ROBERTA CIOCCO, MS, OT • MICHELLE HSIA, MS, OTR/L • TAMI KONIECZNY, MS, BS

Among the more challenging pediatric hand presentations are upper limb deficiencies. These can result from congenital or acquired causes. Each of these deficiencies brings its own unique challenges, which will be discussed later in this chapter.

The Center for Disease Control and Prevention estimates 4 out of every 10,000 babies or about 1500 babies per year are born with upper limb reductions.[1] Limb reduction can be due to genetic factors, exposure to chemicals, viruses, taking certain medications while pregnant, or by amniotic tissue becoming tangled with arms or legs. Additionally, other birth defects of organs and tissue, typically heart and kidneys, can be associated with limb deficiencies.[2] The child may face varying degrees of challenge because of limb reduction. These challenges are dependent on the extent and location of the reduction. Some limitations could include delays in normal development of motor skills, limitations in performing activities of daily living (ADLs), and possible impact of social–emotional well-being due to their appearance.

Acquired limb amputations are caused by either trauma or disease. Trauma causes twice as many amputations as disease.[3] Over 90% of amputation injuries involve fingers. For children age 0–2 finger amputations increase to 95.2%.[4] The most common cause of finger amputations in pediatrics is a result of being "caught between" objects such as a door. Other traumatic causes of limb loss in childhood include recreation, thermal injuries, household accidents, railroad accidents, gunshot or explosion, and vehicular. Diseases that may result in upper limb loss include tumors, blood vessels or nerve abnormalities, and severe infections (Table 6.1).[5]

Multiple limb amputations are a rare occurrence. Amputations of all four limbs, or quadrimembral amputee, are even rarer (less than 1%) in pediatrics. Causes of four limb amputations include electrical burns, complications of renal disease, and ischemic gangrene resulting from septic conditions.[6] Prosthetic implications and considerations are highly dependent on the level of amputation and current level of physical and cognitive functioning.

LEVEL OF AMPUTATION

The length of the residual limb can impact performance of functional activities. Amputations of the upper extremity are described by location. Upper extremity amputations can be partial or full, as well as unilateral or bilateral. The separation of the carpal bones from the radius and ulna is called as a wrist disarticulation. Amputations through the radius and ulna are referred to transradial (below the elbow) amputations. This can further be classified as long, medium, or short residual limb. When the ulna and radius are removed, but the humerus remains intact, this is called an elbow disarticulation. Transhumeral (above the elbow) amputation can be classified as long, mid, or short transhumeral amputation. Length of the residual limb impacts decision-making for prosthetic devices and will be discussed later in this chapter. Shoulder disarticulation is when there is less than 30% of the humerus remaining. Scapulothoracic amputation is when part or all of the clavicle and scapula are removed.[7]

TRANSVERSE VERSUS LONGITUDINAL DEFICIENCIES

The International Society for Prosthetics and Orthotics developed a classification for congenital limb deficiencies. These deficiencies have been categorized as transverse or longitudinal. In the case of transverse deficiencies, "the limb has developed normally to a particular level beyond which no skeletal elements exists, although there may be digital buds."[8] These are named

TABLE 6.1
Most Common Causes of Pediatric Traumatic Amputations (0–17 Years Old).[4]

Mechanism	Percent	Example
Caught between	16.3%	Doors Primarily digits
Machinery	15.6%	Farm equipment Table saws—school wood shop Power lawn mowers—lower limb
Motor vehicle collisions	8%	Shoulder/upper arm—61% Forearm/elbow—31% Hand/wrist—13.8%
Firearms	6.1%	Primarily lower extremities, but can be fingers
Off-road vehicles	6.1%	

where the limb terminates (example: carpal, forearm, shoulder) and further described as total, partial, upper, middle, or lower third[8].

A longitudinal deficiency is a "reduction or absence of an element within the long axis of the limb."[8] There can be normal skeleton distal to the affected bones. When describing longitudinal deficiencies, the affected bones are named, beginning proximally and moving distally. Bones not named are considered normal. To further classify, bones are identified as totally or partially absent. In the case of partially absent, location can be added. The digits affected should be related to metacarpals and phalanges and numbered from the radial side (thumb = 1). The term "ray" can be used to describe these relationships.

PROSTHETIC ACCEPTANCE AND REJECTION

There are several studies looking at factors impacting acceptance and rejection of upper extremity prosthetic devices.[9–12] The physical factors influencing acceptance of the device include: fit, comfort, weight of the device, repeated mechanical failure, lack of tactile sensation, and/or whether the prosthesis is unnatural looking (hook).[8] The psychosocial factors impacting acceptance of the device include negative reactions by others, low self-esteem, lack of acceptance of disability,

unrealistically high expectations, and poor initial prosthetic experiences.

Studies in adults suggest that early training with an experienced clinician, proper fitting, and functional training with an experienced team are critical to prosthetic acceptance.[9] The level of amputation is also a contributing factor in accepting a prosthesis. Shoulder disarticulation has the highest rate of rejection at 60%. Next is transhumeral rejection rate at 57% and transradial at 6%.[9] The average rate of rejection is approximately 35%–45%.[10] Individuals with multi-limb amputations tend to have higher rejection rates of their upper limb prosthetic(s).[13] They can adapt amazingly well, but continue to experience deficits with completing some aspects of ADLs, such as opening containers for self-feeding and toileting skills.

A study by Vasluian et al. found the most common reasons to wear a prosthetic were cosmesis, improved function, manipulation, specific activities, muscle development, locomotion, posture, and balance.[10] The subjects who did not use their prostheses identified cosmesis (did not look normal), being more functional without the prosthesis, technical and interface reasons, too heavy, discomfort and physical fatigue, and pain as reasons to not use a prosthetic device.[10] Children often learn to adapt and use their deficient limb functionally without a device (see Image 6.1).

A consideration that should be discussed with the child and family are the potential long-term effects on the musculature of the dominant side, or the nonaffected extremity, due to compensation and over use over time.[14,15] It is still unclear if prosthetic use can reduce overuse injuries, but it can be a necessary tool

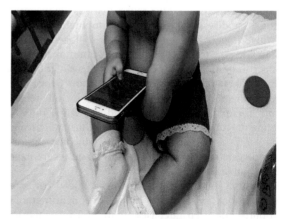

IMAGE 6.1 A 12-month-old child with a congenital short transradial (forearm upper third) limb difference showing adaptability without prosthetic. (Photo courtesy of the Children's Hospital of Philadelphia.)

in adulthood to manage functional tasks in the event of pain or disability of the intact limb.

Developmental Stages and Implications for Fitting

When considering fitting of prosthetics for children and adolescents there are multiple factors to consider, which fall into three main areas: physical, psychosocial, and environmental (Table 6.2).

There are some basic guidelines, but each case should be considered individually, and no one approach works for every case. Generally, it is a very emotional and traumatic time for families whether they are faced with a congenital or traumatic limb difference. The psychosocial adjustment can be just as important as the child's physical attributes to ensure the success of any prosthetic intervention.[10,16] As this is a very unique population, it is imperative to work with a cohesive team with prosthetic experience and knowledge. Disciplines represented on the team could include physiatrist, orthopedic surgeon, prosthetist, occupational therapist, and physical therapist. Often, a social worker, psychologist, or nurse is included in the team. As this is a very unique population, it is important to have practitioners with upper limb prosthetic experience and knowledge. Education of the family and child is key and referrals to the team should happen as soon as possible.[17] The team should present all options and answer questions as early as possible, so that informed decisions can be made. Different from

TABLE 6.2 Factors to Consider.		
Physical	**Psychosocial**	**Environmental**
Age	Developmental	Functional
Level of	status	demands
amputation	Cognition	Access to
Number of	Values	prosthetic
missing limbs	Adjustment or	services and
Skin condition	acceptance by	maintenance
Edema	child and parent	Climate/Weather
Residual	Interests	Cultural
strength	Roles and	influences
Range of motion	responsibilities	Places in which
and excursion	Financial	the child lives,
Pain	resources	plays, and
Muscle sites	Family readiness	participates in
available for	and "buy in"	school and
myoelectric		community
control		
Size of the child		

the treatment of adults, children's needs and abilities are constantly changing through their developmental progression. Consideration needs to be made of a child's physical capacity, cognitive skills, attentional skills, functional demands, interests, and psychosocial needs. These factors will often change over time. For example, the goal for a 2-year old with a below elbow amputation would be basic grasping abilities required for two-handed play. A body-powered or myoelectric prosthesis would meet the child's needs. However, a teenage girl who wants to do gymnastics, play the cello, and has significant concerns about cosmesis may require multiple devices to meet her needs. Evidence from one study suggests that the provision of multiple prosthetic options may result in longer periods of wear.[18]

The residual limb length is also an important consideration. Children with above elbow and longer transradial residual limbs, specifically those with wrist or partial hand, tend not to accept prostheses.[19] Similarly, a very short transradial amputation presents significant challenges for fitting. Myosite options may be limited, and suspension and tolerance of the weight of a prosthesis is more difficult. If the amputation is a result of a burn, a myoelectric may not be the best option due to skin integrity and dryness, causing impediment of the myoelectric signal. Prosthetic sockets can be hot and uncomfortable, and with a rapidly growing child, may be a significant hurdle to overcome for prosthetic success. The weight of a prosthesis is also a consideration and often contributes to the success or failure of fitting. Myoelectric prosthetics are heavier and require intimate fit with skin contact for the electrodes. On the other hand, body powered prosthetic users have to deal with either a figure 8 or 9 harness that can be uncomfortable and cause issues with clothing and cosmesis.

The following chart is a general list with guidelines for prosthetic choices related to age. It is important to consider each child individually. This list is not intended to be prescriptive for every case, and does not include every option. The importance of collaboration with a knowledgeable team and the patient and family cannot be over stressed (Table 6.3, Image 6.3).

Rehabilitation for Upper Limb Prosthetic Patients

Rehabilitation will be discussed separately as appropriate for acquired or traumatic amputations versus congenital deficiencies. The main difference is the preprosthetic stage due to the preparation and care needed before prosthetics can be initiated. Later stages should

TABLE 6.3
Prosthetic Choices.

Type of Componentry	Description	Age Range and Most Appropriate Level of Amputee	Advantages	Challenges
Infant/toddler mitt/hand passive	Passive lightweight mitt or foam-filled hand (fisted or open) Usually attached to self-suspending socket	3–18 months short to midlevel transradial 6–24 months transhumeral Long Transradial Partial hand and shoulder disarticulation levels generally less appropriate	Cosmetic May help to provide balance Establishes wearing tolerance May provide a better weight-bearing surface for crawling May improve incorporation of prosthetic into body image	Takes away sensation of residual limb Functionally limiting, a hand or terminal device that can allow passive insertion of toys initially by adult and then by children tends to be preferable for older infants and toddlers
Passive split hook, reverse ADEPT or mechanical hand	A terminal device (TD) attached to a socket that does not have any type of cable but has a passive closing force	6–24 months transradial 12–36 months transhumeral Long Transradial, partial hand and shoulder disarticulation levels generally not appropriate	Allows for passive grasp usually by adult placing objects into TD Facilitates early bimanual incorporation of a prosthesis	Depending on the choice of TD may be less cosmetic Grasp force limited Some limitations on size of object that can be held
Preflexed or Banana elbow	Prosthetic socket that is formed in 30–45 degrees of flexion at elbow level	12–36 months transhumeral	Allows for TD to be in position for midline hand use Has a natural appearance	Limited reach Unable to get hand to face without compensatory shoulder movement
Passive elbow	Friction elbow joint that allows adult or child to position elbow in flexion or extension	Usually an option for younger transhumeral or shoulder disarticulation	Allows for passive positioning of the elbow to put the TD in a greater variety of planes to reach from face to leg Lighter in weight than body powered elbow	Joint less stable Requires use of intact limb or use of a surface to independently push into position
Voluntary opening TD such as Split hook, CAPP, and mechanical hand	TD that is controlled by cable for opening, force of closure provided by a spring or rubber band Suspension figure 8 or 9 harness	Can be used by any child that has skills for learning TD operation (usually 18 months or older)	Easier to control than voluntary closing Split hook allows best visual access during operation for grasp	Grip strength is often limited Rubber bands wear out and need changing Mechanical hand is the most difficult VO TD to use because vision of grasp can be occluded and resistance is greatest for opening

Voluntary closing TD such as ADEPT or mechanical hand	TD that is controlled by cable for closing force	Can be used by any child who has skills for learning TD control (usually 18 −24 months)	May be more difficult to train younger children Requires sustained movement for activation to maintain grasp (there is a locking mechanism that can be added)	Gives proprioceptive feedback for grasp force More control of force Better grasp of cylindrical objects
Myoelectric hand	TD that is controlled by electrical signals from muscles in the residual limb	Possible to be fitted at any age from 12 months to adult. Best age for younger fitting appears to be around 2 ½[20]	Reliable strong grip Cosmetic No harness Can adjust sensitivity of electrodes Options for on off, variable or proportional control Single electrode "cookie crusher" operation mode for younger children[21]	Cost High maintenance Weight can be heavier Does not hold up to sand dirt and heavy activities Requires tight fit without use of stump sock resulting in complaints of heat and sweat Glove durability problematic Requires battery charging
Body-powered elbow	Suspension figure 8 Locking joint is controlled by shoulder extension, abduction and depression Once unlocked elbow is positioned with same action as TD control	Tends to work better for children over 36−48 months Pull tab can be used for younger children for lock	Provides more degrees of freedom for TD positioning Can also get internal rotation to get into midline better for bilateral amputee	More training required Heavier in weight Harnessing more complicated Elbow needs to be locked to operate TD
Myoelectric or switch-activated elbow	Electric elbow that can be operated by either an electrode or physical switch	Can be used with children over 36 −48 months	Less taxing to operate than BP Can be used with electric or body powered TD	Cost Heavy High maintenance Need to charge batteries
Activity-specific prosthesis	Sports specific Musical instrument specific adaptation	Can be used at any age as appropriate activities are identified Adapters are available for a multitude of activities including ski pole, bike, golf club, weight lifting, violin, guitar, fishing rod, and hockey stick	Allows for bimanual function for specific sports or activities that otherwise would be difficult or impossible Can sometimes be interchanged in same socket as TD with a quick disconnect wrist unit	Additional cost that may not be covered by insurance

Continued

TABLE 6.3
Prosthetic Choices.—cont'd

Type of Componentry	Description	Age Range and Most Appropriate Level of Amputee	Advantages	Challenges
Multigrasp hand such as iLimb (Image 6.2) or Bebionic	One of the most advanced myoelectric prosthetics looks and moves more like a natural hand	More available to adult-sized adolescent Recently, iLimb developed an extra small size that may be used with some preadolescent patients	Conforming grip Multiple grip patterns Natural more fluid hand movements	Cost Heavy High maintenance Better for light load work
Pattern recognition	Myoelectric control system that uses multiple sites (up to 8) control and algorithms to control prosthesis[21]	Only available to adult-sized adolescent	Allows user to use more natural multi muscle patterns for activation Allows for more functions with same number of muscles User can recalibrate as needed	May be difficult for nontechnology savvy user/family Training more difficult
iDigit	An advanced myoelectric prosthesis for partial hand amputees	Sizing tends to be a limitation as in the case of the iLimb	Conforming grasp Multiple grasp patterns Light-to-moderate work load	Cost Lack of sensory feedback Batteries need to be charged May be difficult for nontechnology savvy user/family
3D printed partial hand prosthesis	Prosthetic that operates off wrist motion much like a tenodesis splint	Best for child with metacarpals intact	Low cost Good for task-specific activities	May not hold up to wear and tear of child

BP, body powered; *TD*, terminal device.

not vary significantly between the two groups. In either acquired or congenital situations, parent and child education as well as more frequent follow-up are critical to encourage long-term use and success. The importance of a cohesive, experienced clinic team with the ability to follow the child with an amputation cannot be underestimated in importance. Education with respect to available choices including no prosthesis, emotional support, and opportunities for peer support, and consistent follow-up have all been reported to be helpful and valued by patients with limb differences and their families.[10,17,19–21]

Prosthetic needs change throughout childhood, and as the needs of the child change and multiply prosthetic intervention may need to be modified. Rehabilitation may be required at different ages and stages. Intensity of rehabilitation is often variable depending on the situation. Early fitting has been debated but is advocated by most clinical teams if the family is interested. Most studies have found that fitting before 2 years old is preferable[20] for congenital amputees and within 6 months postinjury for acquired amputations.[22] The standard of care for traumatic amputees without complication in adults is fitting with a temporary prosthesis within 30 days.[22] In pediatrics, there may be multiple complications that do not allow this to happen. Funding for prosthetics is more difficult and is often a major complication and reason for time delay. Despite this, there are creative ways to try and establish an early understanding and pattern of prosthetic use for the young

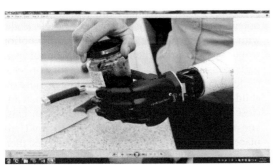

IMAGE 6.2 Myoelectric prosthetic hand and flexion wrist unit: i-limb quantum and flexion wrist. *Photo courtesy of Touch Bionics by Ossur, Foothill Ranch California, USA*

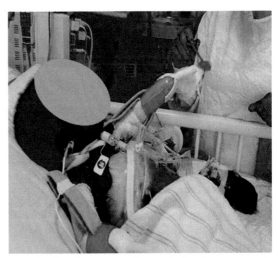

IMAGE 6.4 Temporary thermoplastic temporary play prosthesis for a 12-monthsold traumatic quadrilateral amputee in the acute care setting. (Photo courtesy Children's Hospital of Philadelphia.)

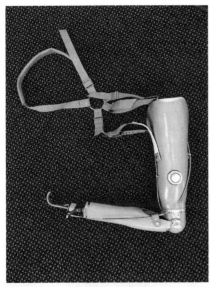

IMAGE 6.3 Left conventional transhumeral prosthesis with figure of 8 harness, cable and housing system, and aluminum voluntary opening terminal device. (Courtesy Ability Prosthetics and Orthotics, Inc., Exton Pennsylvania, USA.)

traumatic amputee. Image 6.4 is a picture of a thermoplastic splint that was fabricated to give a young amputee play-specific function and the experience of wearing a full contact pseudo socket.

Frequency of therapy is usually dictated by the clinical presentation of the amputation, complexity of the prosthesis, age of the child, and family's ability to attend therapy appointments. There is no hard and fast rule, but generally younger children with passive prosthetics are treated for shorter periods of time and

followed with home programs in place. Once a prosthesis is activated, initial training is recommended at least one time a week. A more intensive program, either inpatient or outpatient, may be recommended depending on the situation. Above elbow prosthetics and multilimb amputees require more lengthy and intense rehabilitation. Because specialized prosthetic teams are few and far between, geographic distance often plays into the equation. It may not be feasible to attend weekly outpatient sessions, so either a short admission or home program may be necessary. There has also been success with training children in a group "camp" program. This allows for total immersion in training for a week, much like the constraint programs with hemiplegic patients. Families can be trained fully and long-term support groups can be fostered with peers and families of others in the same situation. Diane Atkins has reported that for a new adult prosthetic user, it takes 5 h to train an adult transradial amputee, 10 h for a transhumeral amputee, 12 h for a shoulder disarticulation amputee, and 20 h for a bilateral amputee.[23] Children often need longer training due to limited attention and cooperation challenges.

Acute Postsurgical Stage for Acquired Limb Deficiency

Priorities during this stage include the steps:

- Edema management, and volume control (shaping). A permanent prosthesis cannot be fabricated until the residual limb is healed and stable.

- Wound care and preparation for the prosthetic both physically and emotionally including desensitization, skin checks, and cleaning
- Range of motion (ROM) and strengthening are important to prepare for the prosthetic fitting, subsequent training, and for life participation in general
- Managing phantom limb pain

Often, there is fear with touch and wound care procedures. Therapists can help to provide emotional support and encouragement to get through these difficult times. Stump shrinkers are more beneficial than traditional ace bandage wrapping; however, there are size limitations, and it may not be possible to fit younger children. Elastic stockinette can work well for compression using a double layer. By cutting a piece twice the length, twisting at the bottom, and rolling back the second layer on to residual limb, it is possible to get good conformity and even pressure.

Residual limb care is important to emphasize and start as early as possible. Due to the dark moist environment of prosthetic sockets, it is important to foster maintenance of a clean, dry residual limb.

Phantom pain can be a persistent problem for traumatic amputees. Although phantom pain is less prevalent and shorter lived in children,[24] it still should be on the therapist's radar. Pharmacological management, desensitization, mirror therapy, and biofeedback are commonly used in isolation or combination.[25,26] Recently, with the development of the surgical procedure of targeted muscle reinnervation (TMR), early studies have reported a significant decrease in phantom pain.[27] TMR will be further discussed in the future trends section of this chapter.

Subacute Preprosthetic Stage for Acquired or Congenital Patients

In this stage, the following areas are priorities:
- Residual limb care continues for the acquired limb loss patient
- If myoelectric fitting is chosen, testing for appropriate myosites is initiated. This is sometimes done by the prosthetist; however, if at all possible, collaboration with the therapist should be encouraged. With children, it may take longer to identify consistent sites. Sites should be reliable with the arm held in different positions (i.e., arm overhead, held out at side, and down resting next to body).
- Training muscles needed for effective myoelectric control or strengthening muscles for body motions needed to operate a conventional prosthesis may be necessary. Surface electromyography (EMG) is often helpful to train the child to isolate particular muscle

groups to activate a prosthetic device. The Myoboy program by Otto Bock allows the patient to practice opening and closing using myoelectric electrodes with a virtual hand (see Image 6.5). Another option would be to use a test hand often made out of spare parts consisting of a myoelectric hand with electrodes attached. This is often motivating because the child can see the actual myoelectric hand open and close and can start to actually participate in grasp and release with the therapist's help to hold and place the hand. In congenital limb differences, there are often small residual digit nubbins. It can be helpful to ask the child to wiggle these to activate muscles for identification of myosites and exercise for control.
- ADL training or retraining—this may require teaching adapted techniques or using adaptive equipment. It is important to be able to accomplish ADL tasks with and without the prosthesis, as there are times when a prosthesis may not be available due to repairs or need for replacement. Dressing sticks can be modified with low temperature plastic to stand on the floor and can serve as an assist for donning and doffing shirts and socks for a high-level bilateral amputee (see Image 6.6). Foot skills are a must for these children to complete most of their daily tasks.

Basic Prosthetic Training for Acquired or Congenital Patients

The main goal of prosthetic training, no matter what the age of the child, is to provide optimal bilateral function.

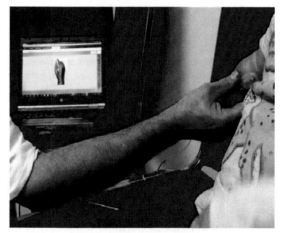

IMAGE 6.5 Myosite testing on a 2 and a half-year-old patient with unilateral congenital transverse radial limb deficiency using the Ottobock Myoboy (Photo courtesy Children's Hospital of Philadelphia.)

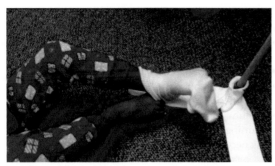

IMAGE 6.6 A 4-year-old girl with bilateral congenital transverse deficiency of proximal humerus donning socks with adapted dressing stick. (Photo courtesy Children's Hospital of Philadelphia.)

Most ADL tasks can be accomplished with one hand so it is important to remember that children will adapt with or without a prosthesis. Training should also be focused on accomplishing tasks with and without the prosthesis. It is important to be mindful of the child's age and abilities, and to match the prosthetic choice and treatment activities with their developmental level.[17]

Factors that impact training include level of amputation, complexity of the prosthesis, functional needs, and learning abilities. Training intensity and duration are often dependent upon these factors and no one approach is necessarily appropriate for every child.

At the initial session, evaluation should include at least the following:

- Assessment of the fit and adjustment of the prosthesis
- Measurement of passive ROM and active ROM with and without the prosthesis
- Administration of at least one functional assessment (refer to the outcomes measure section of this chapter)
- Assessment of skin condition
- ADL assessment
- Assessment of patient's interest and goals

As with any population receiving occupational therapy, prosthetic training goals should be developed with the patient and family. Patient interests should be incorporated whenever possible. Activities should also be developmentally appropriate.

The sequence of training that is utilized in the pediatric population and mimics typical grasp pattern development is as follows:

1. Typically training starts with basic opening and closing tasks with grasp of larger objects (1–2″ diameter)

and release into a large container. Large pegs, pop beads, shape sorters, and stacking rings work well for younger children. Blocks, beanbags, cones, and cups work well for older kids. The control motion that is used for terminal device (TD) activation for a conventional prosthesis is humeral flexion of the prosthetic arm while maintaining opposite arm in shoulder protraction. Myoelectric systems have varying operational control systems from a very simple one site open with automatic close (often called as a cookie crusher system), to pattern recognition systems with multiple electrodes and multiple functions. With young children using a body-powered device, it is necessary to position behind the child and assist with forward reach with the prosthetic arm at the same time stabilizing the opposite arm while reaching for a toy. With voluntary opening systems (i.e., split, hook, Child Amputee Prosthetic Project (CAPP), cookie crusher myoelectric) working on release is the main focus; with a voluntary closing TD, the focus for initial training is on grasp. The challenge for training with a voluntary closing TD is that the child must maintain tension on the harness to keep the TD closed. The benefit to this system is that grasp pressure can be varied and controlled better.

2. Gradually training progresses to grasp of smaller items with increased precision of release. Activities such as pegboards, games that have smaller diameter pieces and require targeted release such as Connect 4 or Kerplunk, work well.

3. At the same time, the therapist should encourage use of the prosthesis as a gross stabilizer. Craft activities, puzzles, paper and pencil, and simple construction tasks are good activity choices for this skill.

4. As precision grasp and release progress, the therapist should also teach the child to preposition (rotation of the TD in horizontal, vertical, or any plane in between) the TD for the optimal grasp pattern. Most terminal devices just passively turn using the other hand. Some myoelectric prosthetics can include wrist rotation.

5. Once grasp and release from a stationary position are mastered, have the child carry items or change arm position while maintaining grasp before release. Obstacle courses can be used or the child can be asked to place items at different height levels.

6. With transhumeral and higher level amputees, the control of the elbow has to be introduced next.
   a. Locking and unlocking of the body-powered elbow tends to be the hardest control motion to teach and having the harness adjusted appropriately is key to the success of this skill.

b. The locking and unlocking the control motion is shoulder extension abduction and depression.
c. Teaching elbow activation for the body-powered elbow is the same control motion as TD activation with the elbow in an unlocked state.
d. The hardest skill to learn is maintaining elbow position while relocking the elbow. This requires holding the position desired with tension on the control cable while quickly elevating and depressing the affected shoulder.
7. Then the last phase of treatment involves incorporation of prosthetic use into self-care and functional activities that are meaningful and appropriate for the child.

Throughout the training process, donning, doffing, and care of the prosthesis need to be taught to parents, caregivers, and children if appropriate. Most young children will require assistance to don the prosthesis; doffing tends to be easier. Even if they cannot fully participate in the care of the prosthesis, it is important for them to learn responsibility for the prosthesis and to learn the donning sequence. They need to know what activities are or are not appropriate when wearing the prosthesis. For example, if a child has a myoelectric, wearing this prosthesis to the beach and playing in sand and water are not recommended. The therapist also needs to help the family develop a meaningful wear schedule to maximize prosthetic skill. This often is individualized and is dependent on factors such as level of amputation, age, skin condition, and environmental temperature or conditions. As with any splint or orthotic, gradual increase of wear time and frequent skin checks are recommended. Bilateral and high level amputees tend to wear their prostheses less, and they are often used only for task-specific activities. It is recommended for children who are younger to remove the prosthesis for nap times. School age children will often wear their prosthesis in school all day and then remove the prosthesis when they get home. A reasonable goal for good wear is at least 6–8 h a day. However, if the device is useful and the child chooses to wear it less, this can still be considered a successful prosthetic outcome. Tolerance of the weight of a prosthesis can be difficult. Sometimes when transitioning from body power to myoelectric, it is recommended that the body power prosthesis be gradually weighted to improve acceptance.

Advanced Long-Term Rehabilitation for Acquired or Congenital Patients

Regular check-ins with the team are advised to keep up with changing technology, need for repairs, medical issues, and to advance the child when appropriate. The focus of intervention at this stage is as follows:
- Maintaining maximal active range of motion and strength in all residual muscle groups
- Prevention of overuse in the nonaffected upper limb
- Instruction on continued in care and use of the prosthesis
- Return of the child to the highest level of functioning, using adaptive techniques and equipment as necessary

Outcome Measures

There are a wide variety of tools being utilized with the pediatric prosthetic population in the literature, many of which are nonstandardized. Table 6.4 describes the most widely utilized outcome measures for this population.

In addition, there are a number of patient-reported outcomes measures being utilized, which are becoming more widely known and accepted, that are not mentioned in the earlier list such as the Pediatric Outcomes Data Collection Instrument[35] or the Patient-Rated Outcomes Measurement Information System.[36]

Future Trends for Pediatric Upper Limb Prosthetics

Military injuries have driven the advancement of upper limb prostheses in the field at the time of this publication.[37] In 2005, the US Government launched a program, the Defense Advanced Research Projects Agency, issuing a request to engineer the most advanced prosthetic limb.[38] Often, advancements in the adult population have a trickledown effect into pediatrics. However, much of the upper extremity prosthetic advancements are not suitable for the pediatric population due to size, weight, cost, and the issue of growth in children. A brief description of some of the latest technology will be described.

COMPUTER-AIDED DESIGN

Three-dimensional (3D) printing is widely utilized in medicine and has allowed for a cost-effective and customized upper extremity prosthetic that has been utilized worldwide for many purposes.[39–43] The end result for upper limb prosthetics is similar to thermoplastic splint material that can be completely customized for the patient. In addition, 3D printing can be fabricated from a distance using measurements from a picture,[42] thus making it available to children living

TABLE 6.4
Outcome Measures.

Name of Measure	Type of Measure/ Age Group	Purpose	Structure	Validation
Prosthetic Upper Extremity Functional Status Index[28]	Parent or child report child version. 3–6 years Child or parent report on older child version. 7 years and older	Evaluate the extent a child uses the prosthetic limb for daily activities, ease of task performance, and perceived usefulness of the device	26 bilateral activities in child version 38 bilateral activities in the older child version. 5 questions for each functional task looking at: Does the child do the activity? How does the child do the activity? How well does the child do the activity? Does the child do the activity with or without the prosthetic	Test–retest and interrater reliability established
Child Amputee Prosthetics Project—Functional Status Instruments (CAPP-FSI)[29]	**CAPP-FSIT**—parent report 1–4 years **CAPP-FSIP**—parent report 4–7 years **CAPP-FSI**—parent or child report 8–17 years old	Frequency of use and performance for upper and lower extremity functional prosthetic use	5-Point scale **CAPP-FSIT/ FSIP**—31 upper extremity items and 6 lower extremity items **CAPP-FSI**—34 upper extremity items and 6 lower extremity items	Internal consistency and discriminant validity established
University of New Brunswick Test (UNB) Revised 2012[30]	Observational (video tape) 2–13 years old	Evaluates performance with a prosthesis using developmentally based daily life activities	Assesses spontaneity and skill of prosthetic function using 10 developmentally based age appropriate daily life activities	Interrater reliability established
Unilateral Below Elbow Test (UBET)[29]	Observational (videotaped) −20 min to complete 2–4 years 5–7 years 8–10 years 11–21 years	Evaluation of performance of bimanual tasks of children with unilateral limb deficiency for both prosthesis wearer and nonwearer	9 functional tasks specific to age 2 scales—completion of task and method used —0–4 rating scale 0 = unable to complete 4 = completes without difficulty	Interobserver reliability established
Assessment for Capacity of Myoelectric Control 2.0 (ACMC)[31]	Observational Child, adolescent, and adult	Assessability to control a myoelectric hand during functional tasks	22 items assessing 6 different aspects: 1. grip force 2. coordination of both hands	Scale validity Person response validity Test–retest reliability—satisfactory for monitoring change

Continued

TABLE 6.4
Outcome Measures.—cont'd

Name of Measure	Type of Measure/ Age Group	Purpose	Structure	Validation
			3. need for external support 4. Different positions and motions 5. Repetitive grasp and release 6. Need for visual feedback 4-Point rating scale (0–3) 0 = not capable 3 = extremely capable	
TESTS BELOW ARE NOT PECIFIC TO CHILDREN WITH LIMB DEFICIENCY				
Box and Blocks Test[32–34]	3 years–adult	- Gross manual dexterity - Prevocational test for handicapped people	- Number of cubes transferred in 1 min	Not normed for children with upper limb deficiency - Test–retest reliability

in remote areas with limited resources. This type of prosthetic is well suited for activities that involve manipulation of lighter objects using lateral and spherical prehensile patterns.[40] However, durability may be as issue with children, as they are often very hard on their prosthetics.

OSSEOINTEGRATION

Osseointegration, approved by the Food and Drug Administration in 2003, allows for a prosthesis to be anchored into a bone, eliminating the use of a socket that can limit range of motion for some users (see Image 6.7). It is a two-stage surgical procedure, performed 6 months apart. In that time, the patient cannot wear a prosthetic or put any weight on the bone. This procedure can only be performed on a skeletally mature person with adequate bone quality.[44] In addition, before this is considered, a potential recipient must have proven difficulty with a conventional prosthesis, and must commit to the extensive rehabilitation required. Cosmetic, body powered, myoelectric, and hybrid prosthetics have

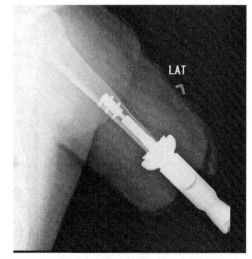

IMAGE 6.7 Radiograph of an osseointegrated implant (custom Compress transdermal system, Zimmer-Biomet Inc. Warsaw Indiana, USA). Surgical clips are visible from targeted muscle reinnervation procedure, performed concurrently. (Courtesy Jonathan A. Forsberg MD PhD, Orthopedic Oncology, Johns Hopkins University".)

been used with good success due to the stable fixation.[44]

TARGETED MUSCLE REINNERVATION SURGERY

TMR is a surgical procedure utilized since 2002 with myoelectric prosthetic users to enhance their functional abilities.[45] TMR is utilized for traumatic amputations only at this time.[45] TMR salvages a nerve from the amputated limb, and repositions it to a more proximal innervated muscle to provide additional myosites. The user then has to learn to recognize signals from EMG and create movement patterns from that information. This technique has been shown to help combat phantom pain because the nerves have been relocated for an alternate purpose.[27]

SENSORY FEEDBACK

Currently, the end user relies heavily on visual feedback to operate their prosthetic; both to control movement patterns and force on objects.[46] There are currently various ways that sensory pathways are being looked at to allow for greater sensory feedback to the user in real time. Researchers are working to determine best modality-matched sensation, such as vibration, touch, proprioception, and temperature somatic receptors, for sensory substitution.[46] The number of signals that can be used and interpreted is a challenge, and one would presume that the pediatric population may experience an even greater challenge interpreting multiple pieces of information simultaneously. Now, research in this area is focused on the adult population.

VASCULARIZED COMPOSITE ALLOTRANSPLANTATION

A vascularized composite allotransplantation (VCA) procedure is when multiple tissue types are transplanted at the same time, including bones, skin, vessels, and/or tendons. VCA has proven successful in the adult population, with approximately 150 cases of hand transplantation from 1998 to date of this chapter worldwide. Hand transplant has been utilized for unilateral and bilateral upper extremity traumatic amputations. There was one case of conjoined twins with limb transfer from one to another and one case of infant transplant from deceased identical twin sibling.[47] To date of this publication, there is one known successful pediatric bilateral upper extremity hand transplantation case, which was performed at Children's Hospital of Philadelphia in 2015.[47] This child was an ideal

candidate as he already had a living donor kidney transplant, and was therefore on immunosuppression treatment. Transplantation can allow for increased independence with ADLs and functional bimanual activities, particularly the ability to perform peri care, self-feed, and participate in play with peers. Hand transplantation can allow for greater self-confidence and self-esteem, by providing a less visible disability. Return of partial sensation of the hands has been verified in this case, by pairing sensory testing with neuroimaging.[48] There are many ethical considerations with VCA procedures, particularly in the pediatric population. VCA requires a long rehabilitation process, and parents and family members must be fully invested in the lifelong commitment. During the acute phase, there is a significant loss of function before gain. Tasks that the child was once able to perform in a modified manner with their residual limbs, will now require assistance from a caregiver until function restores. VCA is not guaranteed to be successful. In addition, unknown long-term side effects of the immunosuppressive drug therapy remain unknown. Different from solid organ transplant, hand transplants are not lifesaving, but are considered to be life altering. There are also concerns for compliance issues in children as they enter into adolescence with adherence to prescribed pharmaceutical management. The importance of extensive psychological evaluation cannot be understated (Image 6.8).

CONCLUSION

In conclusion, there is great variation in the limb difference population and each child has his or hers own unique strengths and needs. Prosthetic intervention varies based on the individual needs and goals and can be

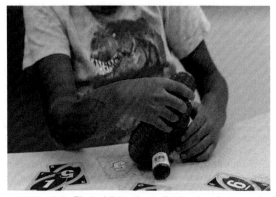

IMAGE 6.8 First bilateral pediatric hand transplant recipient, after receiving donor limbs. (Photo courtesy Children's Hospital of Philadelphia.)

different through the ages and stages. Technology innovations tend to trickle down to the pediatric population once established in the adult practice due to the size restrictions and increased complexity of dealing with developing children. There are some general guidelines for intervention commensurate with the various ages and levels of amputation. Early fitting if appropriate and desired by the family is generally agreed to be recommended before 2 years old or within 6 months from onset of trauma. Most important is to have a knowledgeable and comprehensive team to follow the child on a regular basis and provide family education so patient and parents can make informed choices.

REFERENCES

1. Reference CDC, Canfield MA, Honein MA, et al. National estimates and race/ethnic-specific variation of selected birth defects in the United States, 1991-2001. *Birth Defects Res A.* 2006;76(11):747−756.
2. Kozin SH. Upper-extremity congenital anomalies. *J Bone Joint Surg Am.* 2003;85(8):1564−1576.
3. Tooms RE. *Atlas of Limb Prosthetics: Surgical, Prosthetic, and Rehabilitation Principles.* 2nd ed. Illinois: American Academy of Orthopedic Surgeons; 2002 [Chapter 32].
4. Hostetler SG, Schwartz L, Shields BJ, Xiang H, Smith GA. Characteristics of pediatric traumatic amputations treated in hospital emergency departments: United States, 1990-2002. *Pediatrics.* 2005;116(5):e667−e674.
5. Ramierz C, Menaker J. *Traumatic Amputations;* 2017. https://www.ahcmedia.com/newsletter/27/issues/76297/.
6. Yoshimoto K, Okuma Y, Nakamura T, et al. Limb fitting for quadruple amputees: report of two cases of symmetrical peripheral gangrene caused by pneumococcal purpura fulminans. *Prosthet Orthot Int.* 2013;37(6):489−494.
7. Zenie JR. Prosthetic options for persons with upper-extremity amputation. *Phys Med Rehabil.* July 12, 2016.
8. Day HJB. The ISO/ISPO classification of congenital limb deficiency. *Prosthet Orthot Int.* 1991;15:67−69.
9. Resnik L, Meucci MR, Lieberman-Klinger S, et al. Advanced upper limb prosthetic devices: implications for upper limb prosthetic rehabilitation. *Arch Phys Med Rahabil.* 2012;93:710−717.
10. Vasluian E, deJong IGM, Janseen WGM, et al. Opinions of youngsters with congenital below-elbow deficiency, and those of their parents and professionals concerning prosthetic use and rehabilitation treatment. *PLoS One.* 2013;8(6):e67101.
11. Fisk JR. *Atlas of Limb Prosthetics: Surgical, Prosthetic, and Rehabilitation Principles.* 2nd ed. Illinois: American Academy of Orthopedic Surgeons; 2002 [Chapter 31].
12. Biddiss EA, Chau TT. Upper limb prosthesis use and abandonment: a survey of the last 25 years. *Prosthet Orthot Int.* 2007;31(3):236−257.
13. Marquardt E. *Atlas of Limb Prosthetics: Surgical, Prosthetic, and Rehabilitation Principles.* 2nd ed. Illinois: American Academy of Orthopedic Surgeons; 2002 [Chapter 36A].
14. Ostlie K, Franklin RJ, Skjeldal OH, Skrondal A, Magnus P. Musculoskeletal pain and overuse syndromes in adult acquired major upper-limb amputees. *Arch Phys Med Rehabil.* 2011;92:1967−1973. https://doi.org/10.1016/j.apmr.2011.06.026. e1.
15. Jones LE, Davidson JH. Save that arm: a study of problems in the remaining arm of unilateral upper limb amputees. *Prosthet Orthot Int.* 1999;23:55−58. https://doi.org/10.3109/03093649909071611.
16. Varni JW, Setoguchi Y, Rappaport LR, Talbot D. Psychological adjustment and perceived social support in children with congenital/acquired limb deficiencies. *J Behav Med.* 1992;15:31. https://doi.org/10.1007/BF00848376.
17. Patton JG. *Developmental Approach to Pediatric Prosthetic Evaluation and Training. Comprehensive Management of the Upper-Limb Amputee.* New York, NY: Springer; 1989:137−149. New York https://doi.org/10.1007/978-1-4612-3530-9_13.
18. Crandall RC, Tomhave W. Pediatric unilateral below-elbow amputees: retrospective analysis of 34 patients given multiple prosthetic options. *J Pediatr Orthop.* 2002;22(3):380−383.
19. Biddiss E, Chau T. Multivariate prediction of upper limb prosthesis acceptance or rejection. *Disabil Rehabil Assist Technol.* 2008.
20. Shaperman J, Landsberger SE, Setoguchi Y. Early upper limb prosthesis fitting: when and what do we fit. *JPO J Prosthet Orthot.* 2003;15(1):11−17.
21. Roche AD, Rehbaum H, Farina D, et al. *Curr Surg Rep.* 2014;2:44. https://doi.org/10.1007/s40137-013-0044-8.
22. Brenner CD, Brenner JK. The use of preparatory/evaluation/training prostheses in developing evidenced-based practice in upper limb prosthetics. *JPO J Prosthet Orthot.* 2008;20.
23. Atkins DJ. *Prosthetic Training. Atlas of Amputations and Limb Deficiencies: Surgical, Prosthetic, and Rehabilitation Principles.* Rosemont, IL: American Academy of Orthopaedic Surgeons; 2004:275−284.
24. Burgoyne LL, Billups CA, Jirón JL, et al. Phantom limb pain in young cancer-related amputees: recent experience at St Jude children's research hospital. *Clin J Pain.* 2012;28(3):222−225.
25. Thomas S. Effectiveness of electromyographic biofeedback, mirror therapy, and tactile stimulation in decreasing chronic residual limb pain and phantom limb pain for a patient with a shoulder disarticulation. *J Prosthet Orthot.* 2015;27.
26. Richardson C, Kulkarni J. A review of the management of phantom limb pain: challenges and solutions. *J Pain Res.* 2017;10:1861−1870. https://doi.org/10.2147/JPR.S124664.
27. Souza JM, Cheesborough JE, Ko JH, Cho MS, Kuiken TA, Dumanian GA. Targeted muscle reinnervation: a novel approach to postamputation neuroma pain. *Clin Orthop*

Relat Res. 2014;472:2984−2990. https://doi.org/10.1007/s11999-014-3528-7.

28. Wright VF, Hubbard S, Naumann S, Jutai J. Evaluation of the validity of the prosthetic upper extremity functional index for children. *Arch Phys Med Rehabil.* 2003;84:518−527.

29. Bagley AM, Molitor F, Wagner LV, Tomhave W, James MA. The Unilateral below Elbow Test: a function test for children with unilateral congenital below elbow deficiency. *Dev Med Child Neurol.* 2006;48:569−575.

30. Wright FV. Prosthetic outcome measures for use with upper limb amputees: asystematic review of the peer − reviewed literature. *Am Acad Orthot Prosthet.* 1970-2009.

31. Linder HYN, Langius-Eklof A, Hermansson LMN. Test-retest reliability and rater agreements of assessement of capacity for myoelectric control version 2.0. *JRRD.* 2014;51:635−644.

32. Jongbloed-Pereboon M, Nijhuis-vander Sanden MWG, Steenbergen B. Norm scores of the box and block test for childern ages 3-10 years. *Am J Occup Ther.* 2013;67:312−318.

33. Mathiowetz V, Federman S, Wiemer D. Box and block test of manual dexterity: norms for 6-19 Year olds. *Can J Occup Ther.* 1985;52:241−245.

34. Mathiowetz V, Volland G, Kashman N, Weber K. Adult norms for the box and block test of manual dexterity. *Am J Occup Ther.* 1985;39:386−391.

35. Lerman J, Sullivan E, Barnes D, Haynes R. The pediatric outcomes Data collection instrument (PODCI) and functional assessment of patients with unilateral upper extramity deficiencies. *J Padiatr Orthopaed.* 2005;25:405−407.

36. Cella D, Yount S, Rothrock N, et al. The Patient-Reported Outcomes Measurement Information System (PROMIS): progress of an NIH Roadmap cooperative group during its first two years. *Med Care.* 2007;45(5 suppl 1):S3−S11.

37. Gonzalez-Fernandez M. Development of upper limb prostheses: current progress and areas of growth. *Arch Phys Med Rehabil.* 2014;95:1013−1014.

38. Burck J, Biegelow J, Harshbarger S. Revolutionizing prosthetics: systems engineering challenges and opportunities. *Johns Hopkins APL Tech Dig.* 2011;30(3).

39. Zuniga JM, Carson AM, Peck JM, Kalina T, Srivastava RM, Peck K. The development of a low-cost three-dimensional printed shoulder, arm, and hand prostheses for children. *Prosthet Orthot Int.* 2017;41(2):205−209.

40. Burn MB, Ta A, Gogola GR. Three-dimensional printing of prosthetic hands for children. *J Hand Surg Am.* 2016;41(5):e103−e109.

41. Zuniga J, Katsavelis D, Peck J, et al. Cyborg beast: a low-cost 3d-printed prosthetic hand for children with upper-limb differences. *BMC Res Notes.* 2015;8:10.

42. Lee KH, Bin H, Kim K, Ahn SY, Kim BO, Bok SK. Hand functions of myoelectric and 3D printed pressure-sensored prosthetics: a comparitive study. *Ann Rehabil Med.* October 2017;41(5):875−880.

43. Zuniga JM, Peck JL, Srivastava R, et al. Functional changes through the usage of 3D-printed transitional prostheses in children. *Disabil Rehabil Assist Technol;* 2017. https://doi.org/10.1080/17483107.1398279.

44. Jonsson S, Caine-Winterberger K, Branemark R. Osseointegration amputation prostheses on the upper limbs: methods, prosthetics, and rehabilitation. *Prosthet Orthot Int.* 2011;35(2):190−200.

45. Lipschutz RD. Impact of emerging technologies on clinical considerations: targered muscle reinnervation surgeries, pattern recogntion, implanted electrodes, ossesointegration, and three-dimensional printed solutions. *Am Acad Orthotists Prosthetists.* 2017;12.

46. Hsiao SS, Fettiplace M, Darbandi B. Sensory feedback for upper limb prostheses. *Prog Brain Res.* 2011;192. ISSN: 0079-6123.

47. Amaral S, et al. 18-month outcomes of heterologous bilateral hand transplantation in a child: a case report. *Lancet Child Adolesc Health;* 2017. https://doi.org/10.1016/S2352-4642 (17) 30035-4.

48. Gaetz W, Kessler SK, Roberts TPL, et al. Massive cortical reorganization is reversible following bilateral transplants of the hand: evidence from the first successful bilateral pediatric hand transplant patient. *Ann Clin Transl Neurol.* 2017.

FURTHER READING

1. Routhier F, Vincent C, Morissette M-J, Desaulniers L. Clinical results of an investigation of paediatric upper limb myoelectric prosthesis fitting at the Quebec rehabilitation institute. *Prosthet Orthot Int.* 2001;25(2):119−131. https://doi.org/10.1080/03093640108726585.

2. Shida J, Bagley A, Molitor F, et al. *Predictors of Continued Prosthetic Wear in Children with Upper Extremity Prostheses.* 2005.

CHAPTER 7

Congenital—Syndactyly

MEAGAN PEHNKE, MS, OTR/L, CHT, CLT • SANDRA SCHMIEG, MS, OTR/L, CHT • APURVA S. SHAH, MD, MBA

PERTINENT ANATOMY AND CLASSIFICATIONS

Fine motor function of the hand is based on independent digital motion. Supple web spaces facilitate digital abduction, flexion, and extension for activities of daily living. Normal interdigital abduction ranges from 70–80 degrees at the first web space (between the thumb and index finger) to 30–40 degrees at the remaining (second, third, and fourth) web spaces. The second, third, and fourth web spaces or commissures gently slope at an approximate 45 degrees angle from proximal-dorsal to distal-palmar starting at the metacarpophalangeal (MCP) joint and ending just proximal to the midpoint of proximal phalanx. The second and third commissures are typically U-shaped and the fourth web space is typically V-shaped. The natatory ligaments help to form the web contour at the junction between the glabrous and nonglabrous skin.

During embryogenesis, the hand and upper extremity develop from the upper limb bud that emerges from the lateral body wall at 26 days of gestation.[1–3] Upper limb development generally proceeds in a proximal-to-distal fashion with the hand plate appearing by day 37.[1–3] During typical development, the hand plate forms individual rays between days 41 through 54 of gestation.[1–3] Complete separation of the digits occurs through apoptosis, or programmed cell death, of the interdigital tissue, which occurs in a distal-to-proximal fashion.[1–3] Syndactyly, or "webbed fingers," is a congenital anomaly that results from a failure of interdigital apoptosis, leading to residual skin, soft tissue, and sometimes bone connecting adjacent digits (Fig. 7.1A–C).

Syndactyly is the second or third most common congenital hand anomaly, and it occurs in approximately 1.3–1.9 per 10,000 live births.[4,5] It more commonly occurs in males (3:2) and has a racial predilection toward whites more than African Americans.[4,5] Morphologically, syndactyly occurs bilaterally more often than unilaterally (7:3).[5] Syndactyly has a predilection for specific web spaces with the third web space (between the long and ring fingers) being most common. The "5-15-50-30" rule can be used to remember the frequency of web space involvement from first to fourth.[6] Although most cases are sporadic, up to 50% of syndactyly cases can be hereditary, with the most common pattern being autosomal dominant with variable penetrance.[5,6] Most commonly, syndactyly presents as an isolated malformation, but it can also be found in association with other skeletal anomalies or syndromes such as symbrachydactyly, cleft hand, ulnar longitudinal deficiency, synpolydactyly, acrocephalosyndactyly (Apert, Crouzon, and Pfeiffer syndromes), acrocephalopolysyndactyly (Carpenter and Noack syndromes), oculodentodigital dysplasia, and orofaciodigital dysplasia.[5–8] Although amniotic band syndrome represents a separate entity, as the etiology is due to intrauterine scarring rather than a true malformation, syndactyly can also occur in this syndrome and presents as acrosyndactyly (Fig. 7.2A–C). In these cases, there is a soft tissue only connection at the distal tips of the involved digits with a separation or fenestration proximally.

In 2010, the International Federation of Societies for Surgery of the Hand classification was modified into the Oberg, Manske, and Tonkin (OMT) classification to incorporate an improved understanding of the genetic and molecular basis of congenital hand and upper limb anomalies.[1] The OMT classification placed syndactyly into Group I, or "malformation", and into the subtype "failure of hand plate formation/differentiation." However, syndactyly is more commonly described by

Pediatric Hand Therapy. https://doi.org/10.1016/B978-0-323-53091-0.00007-5

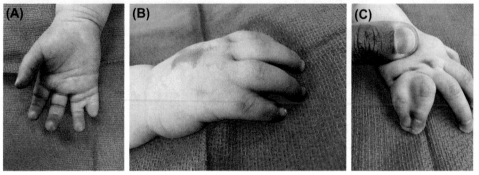

FIG. 7.1 (A-B) Simple incomplete syndactyly of fourth web space. (C) Complete complex syndactyly of fourth web space which developed progressive proximal interphalangeal joint contracture of ring finger.

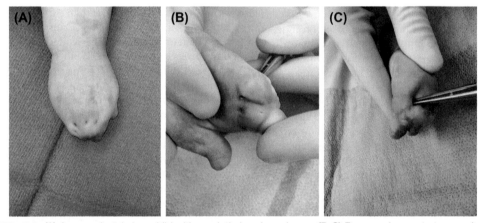

FIG. 7.2 (A) Acrosyndactyly in a child with amniotic band syndrome. (B-C) Forceps demonstrates proximal fenestrations distinguishing this condition from acrocephalosyndactyly such as Aperts.

the clinical morphology of the involved digits. The extent of digital involvement can be described as "complete" syndactyly if the connection extends the entire length of the digits (from commissure to fingertip) or "incomplete" syndactyly if the distal portion of the digits are separate (Fig. 7.1A–C). Syndactyly can be further characterized by the type of tissue involved in the connection between digits. In "simple" syndactyly, the involved digits are connected by skin and soft tissue. Simple syndactyly can also present with a common nail plate shared by the two adjoined digits—termed synonychia. In simple syndactyly, the joints, ligaments, and tendons are typically normal. "Complex" syndactyly involves an osseous connection between adjacent phalanges, in addition to the soft tissue connections. "Complicated" syndactyly refers to the interposition of accessory phalangeal or abnormal bones between digits, and can also involve anomalous nerves, tendons, and/or muscles. Other classification systems have been described for syndromic syndactyly including the

Upton classification specifically for Apert syndrome with Type 1 (spade hand), Type 2 (mitten hand), and Type 3 (rosebud hand), in addition to further subdivision based on angular and rotational deformities.[8]

SYNDACTYLY: PREOPERATIVE EVALUATION

In most cases, syndactyly is detected at birth, and early consultation with a hand surgeon is sought. The diagnosis of syndactyly is obviously not subtle, but, occasionally, mild simple incomplete syndactyly is not recognized by parents or brought to the attention of a hand surgeon. Simple inspection will reveal the extent of the syndactyly (simple vs. complete) and the presence or absence of a synonychia. Careful observation will often allow the treating provider to distinguish between simple, complex, and complicated syndactyly. The degree of active and passive MCP joint and interphalangeal (IP) joint motion should be measured with a goniometer and recorded. Poorly formed flexion or extension creases generally indicates restricted or absent joint motion and suggests complex or complicated syndactyly. Standard plain radiographs of the affected hand should be obtained at 6–12 months old to further characterize the type of syndactyly. In most cases, a single posteroanterior radiograph is sufficient to delineate the osseous elements and determine whether there is fusion of adjacent phalanges.

In the case of syndactyly associated with a syndrome, examination of the remainder of the extremity, chest wall, feet, and head will reveal additional abnormalities. Poland syndrome is one of the most common syndromes that has syndactyly and typically presents with unilateral symbrachydactly and pectoralis major deficiency.[7] Genetic evaluation and counseling should be sought for all cases of syndactyly presenting as part of a syndrome. In select cases, a preoperative electrocardiogram (EKG) may be warranted to screen for prolonged QT interval that occurs in Timothy syndrome and can cause ventricular tachyarrhythmia leading to cardiac arrest.[9] This extremely rare syndrome is also associated with a flattened nasal bridge, low-set ears, a small upper jaw, a thin upper lip, small misplaced teeth, developmental delay, and autism—in addition to ulnar-sided syndactyly. Due to the rarity of this syndrome, routine screening with an EKG is not necessary.[9]

Surgical reconstruction is recommended for most cases with the occasional exception of a mild, simple incomplete syndactyly that does not impact function. In addition, there are rare cases of complex or complicated syndactyly in which surgical reconstruction is not recommended.[6] These contraindications include digits with substantial instability or absent anatomic structures that would inhibit digit function if surgically separated.[6,10,11] Caution should also be exercised when a "super digit" is encountered.[12] This term is used to describe a single oversized digit supported by two metacarpals (Type I) or a single metacarpal that supports two or more digits distally (Type II). In these cases, although surgical separation may be technically feasible and could improve cosmesis, hand function could be compromised due to the unpredictability of postoperative alignment, motion, and function.[6,12–14]

The timing of surgical reconstruction remains controversial, but is primarily based on the pattern of web space involvement and the type of syndactyly. Syndactyly involving border digits (small ring or thumb–index) and some forms of complex syndactyly may benefit from earlier release at 6–12 months old.[6,10,11,13–15] When border digits are involved, earlier surgery is recommended to avoid a flexion contracture

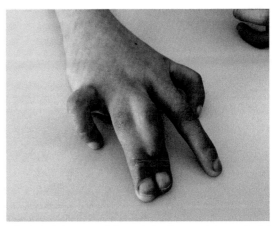

FIG. 7.3 Late presentation of simple complete syndactyly of third web space with middle finger proximal interphalangeal joint contracture.

and angular deformity, which occur due to disparate length and growth of the syndactylized digits[6,10,11,13–15] (Figs. 7.1C and 7.3). In general, syndactyly reconstruction before 12 months old has been associated with a higher incidence of scar contracture and web creep. For this reason, in the absence of a progressive flexion contracture or angular deformity, surgery can be timed between 18 months and 3 years old without compromising ultimate fine motor function. In younger children with bilateral deformity, both hands may be treated concurrently. This decreases overall anesthetic exposure and is optimally performed with two surgical teams performing simultaneous procedures on both hands. Staged reconstruction for bilateral syndactyly may be preferred by the surgeon or family. When adjacent web spaces are involved, most surgeons recommend staged reconstruction to minimize the risk of digital ischemia or loss.[10,13,14,16]

Syndactyly of the thumb–index web space is the least common, but associated with the greatest surgical complexity.[6,14] This is due to the large length discrepancy between the thumb and index finger as well as the complex motion of the thumb.[10,14,17] Patients often present with web space narrowing and a thumb flexion contracture preoperatively that requires surgical reconstruction initially to separate the digits, but also to both deepen and adequately widen the space to allow normal position and function of the thumb[10,14,17] (Fig. 7.4A–D).

A preoperative therapy evaluation and treatment are not often indicated in children with syndactyly. A therapist may be consulted if contractures or angular

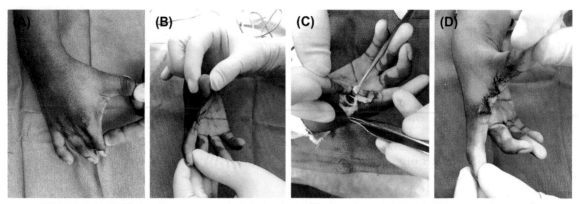

FIG. 7.4 (A-D) First web space syndactyly treated with four flap z-plasty. In figure c, photograph demonstrates thick fascial bands of the adductor pollicis and first dorsal interosseous which were released.

deformities are present, and preoperative intervention including orthotics or caregiver education on stretching would support surgical goals and anticipated outcome. A general screen of functional hand use, grasp patterns, and developmental skills could be beneficial in challenging cases to determine if any adaptations or intervention would be beneficial to support age appropriate activity (Figs. 7.1C and 7.3).

SURGICAL STEPS

Syndactyly reconstruction is one of the most common procedures performed in congenital hand surgery. Reconstructive surgery is performed under general anesthesia with the patient supine on a standard operating table with the upper limb positioned on a hand table. A tourniquet is used for skin incision and flap elevation to optimize visualization and limit the risk of inadvertent injury to the neurovascular bundles. The specific surgical technique for release varies based on the particular web space under reconstruction and the morphology of the involved digits. Although the specific surgical approach and flap design may vary depending on the specific case and surgeon preference, there are several universal surgical principles (see Box 7.1).

In patients with complete syndactyly, a variety of different surgical incisions have been proposed, but all use a dorsal skin flap measuring two-thirds the length of the proximal phalanx to reconstitute the web commissure with interdigitating zigzag flaps for coverage of the lateral border of each of the involved digits (Fig. 7.5A and B).[6,14-16,18] After marking the skin incision, the tourniquet is inflated and the dorsal skin flaps are raised, while preserving longitudinal veins when possible. The volar skin flaps are raised next, taking care to identify and protect the digital neurovascular bundles. The bifurcation of the common digital artery must be identified. In cases where the bifurcation is atypically distal, the surgeon must decide between an incomplete release or ligation of one of the two proper digital arteries. In general, ligation of a single digital artery is acceptable, but the safety of this maneuver should be confirmed with temporary application of a microvascular clamp on the target vessel and tourniquet deflation to assure that this is no concern for vascular insufficiency. All fibrous connections between the digits are then sharply divided. In complex syndactyly, osseous connections are divided with a scalpel or small osteotome.[19] After a complete release is achieved, the skin flaps are rotated into position, allowed to interdigitate, and secured with absorbable suture. The tourniquet should be deflated to confirm perfusion of both digits and each flap. There is typically a bare spot on the dorsal ulnar aspect of the radial digit and the dorsal radial aspect of the ulnar digit that are covered with full-thickness skin graft from the hypothenar region, volar wrist, upper arm, or groin. The skin grafts should be fenestrated to allow egress of hematoma that could otherwise compromise graft adherence. In cases of incomplete syndactyly, the general approach described earlier may be substituted with simple skin rearrangement utilizing simple z-plasty, four-flap z-plasty, double-opposing z-plasty, or other similar techniques.

Application of the immediate postoperative dressing is one of the most important steps. Nonadherent petroleum-impregnated gauze, such as Xeroform (Kendall/Covidien, Mansfield, MA), should be applied to suture lines and over the full-thickness skin graft. The web space should then be packed with cotton balls soaked in mineral oil. Postoperative immobilization depends on the age and maturity of the patient, but most children are placed into a long arm mitten cast with the elbow

---

BOX 7.1
Surgical Principles in Syndactyly Reconstruction

1. Release border digits early to prevent progressive flexion contracture and angular deformity of the adjacent digit.
2. Staged surgical reconstruction is recommended when multiple adjacent web spaces are involved. Vascular compromise can occur if surgery is performed on both sides of a single digit, and both the ulnar and radial digital arteries are compromised.
3. Ligation of a digital artery may be required to achieve optimal web space depth in cases where the common digital artery bifurcates distally.
4. A robust, local vascularized flap should be used to create the commissure and minimize the risk of scar formation and web creep.
5. Interdigitating lateral zigzag flaps should be used to avoid longitudinal scar contracture.
6. Full-thickness skin grafting should be used to cover bare areas. Avoid split-thickness skin grafting or healing by secondary intention, as this results in excessive scarring and contracture.

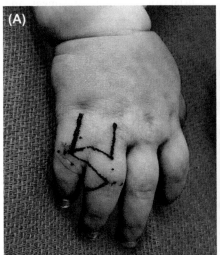 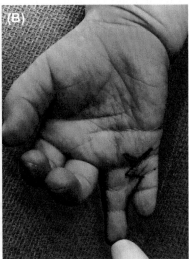

FIG. 7.5 Classic skin flap markings for a simple incomplete syndactyly utilizing a chevron-tipped dorsal rectangular flap to re-create the web commissure.

at 90 degrees of flexion and a supracondylar mold to avoid inadvertent cast removal by the child. The cast and dressings are typically removed 2–4 weeks after surgery and therapy is initiated.

SYNDACTYLY: POSTOPERATIVE EVALUATION

Consultation to therapy for evaluation following syndactyly reconstruction is dependent on the complexity of the surgery and the preference of the surgeon and center. A patient may be referred immediately following cast removal for orthotic fabrication, otherwise a consult may not be made unless the patient presents with later development of complications requiring therapeutic intervention, such as hypertrophic scarring. A thorough evaluation may not be mandatory in most syndactyly reconstruction cases; however, this section highlights measures and outcome assessments most appropriate to assess motion, digital deformity, web creep, and scar integrity. A general assessment of edema, grip/pinch strength, and sensation may be indicated and are not reviewed in further detail. The use of objective outcome measures, when possible, is important for therapists to incorporate into practice to support the role of therapy and use of evidence-based practice.[20]

Range of Motion

The therapist should consider functional impact on prehension patterns specific to the released web space as well as the child's developmental level. Documentation should include functional motion detailing joint position, digit function, as well as types of grasp and pinch patterns utilized with comparison to the contralateral side.[21] It includes details of active digit adduction and abduction of bilateral hands to note any active deficits.[22] Additional observations should include details of the child's ability to perform sufficient composite digit flexion to reach the distal palmar crease, spontaneous hand use, and any observed pain behaviors with motion. In cases of syndactyly of the thumb–index web space, a thorough assessment of thumb motion and function is indicated as the thumb is cited to be responsible for at least 40% of hand functionality.[23] Objective assessment of digit motion can be achieved through measuring the total active motion (TAM) of each digit rather than that of individual joint.[14] TAM is the combined degrees of active flexion of the IP joints minus the degrees of extension deficits at these joints.[14,24] The normal TAM of a digit is approximately 175 degrees.[14,19,24]

Digital Deformity

Digital rotation toward supination or protonation can be measured with a goniometer comparing the plane of the distal phalanx to the plane of the proximal phalanx.[14,19] Digital angulation can be assessed with goniometer placement along the dorsal longitudinal aspects of the joints and corresponding phalanges to determine the degree of deviation.[14,19]

Web Creep

Web creep is a common postoperative complication and is defined as the distal migration of the commissure following a syndactyly reconstruction.[6,10,16,18,25] Web creep can be assessed using a five point scoring system developed by Withey and colleagues[26].[14,22,26] This scale grades web creep based on the location of the web relative to the MCP and proximal interphalangeal joints (see Table 7.1).

Scar Integrity

Detailed documentation of scar integrity allows for ongoing assessment to monitor maturation. The modified Vancouver scar scale is an outcome measure originally developed for assessment of scars following a burn, but has been cited in the literature as a tool to assess scar integrity following syndactyly reconstruction.[14,19,22,27] This scale allows users to quantify the pigmentation, vascularity, pliability, and height of a scar in comparison to a patient's normal skin[14,27,28] (see Table 7.2). The terminology used in this scale provides therapists with more consistent and objective language to describe subjective parameters of scar appearance and mobility. Consistent documentation through serial photographs of scar maturation is beneficial for ongoing assessment and monitoring of potential changes in joint positioning and scar presentation.

TABLE 7.1
Web Creep Scale According to Withey et al.[26].

0	Soft web, abduction mirrors the adjacent web or Equivalent web on the Other Hand
1	No web advancement, but thickening of the web with reduced span
2	Creep of web to 1/3 of the distance between base of the web and PIP crease
3	Creep of the web to 2/3 of the distance between base of the web and PIP crease
4	Creep of the web to the PIP crease

TABLE 7.2
Modified Vancouver Scar Scale.[27,28]

Pigmentation	0—normalminimal variation from normal skin pigmentation 1—hypopigmentation 2—hyperpigmentation * In a scar with mixed pigmentation, the higher rating is chosen
Vascularity	0—normal 1—pink 2—pink to red 3—red 4—red to purple 5—purple
Pliability	0—normal 1—supple—flexible with minimal resistance 2—yielding—scars give way to pressure with a moderate resistance, do not move as a solid mass of scar 3—firm—moves as a solid, inflexible unit 4—banding—"ropes" of scar tissue that blanches with stretch, does not limit range of motion 5—contracture—limits range of motion
Height	0—flat scars, flush with normal skin 1—<2 mm 2—2–5 mm 3—>5 mm

SYNDACTYLY: POSTOPERATIVE IMMOBILIZATION

Factors surrounding the surgical complexity and specific anatomic structures involved in the reconstruction determine the length of postoperative immobilization. If the reconstruction involves skin grafting only, a bulky postoperative dressing is applied, as noted earlier, with an overlying long arm mitten cast to prevent shearing and graft failure.[11,16,18,29] The cast is typically removed after 2−4 weeks depending on the individual case.[10,30,31] Reconstruction involving pinning may require increased immobilization to allow sufficient healing. Following a thumb−index web space reconstruction, 4−6 weeks of immobilization is sometimes recommended before pin removal due to the high complexity of the reconstruction with the goal of maintaining a broad web space.[17] Further immobilization through orthotic intervention is not always indicated and is rather dependent on surgeon and center preferences, as well as the surgical complexity.[32]

SYNDACTYLY: POSTOPERATIVE ORTHOTICS

The primary goal of orthotic intervention following an initial therapy referral is often for protection of the postoperative hand. The secondary roles of a postoperative orthotic focus on scar management and positioning to prevent complications of digital deformity and web creep. A child's age and tolerance to orthotic wear plays an important role in decision making. Fabrication of hand- or forearm-based orthotic is dependent on the complexity of the reconstruction and the therapeutic goals. If the child does not require an orthotic for protection of the reconstructed digits, an elastomer web spacer custom mold is sufficient to improve scar appearance and prevent web creep[31] (see Table 7.3).

If an orthotic is indicated for joint positioning and/or protection in the case of a complex syndactyly reconstruction, a static volar forearm-based orthotic in slight wrist extension, extending to a finger pan with the material pushed within the web space with the IP joints positioned in extension and MCP joint abduction is recommended.[33,34] (Fig. 7.6). Use of orthotic intervention is most effective to maintain joint position in extension and abduction, to correct flexion contracture as well as to prevent prolonged positions that encourage deformity formation.[34] The therapist should carefully consider positioning to maintain neutral digit positioning as well as monitor for any angulation or rotation and intervene as appropriate.[34] The orthotic design following thumb−index syndactyly reconstruction

should position the web space in full abduction to maintain the surgically achieved depth and width. This can be achieved through a hand-based c-bar or a forearm-based thumb spica with a c-bar orthotic.[17,32] Creativity in orthotic design, including strap placement, use of separate digit straps, use of d-rings, or use of a clamshell dorsal splint component, may be needed to increase difficulty of independent removal in the young child, as well as to support optimal joint positioning and control deviation.

Maintaining web space depth and preventing thick scar formation are also critical to support functional digital motion and hand use.[16] Orthotics or web spacers provide support to the reconstructed web space and can help in prevention of web creep development.[31,33,34] Positioning within the orthotic should support and maintain contact against the reconstructed web space.[14] Compression over a healing graft and scar has been shown to be beneficial in prevention or minimization of hypertrophic scar formation.[27,35] Addition of a custom elastomer insert or silicone sheet within the orthotic provides needed compression against the scars and graft. Perforated thermoplastic material is valuable to more securely affix the custom molded elastomer spacer or pad the young patient.[32]

The length of recommended wear time is dependent on scar maturation and the complexity of the surgery. The protective orthotic is worn at all times initially, except for supervised removal during bathing and exercise. Following thumb−index reconstruction, continued daytime wear is encouraged if the child presents with limited active thumb abduction and opposition, to minimize the development of contractures impacting the passive width and depth of the newly formed web space.[32] The orthotic can be weaned gradually during daytime sedentary activities with improved active motion and comfort, but should be continued overnight for ongoing scar management.[33] In the young child, orthotic wear may be primarily indicated to protect the healing graft and scar. In this instance, weaning from daytime wear would be indicated once sufficient healing is achieved. Overnight orthotic wear should be continued for scar management and maintenance of web space depth for an additional 6−12 months[17,33] (see Table 7.3).

Alternatively, if ongoing poor tolerance to orthotic wear persists, despite efforts for modification, or in cases of complex scar or web creep development, a custom compression garment may be an optimal long-term solution to manage scar integrity once there is no longer protection or positional needs (Fig. 7.7). Custom compression garments allow longer wear

TABLE 7.3
Syndactyly Postoperative Orthotic Immobilization.

	Goals of Orthotic	Orthotic Design	Wear Schedule
Simple syndactyly	■ Protection (as needed)	No protection/positional needs:	Overnight 6–12 months, until scar maturation achieved
	■ Positional: contractures, stiffness, angulation, rotation	■ Elastomer web space custom mold affixed with tape or self-adherent wrap (e.g., 3M Coban)	
	■ Prevent web creep	■ Custom compression garment	
	■ Protect graft and surgical site in young patient	Protection/positional needs:	All times, except supervised exercise and bathing
	■ Scar integrity	Hand or forearm based	Gradual wean during day with sufficient graft/scar healing
		■ Slight wrist extension	Overnight 6–12 months, until scar maturation
		■ Finger pan with the material pushed within web space	
		■ IP joints in extension and MCP abduction	
		* Addition of a custom elastomer insert or silicone sheet against graft/scar	
		* Can transition to custom compression garment when no protection/positional needs	
Complex syndactyly	■ Protection	Hand or forearm based	All times, except supervised exercise and bathing
	■ Positional: contractures, stiffness, angulation, rotation	■ Slight wrist extension	Gradual wean during day with sufficient graft/scar healing
	■ Prevent web creep	■ Finger pan with the material pushed within web space	
	■ Protect graft and surgical site in young patient	■ IP joints in extension and MCP abduction	
	■ Scar integrity	* Addition of a custom elastomer insert or silicone sheet within orthotic against graft/scar	Overnight 6–12 months, until scar maturation
		* Can transition to custom compression garment when no protection/positional needs	

TABLE 7.3
Syndactyly Postoperative Orthotic Immobilization.—cont'd

	Goals of Orthotic	Orthotic Design	Wear Schedule
Thumb—index syndactyly	■ Protection	Hand-based c-bar	All times, except supervised exercise and bathing
	■ Position web space full abduction	■ Thumb in full abduction	Gradual wean during day with sufficient graft/scar healing
	■ Maintain depth/width of web space, prevent web creep		Continue daytime wear if limited active thumb motion to prevent contracture
	■ Protect graft and surgical site in young patient	Forearm-based thumb spica with c-bar	Overnight 6–12 months, until scar maturation
	■ Scar integrity	■ Slight wrist extension	
		■ Thumb in full abduction	
		* Addition of a custom elastomer insert or silicone sheet within orthotic against graft/scar	
		* Can transition to custom compression garment when no protection/positional needs	

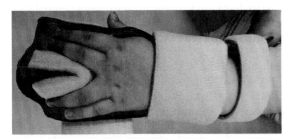

FIG. 7.6 Protective postoperative splint for complex syndactyly. Splint material pulled through web space with additional foam web spacer.

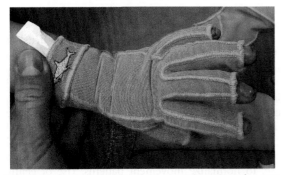

FIG. 7.7 Custom measured compression glove for scar management.

time without inhibiting hand function. Garments can be fabricated with silicone sewn into the desired locations to support scar maturation and/or improve the appearance of raised scars.

SYNDACTYLY: POSTOPERATIVE REHABILITATION

The goals of hand therapy following surgical reconstruction are to maximize a child's ability to grasp, pinch, and manipulate objects in a functional and meaningful way.[30,33] These goals are achieved through interventions that address scar integrity as well as maintain the reconstructed web space, joint position, and improve digit motion to maximize development of fine motor skills.[30,33,34] In the typical hand, available motion includes up to 30–40 degrees of active interdigital abduction with 70–80 degrees at the index—thumb web space available.[6,29] Achieving supple skin at the web space is critical in allowing this functional motion of the reconstructed web space.[6,29] There are limited postoperative therapy recommendations and protocols found in the literature. We have described a general postoperative protocol that can be used to guide treatment, but this may vary among surgeons and centers (see Table 7.4).

TABLE 7.4
General Postoperative Syndactyly Reconstruction Protocol.

Positional and/or protective orthotic fabricated for day and/or overnight wear

Caregiver education on hand washing, graft/surgical scar care, edema management, and desensitization

Encourage active motion through play-based activities—grade object size to encourage functional, age appropriate grasp patterns (encourage opposition, abduction, flexion/extension)
* Avoid valgus/varus stress with collateral ligament reconstruction (per surgeon)

Gentle passive motion initiated once comfortable and pain-free active motion achieved

Scar management interventions initiated once all scar and graft sites fully healed; caregiver education on massage and appropriate strategies

Progressive strengthening exercises can be initiated once pain free composite digit flexion and extension achieved

Continue to monitor scar maturation, web creep and digit positioning—orthotic intervention and therapeutic strategies to avoid onset and manage complications

* Timing of intervention may be delayed in case of thumb—index reconstruction dependent on complexity
* Timing of interventions should be confirmed with the surgeon in complex cases

The therapist should initially instruct the caregiver in a home program for edema control, scar management, and gentle active motion exercises. Caregiver education on graft and wound care, as well as hand washing, is important to ensure comfort and compliance. Review of expectations of healing graft and wound appearance can increase caregiver comfort in completing skin care and hygiene to support timely healing and maturation to minimize impact of prolonged healing on scar formation. Once motion or functional deficits resolve, the therapist should continue to follow the patient periodically during scar maturation to monitor progress and potential complications. Jordan and colleagues[13] recommended that the surgeon continues to follow the patient to assess for complications of scar healing and joint deformity that warrant further intervention until full skeletal maturity is achieved. In the onset of a complication, such as scar hypertrophy, additional therapeutic intervention may be indicated and is highlighted later in this chapter.[29,31]

Postoperative Precautions

General postoperative precautions are not identified in the literature following syndactyly reconstruction. These may be patient specific and should be confirmed with the hand surgeon, particularly in complex cases. Precautions may include avoidance of valgus/varus stress to a joint if collateral ligament and/or tendon reconstruction was completed. In the younger patient, it is important to keep the graft and surgical site covered and protected to avoid compromised healing and scar integrity, especially when unsupervised.

Complex Versus Simple Syndactyly Considerations

As cited by Manske and Goldfarb,[14] several studies indicate higher complications and less favorable outcomes following reconstruction of complex compared to simple syndactyly. Patients who undergo surgery for a simple syndactyly do not typically require ongoing formal therapy following surgical separation, but may benefit from intervention to prevent or manage complications.[6,29]

Thumb—Index Web Space Reconstruction Considerations

The timing of therapeutic interventions may be delayed in the case of a thumb—index web space reconstruction due to the complexity and involvement of reconstructed structures. The thumb plays an important role in fine motor skills due to greater complexity of motion through rotation and opposition.[20] However, there may be limited functional impact in patients who underwent reconstruction within the typical timing of reconstruction before 6 months old.

If the child presents with functional deficits or delayed reconstruction, the therapist should focus on improving thumb motion to facilitate developmentally appropriate grasp patterns. Play-based activities should incorporate digit abduction, flexion, and opposition, especially if greater complexity and limited preoperative motion of the thumb was present. The therapists and caregivers should discourage previously established compensatory patterns, such as raking without thumb use, to normalize movement patterns. Use of gently placed self-adherent (e.g., 3M Coban or Fabrifoam) wrap of the ulnar side digits can be helpful in encouraging an isolated pinch during self-feeding and play-based activities, if reliance on raking patterns is present. Use of a thumb opponens strap, abduction strap, or therapeutic tape to encourage palmar abduction, flexion, and opposition may be beneficial to facilitate motion patterns for functional thumb use.

Edema Management

Delayed resolution of postoperative edema has the potential to impact joint motion, tissue mobility and the quality of scar healing.[36] The best initial treatment of edema is early prevention and management in the acute inflammatory phase through conservative strategies including elevation, ice, compression, and gentle active motion.[37] Implementing a combination of conservative interventions, as well as gentle motion that facilitates tendon gliding and gentle muscle contraction, is recommended.[36,37]

Traditionally, retrograde massage, moving in a distal-to-proximal direction, has been used to manage postoperative edema in the upper extremity during the subacute and chronic phases of healing.[36] This intervention uses a firmer massage technique than appropriate to efficiently facilitate the lymphatic system to manage persistent edema lingering into the subacute and chronic stages.[36,37] Alternatively, the use of a lighter technique, manual edema mobilization, provides gentle traction to the skin, starting and ending proximally, and is considered a more effective intervention.[36,37] It is the authors' preference to encourage overhead active motion in play to facilitate proximal lymphatics to aide in the management of distal edema, particularly in the younger child that does not tolerate handling. Further education and training in this area is recommended for effective implementation into practice. Therapeutic taping is another intervention strategy that may be effective for the management of lingering edema.[36,37] The tape is proposed to provide a lift of the skin to open tissue space to support lymphatic anatomy for lymph drainage.[36,37] This may be a beneficial strategy to manage edema in a child that does not tolerate massage or with a presentation of ongoing, persistent edema (see Table 7.5).

Desensitization

The therapist should provide caregiver education on desensitization techniques to decrease hypersensitivity and encourage spontaneous hand use following surgery and immobilization. Implementation of desensitization techniques are recommended numerous times throughout the day and incorporated into functional activities, such as hand hygiene, bathing, and play. Techniques can be progressed as tolerated with avoidance directly over the surgical area, until full healing and tolerance to the surrounding area is achieved, with the focus on more proximal areas of the hand and surrounding skin initially. Use of household objects in the desensitization home program may include cotton balls, wash cloths, brushes, various cloth textures, or a gentle vibration massager. Desensitization is an important prerequisite for acceptance of scar management strategies (see Table 7.5).

Range of Motion and Functional Hand Use

A web space that allows digit flexion, extension, abduction, and adduction is essential for functional digital motion during daily activities.[6,29] Active motion and functional hand use within comfort are encouraged early following cast removal.[14,30,33] The protective orthotic should be removed several times a day to encourage gentle active motion to promote functional grasp and pinch patterns.[16,30,33] The therapist should incorporate graded play-based activities using a variety of different sized and shaped objects to encourage grasp patterns and digital motion. Limitations in active and passive digit flexion are most effectively managed with exercise and play-based activity, while flexion contractures are most effectively managed through orthotic intervention.[34] Patients may demonstrate the ongoing use of learned compensatory patterns that may require adaptations and intervention to discourage. It is important to consider the functional movement and role of the reconstructed web space and provide therapeutic intervention accordingly.

Progression to gentle passive motion of the operative digits and web space can be initiated as needed.[33] Passive motion and progressive orthotic intervention for contractures can be initiated once the child demonstrates comfortable active motion and tolerates handling. Progressive strengthening activities can be initiated as needed once the child is able to perform full composite digital flexion and extension without signs of pain or discomfort (see Table 7.5).

Scar Management

Hypertrophic scars result in increased thickness and loss of pliability of the skin that can impact joint motion.[34,35] Keloid scar formation is a rare complication; however, there is a higher incidence of formation when accompanied by a digital overgrowth or enlargement condition, such a macrodactyly.[18,38] Development of a keloid or hypertrophic scarring in the hand can result in issues with soft tissue mobility and

TABLE 7.5
Syndactyly: Postoperative Therapeutic Intervention.

	Goals	Strategies
Edema management	■ Facilitate tendon gliding and gentle muscle contraction ■ Promote joint motion, tissue mobility ■ Improve quality of scar healing ■ Improve comfort ■ Improve active motion	* Early conservative strategies ■ Elevation ■ Ice ■ Compression ■ Gentle active motion ■ Proximal active motion ■ Lingering edema in subacute and chronic stages: manual edema mobilization—light skin traction, proximal to distal-to-proximal (additional education and training recommended)
Desensitization	■ Decrease guarding ■ Preparatory for scar massage ■ Improve spontaneous hand use and active motion	* Start proximal to surgical area, work progressively toward surrounding tissue ■ Household items—cotton balls, wash cloth, various textures ■ Gentle massage and tickles ■ Vibration massage ■ Encourage clapping and bimanual hand use ■ Sensory bins with progressively coarser textures ■ Hand under running water

Scar management	■ Monitor scar maturation
	■ Prevent hypertrophic scar formation
	■ Maximize cosmesis, motion and digit position
	* Preventative approach important
		■ Early edema management crucial
		■ Initiate once closure of surgical incisions and graft healing (3–4+ weeks, per MD)
		■ Lotion massage—crisscross, rolling, circles; 3–5 times a day, 3–5 minutes
		■ Therapeutic taping—longitudinal application to reduce tension on scar
		■ Custom elastomer mold affixed with self-adherent wrap or tape
		■ Orthotic with elastomer or silicone sheet insert
		■ Compression garment
		  • Silicone can be sewn into garment by manufacturer; or include custom elastomer mold or silicone sheet
		  • Glove with open finger tips (should cover full length of scar); can shorten glove at uninvolved digits for greater ease of donning
		  • Compression class I (20–30 mmHg)
		  • A tracing or photo copy of the child's hand with a scale and detailed anatomy drawings of scar location

Range of motion and strength	■ Promote functional pinch and grasp patterns ■ Improve functional hand use ■ Facilitate developmental fine motor and bimanual skills ■ Discourage compensations	■ Encouragement of age appropriate grasp and pinch patterns • Age appropriate self-help skills—pretend play ■ Active motion—consider function of web space

TABLE 7.5
Syndactyly: Postoperative Therapeutic Intervention.—cont'd

Goals	Strategies
■ Prevent joint stiffness and contractures	• Stickers, finger puppets • Tracing hand to encourage digit abduction • Tool use—various sized objects/modalities (water "painting" with sponge, large brush, wash cloth) • Container play with balls, cups and objects that require circumferential or cylindrical grasp; grade object size to encourage abduction • Water play • Isolated digit movement • Object manipulation—rotation, translation, shift ■ Discourage compensatory patterns • Gentle wrap (3M Coban, Fabrifoam) to ulnar digits to isolate pinch • Blocking splint to encourage MP flexion if guarding and hyperextension positioning • Thumb opponens or abduction strap to encourage specific movement patterns • Therapeutic tape ■ Passive motion—progress as tolerated • Use of distraction- preferred activities, counting, incorporate in active play • incorporate stretch to long digit flexors and extensors; assess intrinsic tightness • flexion contracture best managed with orthotic ■ progressive strengthening • Water toys- squirt toys, bottles, turkey baster, eye dropper • Ball poppers, stress balls • Velcro connected toys/puzzles to encourage both grasp and pinch strengthening • Digit adduction/abduction in putty, sand, play doh • Open rubber bands, hair ties with digit abduction to place around ball or tube

contractures that ultimately impact function[6,38] (Fig. 7.8). Surgical intervention to excise the scar or corticosteroid treatment may be indicated if conservative management is not successful.[6]

The timely implementation of preventative scar management strategies plays a critical role in optimizing outcomes of scar integrity. Early edema management is a key preventative factor to avoid delayed scar healing, as this can result in accelerated scar tissue development, increased adhesions, and limitations in tendon gliding and soft tissue mobility. Aggressive orthotic positioning and passive motion that applies tension along scars should be avoid during the initial stages of scar healing.[31] Therapeutic scar management interventions can be initiated once the surgical areas have fully healed.[30]

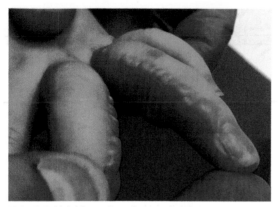

FIG. 7.8 Keloid scarring after syndactyly re-construction.

Conservative therapeutic interventions that best manage scar integrity include scar massage, custom elastomer molds, silicone gel sheets, therapeutic taping, and pressure garments.[10,16,30,31,35] Silicone sheets or custom elastomer molds can be easily affixed within an orthotic during overnight wear. Therapeutic tape with paper off tension applied longitudinally over a thickened scar, once full scar closure is achieved, may be a useful intervention to minimize scar appearance while allowing functional movement of the hand.[31,34] When a scar is raised comparatively to the surrounding skin, compression therapy is the most effective means to decrease the height of the scar and can be initiated once the patient is able to tolerate pressure over the surgical area.[35] The use of a custom compression glove in the young child discourages self-removal and maintains an elastomer or silicone insert in place while decreasing the risk as a choking hazard when affixed within a glove.[34] It is our experience that garments can be difficult for families to don in young patients and helpful modifications such as a zipper closure or shortened finger length at the uninvolved digits improves the ease of donning when used for scar management. Sharp et al.[35] recommended a compression class I with 20–30 mmHg and garment wear scheduled of 23 hours a day until the scar is fully matured (1–2 years). Garments typically need to be replaced every 3–6 months to ensure sufficient pressure as well as to accommodate for patient growth. It is important to consider that insurance coverage of garments varies substantially, and there may be high out-of-pocket expenses for families (Fig. 7.7) (see Table 7.5).

COMPLICATIONS AND OUTCOMES

The literature describes less favorable results in the surgical reconstruction of complex syndactyly, syndactyly of digits of dissimilar length, and in delayed presentation of the older child at the time of reconstruction.[15] Complex syndactyly reconstruction has a higher reoperation rate due to increased scarring and joint contracture impacting digital motion.[16] These cases also have a greater incidence of joint instability and angular or rotational deformities.[15,18,19] Delayed timing of treatment and surgical intervention in the older child is also associated with less favorable aesthetic outcomes.[14,15] Postoperative complications requiring therapeutic intervention are often delayed and occur during patient growth.[10] This can include web creep, hypertrophic scarring, keloid formation, and digit deformity.[10,13] Referral to hand therapy to manage these complications may be indicated.[34] Web creep is the distal migration of the commissure that occurs with the child's growth during scar maturation.[6,10,16,18,25] The incidence of web creep has been reported to vary from 2% to 24% of cases.[11,22,39] Outcome studies indicate a higher incidence of web creep in complex syndactyly release compared to that of simple syndactyly, with contributing factors related to greater surgical complexity including complications with graft adherence, the use of split thickness versus full thickness graft, and placement of longitudinal incisions at the base of the digit during flap design.[6,13,16] Dependent on the severity of the postoperative complications and the impact on functional hand use, additional surgery may be indicated secondary to joint instability, scar contracture, or poor aesthetic outcomes.[13,16,18,19]

REFERENCES

1. Oberg KC, Feenstra JM, Manske PR, Tonkin MA. Developmental biology and classification of congenital anomalies of the hand and upper extremity. *J Hand Surg Am.* 2010; 35(12):2066–2076.
2. Al-Qattan MM, Yang Y, Kozin SH. Embryology of the upper limb. *J Hand Surg Am.* 2009;34(7):1340–1350.
3. Al-Qattan MM, Kozin SH. Update on embryology of the upper limb. *J Hand Surg Am.* 2013;38(9):1835–1844.
4. Goldfarb CA, Shaw N, Steffen JA, Wall LB. The prevalence of congenital hand and upper extremity anomalies based upon the New York congenital malformations registry. *J Pediatr Orthop.* 2017;37(2):144–148.
5. Ekblom AG, Laurell T, Arner M. Epidemiology of congenital upper limb anomalies in 562 children born in 1997 to 2007: a total population study from Stockholm, Sweden. *J Hand Surg Am.* 2010;35(11):1742–1754.
6. Waters PM, Bae DS. Syndactyly. In: *Pediatric Hand and Upper Limb Surgery: A Practical Guide.* Philadelphia: Wolters Kluwer Health; 2012:12–25.
7. Buckwalter VJASA. Presentation and treatment of Poland anomaly. *Hand (N Y).* 2016;11(4):389–395.

8. Upton J. Apert syndrome. Classification and pathologic anatomy of limb anomalies. *Clin Plast Surg.* 1991;18(2): 321−355.

9. Nuzzi LC, Pike CM, Lewine EB, et al. Preoperative electrocardiograms for nonsyndromic children with hand syndactyly. *J Hand Surg Am.* 2015;40(3):452−455.

10. Kozin SH, Zlotolow DA. Common pediatric congenital conditions of the cand. *Plast Reconstr Surg.* 2015;136(2): 241e−257e.

11. Comer GC, Ladd AL. Management of complications of congenital hand disorders. *Hand Clin.* 2015;31(2): 361−375.

12. Wood VE. Super digit. *Hand Clin.* 1990;6(4):673−684.

13. Jordan DJ, Snashall E, Hindocha S. Syndactyly. In: Laub DR, ed. *Congenital Anomalies of the Upper Extremity: Etiology and Management.* New York: Springer Science and Business Media; 2015:159−177.

14. Manske MC, Goldfarb CA. Syndactyly. In: Abzug JM, Kozin SH, Zlotolow DA, eds. *The Pediatric Upper Extremity.* Vol. 3. New York: Spring Science and Business Media; 2015:277−295.

15. Vekris M, Lykissas M, Soucacos P, Korompilias A, Beris A. Congenital syndactyly: outcome of surgical treatment in 131 webs. *Tech Hand Up Extrem Surg.* 2010;14(1):2−7.

16. Braun TL, Trost JG, Pederson WC. Syndactyly release. *Semin Plast Surg.* 2016;30(4):162−170.

17. Ghani HA. Modified dorsal rotation advancement flap for release of the thumb web space. *J Hand Surg Br.* 2006; 31B(2):226−229.

18. Tonkin MA. Failure of differentiation part I: syndactyly. *Hand Clin.* 2009;25(2):171−193.

19. Goldfarb CA, Steffen JA, Stutz CM. Complex syndactyly: aesthetic and objective outcomes. *J Hand Surg Am.* 2012; 37A(10):2068−2073.

20. Ho ES, Clarke HM. Upper extremity function in children with congenital hand anomalies. *J Hand Ther.* 2005; 18(3):352−364.

21. Ho ES. Measuring hand function in the young child. *J Hand Ther.* 2010;23(3):323−328.

22. Lumenta DB, Kitzinger HB, Beck H, Frey M. Long-term outcomes of web creep, scar quality, and function after simple syndactyly surgical treatment. *J Hand Surg Am.* 2010; 35A(8):1323−1329.

23. Ardon MS, Selles RW, Hovius SE, et al. Stronger relation between impairment and manual capacity in the non-dominant hand than the dominant hand in congenital hand differences; implications for surgical and therapeutic interventions. *J Hand Ther.* 2014;27(3):201−208.

24. Strickland JW, Glogovac SV. Digital function following flexor tendon repair in Zone II: a comparison of immobilization and controlled passive motion techniques. *J Hand Surg Am.* 1980;5(6):537−543.

25. Moss ALH, Foucher G. Syndactyly: can web creep be avoided? *J Hand Surg Br.* 1990;15B(2):193−200.

26. Withey SJ, Kangesu T, Carver N, Sommerlad BC. The open finger technique for the release of syndactyly. *J Hand Surg Br.* 2001;26B(1):4−7.

27. Forbes-Duchart L, Marshall S, Strock A, Cooper JE. Determination of inter-rater reliability in pediatric burn scar assessment using a modified version of the Vancouver scar scale. *J Burn Care Res.* 2007;28(3):460−467.

28. Baryza MJ, Baryza GA. The Vancouver scar scale: an administration tool and its interrater reliability. *J Burn Care Rehabil.* 1995;16(5):535−538.

29. Kozin SH. Syndactyly. *J Am Soc Surg Hand.* 2001;1(1): 1−13.

30. Little KJ, Cornwall R. Congenital anomalies of the hand-Principles of management. *Orthop Clin N Am.* 2016; 47(1):153−168.

31. Moran SL, Tomhave W. Management of congenital hand anomalies. In: Skirven TM, Osterman AL, Fedorczyk JM, Amadio PC, eds. *Rehabilitation of the Hand and Upper Extremity.* Vol. 6. Philadelphia, PA: Elsevier Mosby; 2011: 1631−1646.

32. Dorich JM, Shotwell C. Orthotics and casting. In: Abzug JM, Kozin SH, Zlotolow DA, eds. *The Pediatric Upper Extremity.* Vol. 3. New York: Springer Science and Business Media; 2015:141−169.

33. Fuller M. Treatment of congenital differences of the upper extremity: therapist's commentary. *J Hand Ther.* 1999; 12(2):174−177.

34. Gibson G. Therapy management of children with congenital anomalies of the upper extremity. In: Laub DR, ed. *Congenital Anomalies of the Upper Extremity: Etiology and Management.* New York: Springer Science and Business Media; 2015:59−72.

35. Sharp PA, Pan B, Yakuboff KP, Rothchild D. Development of a best evidence statement for the use of pressure therapy for management of hypertrophic scarring. *J Burn Care Res.* 2016;37(4):255−264.

36. Miller LK, Jerosch-Herold C, Shepstone L. Effectiveness of edema management techniques for subacute hand edema: a systematic review. *J Hand Ther.* 2017;30(4):432−446.

37. Villeco JP. Edema: a silent but important factor. *J Hand Ther.* 2012;25(2):153−162.

38. Muzaffar AR, Rafols F, Masson J, Ezaki M, Carter PR. Keloid formation after syndactyly reconstruction: associated conditions, prevalence, and preliminary report of a treatment method. *J Hand Surg Am.* 2004;29A(2): 201−208.

39. Tonkin MA, Chew EM, Ledgard JP, Al-Sultan AA, Smith BJ, Lawson RD. An assessment of 2 objective measurements of web space position. *J Hand Surg Am.* 2015;40(3): 456−461.

CHAPTER 8

Rehabilitation of the Pediatric Upper Extremity Congenital Part II—Polydactyly

MATTHEW B. BURN, MD • JENNIFER M. CHAN, OTR/L, CHT • AMY L. LADD, MD

POLYDACTYLY (PREAXIAL AND POSTAXIAL)

Pertinent Anatomy and Classifications

Polydactyly can be divided based on the region of the hand involved into preaxial (radial), central, and postaxial (ulnar)—with variants on these categories (i.e., ulnar dimelia and mirror hand).[1] However, discussion within this chapter will be limited to preaxial and postaxial polydactyly. According to the Oberg, Manske and Tonkin (OMT) classification, polydactyly falls into Group 1 or "malformations" and into the subtype "failure of hand plate formation/differentiation."[2–4] Morphologically polydactyly types can be described based on the duplicated digits' location, size, individual component development, mobility, and joint stability.[1]

Preaxial polydactyly—also called thumb duplication, thumb polydactyly, radial polydactyly, split thumb—occurs in 1 per 3000–10,000 live births, most commonly in males, and is more common in children of Asian and Native American descent. An ethnic predilection between Caucasians and African Americans is controversial with some sources citing a higher occurrence in Caucasians, while others report equal representation.[1,5] The etiology is commonly attributed to delayed involution of the apical ectodermal ridge on the radial side of the hand.[5] It is often unilateral and from sporadic mutations.[5,6] Triphalangism is an exception that is more likely to be hereditary, associated with autosomal dominant inheritance, and associated with systemic syndromes that benefit from referral to a geneticist—including Blackfan—Diamond anemia, Holt—Oram syndrome, Bloom syndrome, Carpenter syndrome, and Ullrich-Feichtiger syndrome.[1,5] Although many classification systems have been described, the most common clinically utilized system was described by Wassel and is based on the level of the duplication.[1,5,7] Starting at the tip of the digit and moving

from distal to proximal, Type I involves a split in the midportion of the distal phalanx, Type II involves a split at the distal interphalangeal joint, and so on (Fig. 8.1).[1] Odd classification numbers involve bifurcation of the duplicated thumbs within the phalanx or metacarpal, while even numbers bifurcate at a joint.[8] Triphalangism, or Type VII, usually bifurcates the metacarpophalangeal (MCP) joint (similar to Type IV) but one of the duplicated thumbs has three phalanges rather than two (Fig. 8.2).[1] Type IV is the most common, making up 33%—46% of cases, followed by Type VII (20%—30%) and Type II (9%—28%). Type V (5%—10%), Type III (6%—14%), Type VI (3%—14%), and Type 1 (0%—3%) are less common.[7–10] Of note, Wassel did not include a category for thumb triplication or for a rudimentary preaxial thumb or "nubbin" attached only by skin and neurovascular pedicle (Fig. 8.3).[8]

Postaxial polydactyly occurs more often (10:1) in African Americans (1 per 139—300 live births) and is less common in Caucasians (1 per 1340—3000 live births).[5] It is more commonly hereditary, inherited in an autosomal dominant pattern with incomplete penetrance, with one of the child's parents noting a history of similar features as a child, especially in African American children.[1] When the child is Caucasian, it is more likely to be associated with various syndromes with systemic malformations such as Trisomy 13, Ellis-van Creveld syndrome, Laurence—Moon—Bardet—Biedl syndrome, and Meckel syndrome.[1] When it is syndromic, the inheritance pattern is often autosomal recessive, and these patients should be referred for a genetics workup, an echocardiogram, and a renal ultrasound.[1,5] Temtamy and McKusik described a classification system for postaxial polydactyly where Type A is a partially developed extra digit that articulates with either the fifth metacarpal or its own additional metacarpal, while Type B is a rudimentary digit

Pediatric Hand Therapy. https://doi.org/10.1016/B978-0-323-53091-0.00008-7

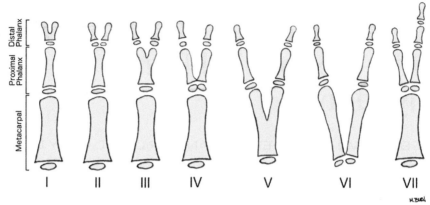

FIG. 8.1 Diagram illustrating the Wassel classification for preaxial or thumb polydactyly.

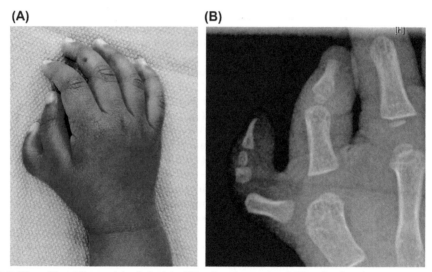

FIG. 8.2 Wassel type VII preaxial polydactyly. Often the ulnar and radial thumbs do not appear as symmetric as that shown in Fig. 8.1 either clinically **(A)** or radiographically **(B)**.

connected only by a skin bridge and a neurovascular pedicle.[1,5] Although postaxial polydactyly is more common in African Americans, this is only true for Type B postaxial polydactyly while Type A does not have racial predilection.[1] Stelling and Turek proposed a modification of this classification with Type B being reclassified as Type 1, and Type A being divided into Type 2 (if the extra digit articulates with the fifth metacarpal) and Type 3 (if the extra digit contains its own metacarpal).[11]

Preoperative Evaluation

Genetic counseling should be sought for all cases of syndromic involvement. Preoperative consultation with a hand therapist can be beneficial for children with polydactyly who have substantial functional deficits. By observing the child's extra digit in resting stance and during play or object manipulation, one can notice preferential use of one of the duplicated digits (usually the ulnar-most thumb in preaxial polydactyly) that is the most functional portion that should be maintained during surgery.[12] If there is unilateral involvement, the therapist observes the noninvolved side to assess the baby or child's "normal" grasp and pinch. Lack of functional pinch and grip patterns can be a sign of substantial joint instability, which should be documented and communicated to the surgeon. Both passive and active ROM can be measured, documented, and compared to the contralateral side, which can assist in preoperative counseling, as a joint (i.e., interphalangeal joint in a Type IV preaxial polydactyly) that does not bend preoperatively will likely

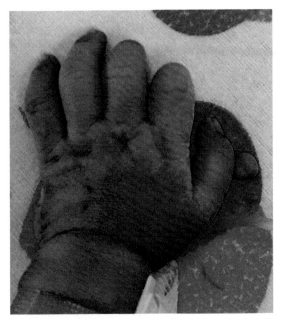

FIG. 8.3 Rudimentary preaxial polydactyly or "nubbin."

not bend postoperatively. Use of developmental assessment tools such as the HELP and PDMS scales can provide an overview of function in various areas of development including fine and gross motor skills and adaptive/self-help areas, while the Pediatric Outcomes Data Collection Instrument (PODCI) can provide a measure of surgical outcomes (see Tables 8.1—8.3).[13-18] The Hawaii Early Learning Profile (HELP) provides an overview of function in various areas of development including fine and gross motor skills and adaptive/self-help areas (see Table 8.1).[13,14] For a more thorough assessment of fine motor abilities, the Peabody Developmental Motor Scales (PDMS) is recommended (see Table 8.2).[15] According to the PDMS, a baby begins to grasp placed toys in the hand at 3—6 months and uses fingers and thumbs to grasp at 6—9 months. The ability to use tip-to-tip pinch of a small object occurs around 9 months. The PODCI questionnaire is a patient-based instrument for monitoring surgical outcomes in pediatric patients across a wide range of ages (see Table 8.3).[16,17]

Preaxial polydactyly, as the thumb represents 40% of overall hand function, may substantially affect the pediatric patient's fine motor skills, upper limb gross motor function, such as ball skills, and ability to perform age appropriate self-care and other activities of daily living.[19] It is less common for postaxial polydactyly to interfere with functional hand use. Functional grasp can be evaluated using 1½-to-2″ spherical and cylindrical objects, while smaller ¼-½″ objects, such as small pieces of

food, can evaluate pinch. The use of resistive objects and toys, such as suction balls, accordion tubes, playing gentle tug-of-war with cylindrical toys or the caregiver's finger, allows observation of stability and interphalangeal (IP) joint function (Fig. 8.4). Some authors favor a preoperative orthosis as a method to improve angular and rotatory deformities.[20] Improvement in postoperative IP joint motion has been reported with preoperative splinting.[21]

Few parents elect to retain a child's duplicated digit (either thumb or small finger) due to the aesthetics and social stigma.[5] However, contraindications to surgery may include medical conditions precluding surgery and/or anesthesia. The timing of surgery is not well established, but the child's (1) anesthesia risk decreases at 1 year old, (2) hand doubles in size by 2 years old (allowing for easier identification of anatomy), and (3) more refined fine motor skills are not developed until 3 years old.[5,22] Thus, most recommend operative intervention between 18 and 32 months of age.

In patients with Type A postaxial polydactyly and any preaxial polydactyly, preoperative radiographs should be obtained to assist in surgical planning.[1] Surgical reconstruction of preaxial polydactyly can be complex. Although simple ablation has been suggested for nonrudimentary preaxial polydactyly, the results are more often than not unsatisfactory with angular deviation and/or ligamentous instability.[6] Although the term "duplication" is used, a better term would be "split" or "bifurcated" thumb as neither of the two thumbs has normal anatomy nor are they of normal size when compared to the patient's normal contralateral thumb (Fig. 8.5).[1,5] In nearly all cases, the remaining thumb is hypoplastic with typical underdeveloped or aberrant anatomical structures. Preoperative discussion regarding this residual hypoplasia allows for appropriate postoperative expectations, especially the understanding that surgical ablation of the duplicated thumb will not result in a normal sized and appearing retained thumb.[5,6]

For Type B postaxial polydactyly and the uncommonly seen nubbin in preaxial polydactyly, the treatment method is controversial. Some surgeons recommend simple ligation at birth or sharp amputation at the base of the stalk with pressure hemostasis. This is easily performed in the newborn nursery using a surgical staple or suture causing the tissue to undergo necrosis and fall off in 1—2 weeks without the need for anesthetics.[5] However, this technique can cause superficial neuroma formation that can be symptomatic or a small "nubbin" or "nipple" of tissue that is aesthetically displeasing— which may require formal excision later in life.[5] Others recommend formal surgical excision with an elliptical skin incision to prevent "dog ears" (see later).

TABLE 8.1
Hawaii Early Learning Profile (HELP).

Age range
- HELP (0–3 years old)
- HELP for preschoolers (3–6 years old)

Administration
- HELP checklist (685 items in 58 strands)
- HELP for preschoolers checklist (622 items in 46 strands)
- Completed by examiner based on observation and parent report

Developmental Domains Assessed
- Cognitive
- Language
- Gross motor
- Fine motor
- Social emotional
- Self-help

Distributed by
Vort Corporation (www.vort.com)
P.O. Box 60132-W, Palo Alto, CA 94306

Source: Slentz KL, Early DM, McKenna M. A Guide to Assessment in Early Childhood. http://www.k12.wa.us/EarlyLearning/pubdocs/assessment_print.pdf. 2008. Accessed June 30, 2018.

TABLE 8.2
Peabody Developmental Motor Scales, Second Edition (PDMS-2).

Age range
- 0–6 years old

Administration
- Completed by examiner with direct assessment of the child
- Each item on which the child met the criterion for mastery is marked on the profile of Item Mastery section, enabling examiner to compare the child's performance on the items he or she has mastered with that of the normative sample.

Domains Assessed
- Reflexes (8 items)
- Stationary (30 items)
- Locomotion (89 items)
- Object manipulation (24 items)
- Grasping (26 items)
- Visual-motor integration (72 items)
- Fine motor
- Gross motor
- Total motor quotients

Distributed by
PRO-ED, Inc. (www.proedinc.com)
8700 Shoal Creek Boulevard, Austin, TX 78757

Source: Slentz KL, Early DM, McKenna M. A Guide to Assessment in Early Childhood. http://www.k12.wa.us/EarlyLearning/pubdocs/assessment_print.pdf. 2008. Accessed June 30, 2018.

Surgical Steps

Nonfunctional pre- and postpolydactyly

For the neonate with a rudimentary pre- or postaxial polydactyly, rather than tying the digit off, our preference is to remove this surgically in the newborn nursery or in the clinical setting within a few weeks of birth. In the newborn nursery, the circumcision tray has most of the instruments the hand surgeon needs. In either setting, a nurse or assistant (sometimes a family member) can administer sugar drops to the newborn, and a fraction

---

TABLE 8.3
Pediatric Outcomes Data Collection Instrument (PODCI).

Age range
- 2–21 years old

Administration
- Between 2 and 11 years old, parents of the child complete a parent-specific version of the questionnaire based on their child's observed function
- Between 12 and 21 years old, the child's parents and the patient themselves complete specific versions of the questionnaire
- Each functional dimension is scored from 0-to-100 with 100 representing the highest level of function or happiness

Functional Dimension Assessed
- Upper extremity function (scored 0–100)
- Transfer and basic mobility (scored 0–100)
- Sports and physical function (scored 0–100)
- Comfort/pain (scored 0–100)
- Global function (an average of the previous four scores, scored 0–100)
- Happiness with physical condition (scored 0–100)

Developed by the
- American Academy of Orthopaedic Surgeons (AAOS)
- Pediatric Orthopaedic Society of North America (POSNA)
- American Academy of Pediatrics (AAP)
- Shriners Hospitals for Children

Public domain available free of charge through the American Academy of Orthopaedic Surgeons (www.AAOS.org)

Sources: Lerman JA, Sullivan E, Barnes DA, Haynes RJ. The Pediatric Outcomes Data Collection Instrument (PODCI) and functional assessment of patients with unilateral upper extremity deficiencies. J Pediatr Orthop. 2005 May–Jun; 25(3):405–7; Daltroy LH, Liang MH, Fossel AH, Goldberg MJ. The POSNA pediatric musculoskeletal functional health questionnaire: report on reliability, validity, and sensitivity to change. Pediatric Outcomes Instrument Development Group. Pediatric Orthopaedic Society of North America. J Pediatr Orthop. 1998 Sep–Oct; 18(5):561–71.

---

of anesthetic is injected into the stump. After making a small skin ellipse, the surgeon traces the neurovascular bundle proximally and both crushes and cauterizes the stump to minimize a potential neuroma formation.[5] Absorbable suture and skin adhesive provides a simple solution for the newborn. The older infant will typically require removal in the operating room with anesthesia.[5]

Preaxial polydactyly

The goal of surgery is to produce a single, stable thumb aligned with the mechanical axis of the remaining digit.[1] Surgical planning is based on the level of the duplication (i.e., Wassel I, II, III, etc.) and also the morphology of the two thumbs, which can be divergent, parallel, or "zigzag" (divergent and convergent) (Fig. 8.1).[5] Greater deformity suggests abnormal osseous alignment and tendon insertions, which lead to a higher rate of recurrent deformity especially if these deforming forces are not addressed intraoperatively.[5] The presence of IP joint stiffness preoperatively may suggest the presence of a pollex abductus (present in 20%), which is an abnormal connection between the flexor pollicis longus and extensor pollicis longus.[5]

Surgery is performed with the patient supine on a standard operating room table with a hand table utilizing general anesthesia—in addition to a tourniquet and loupe magnification for visualization. A "tennis racquet" shaped incision is made either circling the perionychium (i.e., Wassel I, II) or the base of the thumb to be removed. Subcutaneous tissue and skin from the thumb to be removed can be maintained to add bulk to the retained thumb. Excess, unnecessary, retained skin and soft tissue can always be excised at the end of the procedure during closure. This racquet incision is extended proximally (to allow shaving of the proximal articular surface or osteotomy of the proximal shaft) and distally (to allow insertion of the abductor complex and radial collateral ligament onto the retained thumb) with a straight or zigzag type pattern as needed.[5] Careful dissection allows identification of the neurovascular structures within the excised thumb, which are ligated (digital vessels) or treated with traction neurotomy (digital nerves). The ulnarmost thumb usually has at least one digital artery, and has two digital arteries in 21% of patients, but the radial-most thumb has a 5% chance of having no digital artery.[9] This small risk should be considered if one is planning to ablate the ulnar-most thumb.[9] The insertion of the radial collateral ligament (RCL), abductor pollicis brevis (APB, in Wassel IV+) or abductor pollicis longus (APL, in Wassel VI only), and a periosteal sleeve

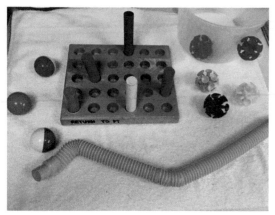

FIG. 8.4 Other tools (toys) in the armamentarium of occupational therapy to encourage motion as well as strengthen grip and pinch.

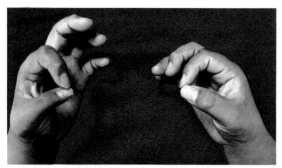

FIG. 8.5 Seven year follow-up of left Wassel IV thumb preaxial polydactyly reconstruction. This image demonstrates the patients' normal right thumb in comparison with their reconstructed left thumb.

extending distally are carefully elevated from the thumb to be ablated before making an arthrotomy and ablating the thumb.[1,5] If necessary (Wassel II, IV, VI, VII), a chondroplasty of the widened articular surface can be performed with a Beaver mini-blade. An anomalous connection between the flexor and extensor tendons to the thumb (pollex abductus) may need to be released and/or transferred to the retained thumb (rebalanced).[1,6] It may be necessary to stabilize the remaining thumb with a transarticular wire while the reconstructed ligament heals (Fig. 8.6A and B) or, in severe deformity, an osteotomy is performed to realign the distal portion of the digit.[5,22] The previously retained sleeve (RCL, APB, periosteum) is reinserted onto the radial base of the retained thumb utilizing suture into the periosteum.[1] The skin flaps are trimmed as necessary before closure

with 5-0 or 6-0 absorbable suture.[5] Postoperative immobilization depends on the age or maturity of the patient, but most children are placed into a long arm club-type cast immediately postoperatively with a gentle supracondylar mold. Some prefer a dressing that allows the thumb tip to be seen (i.e., thumb spica) so that thumb "disappearance" due to cast migration can be noticed.

Of special note is the Bilhaut-Cloquet procedure, which can be utilized for Wassel II when both thumbs are of near equal size and appearance.[5] A central wedge of tissue (including pulp, nail bed, and distal phalanx) can be removed from both the radial and ulnar thumbs.[1] Following removal, the remaining ulnar and radial portions of their respective duplicated thumbs are combined to recreate a single thumb.[1,23] Critics of this technique suggest that it leads to increased thumb IP joint stiffness and a central longitudinal nail ridge. Another option is to excise the radial-most nail-plate, nail bed, and distal phalanx, while retaining the skin and soft tissue as a flap used to add bulk to the retained ulnar-most thumb.[5] Rarely the radial-most thumb will be more developed and thus retained, while the ulnar-most thumb is excised.[5] Even rarer a surgeon may decide to perform an "on-top plasty" where the distal portion of the radial-most thumb is retained and transferred to the proximal portion of the ulnar-most thumb.[5]

Postaxial polydactyly

Surgical management of a well-developed postaxial polydactyly mirrors that of preaxial polydactyly as described earlier, but with an ulnar sided incision, maintenance of the ulnar collateral ligament (if at or distal to the MCP joint) with a periosteal sleeve, and of the abductor digiti quinti, as it is often attached to the ulnar-most digit.[1,5]

Postoperative Rehabilitation

At the first postoperative follow-up visit 2–3 weeks from surgery, the postoperative cast is removed and the wound is inspected.[5,6] Children are placed into a new cast until 4–6 weeks postoperatively when the wires are removed. Some authors prefer that the patients' first follow-up occurs at 5 weeks postoperatively.[22] After pin removal, children are immobilized full-time, except for during therapy sessions or for hygiene, in a thumb spica orthosis—either hand-based or, especially in younger children, forearm-based (Fig. 8.7A and B).[24,25,26] The orthosis is worn at nighttime only starting at 6–8 weeks and continuing until 3 months postoperatively.[24–27]

Therapy starts with gentle active ROM exercises at 4 weeks postoperatively, advances to gentle active assisted or passive ROM exercises at 6–8 weeks

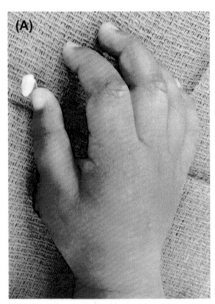
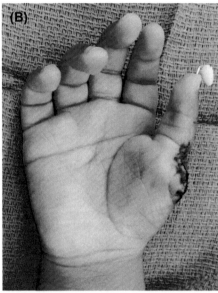

FIG. 8.6 The appearance of a Wassel IV thumb postoperatively viewed from a dorsal **(A)** and volar **(B)**.

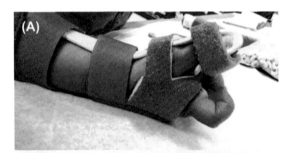
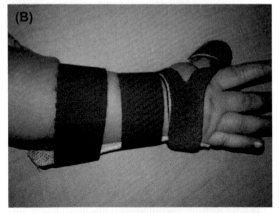

FIG. 8.7 Forearm-based thumb spica orthosis used for protection following thumb reconstruction maintaining thumb palmar **(A)** and radial **(B)** abduction.

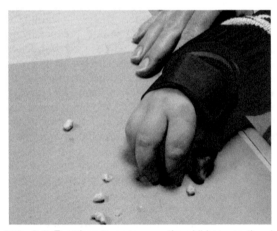

FIG. 8.8 Exercises to encourage the child to use thumb interphalangeal (IP) joint motion.

postoperatively (especially if limited gains have been attained actively), followed by functional grasp and pinch rehabilitation. An exercise orthosis blocking the thumb MCP joint, thereby facilitating thumb IP joint motion, may be fabricated for use during fine motor activities, such as self-feeding finger foods (Fig. 8.8). Functional activities involving the use of large objects and smaller objects to facilitate grip and pinch, respectively, should be encouraged. The child may require motor retraining to spontaneously use their new thumb. Scar management is initiated when the wounds are completely closed, including sun protection (i.e., sunblock, dressings), scar massage, and elastomer silicone scar pads worn at night, secured in place using the orthosis. At approximately 8 weeks postsurgery, strengthening activities may be provided. Patients are monitored at least yearly until skeletal maturity for recurrent deformity.[1]

Complications/Outcomes

For reconstruction of preaxial polydactyly and Type A postaxial polydactyly, the most common complication is residual or recurrent deformity and imbalanced growth.[1] Thumb angulation can occur at the IP joint alone (mostly in Wassel II), MCP joint alone (mostly in Wassel IV), or at the IP and MCP joints as a Z-type deformity.[12,20,28] Lee reported 32% (44/139 cases) of Wassel type IV reconstructions developed greater than 20 degrees of joint angulation at either the IP and/or MCP joints postoperatively.[29] Stutz, at a minimum of 10-year follow-up, found that 23% (10/43 thumbs) required revision surgery—most commonly at the thumb IP joint.[30] This, with emphasis on the possibility of future revision surgeries, should be discussed with patients and family preoperatively. Other complications of polydactyly reconstruction include residual instability of the affected joints, symptomatic scarring, joint stiffness, and/or pinch weakness.[1,20,31] Thumb IP joint motion for preaxial polydactyly reconstruction may be limited to 0–30 degrees.[5] Pinch weakness may result from persistent instability, smaller thumb size, and/or motor unit abnormalities.[12]

Although some authors have reported no adverse results from suture ligation of Type B polydactyly, others have reported a 16%–24% risk of bleeding, infection, symptomatic or cosmetically unappealing scarring, incomplete excision/residual growth, and/or symptomatic neuroma formation (compared to a 4% risk with surgery) and a residual 1–6 mm bump in up to 43%.[1,5,32–34] Revision formal surgical excision, after failed suture ligation, has been shown to have good results.[1]

REFERENCES

1. Little KJ, Cornwall R. Congenital anomalies of the hand—principles of management. *Orthop Clin N Am.* 2016;47(1):153–168. https://doi.org/10.1016/j.ocl.2015.08.015.
2. Manske MC, Goldfarb CA. Chapter 13: syndactyly. In: Abzug JM, Kozin SH, Zlotolow DA, eds. *The Pediatric Upper Extremity.* New York; Heidelberg: Springer; 2015: 277–295.
3. Oberg KC, Feenstra JM, Manske PR, Tonkin MA. Developmental biology and classification of congenital anomalies of the hand and upper extremity. *J Hand Surg.* 2010; 35(12):2066–2076. https://doi.org/10.1016/j.jhsa.2010.09.031.
4. Tonkin MA, Tolerton SK, Quick TJ, et al. Classification of congenital anomalies of the hand and upper limb: development and assessment of a new system. *J Hand Surg.* 2013;38(9):1845–1853. https://doi.org/10.1016/j.jhsa.2013.03.019.
5. Waters PM, Bae DS. Chapter 4: preaxial polydactyly. In: *Pediatric Hand and Upper Limb Surgery: A Practical Guide.* Philadelphia: Wolters Kluwer Health/Lippincott Williams & Wilkins; 2012:32–42.
6. Baek GH. Chapter 15: duplication. In: Abzug JM, Kozin SH, Zlotolow DA, eds. *The Pediatric Upper Extremity.* New York; Heidelberg: Springer; 2015: 325–368.
7. Wassel HD. The results of surgery for polydactyly of the thumb. A review. *Clin Orthop.* 1969;64:175–193.
8. Al-Qattan MM. The distribution of the types of thumb polydactyly in a Middle Eastern population: a study of 228 hands. *J Hand Surg Eur.* 2010;35(3):182–187. https://doi.org/10.1177/1753193409352417.
9. Kitayama Y, Tsukada S. Patterns of arterial distribution in the duplicated thumb. *Plast Reconstr Surg.* 1983;72(4): 535–542.
10. Naasan A, Page RE. Duplication of the thumb: a 20-year retrospective review. *J Hand Surg.* 1994;19(3):355–360.
11. Withey SJ, Kangesu T, Carver N, Sommerlad BC. The open finger technique for the release of syndactyly. *J Hand Surg Edinb Scotl.* 2001;26(1):4–7. https://doi.org/10.1054/jhsb.2000.0575 45.
12. Dobyns JH, Lipscomb PR, Cooney WP. Management of thumb duplication. *Clin Orthop.* 1985;195:26–44.
13. Parks S. *Inside HELP – Administration and Reference Manual for the Hawaii Early Learning Profile (HELP).* Palo Alto: VORT Corporation; 1992.
14. Ashworth S, Estilow T, Humpl D. Chapter 8: occupational therapy evaluation and treatment. In: *The Pediatric Upper Extremity.* New York; Heidelberg: Springer; 2015: 171–195.
15. van Hartingsveldt MJ, Cup EHC, Oostendorp RAB. Reliability and validity of the fine motor scale of the Peabody developmental motor scales-2. *Occup Ther Int.* 2005;12(1): 1–13.
16. Lerman JA, Sullivan E, Barnes DA, Haynes RJ. The Pediatric Outcomes Data Collection Instrument (PODCI) and functional assessment of patients with unilateral upper extremity deficiencies. *J Pediatr Orthop.* 2005;25(3): 405–407.
17. Daltroy LH, Liang MH, Fossel AH, Goldberg MJ. The POSNA pediatric musculoskeletal functional health questionnaire: report on reliability, validity, and sensitivity to change. Pediatric Outcomes Instrument Development Group. Pediatric Orthopaedic Society of North America. *J Pediatr Orthop.* 1998;18(5):561–571.

18. Folio MR, Fewell RR. In: *Peabody Developmental Motor Scales*. 2nd ed. An International Publisher; 2000. Austin: Pro-Ed.

19. Townsend DJ, Lipp EB, Chun K, Reinker K, Tuch B. Thumb duplication, 66 years' experience–a review of surgical complications. *J Hand Surg.* 1994;19(6):973−976. https://doi.org/10.1016/0363-5023(94)90099-X.

20. Chapter 128-management of congenital hand anomalies. In: Skirven TM, ed. *Rehabilitation of the Hand and Upper Extremity*. 6th ed. Philadelphia, PA: Elsevier/Mosby; 2011.

21. Fuller M. Treatment of congenital differences of the upper extremity: therapist's commentary. *J Hand Ther.* 1999; 12(2):174−177. https://doi.org/10.1016/S0894-1130 (99)80021-0 38.

22. Kozin SH, Zlotolow DA. Common pediatric congenital conditions of the hand. *Plast Reconstr Surg.* 2015;136(2): 241e−257e.

23. Baek GH, Gong HS, Chung MS, Oh JH, Lee YH, Lee SK. Modified Bilhaut-Cloquet procedure for Wassel type-II and III polydactyly of the thumb. *J Bone Joint Surg Am.* 2007;89(3):534−541. https://doi.org/10.2106/JBJS.F.0 0812.

24. Goldfarb CA. Congenital hand differences. *J Hand Surg.* 2009;34(7):1351−1356. https://doi.org/10.1016/j.jhsa. 2009.06.014.

25. Tonkin MA. Failure of differentiation part I: Syndactyly. *Hand Clin.* 2009;25(2):171−193. https://doi.org/10.101 6/j.hcl.2008.12.004.

26. Dorich JM, Shotwell C. Chapter 7: Orthotics and casting. In: *The Pediatric Upper Extremity*. New York; Heidelberg: Springer; 2015:141−169.

27. Goldfarb CA, Steffen JA, Stutz CM. Complex syndactyly: aesthetic and objective outcomes. *J Hand Surg.* 2012; 37(10):2068−2073. https://doi.org/10.1016/j.jhsa.2012 .06.033.

28. Baek G. Chapter 19: radial polydactyly. In: *Congenital Anomalies of the Upper Extremity: Etiology and Management*. New York: Springer; 2015:241−260.

29. Lee CC, Park HY, Yoon JO, Lee KW. Correction of Wassel type IV thumb duplication with zigzag deformity: results of a new method of flexor pollicis longus tendon relocation. *J Hand Surg Eur.* 2013;38(3):272−280. https://doi.org/10.1177/1753193412460809.

30. Stutz C, Mills J, Wheeler L, Ezaki M, Oishi S. Long-term outcomes following radial polydactyly reconstruction. *J Hand Surg.* 2014;39(8):1549−1552. https://doi.org/ 10.1016/j.jhsa.2014.05.006.

31. Goldfarb CA, Calhoun VD, Dailey L, Manske PR. *Hand and Upper Extremity Therapy: Congenital, Pediatric and Adolescent Patients : Saint Louis Protocols*. 2012.

32. Rayan GM, Frey B. Ulnar polydactyly. *Plast Reconstr Surg.* 2001;107(6):1449−1454. discussion 1455-1457.

33. Watson BT, Hennrikus WL. Postaxial type-B polydactyly. Prevalence and treatment. *J Bone Joint Surg Am.* 1997; 79(1):65−68.

34. Katz K, Linder N. Postaxial type B polydactyly treated by excision in the neonatal nursery. *J Pediatr Orthop.* 2011; 31(4):448−449. https://doi.org/10.1097/BPO.0b013e31 821addb.

CHAPTER 9

Congenital II: Radial Longitudinal Deficiency and Thumb Hypoplasia

SCOTT OISHI, MD • AMY LAKE, OTR, CHT • NICHOLAS PULOS, MD

PERTINENT ANATOMY AND CLASSIFICATIONS

The upper limb develops early and rapidly during development, beginning at approximately 28 days after fertilization and completed by day 56. Development in three axes involves the apical ectodermal ridge, the zone of polarizing activity, and the dorsal ectoderm through a complex feedback mechanism, regulated by fibroblast growth factor, sonic hedgehog, and the wingless-type pathway. Disruption in any of these during development can lead to longitudinal, central, or transverse deficiencies.[1]

The etiology of many of the hand differences we see clinically are not fully recognized. However, Ogino and colleagues induced radial and ulnar longitudinal deficiencies in a rat model by administering a chemotherapy agent at different points in fetal development of the upper limb. Interestingly, high rates of fetal demise occurred at a similar time point as the induction of ulnar longitudinal deficiencies, suggesting a mechanism for the 10:1 ratio in the incidence of radial-to-ulnar longitudinal deficiencies seen clinically.[2,3] Transverse deficiencies have not been induced in an animal model, but are thought to be due to subclavian artery disruption during early development.[4]

Radial longitudinal deficiency (RLD) is the most common upper limb longitudinal deficiency, with an incidence reported between 1:5000 and 1:100,000 live births and a 3:2 ratio of males to females. Bilateral cases present equivalently to unilateral cases; however, the right is more often affected than the left.[5] Clinical presentation is greatly varied from mild shortening to complete absence of the radius and with, or without, thumb hypoplasia. In the classification system proposed by Swanson, RLD falls under IB1, failure of formation, longitudinal arrest, and radial ray.[6] In the expanded Oberg–Manske–Tonkin classification system, RLD is classified as I.A.2.i if there is thumb hypoplasia and forearm involvement and I.B.2.i if there is thumb hypoplasia without forearm involvement.[7]

Bayne and Klug initially classified RLD into four types.[8] As understanding of the disease process evolved, this was expanded to include types 0/N[9] for patients with a normal distal radius as well as type V, reflecting proximal involvement of the radius as seen with phocomelia[10] (Table 9.1). The thumb involvement in radial longitudinal deficiency was classified by Blauth into types I–V.[11] Manske subsequently added subtypes IIIA and IIIB to reflect the stability of the carpometacarpal joint, which importantly helps drive our reconstructive algorithm.[12] (Table 9.2).

PREOPERATIVE EVALUATION AND TREATMENT

A thorough history and complete physical examination of the patient is imperative. In addition to the upper extremities, the initial evaluation should include an assessment of the lower extremities, hips, back, head, and neck area. Although most cases of RLD are the result of sporadic mutations, some are related to underlying inherited conditions including Holt–Oram syndrome, thrombocytopenia absent radius, Fanconi's anemia, and Blackfan–Diamond anemia[5] (Table 9.3). The frequency of association with a syndrome has been reported to range from 33% to 44% and nearly three quarters of patients have an accompanying medical or musculoskeletal anomaly.[13] Therefore, it is imperative that the surgeon be aware of associated conditions and make certain that appropriate tests are completed at presentation, as often he or she is the first provider to accurately make the diagnosis (Table 9.4).

Evaluation of the upper limb typically reveals some degree of radial deviation at the wrist and varying degrees of thumb hypoplasia. Importantly, there is little or no correlation between the severity of the thumb

TABLE 9.1 Modification of Bayne and Klug Classification of Radial Longitudinal Deficiency.[9]				
Type	**Thumb**	**Carpus**	**Distal Part of Radius**	**Proximal Part of Radius**
N	Hypoplastic or absent	Normal	Normal	Normal
0	Hypoplastic or absent	Absence, hypoplasia, or coalition	Normal	Normal, radioulnar synostosis, or congenital dislocation of radial head
1	Hypoplastic or absent	Absence, hypoplasia, or coalition	>2 mm shorter than ulna	Normal, radioulnar synostosis, or congenital dislocation of radial head
2	Hypoplastic or absent	Absence, hypoplasia, or coalition	Hypoplasia	Hypoplasia
3	Hypoplastic or absent	Absence, hypoplasia, or coalition	Physis absent	Variable hypoplasia
4	Hypoplastic or absent	Absence, hypoplasia, or coalition	Absent	Absent

hypoplasia and radius involvement. Active and passive range of motion of the shoulder, elbow, wrist, and fingers should be recorded as well as the resting position of the radius and degree of obtainable passive correction. In the initial evaluation of a newborn with radial longitudinal deficiency, radiographs may not provide much additional information and are usually deferred until 6–12 months old.

Therapeutic intervention for these children begins within the first few months of life with passive stretching. As soon as these children are medically stable, a referral for occupational therapy should be made. Therapists lay early groundwork to promote best outcomes of complex surgeries and overall future functional independence. Potential functioning is optimized through interventions such as Active/Passive Range of Motion (A/PROM), developmentally appropriate activities of daily living (ADLs), engaging children in age appropriate play, and instructing parents how to safely stretch each joint of their child's upper extremity. Parents, often, are hesitant and timid to stretch their child without a good understanding of their child's anatomy, joint location, and attainable goals for increased range of motion (ROM). Each child is unique in their presentation, and thus a standardized approach is insufficient. It is important to understand the extent of each child's individual abilities and functions, as many will need assistive devices or alternative techniques to become independent with ADLs early on.

During the initial therapy evaluation, as well as subsequent visits, it is important that the following items be noted:

1. Is there a shoulder joint? How much ROM is available?
2. Is there an elbow joint? How much ROM is available?
3. What is the ROM of the wrist at rest? (How radially deviated is the wrist?)
4. What is the available passive ulnar deviation of the wrist (typically a negative number)?
5. Does the patient have a thumb?
6. Is the thumb helpful in functional tasks?
7. What position is the index finger in (Has it started to pronate)?
8. How does the child hold objects (rattle, bottle, toys, etc.) … is it between the thumb and fingers, index and long, or ring and small?
9. Look at Function—depending on the age of the child … is the child developmentally on target or are they having difficulty with certain tasks?
10. Is there a need for an orthosis? (The need for orthotic fabrication depends on anatomy and presentation of the upper extremity. Orthoses will be discussed further in regards to specific joints throughout this chapter.)

All of these questions help the therapist plan therapeutic interventions to increase ROM, improve

TABLE 9.2
Modified Blauth Classification.[11,11a]

Feature	Type I	Type 2	Type 3A	Type 3B	Type 4	Type 5
Thumb size	Normal or small	Normal or small	Small	Small	Very small	Absent
First web	Normal size and location	Distal and tight	Distal and tight	Distal and tight	APB, OP, FPB, and adductor absent	APB, OP, FPB, and adductor absent
Intrinsic muscles	APB and OP hypoplastic	APB and OP hypoplastic or absent	APB and OP absent or severely hypoplastic	APB and OP absent or severely hypoplastic	APB, OP, FPB, and adductor absent	APB, OP, FPB, and adductor absent
Extrinsic muscles	Normal	Normal or nearly normal	Abnormal: FPL and/or EPL absent or FPL −EPL connection or pollex abductus	Abnormal: FPL and/or EPL absent or FPL −EPL connection or pollex abductus	Absent	Absent
Ligaments	Normal	MP UCL lax	MP UCL and possibly RCL lax	MP UCL and possibly RCL lax	Absent	Absent
Bones and joints	All bones present, may be hypoplastic	All bones present, may be hypoplastic	All bones present, may be hypoplastic	Proximal metacarpal absent	Metacarpal, trapezium, and scaphoid absent	Phalanges, metacarpal, trapezium, and scaphoid absent

APB, abductor pollicis brevis; *EPL*, extensor pollicis longus; *FPB*, flexor pollicis brevis; *FPL*, flexor pollicis longus; *MP*, metacarpophalangeal; *OP*, opponens pollicis; *RCL*, radial collateral ligament; *UCL*, ulnar collateral ligament.

function, and help the surgeon plan for future surgery as the child grows.

It is important to assess all of these data points on a regular basis and communicate such with the treating surgeon so that changes in ROM and function are observed throughout development and patterns of decline or concern can be appropriately addressed.

As children grow, orthotic fabrication may become an important component of treatment. However, parent readiness, understanding of the purpose of the orthosis, and follow through is paramount before initiating an orthosis. Activities of daily living are also addressed at each of these stages, and children are instructed on the use of adaptive equipment or educated on an alternate method if completion is unobtainable.

Newborns less than 6 months old are typically easy to fabricate orthoses on; however, these orthoses are exceptionally small and require patience and precision to fabricate correctly. Encouraging caregivers to hold their baby during the fabrication process while maintaining a quiet and dimly lit atmosphere helps to soothe the child. It is important to remember that crying is a normal form of communication at this age.[14] The typical orthoses for radial dysplasia may be something soft, such as cylindrical foam strapped onto the wrist radially, to act as a block for prevention of radial deviation (Picture 9.1A and B), or a custom-molded orthosis to hold the wrist into an ulnar-deviated stretch (Picture 9.2A and B). The primary activity of daily living at this age is feeding and parents rarely need assistance, as it is still age appropriate for children to breast or bottle feed. Grasping and reaching for toys is observed during this time, and alterations in the size of the toy or distance from reach can be easily adjusted (Picture 9.3).

Infants 6−18 months old are more difficult to fabricate orthoses on, as they become more aware of strangers with their fight or flight response. Orthoses at this age may also become choking hazards if fabricated too small. Distraction becomes important during the fabrication process, so including the caregivers is a

TABLE 9.3
Common Syndromes Associated With Radial Longitudinal Deficiency.

Associated Syndrome	Presentation	Inheritance Pattern
Holt–Oram	Radial longitudinal deficiency and a cardiac anomaly, most commonly a ventricular septal defect.	Autosomal dominant
TAR	Thrombocytopenia that manifests during infancy and can be fatal. Will resolve spontaneously with age.	Autosomal recessive
Fanconi anemia	Presents after age 3, commonly around 8–9 years old, with aplastic anemia. Historically, this condition was fatal; however, bone marrow transplants have been performed successfully to treat the anemia and prolong the life expectancy[5]	Autosomal recessive
VACTERL association	A sporadic collection of anomalies consisting of vertebral deformity, anal atresia, cardiac anomalies, tracheoesophageal fistula, renal agenesis, and limb deformities	Sporadic

must, not only with distraction but also often for a second set of hands to hold a stretch.[14] At this age, custom-molded orthoses that stretch the wrist into ulnar deviation, as well as thumb opposition orthoses for thumb abduction, are utilized. Orthoses to prevent radial deviation are best molded past the elbow just distal to the axilla. A longer orthosis allows pressure to be distributed over a larger surface area, decreasing the risk of pressure points distally and proximally and increasing comfort. This length also helps to prevent the child from removing the orthosis (Picture 9.4). Distally, the orthosis should extend down to the fingers with a cut out area for the thumb if present. Increasingly, feeding becomes important to both the child

and the parent. Adapted equipment, such as curved silverware, scoop dishes with suction, and universal cuffs, can be helpful for the child to feel independence. Often, simply switching to plastic silverware that is lighter in weight and easier to hold is sufficient. This is also a prime time to observe pinch-and-grasp patterns and ask parents which grasp they are observing in the home setting most often (Picture 9.5A–C).

Children 18 months to 4 years old have a resistance to control, making this the most difficult age to fabricate orthoses. It is important to distract, but also to realize that this group works well with rewards. Making orthotic fabrication a game with appropriate choices and a reward at the end, such as a sticker, is often a sufficient strategy.[14] Orthoses remain customized to the patient, typically worn only at night, and are remolded as the child grows. ADLs for young children include simple dressing maneuvers for toilet training. Difficulties pulling up and down pants due to weak grasp or insufficient arm length are two common complaints. Sewing loops in the pants and placing hooks on the wall allow the upper arms to complete these tasks instead of relying on small muscles in the hand and fingers for pinch and grasping. There are several toilet aid options on the market to assist with reach, and parents are increasingly investing in bidets to ease this task at home.

As children enter school, they become more flexible in their thinking and begin to follow directions. They tend to love being involved in the orthosis fabrication process. Engaging them with choices, such as orthosis and strap color to assist in the orthotic creation, gives them more ownership.[14] Orthoses are typically worn at night to continue with stretching of the wrist. Activity-specific orthoses for sports and recreation, which protect joints during activity, are also used during this time (Picture 9.6). ADLs in this age group involve more fine motor tasks such as buttoning, zipping, and school-related activities, such as cutting and writing. There are several options such as button hooks, zipper pulls, spring-loaded easi-loop scissors, and writing aids to help with these activities (Picture 9.7). Children can benefit from pencil grips, cylindrical foam build-ups, or even a simple hair band to assist with holding a pencil in the hand. Children are also riding bikes, playing sports and doing extracurricular activities that sometimes warrant the use of an assistive device or a special fabricated prosthetic to complete the task.

Typically, additional orthotic fabrication does not become necessary again until adolescence, when patients are socially dependent on their peers, generally

TABLE 9.4
Radial Longitudinal Deficiency Evaluation.

- Careful examination of the entire patient
- Scoliosis screening
- Complete Blood Count (CBC), renal ultrasound, echocardiogram
- +/− Diepoxybutane-induced chromosomal breakage assay

distrust adults, and have a more fragile body image. It is important to educate the patient on the purpose of the orthosis and consequences of noncompliance. Orthotic fabrication only works if the adolescent buys in to the treatment.[14] Typical orthoses at this age are intended for support during activity rather than focused on stretching. Often, these kids also need more supportive options to complete tasks, such as extracurricular activities in music, sports, art, or even weight lifting (Picture 9.8A and B).

In addition to physicians and hand therapists, support groups, child-life specialists, and child psychologists play an important role in helping patients and their parents cope with the significant societal issues many of these individuals face. To meet this need, the authors started a hand camp, inviting children and parents to meet other individuals with congenital hand differences, to assist with fostering independence and self-confidence through recreation and team building activities.

SURGERY AND SURGICAL STEPS
Radial Longitudinal Deficiency

Patients with type I or II radial longitudinal dysplasia typically do not require surgical intervention to address the wrist. Patients with more severe dysplasia may benefit from surgical intervention with options ranging from soft-tissue rebalancing alone to full centralization/radialization of the wrist or even vascularized toe transfer.

Ekbolm demonstrated that range of motion, forearm length, grip, and key pinch strength are more important than radial angulation for daily activity and participation.[15] Thus, serial examinations and response to appropriate nonsurgical treatments are an important component of the preoperative assessment. Centralization may lead to undergrowth of an already shortened ulna.[16] Moreover, in a child who grasps objects between his or her ring and small finger, it may actually worsen hand-to-mouth function. Severe radial dysplasia with

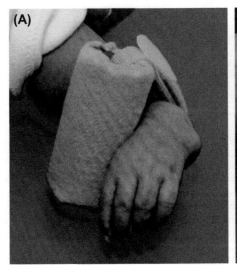 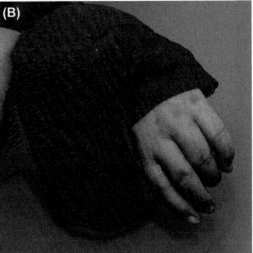

PICTURE 9.1 **(A)** Cylindrical foam covered with moleskin can be used early on to begin stretching with children who have a radially deviated wrist. **(B)** The entire orthosis is covered with coban to help keep cylindrical foam in place.

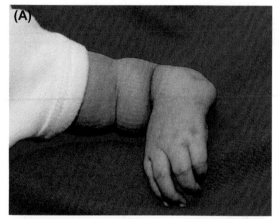

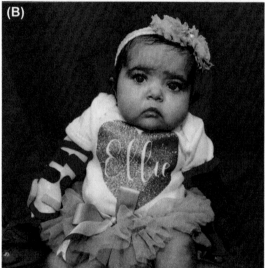

PICTURE 9.2 **(A)** Radial deviation at wrist often requires an orthosis at night to help increase/maintain motion and prevent further deviation. **(B)** An orthosis to help stretch wrist out of radial deviation can be held on with straps or coban depending on the age of patient and parent preference. Either technique to keep splint in place can be utilized effectively with proper education.

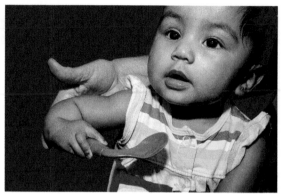

PICTURE 9.3 Once child is ready to begin age appropriate eating, curved silverware can increase independence.

and flexor carpi radialis are transposed to the ulnar side.[19] With either procedure, wrist deformity tends to occur[20] without substantial improvement in function.[15]

In our practice, soft-tissue release with a bilobed flap reconstruction has provided the most reliable and effective results.[21] This procedure is typically performed between 18 months and 2 years old. In this procedure, constricting or deforming soft-tissue structures are released with creation of a biloped flap for skin closure. Although this procedure may be combined with other surgical procedures to address mild thumb hypoplasia, including webspace deepening and opponensplasty

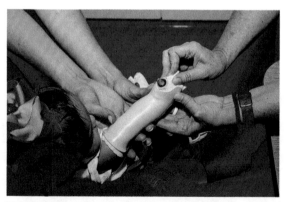

PICTURE 9.4 An orthosis that extends from the proximal shoulder distally to the fingers allows for pressure to be distributed over a larger surface area. This allows greater leverage to maintain placement and increase motion. When the thumb is present, a cut out area for the thumb to pass through is preferred. Additionally, using either a prefab neoprene thumb orthosis adds padding and correct positioning of thumb within the confines of the radially based custom orthosis.

poor elbow or finger function is a contraindication to surgical intervention.

Centralization was first described by Sayre in 1893.[17] Although several modifications have been described, many create a notch in the carpus to align the third metacarpal with the ulna. Gradual distraction of the soft tissues before centralization may be necessary to mitigate the often-severe soft-tissue contractures.[18] Buck-Gramcko describe the radialization procedure, where the second metacarpal is aligned with the ulna in slight ulnar deviation, and the extensor carpi radialis

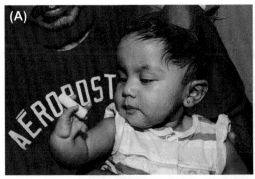
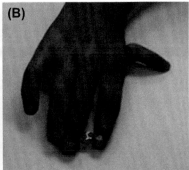
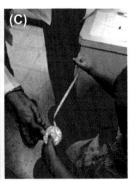

PICTURE 9.5 Observing grasp pattern during intentional play is important information to share with the physician for surgical planning. **(A)** Child using a small to ring pinch grasp. **(B)** Utilization of index to long for preferred pinch. **(C)** Note if and how the thumb is utilized during activity.

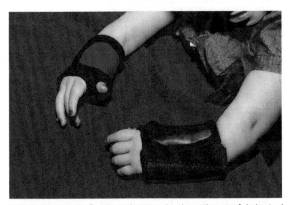

PICTURE 9.6 Custom thermoplastic orthoses fabricated over neoprene orthoses or directly on the wrist can help support the wrist during sport and recreation activities.

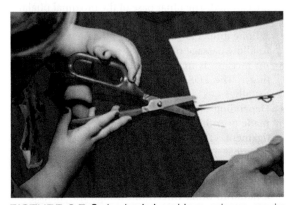

PICTURE 9.7 Spring-loaded easi-loop scissors require less strength, give options for various hand placements, and allow the child to use one or two hands for utilization.

(see later), we prefer to perform pollicization or thumb reconstruction procedures for types IIIB to V thumbs in a staged manner.

Importantly, there is minimal risk for distal ulnar physeal injury, minimizing the risk for further shortening.[22] Additionally, this procedure does not preclude a vascularized bone transfer from the second metatarsal phalangeal joint, as described by Vilkki,[23] to be performed later. This results in a straighter wrist while preserving wrist motion. Although some degree of radial deviation recurrence is expected, we have found that many patients are satisfied with the soft-tissue release alone and do not proceed with the vascularized bone transfer.

Surgical steps—bilobed flap reconstruction

- Before surgery, the patient must undergo adequate soft-tissue stretching with orthoses, serial casting, or, in the most severe cases, external fixator distraction.
- The procedure is performed under general anesthesia.
- A bilobed flap is drawn to take advantage of the redundant tissue on the ulnar side of the wrist. Though a dorsal or volar approach may be used, we employ a volar approach for more direct access to tight structures and less conspicuous scars.
- Under tourniquet control, full-thickness skin flaps are elevated. The finger flexor tendons, median and superficial radial nerves, which may be in an aberrant location, are identified and preserved.
- All tight structures along the radial wrist are released including fascial bands and tendons with pure radial deviation moments, which may be transposed to the ulnar side of the wrist.

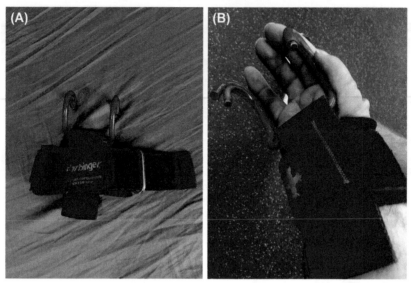

PICTURE 9.8 **(A)** Commercially available Harbinger lifting hooks can be used to assist with weight lifting. **(B)** Wrist support on hand in position to accept weight.

- After adequate release, the wrist is placed in a neutral position and pinned with a 0.062-inch Kirschner wire (K-wire) carefully placed so as not to cross the ulnar physis.
- Skin flaps are rotated and sutured in place with absorbable suture.
- The tourniquet is deflated before long arm-cast application to ensure adequate perfusion of the fingers.
- A long arm cast is maintained for 3–4 weeks at which point the pin is removed and the patient is placed in a removable orthosis.

Thumb Hypoplasia

By definition, type I thumbs have all structures and therefore do not usually require reconstruction. However, they may benefit from a 4-flap Z-plasty of the first webspace. Due to the hypoplastic thenar musculature, type II hypoplastic thumbs often benefit from an opponensplasty, with or without metacarpophalangeal (MP) ligament reconstruction depending on the stability of the joint. This surgery is typically performed at age 4–5, once a child is able to follow specific therapy instructions. Preoperatively, these children are evaluated by the therapist to assess thumb function. It is important preoperatively to assess thumb use and tendencies of grasp and release. We

prefer a flexor digitorum superficialis (FDS) ring transfer over a Huber transfer utilizing the abductor digiti minimi, as the former provides additional tissue for joint reconstruction.

Surgical steps—opponensplasty

- The procedure is performed under general anesthesia.
- A 45° 4-flap Z-plasty is designed along the first webspace
- Under tourniquet control, full-thickness skin flaps are elevated. The ulnar base of the proximal phalanx and distal metacarpal neck is exposed.
- A bone tunnel is made through the metacarpal neck to allow passage of the FDS ring finger tendon.
- An incision is made over the A1 pulley of the ring finger. The FDS tendon is isolated and transected distally.
- Depending on the pulley to be used, an incision is made over the volar ulnar wrist or transverse carpal ligament. The tendon is retracted through this proximal incision and then rerouted around its pulley toward the radial incision.
- The tendon is passed through the bone tunnel in a radial-to-ulnar direction through the metacarpal and may be secured to the ulnar base of the proximal phalanx to reconstruct the ulnar

collateral ligament (UCL). Alternatively, the slips can be split to allow reconstruction of both the UCL and radial collateral ligament (RCL). Tendon ends are secured the proximal phalanx with suture anchors placed distal to the proximal phalanx physis.

- The Z-plasty flaps are rotated to lengthen the first webspace and sutured in place with absorbable suture.
- A 0.045 K-wire is placed across the MP joint to stabilize the thumb.
- The tourniquet is deflated before long arm-cast application to ensure adequate perfusion of the fingers.
- A long arm cast is maintained for 4 weeks at which point the pin is removed and the patient is placed in a removable orthosis.

Although type IIIA thumbs benefit from reconstruction as described earlier, index finger pollicization is our treatment of choice for type IIIB thumbs, due to gross instability of the Carpometacarpal (CMC) joint. Types IV and V thumb hypoplasia are similarly treated with an index finger pollicization. This procedure is typically performed between 18 months and 2 years old. Just as in the treatment for radial longitudinal deficiency, critical assessment of hand function by the surgeon and therapist is necessary before commencing with pollicization. There is not a validated functional evaluation tool to assess thumb use at this age. Therefore, play activities to engage the patient to pick up small to large items (i.e., bean, block and cylinder type objects) are encouraged to see if the patient utilizes the thumb, ignores the thumb, uses a scissor grasp between the index and long or between the ring and small digits. In the case of a stiff index finger, where the child preferentially pinches between the ring and small fingers, pollicization is unlikely to provide much benefit and is not warranted. If the patient is an index/long pincher and the index has started to pronate, indicating that it is already being treated as a potential thumb, then this child would be a good candidate for a pollicization.

A thorough explanation of the procedure by both the surgeon and the therapist to care givers is an important part of the preoperative visit. It should be explained that the index finger will be moved into the thumb position and that the base of the index finger is shortened, rotated, and repositioned to look more like a thumb, reinforcing that it will never be "normal." Occasionally, a vascularized composite second toe transfer is preferred for cultural reasons.

Surgical steps—pollicization

- The procedure is performed under general anesthesia.
- A skin incision is designed to incorporate glabrous skin of the index finger to create a first webspace.
- Under tourniquet control, full-thickness skin flaps are elevated on the volar surface. The radial neurovascular bundle is identified and protected
- Dissection proceeds ulnarly to identify the common digital nerve and vessels to the index and long finger. The artery to the long finger is tied off and proximal microsurgical dissection of the digital nerve allows for mobilization of the pollicized digit.
- The A1 and A2 pulleys are incised to prevent kinking of the flexor tendon, and the intermetacarpal ligament is divided.
- Thin skin flaps are elevated on the dorsal side to preserve veins.
- The first dorsal and second volar/dorsal interossei are released from their insertion on the index digit and tagged for later reconstruction.
- The distal index finger metacarpal physis is incised with #15 blade. A bone cutter is used to osteotomize the metacarpal proximally at the metaphyseal flare. After removing the segment of metacarpal, the base is contoured to allow proper position of the pollicized digit.
- The metacarpal is secured to the carpus with a 0.035″ K-wire holding the digit in radial abduction, palmar abduction, and pronation.
- The first dorsal interossei are repaired to the radial band and the second dorsal/volar interossei are repaired to the lateral band, recreating thumb abductor and adductor function, respectively.
- The skin flaps are inset, removing any redundant skin. The tourniquet is deflated before long arm-cast application to ensure adequate perfusion of the digit.
- A long arm cast is maintained for 4 weeks at which point the pin is removed and the patient is placed in a protective orthosis.

INDICATIONS FOR IMMOBILIZATION/ MOBILIZATION

Presurgery orthotic wear is important for kids born with radial longitudinal dysplasia to stretch the soft tissues in the wrist and hand to increase ROM as well as after surgery to maintain a position obtained in surgery, protect newly repaired or altered structures, and to continue to stretch into a more functional position.

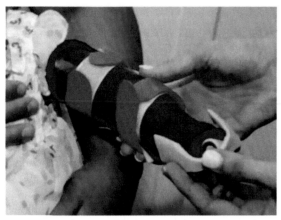

PICTURE 9.9 A radially based orthosis is fabricated from the axilla distally to the tips of the fingers for maximum stretch, distributed pressure, and prevention of child-directed doffing.

Radial Longitudinal Deficiency
Postoperative therapy following a bilobed flap

Once the cast is removed, the patient is referred to therapy for fabrication of a custom radial positioned orthosis and instruction on skin/scar care and gentle A/PROM of the wrist, elbow, and fingers. The orthosis (Picture 9.9) is worn for 6 weeks continually except for bathing and a home exercise program (HEP) and then at night only for an additional 6 weeks or longer if needed. The orthosis extends past the elbow, not only for improved comfort but also for a better stretch due to extending the force of the orthosis over a greater surface area, which in turn decreases the amount of pressure needed to stretch the joint. The longer length also helps to keep the orthosis on the child better and is more difficult for children to remove. It is important for the therapist to take resting as well as A/PROM measurements of the wrist, and to take elbow and finger ROM measurements. When measuring the radial deviation of the wrist, it is important to use the method described by Manske[24] in which one goniometer arm extends along the long finger metacarpal axis and the adjacent arm lies along the longitudinal axis of the distal ulna, with the center of the goniometer at the level of the wrist (Picture 9.10A and B). The resting angle is measured in degrees of radial deviation and passive and active ulnar deviation is typically a negative number if the therapist/patient is unable to reach a neutral wrist position. ADLs are also addressed and depending on whether the condition is bilateral or unilateral, adaptive equipment may be necessary, especially for eating at this age.

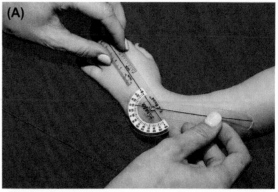

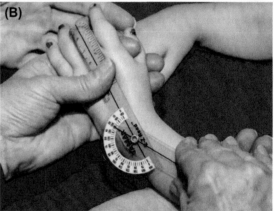

PICTURE 9.10 **(A)** To measure resting angle of wrist in radial deviation place one goniometer arm along the long finger metacarpal and the other arm along the longitudinal axis of the distal ulna with the center of the goniometer at the wrist. **(B)** To measure passive motion, an ulnar-deviated passive stretch is given to the wrist and a new measurement is taken (Please note that this measurement is often a negative number if the wrist is unable to reach a neutral position.).

Thumb Hypoplasia
Postoperative therapy following opponensplasty

Following cast removal and pin pull, the patient is seen by the therapist. Children, being 4–5 years old, are better able to follow directions and understand the process of orthotic fabrication, skin/scar care, and the importance of a home exercise program. We call the exercises program muscle school and compare it to going to school and needing a teacher. We tell the children their thumb needs to go to school and they will be the teacher, teaching their thumb how to work. Much like a pollicization, these children need opportunities to oppose the surgical thumb to the other digits on that hand. If the child had an FDS opponensplasty then offering times for the thumb to oppose to the ring digit will maximize the thumbs ability to learn its new job of opposition instead of flexing the ring digit. In addition, meal, bath, and play times are best utilized for this HEP of "muscle school." Children at this age are typically interested in the process, enjoy being called a teacher, and have caregivers attached to be the "principal" if needed. It is important to review skin/scar care with parents and the importance of daily scar massage. These kids typically fit into a prefab short basic opponens (SBO) orthosis, however, will occasionally need a custom SBO or elastomer insert to maintain proper position of thumb opposition. The orthosis will be utilized at all times for 4 weeks except for bathing and the HEP, then four additional weeks just at night (Fig. 9.1).

Patient Education

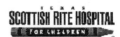

Home Therapy After Opponensplasty

You have had an operation on your thumb called an opponensplasty. Now that your cast has been removed, it is time to start your therapy program. Therapy after your cast comes off is an important part of the success of your operation, and this is the part where you can make a difference! Your therapist will go over the information below with you and make sure you understand what you can do to get the best possible result from your operation.

1. **Skin Care**
   - Wash your hand in warm, soapy water and pat dry with towel three times a day.
   - Next apply lotion or hand cream to the entire hand to moisturize and help remove the old and dry skin. Avoid lotions with vitamins or perfume.
   - Continue this wash/dry/lotion routine until the skin on the hand that had the operation looks like the skin on your other hand — usually one to two weeks.

2. **Scar Care**
   - "Make friends" with your hand. Begin by lightly touching the scar area with your finger, a cotton ball or washcloth many times during the day.
   - As soon as you can tolerate it and for sure by one week after your cast comes off, begin massaging your scar using light to moderate pressure in a circular motion with your thumb or fingers. Massage for one to three minutes three times a day. A little lotion makes this easier.

3. **Splint Use and Care**
   - A therapist will fit your child with a protective and removable hand splint.
   - When you are not washing or exercising the hand, you should be wearing the splint.
   - For the first_____weeks you will wear your splint continuously except for bathing and exercise. Then for the next_____weeks you will wear your splint at night and during strenuous activity.
   - Clean the splint as needed to minimize odor and discomfort. Hard splints can be cleaned using rubbing alcohol and a cotton ball. Soft splints can be washed with soap and water and air-dried.
   You have a_____soft splint (wash with soap and water as needed and air-dry)
   You have a_____hard splint (clean with rubbing alcohol and cotton ball daily)

4. **Exercises: "Muscle School"**
   - The transferred muscle has to "learn" a new function. Here is how the transferred muscle learns some new tricks.
   - Actively bring your thumb and ring finger to touch each other 10 times.
   - Pick up small objects, such as cotton balls, using only your thumb and ring finger. As you start getting more motion, you should progress onto picking up marbles and pennies.
   - Do "muscle school" for five minutes three times a day.

FIG. 9.1 Educational snapshot of home therapy after opponensplasty.

Postoperative therapy following pollicization
Once the cast is removed and the pin is pulled, patients are seen by a therapist. This can be a traumatic time for both the child and the parent. A handout with all information you go over is imperative so caregivers can reference what you said during this often-overwhelming visit. It is important to go over skin and scar care as well as a HEP of oppositional activities to get the new pollicized digit to begin working. These kids need to be in an orthosis for 4 weeks all the time

Patient Education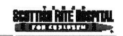

2222 WELBORN STREET | DALLAS, TEXAS 75219 | 214-559-5000 | SCOTTISHRITEHOSPITAL.ORG

Home Therapy After Pollicization

Your child had an operation to move the index finger into the thumb position. This is called a pollicization. Now that the cast has been removed, it is time to start the therapy program. Therapy after the cast comes off is an important part of the success of the operation. This is the part where you can make a difference for your child!

1. Skin Care
  • Wash the hand in warm, soapy water and pat dry with a towel three times a day.
  • Next apply lotion or hand cream to the entire hand to moisturize and help remove the old and dry skin. Avoid lotions with vitamins or perfume.
  • Continue this wash/dry/lotion routine until the skin on the hand that had the operation looks like the skin on the other hand — usually one to two weeks.

2. Scar Care
  • "Make friends" with the hand. Begin by lightly touching the scar area with your finger, a cotton ball or washcloth several times during the day.
  • One week after the cast comes off, begin massaging the scar using light to moderate pressure in a circular motion with your thumb or fingers. Massage for one to three minutes three times a day with lotion.

3. Splint Use and Care
  • Your therapist will fit your child with a protective and removable hand splint.
  • When you are not washing or exercising the hand, your child should be wearing the splint. This splint will be needed for about two weeks.
  • Clean the splint as needed to minimize odor and discomfort. Hard splints can be cleaned using rubbing alcohol and a cotton ball. Soft splints can be washed with soap and water and air-dried.

  You have a_____ soft splint (wash with soap and water as needed and air-dry) You have a__ hard splint (clean with rubbing alcohol and cotton ball daily)

4. "Thumb School" (Starts one week after the cast comes off)
  • The new thumb has to "learn" how to function in its new position, and only you can teach it. Here is how you teach the new thumb some new tricks!
    – Touch the tip of the new thumb to the tip of each finger 10 times – it's okay to help with your hand or your child's other hand.
    – Work on opening the thumb (extending) as much as possible.
    – Pick up small objects, such as cotton balls, using only the tip of the new thumb and one other finger. Progress to picking up marbles and pennies.

9/08
REVIEWED: 3/16   THIS MATERIAL IS FOR EDUCATIONAL USE. DISCUSS ANY QUESTIONS AND CONCERNS WITH YOUR HEALTH CARE PROVIDER.

FIG. 9.2 Educational snapshot of home therapy after pollicization.

and for another 4 weeks just at night. Typically, these children fit nicely into a prefabricated benik SBO orthosis that can be modified easily for proper fit. Due to the age of the child at the time of surgery, neoprene usually does well at holding the surgical position. If you feel this is not enough support, then a custom SBO orthosis can be fabricated (see Fig. 9.2 for home therapy after pollicization). Occasionally children are brought back 2 weeks later, after the chaos of cast removal and the initial post-op visit has subsided to get an elastomer insert or scar pad to soften the scar and better maintain thumb position. Parents are told that the tip of the thumb interphalangeal joint would not typically flex for at least 6 months. Activities to encourage thumb use are typically completed at bath, meal, and play times. Different sized toys and food items entice the patient to use the new thumb to grasp and pinch objects. Food can be very motivating especially if you offer the nonsurgical hand a food item first and then offer the same item to the surgical side. At this age, it is easy for children to forget about their surgery and begin to use the new thumb in functional and play activities. Occasionally, patients choose to scissor between the long and ring fingers instead of using the new pollicized thumb. If this occurs instruct the parents to buddy tape those digits together to encourage thumb use.

CONCLUSIONS

Radial longitudinal deficiency presents as a clinical spectrum dysplasia. As Adrian E. Flatt noted, "*A radial clubhand is not a normal hand set on an abnormal wrist, rather, it is a profoundly abnormal hand joined to a poor limb by a bad wrist.*" Early treatment for patients with radial longitudinal deficiency includes stretching and orthotic fabrication of the wrist. Surgical procedures for realignment of the wrist and to improve thumb function are often performed before the child reaches school age. Therapy must take into account not only the pathology and surgical procedure performed, but also the aptitude of the child to participate in the treatment plan in a meaningful way using adapted techniques and equipment when needed. Additionally, therapy must consider the willingness of the caregivers to adhere to an orthosis wear schedule and daily home exercise program to gain maximum functional potential.

REFERENCES

1. Dy CJ, Swarup I, Daluiski A. Embryology, diagnosis, and evaluation of congenital hand anomalies. *Curr Rev Musculoskelet Med*. 2014;7:60–67.
2. Ogino T, Kato H. Clinical and experimental studies on ulnar ray deficiency. *Handchirurgie*. 1988;20:330–337.
3. Kato H, Ogino T, Minami A, Ohshio I. Experimental study of radial ray deficiency. *J Hand Surg Br*. 1990;15B:470–476.
4. Bavinck JN, Weaver DD. Subclavian artery supply disruption sequence: hypothesis of a vascular etiology for Poland, Klippel-Feil and Mobius anomalies. *Am J Med Genet*. 1986;23(4):903–918.
5. Wall LB, Ezaki MB, Oishi SN. Management of congenital radial longitudinal deficiency: controversies and current concepts. *Plast Reconstr Surg*. 2013;132(1):122–128.
6. Swanson AB. A classification for congenital limb malformations. *J Hand Surg Am*. 1976;1:8–22.
7. Tonkin MA, Tolerton SK, Quick TJ, et al. Classification of congenital anomalies of the hand and upper limb: development and assessment of a new system. *J Hand Surg*. 2013;38A:1845–1853.
8. Bayne LG, Klug MS. Long-term review of the surgical treatment of radial deficiencies. *J Hand Surg Am*. 1987;12(2):169–179.
9. James MA, McCarroll Jr HR, Manske PR. The spectrum of radial longitudinal deficiency: a modified classification. *J Hand Surg Am*. 1999;24(6):1145–1155.
10. Goldfarb CA, Manske PR, Busa R, Mills J, Carter P, Ezaki M. Upper-extremity phocomelia reexamined: a longitudinal dysplasia. *J Bone Joint Surg Am*. 2005;87(12):2639–2648.
11. Blauth W. The hypoplastic thumb. *Arch Orthop Unfall-Chir*. 1967;62(3):225–246.
11a. James MA, McCarroll HR, Manske Jr and PR. Characteristics of patients with hypoplastic thumbs. *J Hand Surg Am*. 1996;21(1):104–113.
12. Manske PR, McCarroll Jr HR, James M. Type III-A hypoplastic thumb. *J Hand Surg Am*. 1995;20(2):246–253.
13. Goldfarb CA, Wall L, Manske PR. Radial longitudinal deficiency: the incidence of associated medical and musculoskeletal conditions. *J Hand Surg Am*. 2006;31:1176–1182.
14. Lake A. Hand therapy for children with congenital hand differences. *Tech Hand Surg*. 2010;14:78–84.
15. Ekblom AG, Dahlin LB, Rosberg HE, Wiig M, Werner M, Arner M. Hand function in adults with radial longitudinal deficiency. *J Bone Joint Surg Am*. 2014;96(14):1178–1184.
16. Sestero AM, Van Heest A, Agel J. Ulnar growth patterns in radial longitudinal deficiency. *J Hand Surg Am*. 2006;31(6):960–967.
17. Sayre RH. A contribution to the study of club-hand. *Trans Am Orthop Assn*. 1893;6:208–216.
18. Kessler I. Centralisation of the radial club hand by gradual distraction. *J Hand Surg Br*. 1989;14(1):37–42.
19. Buck-Gramcko D. Radialization as a new treatment for radial club hand. *J Hand Surg Am*. 1985;10(6 Pt 2):964–968.

20. Damore E, Kozin SH, Thoder JJ, Porter S. The recurrence of deformity after surgical centralization for radial clubhand. *J Hand Surg Am.* 2000;25(4): 745–751.

21. Vuillermin C, Wall L, et al. Soft tissue release and bilobed flap for severe radial longitudinal deficiency. *J Hand Surg Am.* 2015;40(5):894–899.

22. Vuillermin C, Butler L, Ezaki M, Oishi S. Ulna growth patterns after soft tissue release with bilobed flap in radial longitudinal deficiency. *J Pediatr Orthop.* 2018;38(4): 244–248.

23. Vilkki SK. Vascularized metatarsophalangeal joint transfer for radial hypoplasia. *Semin Plast Surg.* 2008;22(3): 195–212.

24. Manske PR, McCarroll HR, Swanson K. Centralization of the radial club hand: an ulnar surgical approach. *J Hand Surg Am.* 1981;6(5):423–433.

CHAPTER 10

Arthrogryposis

DAN A. ZLOTOLOW, MD

INTRODUCTION

Arthrogryposis, also known as arthrogryposis multiplex congenita (AMC) is a rare diagnosis that applies to all children with congenital joint contractures affecting more than one limb. Multiple conditions fall within the AMC umbrella, including progressive neuromuscular disorders such as spinal muscular atrophy, idiopathic disorders such as amyoplasia, and inheritable nonprogressive disorders such as Beal's syndrome and other distal arthrogryposes (DAs). All told, there are over 300 myriad disorders that fit under the AMC umbrella.[1] Having a single chapter on "Arthrogryposis" is akin to having a single chapter on "Fractures." Each of the 300+ variations have their own personality, prognosis, and management. This chapter will therefore focus on the most common types, and could not possibly cover all phenotypes or genotypes.

Amyoplasia is the single most common type, accounting for around 30% of cases. Presentation can range from bilateral mild joint stiffness to complete skeletal muscle aplasia and gastroschisis requiring permanent ventilatory support and tube feeds. Most children, however, are born within a narrow range of the typical phenotype, with the shoulders adducted and internally rotated, elbows extended, forearms in neutral, wrists in flexion, and fingers in flexion with the thumbs in the palm (Fig. 10.1A). Because the posture of the arm is nearly identical to the "waiter's tip" (Fig. 10.1B), amyoplasia isolated to the upper extremities is most commonly misdiagnosed as a bilateral brachial plexus birth injury (BPBI), or Erb's palsy. Clinically, the two diagnoses can be differentiated by the restriction of passive motion in amyoplasia. Children with a BPBI should have full passive motion up to 2 months of age, when shoulder internal rotation and elbow flexion contractures begin to develop. Lower limb involvement is also common in amyoplasia with club feet present in most cases. Another distinct common feature of amyoplasia is a stork-bite hemangioma around the bridge of the nose and/or the occiput (Fig. 10.2), which is thought to be associated with maternal estrogen levels.[2] The etiology of amyoplasia remains unknown, but there is speculation of primary muscular versus anterior horn cell aplasia or apoptosis. Theories of extrinsic causes for amyoplasia such as oligohydramnios and bicornuate uterus are falling out of favor.[3] A genetic cause or predisposition has yet to be found. We have never seen both of a set of identical twins affected with amyoplasia, suggesting that genetics is unlikely to play a role.

Different from amyoplasia, the DAs (Fig. 10.3), of which there are now over 10 types (Table 10.1), do have a predominantly autosomal dominant genetic etiology. Presentation is again quite variable, with some forms of Escobar syndrome resulting in fetal demise and other types such as Sheldon-Hall typically having excellent upper limb function and a normal lifespan.

Regardless of etiology, the role of the therapist in caring for these patients is threefold: (1) assessing the child's function and functional goals, (2) assisting with surgical planning, and (3) providing pre- and postoperative therapy. The treatment goals are to maximize joint motion, compensatory strategies, and overall independence.

CLASSIFICATION

There are three basic subtypes to AMC: (1) amyoplasia, (2) distal arthrogryposes, and (3) congenital neuromuscular conditions. Within these subtypes, amyoplasia encompasses a wide range of presentations but these variations are believed to be due to severity of involvement rather than to a different etiology or subdiagnosis. The DAs are distinct inheritable disorders that may have variable phenotypes within each genotype, but are overall consistent with their patterns of involvement. Beal's syndrome, for example, presents with characteristic camptodactyly and arachnodactyly (contractural arachnodactyly) in nearly all patients, but the degree of contracture varies widely from patient to patient. The third and least common category includes the most distinct disorders, with well over 300 central nervous system and neuromuscular disorders (Table 10.2).

Pediatric Hand Therapy. https://doi.org/10.1016/B978-0-323-53091-0.00010-5

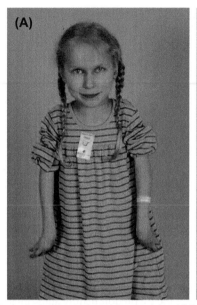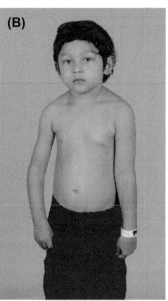

FIG. 10.1 The typical presentation of the arm of a child with amyoplasia (A) is similar to that of a child with a brachial plexus birth injury (B). The two can be differentiated by the absence of congenital contractures in plexus injuries. Plexus injuries also tend to not have bilateral involvement.

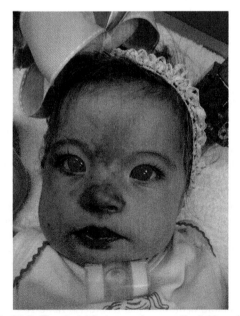

FIG. 10.2 The stork bite hemangioma on the bridge of the nose is present in most children with amyoplasia, but its absence does not rule out the condition.

There is currently no schema by which to classify the severity of involvement, and despite what some have suggested,[4] we have found no identifiable pattern of involvement. Some children have normal lower extremities and very limited upper limb function. Others have the exact opposite. Side-to-side differences are less dramatic. If a patient has asymmetric involvement, some have suggested a central neurologic insult and have recommended imaging of the brain and cervical spine.[5] Despite a classic presentation as described earlier, exceptions are the rule and each child has to be assessed individually.

INITIAL VISIT ASSESSMENT AND EARLY MANAGEMENT

We recommend an initial visit to a therapist or surgeon within the first 2 months of life. Because of the rarity of the diagnosis, families are often misinformed or unaware of the diagnosis and are often hurting emotionally. The primary goal of the initial visit is to explain and/or confirm the diagnosis and answer all the questions asked by the family. It is important for families to understand that most conditions with congenital contractures improve over time, that there is hope that their child will be able to be independent, and that they are a critical part of the care team. For the family,

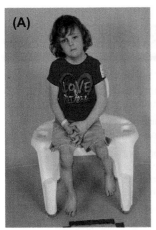 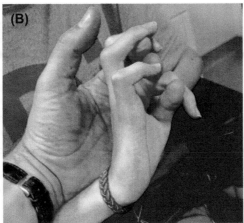 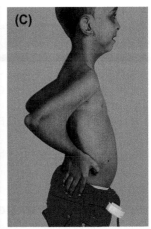

FIG. 10.3 Distal arthrogryposes include Sheldon-Hall (A), Beal's (B), and Escobar (C) syndromes.

this initial interaction with the medical team, who will usher them through their grieving period and into a place where the family can become meaningful participants in their child's care, is critical for building a long-term relationship that best serves the patient.

In neonates, the examination is mostly observational: watch for spontaneous active motion of the limbs as the child lies on an examination table or in their caretaker's arms. Each upper extremity joint complex is assessed for active and passive range of motion. Look for shoulder position and motion, particularly rotation. Determine passive and active elbow, forearm, wrist, and hand motion. In the older child, test grasping ability, writing method, and strength throughout the limb(s). When a child is of age to engage in perineal care, determine if this is best done around the back, or through the legs. Resist the temptation to intervene early with functional aids or functional tricks; allow the child to develop their own compensatory movement patterns. Counsel the family to provide as minimal assistance to the child as possible. Let the child figure things out for themselves whenever possible. Once the child asks for support, provide tips and tricks first, and specialized equipment later.

Most children with amyoplasia will have shoulder internal rotation contractures with a deficit of passive and active external rotation. This will result in a crossover grasp pattern (Fig. 10.4). Elbow extension contractures are more common (Fig. 10.1), but flexion contractures can also occur. Generally, children with both active elbow flexion and extension will have minimal contractures. Children with elbow flexion contractures typically have weak or absent triceps function. Conversely, extension contractures are most often the result of weak or absent elbow flexors. It is rare, but not unheard of, for a child to have no active elbow flexion and retain passive motion. Children with DAs most commonly have a functional active elbow arc of motion in both flexion and extension. The exception is Escobar syndrome, which presents with elbow flexion contractures and pterygia (Fig. 10.3).

Much has been written about the forearm protonation contractures of children with AMC, despite protonation contractures being just as common as supination contractures, and both being relatively uncommon. Most children have a limited arc of forearm motion, both passive and active, that is centered around neutral. Analogous to elbow contractures, forearm contractures follow the principle that the joint will contract in the position of action of the active muscles. Children with AMC typically have no biceps, no supinator, no pronator teres, and no pronator quadratus, so their forearms remain in a neutral position.

The wrist in amyoplasia is most often in flexion and ulnar deviation (Fig. 10.1), but can also be in extension and/or ulnar deviation. By contrast, wrist extension is the norm, but not the rule in DAs (Fig. 10.5A). Nearly all children will have limited passive and active motion regardless of diagnosis or wrist position. Wrist extension contractures in DAs are often accompanied by ulnar deviation of the finger metacarpophalangeal (MP) joints, particularly when the wrist is in radial deviation. In amyoplasia, if the wrist is in flexion and the patient retains active extrinsic finger extension (extensor indicis proprius, extensor digitorum communis, extensor digiti minimi), the MP joints will posture in extension. Some children will be born with or quickly develop MP joint hyperextension contractures.

TABLE 10.1
Distal Arthrogryposis Types.

Distal Arthrogryposis Types	Other Name(s)	Label	Characteristic Findings
Distal arthrogryposis type 1	Common or typical	DA1	Camptodactyly, clasped thumb, clubfoot
Distal arthrogryposis type 2A	Freeman–Sheldon syndrome	DA2A	Whistling face, camptodactyly, clasped thumb, clubfoot, scoliosis
Distal arthrogryposis type 2B	Sheldon-Hall syndrome	DA2B	Prominent nasolabial folds, downslanting palpebral fissures, small mouth, camptodactyly, clasped thumb, clubfoot
Distal arthrogryposis type 3	Gordon syndrome	DA3	Short stature, cleft palate
Distal arthrogryposis type 4	Scoliosis	DA4	Scoliosis, camptodactyly
Distal arthrogryposis type 5	Ophthalmoplegia, ptosis	DA5	Ptosis, strabismus, restrictive lung disease
Distal arthrogryposis type 6	Sensorineural hearing loss	DA6	Hearing loss, camptodactyly
Distal arthrogryposis type 7	Trismus-pseudocamptodactyly	DA7	Trismus, pseudocamptodactyly, short stature
Distal arthrogryposis type 8	Autosomal dominant multiple pterygium syndrome, Escobar	DA8	Multiple pterigia, camptodactyly, scoliosis, ptosis, downslanting palpebral fissures
Distal arthrogryposis type 9	Beals syndrome (congenital contractural arachnodactyly)	DA9	Camptodactly, arachnodactyly, kinked upper earlobe, tall stature
Distal arthrogryposis type 10	Congenital plantar contractures	DA10	Plantar contractures

Adapted from Bamshad M, Van Heest AE, Pleasure D. Arthrogryposis: a review and update. J Bone Joint Surg. 2009; 91(Suppl 4):40–46.

The interphalangeal finger joints will typically be stiff or even ankylosed, with absent or diminished flexion creases. The lack of fingers creases is the telltale sign of a stiff or ankylosed joint. Camptodactyly, a flexion contracture of the proximal interphalangeal (PIP) joint, is common, particularly in the central two fingers (Fig. 10.6). The thumb can present with isolated MP or carpometacarpal (CMC) joint flexion contractures, or a combination of both (Fig. 10.7). Clasp thumb, extension of the CMC and flexion of the MP joints (Fig. 10.5), though considered to be common in AMC, is predominantly seen in DAs and rare in amyoplasia. Most patients with amyoplasia will have flexion at both thumb MP and CMC joints to some degree, but the CMC flexion contracture will be the primary deformity (Fig. 10.8).

Initial treatment is always passive range of motion exercises with an emphasis on a home stretching program. It is not possible to rely solely on the therapy provided by a professional once to a few times a weeks. As we tell our patients, passive stretching is like eating: it is

good to be fed a few times a week, but better to feed yourself three times a day. Some of the best results I have seen are from caretakers who had the time and

TABLE 10.2
Examples of Central Nervous System and Neuromuscular Disorders That Cause Arthrogryposis.

Central Nervous System	Neuromuscular
Moebius syndrome	Maternal myasthenia gravis
X-linked spinal muscular atrophy	Maternal Botox administration
Infantile spinal muscular atrophy (Werdnig–Hoffmann disease)	Congenital muscular dystrophy
	Emery–Dreifuss muscular dystrophy

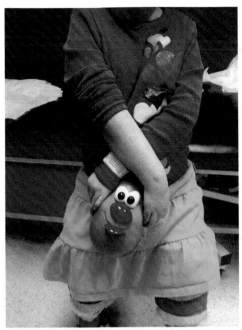

FIG. 10.4 Children with amyoplasia will often have internal rotation contractures of the shoulder that require a crossover grasp pattern for bimanual function. This is a poor compensation strategy because the thumb and palm are obscured from the patient's line of sight.

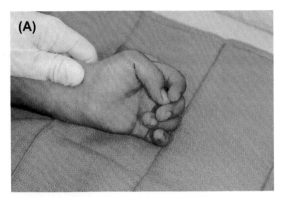

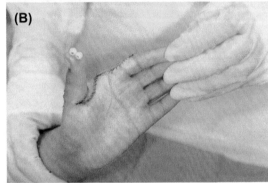

FIG. 10.5 The typical presentation of the thumb in patients with distal arthrogryposes is a clasp thumb (A). Correction of the deformity often requires a stiletto index rotation flap and metacarpophalangeal joint chondrodesis (B).

discipline to range the child every hour on the hour while awake. Although this intense a therapy regimen is unattainable for most, it does demonstrate that, at least in some cases, more therapy is better. As a guideline, we tell our deputized therapists to move every joint that does not move by itself.

Neonates are often too small and some too contracted to be fitted with splints. Even when splints become technically possible, somewhere between 3 and 6 months, we prefer to splint only at night and naptimes to allow unencumbered motion during the day for cognitive and muscle mass development. Common splints include wrist and finger extension, thumb spica wrist extension, and elbow flexion hourglass splints (Fig. 10.9). Dynamic splints are poorly tolerated and have questionable value when considering the cost.

REFERRAL TO AN UPPER LIMB SPECIALIST

Because of the rarity of AMC, it is uncommon for the local therapist, pediatric orthopedist, or upper extremity surgeon to have ever cared for a child with this diagnosis. The information in most textbooks or featured online is either outdated, incorrect, misleading, or

incomplete. Additionally, the scarcity of patients has forced expertise to coalesce around a handful of centers worldwide. Were it not for a robust patient support group (https://amcsupport.org), patients and families would have no referral network to access specialists who are proficient at diagnosing and treating these conditions. Patients whom I see at a late age have often been neglected, told erroneously that there was nothing that could be done to help them, or even worse, received multiple well-intentioned but ill-performed, ill-conceived, or unindicated surgeries. There is little margin for error with these patients due to their often severely limited limb motion, and one mistake can cause an irreversible loss of future independence for the child.

We therefore recommend a referral to a center specializing in AMC (listed in www.amcsupport.org) at or before 6 months of age, before surgical decisions need to be made. The time between 6 and 12 months is critical, because gains made during this time will influence the long-term prognosis and management plan. We are fairly aggressive in our attempts to

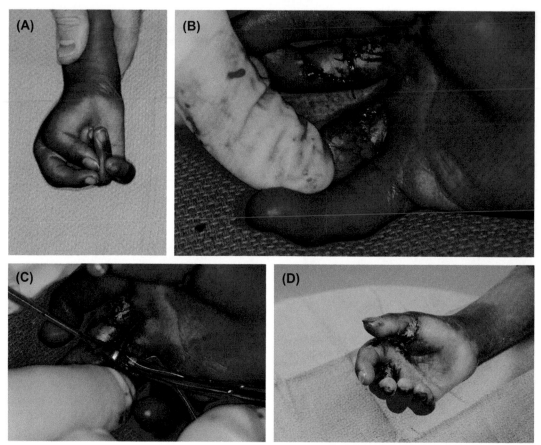

FIG. 10.6 Camptodactyly, defined as a flexion contracture of the proximal interphalangeal joint, is common in all forms of arthrogryposis (A). Release of the contracture can be accomplished with a volar Z-plasty (B) and flexor digitorum superficialis tenotomy (C). The correction is rarely complete (D), and can recur over time.

achieve at least 90 degrees of passive elbow flexion by 12 months of age, because the best results from a surgical elbow release are achieved between 12 and 24 months of age (Zlotolow 2019). Children who have at least 20 degrees of passive elbow flexion are prescribed a daily stretching routine as well as night and naptime hourglass splints. Self-adhesive bandages such as Coban (3M, St. Paul MN) can also be used to apply a steady flexion force to the elbow (https://youtu.be/7QG8_ThW22Y). For children with less than 20 degrees of passive elbow flexion, it is difficult to determine the orientation of the elbow joint without an X-ray, and we discourage passive elbow range of motion exercises in those elbows. We have seen stretching in varus/valgus instead of flexion/extension lead to attenuation of the collateral ligaments about the elbow.

SURGICAL INTERVENTIONS AND POSTOPERATIVE REHABILITATION

For children who do not adequately achieve the requisite range of motion for functional independence using nonsurgical techniques, surgical intervention can be a useful adjunct treatment. The timing of surgery is controversial. So far, only an elbow release has been shown to benefit from earlier intervention, with the best results before 2 years old.[6] Otherwise, there is some suggestion that other procedures may actually have improved outcomes if delayed past the age of 7 or 8.[7,8]

Because passive elbow flexion past 90 degrees and elbow extension within 30 degrees of full motion are so critical to future independence, we prioritize achieving elbow flexion while maintaining adequate elbow extension. We therefore do not recommend, as others have suggested and many centers practice, to

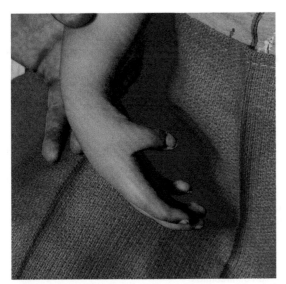

FIG. 10.7 Children with amyoplasia often have a "thumb to nowhere" that is in the palm and underpronated, compromising pinch and grasp.

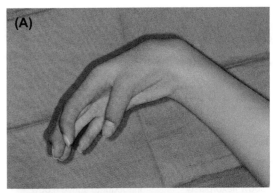

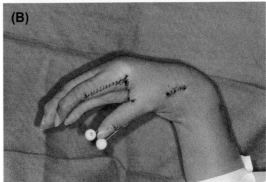

FIG. 10.8 For children with primarily a thumb carpometacarpal joint flexion and supination contracture (A), a thumb reorientation osteotomy can be performed just distal to the thumb metacarpal physis a stiletto index rotation flap to reorient the thumb into a "sock puppet" type position for better pinch and grasp (B). Note that the thumb correction can be performed even when the wrist is not able to be improved, but that adequate finger and thumb active motion are required to benefit optimally from the operation.

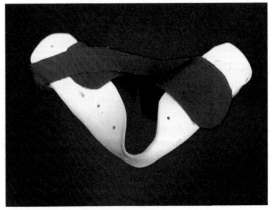

FIG. 10.9 The "hourglass" splint is our workhorse for progressive passive stretching of the elbow into flexion.

perform concomitant procedures along with an elbow release. We typically will wait to perform corrective surgery for the forearm, wrist, and hand until the child is older and the risk of deformity recurrence is likely lower (Table 10.3). One notable exception is a humeral rotational osteotomy to correct the shoulder internal rotation contracture. We have demonstrated that concomitant ipsilateral humeral rotational osteotomy and release is possible,[9] but results in a worse outcome regarding elbow flexion/extension.[10] However, it is unclear if staging the release and osteotomy result in a better outcome, or if the order of the procedures matters. In general, we prefer to rotate the humerus first if the shoulder has a 90-degree or greater internal rotation contracture, because the torso itself becomes a block to elbow flexion in these children, complicating postoperative rehabilitation of an elbow release. In children who require both an osteotomy and a release bilaterally, we will perform a release on the dominant side and an osteotomy on the nondominant side simultaneously using two surgical teams to minimize surgical and anesthesia time and to lessen the number of times under the child requires anesthesia.

Humeral Rotational Osteotomy

The determination of how much to rotate the humerus is made in concert with the family, the patient, the therapist, and the surgeon: if the external rotation is too much, the child may lose through-legs perineal care; if

TABLE 10.3
Surgical Timing.

Intervention	Indications	Timing	Exceptions
Humeral rotational osteotomy	Internal rotation contracture of the shoulder	Open	Before elbow release to facilitate postrelease rehabilitation. Recurrence may be less in older patients.
Elbow release	Elbow extension contracture >90 degrees	12–24 months	Delay if >75 degrees of flexion at 12 months and improving
Elbow flexorplasty	Inadequate active elbow flexion but passive flexion greater than 90 degrees	After 4 years old or when child able to cooperate with therapist instructions	Contraindicated in limb used for perineal care because or flexion contracture risk
One-bone forearm	Pronation or supination contracture that limits function	Open, but always after correction of shoulder internal rotation and elbow extension contractures	None
Carpal wedge	Inadequate wrist extension	Open, but better after age 7	May be done early to improve finger MP hyperextension contractures. Not for patients that (1) weight bear on dorsal wrist, (2) require wrist flexion to reach mouth or perineum, (3) lack finger MP extension
Thumb MP fusion	Fixed thumb MP flexion contracture (clasped thumb)	Open	None
Thumb reorientation osteotomy	Fixed thumb CMC flexion contracture	After age 7	May be done early to improve thumb function during development, but will require revision. Should be done after carpal wedge if one is indicated.
Camptodactyly release	Fixed finger PIP flexion contracture >30 degrees	May be best before 24 months old	None

not enough, the child will not have the hands to face each other for bimanual tasks. A variety of surgical approaches have been proposed,[11] but the medial or anterolateral approaches are most common.[12] The bone is cut, the humerus is rotated until the shoulder sits in neutral to slight internal rotation, and the osteotomy is affixed with a bone plate and screws. A fracture brace is measured before surgery and fitted 3 weeks after surgery. Wear is full time except for bathing until union is confirmed on radiographs. The child can resume their regular rehabilitation schedule after the brace is discontinued. There is a higher risk of fracture for a further

6 weeks, so we recommend limiting to only supervised self-ambulation until 12 weeks after surgery.

Elbow Release

We will only perform an elbow release on one side at a time and if there is less than a 30-degree flexion contracture on the contralateral side. Although the risk of a postoperative elbow flexion contracture is low, the result of loss of sufficient elbow extension to be independent in the bathroom can be devastating. The procedure is performed through a posterior approach (Fig. 10.10). The ulnar nerve is transposed subcutaneously, the triceps

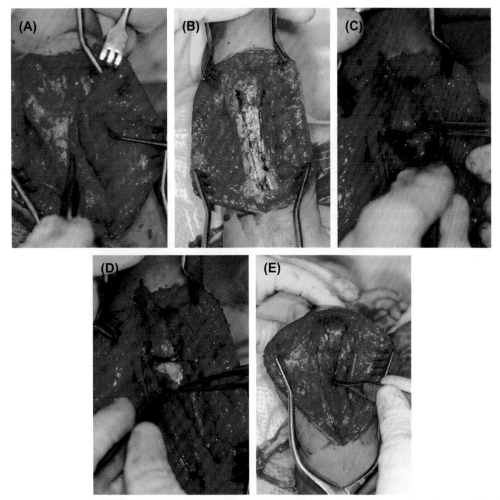

FIG. 10.10 A posterior elbow release can typically grant 30–100 degrees of passive motion when combined with ulnar nerve transposition (A) and triceps lengthening. The triceps is lengthened through a V-shaped incision in the tendon (B). After the capsule is released (C) and the medial head of the triceps is elevated off the bone (D), the triceps is lengthened via a V-to-Y repair (E).

tendon is lengthened in a V-to-Y fashion, the posterior elbow capsule is removed, and the medial head of the triceps is elevated off the bone (https://youtu.be/P0lPEuBMTN8). The patient is placed in a posterior plaster elbow splint for 2 weeks. They then return for a 3-day intensive therapy outpatient stay, with morning and afternoon sessions. Both flexion and extension orthoplast splints are fabricated at that time. Weekly supervised therapy sessions follow. The bulk of the therapy falls upon the caretakers. The results of surgery correlate directly to the efforts put forth by the family during the critical 3 months after surgery. If the patient does not have an arc of at least 30–100 degrees of motion at 3 months, they are brought in for a manipulation under anesthesia and reinitiate the intensive outpatient therapy protocol for 3 days thereafter.

Elbow Flexorplasty

Patients who have adequate passive elbow flexion beyond 90 degrees and do not rely on the ipsilateral hand for perineal care may be considered for an elbow flexorplasty. Our technique of choice is the bipolar latissimus flexorplasty, but other options have been suggested.[13–18] The latissimus must be easily palpable with a strong voluntary contraction to be considered for transfer. Absence of a pectoralis major is a contraindication because the patient will lose shoulder adduction and internal rotation if the pectoralis is absent and the latissimus is removed. The technique is complicated and requires harvesting of the entire latissimus muscle on its neurovascular pedicle (Fig. 10.11). The muscle is then shuttled through the deltopectoral interval to the anterior shoulder while avoiding tension on the neurovascular pedicle. Proximally, the latissimus insertion is affixed to the coracoid using transosseous sutures. The muscle is then tunneled under the skin and affixed to the biceps if the patient has active protonation and lacks supination, or to the proximal ulna if there is no active protonation. The tension is set so that the transfer is tight at 30 degrees shy of full elbow extension. A skin paddle overlying the muscle is routinely taken to monitor the flap viability. The arm is then placed in a 90-degree flexion splint for 4—6 weeks, depending on the quality of the distal fixation. Sensory innervation of the skin paddle is variable postoperatively, with some patients reporting sensation in their back when their paddle is touched. This referred sensation to the back will relocalize to the arm around 3 months after surgery, and is usually a sign of cortical reorientation of the muscle's function.

The child returns for their initial postoperative visit between 4 and 6 weeks. The splint is removed and a hinged elbow brace is placed. Elbow extension is restricted to 60 degrees and advanced by 15 degrees per week until full extension is achieved. It is common to have a persistent 15—20-degree elbow flexion contracture. Any flexion contracture beyond 30 degrees by 3 months postoperatively should merit a change in the rehabilitation program to emphasize elbow extension.

Weight bearing and resistive exercises are restricted for 3 months after surgery.

One-Bone Forearm

For patients with supination or protonation forearm contractures that limit function, we have found rotational osteotomies of the radius and/or ulna tend to recur over time. Although a one-bone forearm removes all forearm motion, the procedure has the advantage of allowing a permanent positional correction of the forearm. Because the position is permanent, extra care should be taken to ensure that the chosen forearm position is optimal to accomplish the patient's functional goals. Generally, this is a neutral position, but a range from 30 degrees of protonation or supination is often acceptable depending on the use of that limb and input from the therapist. Supination can help with self-feeding and can assist with bimanual tasks if the other hand is in protonation. Slight protonation is best for the hand that is used for perineal care.

The procedure is carried out through a volar radial and a posterior ulnar approach. An ulnar and a radial osteotomy are made, with the ulnar osteotomy just proximal to the radial osteotomy so that there is overlap between the bones. The distal radius is then brought to the proximal ulna, and a plate and screws are used for fixation (Fig. 10.12). Rotation is usually set between 30 degrees of protonation or supination depending on the needs of the patient. A sugar-tong splint is applied for 4 weeks, followed by a Munster splint until union of the osteotomies. There are no special rehabilitation needs.

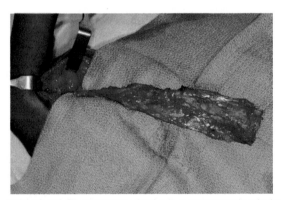

FIG. 10.11 The latissimus dorsi, when present and actively recruitable, has been the most reliable flexorplasty for granting these children active elbow flexion. Flexion contractures of 15—30 degrees are common, and typical active flexion achieved varies between 90 and 120 degrees.

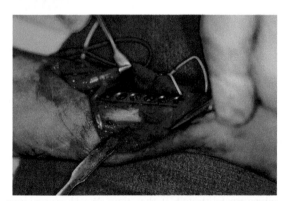

FIG. 10.12 A one bone forearm, where the distal radius is placed on top of the proximal ulna and secured with a plate, has become our go-to surgery for correcting forearm contractures. Although the procedure removes any remaining forearm rotation, it allows for placement of the forearm in the optimal position of approximately 30 degrees of protonation with minimal to no recurrence risk.

Carpal Wedge Osteotomy

Wrist extension improves grasp and pinch and enhances the appearance of the arm, and there are multiple reasons to be cautious before placing the wrist in more extension in patients with AMC. Contraindications include the patient (1) weight bearing on the dorsum of the wrist for scooting, support, or ambulation, (2) requiring wrist flexion to reach their mouth because of insufficient elbow flexion, (3) requiring wrist flexion to reach their perineum, and (4) requiring wrist flexion to have adequate finger extension.

The carpal wedge osteotomy was developed to maintain some wrist motion while realigning the arc of motion into greater extension.[7,19] A carpal wedge is permanent and cannot be repeated. The procedure can also correct a maximum of 50 degrees of flexion and about 20 degrees of ulnar deviation. The results are variable but dependent on the tendon transfer to power active wrist extension. Most commonly, the extensor carpi ulnaris (ECU) tendon is used as a transfer, but the flexor carpi radialis or ulnaris (FCR or FCU) may be used if the ECU is inadequate.

The carpal wedge procedure begins with a release of the tight volar structures through an ulnar longitudinal incision. If the FCU, FCR, or palmaris longus (PL) are tight but there is muscle present, the tendons are fractionally lengthened by incising the tendon within the muscle. If the tendon is present but there is no muscle proximally, the tendon is excised. The ECU is identified and released from its facial attachments.

A transverse elliptical incision is made directly over the wrist, and a small section of skin is removed to provide a dermodesis and remove redundant skin. A wedge of bone is removed from the carpal bones centered over the midcarpal joint if the joint is fused (Fig. 10.13). If not, a more distal wedge can be removed. The wedge is closed to improve wrist extension and radial deviation, and fixation is achieved with multiple transosseous sutures. The ECU is then transferred to the ECRB tendon to augment active wrist extension. The wounds are closed and a short arm cast is placed in maximal wrist extension.

After 4–5 weeks, depending on patient age, the cast is removed and an orthoplast splint is fabricated. If the ECU is used to transfer to the ECRB, minimal retraining is required. If the FCU or FCR was used, more extensive phase reversal training will be needed. We usually have the patients engage in 3 days of twice daily intensive rehabilitation when the cast is removed. Recurrence is common in the long term and nighttime splinting until skeletal maturity is recommended.

Thumb Metacarpophalangeal Fusion

Children with DAs tend to have clasped thumbs, where the CMC joint is in extension and the MP joint is in flexion (Table 10.4). If the MP joint is passively correctable and there is an available tendon for transfer, then an Extensor Indicis Proprius (EIP) (or other available tendon) to Extensor Pollicis Longus (EPL) transfer is performed, usually in combination with a stiletto flap (Fig. 10.5). If the MP joint is fixed in flexion or if there is no tendon available for transfer, then a thumb MP fusion is performed, also in combination with a stiletto flap.

The stiletto flap is a modified Z-plasty that transfers skin from the radial side of the index finger to the first web space and the volar crease of the thumb MP joint, augmenting thumb extension and thumb abduction simultaneously. The Egyptian modification of the stiletto flap (Ghani flap) augments the web space and volar palm further.[20] Release of the fascia overlying the adductor pollicis and the first dorsal interosseous is required to improve the thumb position. If there is no adductor or first dorsal interosseous muscle but the tendon is present, we excise the tendon and fascia.

Once the stiletto flap is inset, a separate dorsal incision is made over the thumb MP joint. The metacarpal head is resected to the level of the metaphyseal flare to shorten the thumb. This allows the thumb MP joint to be extended without placing undue stress on the volar neurovascular bundles. The articular surface of the proximal phalanx is then resected sharply to the level of the ossification center but not beyond to limit the risk of physeal arrest. One or two Kirschner wires are placed in an antegrade out the tip of the thumb, then retrograde to secure the fusion once the joint is reduced into an extended and more pronated position. The incision is then closed and a thumb spica cast or splint is applied.

Union takes about 4 weeks, after which the cast is removed and a thumb spica orthoplast splint is fashioned. This is worn for a further 2 weeks full time except bathing and active range of motion exercises, followed by nighttime splinting for a further 6 weeks.

Thumb Reorientation Osteotomy

Most thumb-in-palm deformities in AMC primarily involve flexion at the CMC joint. The presentation and treatment is quite different than for a clasped thumb (Fig. 10.8). Patients with active Flexor Pollicis Longus (FPL) or Flexor Pollicis Brevis (FPB) function will have the best results. If only the abductor and adductor are working, the reorientation osteotomy will improve the appearance of the hand and improve with large object grasp, but is unlikely to improve pinch. For patients with stiff fingers that cannot flex sufficiently to allow pinch, this procedure is also of limited value. The ideal candidate has a working FPL and good thumb MP motion, index or long finger MP active flexion to at least 45 degrees, but a hypopronated (too supinated) and adducted thumb flexed at the CMC joint.

A stiletto flap is performed as described earlier (https://youtu.be/atL645qeB2k). A separate incision is made on the dorsum of the thumb metacarpal base and carried down to the bone between the EPL and EPB tendons. Typically, a 30 degree dorsal closing wedge is made just distal to the physis with a transverse proximal cut and an angled distal cut to allow for extension and rotation. Two Kirschner wires are then advanced in an antegrade fashion down the metacarpal and out the thumb tip. The osteotomy is then reduced with the thumb placed in an optimal position for tip pinch and grasp, usually in a "sock puppet" position.

A thumb spica cast is maintained for 4 weeks or until bony union. The pins are then removed, and the patient is outfitted with an orthoplast splint in thumb abduction to maintain the first web space at its maximum width. The splint is worn for 4 weeks full time except for bathing and range of motion exercises at least three times daily. Full weight bearing can begin as tolerated.

TABLE 10.4 Modified Thumb Deformity Classification.		
	JOINT POSITION	
Classification	**CMC**	**MP**
Type 1	Extended	Flexed
Type 2	Flexed	Extended
Type 3	Flexed	Flexed

After, a subsequent 4 weeks of nighttime use, the splint can be removed and the child is returned to unrestricted activities. Recurrence of the deformity is common in children younger than 7 years old, but can also occur at older ages as well. We recommend intermittent nighttime splinting until skeletal maturity in younger children or in children with more severe deformities.

Camptodactyly Release

Camptodactyly, a flexion contracture of the PIP joint, is common in patients with both amyoplasia and distal arthrogryposes. However, the contracture does not necessarily inhibit function, and in some patients

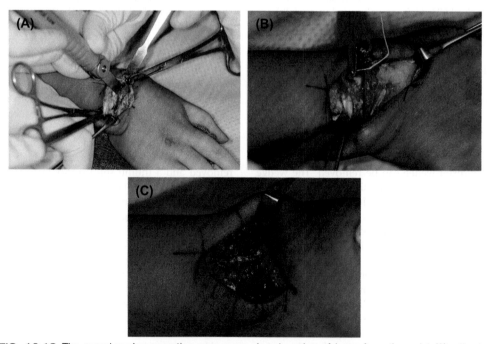

FIG. 10.13 The carpal wedge operation removes a dorsal wedge of bone from the wrist (A), allowing correction of up to 45 degrees of flexion contracture. Fixation can be achieved with suture (B), Kirschner wires, or a combination of the two. We have stopped using wires because of the high complication rate and have so far had no cases of loss of fixation. Some passive motion is preserved at the wrist, but active motion is dependent on the success of a tendon transfer to the extensor carpi-radialis brevis (C).

actually may be beneficial. Some children with minimal finger motion use their contracted finger(s) in the same manner as a static hook on a prosthesis. The camptodactyly allows them to hold onto and manipulate straps and loops. In the index finger, a PIP flexion contracture can be beneficial for key pinch. In other patients, the flexion of the PIP joints prevents them from placing objects in their palm, thus limiting what would otherwise be a functional grasp (Fig. 10.6). Therefore, a camptodactyly release can both improve function, and take away function, even in the same patient. As for all antecedently described procedures, a global preoperative assessment is required to avoid making a misjudgment.

Although a variety of procedures have been described,[21-23] we have only had some success with a simple Z-plasty of the skin at the PIP joint and an flexor digitorum superficialis (FDS) tenotomy. Attempts to use the FDS as a motor to power PIP extension have not been at all successful in our hands, reliably creating extension contractures of the PIP joint. Fusion of the PIP joint is another option for severe deformities that cannot be corrected by any other means.

Our preferred camptodactyly release begins with a Z-plasty centered over the tightest volar portion of the PIP joint (Fig. 10.6). The A3 pulley is then divided and both slips of the FDS are tenotomized, making sure that the cut tendon ends retract past the chiasm of Camper. The Z-plasty is closed in a lengthened fashion with absorbable suture. We do not routinely place a pin to hold the finger in extension, as this can place undue traction on the neurovascular bundles and lead to digital ischemia. The fingers are splinted in as much extension at the PIP joint as the digital vessels will tolerate. After 2 weeks, the operative splint is removed and an orthoplast splint is applied to keep the PIP joint in maximal extension, with the metacarpophalangeal joints and wrist joint in as much extension as possible without compromising PIP extension. The splint is worn for 6 weeks full time except for bathing and range of motion exercises at least three times daily. Full weight bearing can begin as tolerated. After a subsequent 4 weeks of nighttime use, the splint can be removed and the child is returned to unrestricted activities. Recurrence of the deformity is common. We recommend intermittent nighttime splinting until skeletal maturity in younger children or in children with more severe deformities.

CONCLUSION

Children with arthrogryposis, regardless of type or etiology, are challenging to manage and tolerances for error are tight. It is important to make the diagnosis early, and to have the patient be seen as soon as possible by a team that specializes in these conditions. There is much that can be done to help these children, both in adaptive strategies and equipment, as well as in surgical interventions. However, surgical techniques and rehabilitation strategies in these patients can be challenging for any surgeon or therapist. Getting these children to achieve their potential can be frustrating and therefore rewarding. Because they require interventions and observation throughout childhood, patients and their families form deep bonds with their medicals teams, further enhancing the rewards of caring for them.

REFERENCES

1. Fahy MJ, Hall JG. A retrospective study of pregnancy complications among 828 cases of arthrogryposis. *Genet Couns.* 1990;1:3−11.
2. Hall JG, Reed SD, Driscoll EP. Part I. Amyoplasia: a common, sporadic condition with congenital contractures. *Am J Med Genet.* 1983;15(4):571−590.
3. Hall JG. Uterine structural anomalies and arthrogryposis—death of an urban legend. *Am J Med Genet.* 2013;161A:82−88.
4. Oishi SN, Agranovich O, Pajardi GE, et al. Treatment of the upper extremity contracture/deformities. *J Pediatr Orthop.* 2017;37:S9−S15.
5. Fletcher ND, Rathjen KE, Bush P, Ezaki M. Asymmetrical arthrogryposis of the upper extremity associated with congenital spine anomalies. *J Pediatr Orthop.* 2010;30(8):936−941.
6. Richards CJ, Ramirez RN, Kozin SH, Zlotolow DA. Does age contribute to outcomes for elbow release in arthrogryposis? *J Hand Surg.* 2018 (in press).
7. Van Heest AE, Rodriguez R. Dorsal carpal wedge osteotomy in the arthrogrypotic wrist. *J Hand Surg Am.* 2013;38(2):265−270.
8. Zlotolow DA, Tiedeken NC. Reorientation osteotomy for the atypical clasped thumb in children with arthrogryposis. *Tech Hand Up Extrem Surg.* 2014;18:165−169.
9. Zlotolow DA, Kozin SH. Posterior elbow release and humeral osteotomy for patients with arthrogryposis. *J Hand Surg Am.* 2012;37(5):1078−1082.
10. Ramirez RN, Richards CJ, Kozin SH, Zlotolow DA. Combined elbow release and humeral rotational osteotomy in arthrogryposis. *J Hand Surg Am.* 2017;(16):30570−30576. pii: S0363-5023.
11. Zlotolow DA, Catalano LW, Barron OA, Glickel SZ. Surgical exposures of the humerus. *J Am Acad Orthop Surg.* 2006;14(13):754−765.
12. Kozin SH. Medial approach for humeral rotational osteotomy in children with residual brachial plexus birth Palsy. *Oper Tech Orthop.* 2007;17:88−93.
13. Carroll RE, Kleinman WB. Pectoralis major transplantation to restore elbow flexion to the paralytic limb. *J Hand Surg.* 1979;4(6):501−507.

14. Clark J. Reconstruction of the biceps brachii by pectoralis muscle transplantation. *Br J Surg.* 1946;34:180–181.

15. Goldfarb CA, Burke MS, Strecker WB, et al. The Steindler flexorplasty for the arthrogrypotic elbow. *J Hand Surg.* 2004;29A:462–469.

16. Kay S, Pinder R, Wiper J, Hart A, Jones F, Yates A. Microvascular free functioning gracilis transfer with nerve transfer to establish elbow flexion. *J Plastic Recon Aesthetic surg.* 2010; 63(7):1142–1149.

17. Lahoti O, Bell MJ. Transfer of pectoralis major in arthrogryposis to restore elbow flexion: deteriorating results in the long term. *J Bone Joint Surg Br.* 2005;87(6):858–860.

18. Zancolli E, Mitre H. Latissimus dorsi transfer to restore elbow flexion. *J Bone Jt Surg.* 1973;55A:1265–1275.

19. Foy CA, Mills J, Wheeler L, Ezaki M, Oishi SN. Long-term outcome following carpal wedge osteotomy in the arthrogrypotic patient. *J Bone Joint Surg Am.* 2013; 95(20):e150.

20. Abdel Ghani H. Modified dorsal rotation advancement flap for release of the thumb web space. *J Hand Surg Br.* 2006;31(2):226–229.

21. Koman LA, Toby EB, Poehling GG. Congenital flexion deformities of the proximal interphalangeal joint in children: a subgroup of camptodactyly. *J Hand Surg Am.* 1990;15(4): 582–586.

22. Smith PJ, Grobbelaar AO. Camptodactyly: a unifying theory and approach to surgical treatment. *J Hand Surg Am.* 1998;23(1):14–19.

23. Foucher G, Loréa P, Khouri RK, Medina J, Pivato G. Camptodactyly as a spectrum of congenital deficiencies: a treatment algorithm based on clinical examination. *Plast Reconstr Surg.* 2006;117(6):1897–1905.

FURTHER READING

1. Baek GH, Lee HJ. Classification and surgical treatment of symphalangism in interphalangeal joints of the hand. *Clin Orthop Surg.* 2012;4(1):58–65.

2. Bamshad M, Jorde LB, Carey JC. A revised and extended classification of the distal arthrogryposes. *Am J Med Genet.* 1996;65(4):277–281.

3. Benson LS, Waters PM, Kamil NI, Simmons BP, Upton J. Camptodactyly: classification and results of nonoperative treatment. *J Pediatr Orthop.* 1994;14(6):814–819.

4. Brown SHM, Hentzen ER, Kwan A, Ward SR, Fridén J, Lieber RL. Mechanical strength of the side-to-side versus Pulvertaft weave tendon repair. *J Hand Surg Am.* 2010; 35(4):540–545.

5. Ezaki MB, Oishi SN. Index rotation flap for palmar thumb release in arthrogryposis. *Tech Hand Up Extrem Surg.* 2010; 14(1):38–40.

6. Hall JG, Reed SD, Greene G. The distal arthrogryposes: delineation of new entities—review and nosologic discussion. *Am J Med Genet.* 1982;11:185–239.

7. Miller ME, Dunn PM, Smith DW. Uterine malformation and fetal deformation. *J Pediatr.* 1979;94:387–390.

8. Shin AY. 2004–2005 sterling bunnell travelling fellow report. *J Hand Surg Am.* 2006;31(7):1226–1237.

9. Smith DW, Drennan JC. Arthrogryposis wrist deformities: results of infantile serial casting. *J Pediatr Orthop.* 2001; 22(1):44–47.

10. Van Heest A, James MA, Lewica A, Anderson KA. Posterior elbow capsulotomy with triceps lengthening for treatment of elbow extension contracture in children with arthrogryposis. *J Bone Jt Surg.* 2008;90A:1517–1523.

11. Van Heest A, Waters PM, Simmons BP. Surgical treatment of arthrogryposis of the elbow. *J Hand Surg [Am].* 1998;23: 1063–1070.

12. Zlotolow DA, Kozin SH. *Arthrogryposis. Green's Operative Hand Surgery.* Elsevier; 2016.

13. Zlotolow DA. Arthrogryposis elbow extension contracture. In: *Limb Lengthening and Reconstruction Surgery Case Atlas.* Springer; 2015.

14. Zlotolow DA, Kozin SH. In: Abzug JM, Kozin SH, Zlotolow DA, eds. *Arthrogryposis. The Pediatric Upper Extremity.* New York: Springer; 2015.

CHAPTER 11

Brachial Plexus Birth Palsy—Introduction and Initial Treatment

CHERYL ZALIECKAS, OTR/L, MBA • ALEXANDRIA L. CASE, BSE • DANIELLE A. HOGARTH, BS • JOSHUA M. ABZUG, MD

INTRODUCTION

The brachial plexus is the network of nerves most commonly formed by the ventral rami of the spinal nerves C5 to T1, which provide movement and sensation to the entire upper extremity. In some instances, C4 (22% of the population) and T2 (1% of the population) provide contributions to the brachial plexus, which are termed prefixed and postfixed cords, respectively.[1-3] The brachial plexus is divided into the following segments: roots, trunks, divisions, cords, and terminal branches. A mnemonic such as Randy Travis Drinks Cold Beer, can help one to remember the order of the various components of the brachial plexus from proximal to distal. The ventral rami of the spinal nerves C5 to T1 that give rise to the plexus are called as the roots. The C5 and C6 roots unite to form the upper trunk, the C7 nerve root continues to become the middle trunk, and the C8 and T1 nerve roots join to form the lower trunk. Each of the three trunks separates into anterior and posterior divisions. The anterior divisions of the upper and middle trunks combine to form the lateral cord, while the anterior division of the lower trunk forms the medial cord. The posterior divisions of all three cords connect to form the posterior cord. The cords give rise to the terminal branches, which form the peripheral nerves of the upper extremity. More specifically, the ulnar nerve arises from the medial cord, the musculocutaneous nerve arises from the lateral cord, the median nerve arises from a combination of the medial and lateral cords, and the radial and axillary nerves arise from the posterior

cord.[1-3] There are numerous other branches at the various levels of the brachial plexus (Fig. 11.1).

BRACHIAL PLEXUS BIRTH PALSY: HISTORY AND ETIOLOGY

Brachial plexus birth palsy (BPBP) was first reported by William Smellie in 1764. However, at that time it was popularly accepted that the injury to the upper extremity in a newborn was congenital in nature. Over a century later, in 1872, it was confirmed by Duchenne de Boulogne that these injuries to the newborns' upper extremities were not congenital in nature, rather, the result of a traumatic birth process, as Smellie had previously asserted; coining the term obstetrical paralysis. Later in 1877, Erb described injury localized to the upper trunk (C5–C6), now called as Erb's palsy, which accounts for 60% of reported brachial plexus birth palsy injuries.[1,2,4] In 1885, Klumpke reported an isolated injury to the lower trunk (C8 and T1), now called as Klumpke's palsy, which in the literature is reported as the rarest form of injury, accounting for less than 2% of the reported obstetrical brachial plexus birth palsies.[2,5,6]

The widely accepted etiology of BPBP is traction to the brachial plexus during the delivery process, resulting in a peripheral neuropathy with subsequent paresis or paralysis of the upper extremity musculature. Injury to the upper trunk in isolation is most common, however, in approximately 20%–30% of all reported cases of BPBP the middle trunk or C7 root is affected in conjunction with the upper trunk (C5–C6). This injury to

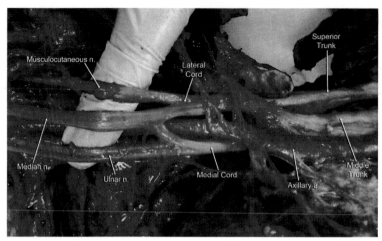

FIG. 11.1 Anatomical image of the brachial plexus. (Courtesy of Joshua M. Abzug, MD.)

C5−C7 is called as an extended Erb's palsy. A total or global brachial plexus palsy is the result of injury to the brachial plexus that affects all of the nerve root levels (C5-T1) at some point along the brachial plexus, and carries the worst prognosis.[1−16]

Infants that sustain BPBPs will present with weakness or paralysis of the muscles served by the injured nerve roots. In general terms, when the nerves originating from the upper trunk are injured, infants will demonstrate limitations in shoulder abduction, external rotation, elbow flexion, supination, and wrist extension. Classically, this presentation of upper extremity shoulder internal rotation, with elbow extension, forearm protonation, and wrist and digit flexion, is called as the "waiter's tip" position. In extended Erb's injuries, additional deficits in shoulder internal rotation, protonation and digit extension are often present, as well as potential ulnar drift. Global plexus injuries result in flaccid paralysis of the upper extremity, while Klumpke's paralysis results in an upper extremity with paralysis of hand function.[1,17]

RISK FACTORS

Although extensive research has revealed explicit risk factors for BPBP that will subsequently be discussed, it is important to note that in many cases of BPBP, known risk factors are not always present.[2,11,18,19] Risk factors associated with BPBP can be related to the infant, the infant's mother, or the actual process of labor and delivery. Risk factors include the following: shoulder dystocia, fetal macrosomia (>4 kg), multiparity, instrument-assisted delivery, maternal gestational

diabetes, previous pregnancies resulting in BPBP, maternal obesity and/or excessive maternal weight gain, advanced maternal age (>35 years old), maternal pelvic anatomy anomalies, use of an epidural, induction of labor, prolonged second-stage of labor, hypotonia and intrauterine torticollis.[1,2,4,5,11,12,17,18,20,21] (Table 11.1) Of these risk factors, shoulder dystocia, macrosomia, and instrument-assisted delivery have been found to increase the risk of BPBP by presenting a 100×, 14×, and 9× greater risk, respectively.[2,11] Shoulder dystocia occurs during a vertex delivery when the infant's anterior shoulder becomes lodged on the mother's pubic symphysis, widening the ipsilateral head−shoulder angle. Alternatively, the posterior shoulder can become lodged on the sacral promontory. It has been reasoned that fetal distress may lead to hypotonia making the brachial plexus more susceptible to injury during the delivery. Of note, cesarean section as a means of delivery does not eliminate the potential for BPBPs, but it does reduce the risk.[2,3,17]

INCIDENCE AND PROGNOSIS

According to a review of the literature on the epidemiology of BPBP, data varies significantly with respect to incidence, with rates as low as 0.19/1000 live births,[5] to as high as 5.1/1000 live births.[11] In a recent epidemiologic study of the Kids' Inpatient Database, a decreasing trend in BPBP was observed between 1997 and 2012, with observed incidences of 1.7 per 1000 live births in 1997 to 0.9 per 1000 live births in 2012.[21] The lack of consistency in the data has been attributed to variations in obstetric care, the average

TABLE 11.1
Risk Factors Associated With BPBP.

Risk Factors Associated with Brachial Plexus Birth Palsy
Shoulder dystocia
Large baby (macrosomia)
Multiparity
Forceps delivery
Vacuum delivery
Gestational diabetes
Previous deliveries resulting in brachial plexus birth palsy
Maternal obesity or excessive maternal weight gain
Advanced maternal age (>35 years old)
Maternal pelvic anatomy anomalies
Use of an epidural
Induction of labor
Prolonged second-stage labor
Hypotonia
Intrauterine torticolis

Data from: Abzug JM, Mehlman CT, Ying J. Assessment of current epidemiology and risk factors surrounding brachial plexus birth palsy. J Hand Surg 2018. S0363—5023(17) 31908—1.

birth weight of infants, and reporting measures according to the region of the world from where the data are being obtained.[11,17]

Reports on the prognosis of BPBP are also incongruent. Previously in the literature, it was consistently reported that BPBP is transient in nature, with 75% —95% of all injuries being classified as "mild" resulting in full spontaneous recovery within the first and second months of life; specifically, when the C5 and C6 nerve roots are the site of initial injury.[1–4,6,10–12,15,17–20,22–24] More recently, the research of Foad and Hoeskma et al. estimates full spontaneous recovery rates in only approximately 66% of the BPBP population.[11,25] For the remaining percentage of the population, where recovery is incomplete, conservative management through occupational and physical therapy interventions to address the residual impairments may not be sufficient, and surgical intervention may be required. Akel et al. (2013) reported that even with conservative management of the injury, more than 15% of patients have permanent disability, or substantially diminished function.[7]

A consistent prognostic indicator within the current literature is the return of function of the upper extremity against gravity within the first 2–3 months of life. It is agreed upon that such return of function leads to complete recovery within the first 1–2 years of life.[3,17] Alternatively, when only partial recovery against gravity is acquired between months three and six, patients will experience long-standing and sometimes permanent loss in total range of motion and strength, decreased limb length and/or girth, as compared to the unaffected upper extremity, and glenohumeral dysplasia, leading to functional impairment. The delay in against-gravity recovery is directly proportional to the long-term risk of incomplete recovery and functional impairments.[16,18] As there are no finite, known clinical indicators relative to the extent of initial injury and specific prognoses, physicians and healthcare team members are cautioned when answering questions about prognosis around the time of injury.

NERVE ANATOMY AND RECOVERY

Attempts to predict recovery require knowledge of the type of nerve lesion sustained and the level or severity of the injury.[3] The peripheral nervous system contains autonomic, sensory, and motor neurons. Each peripheral nerve is made up of three main layers, described from the innermost to outermost layer, they are the nerve fiber or axon covered by the endoneurium and myelin sheath, the nerve bundle (funiculis) or fascicle covered by the perineurium, and the nerve trunk covered by the epineurium. Injuries can occur at each of these layers within the peripheral nerve, and with differing levels of severity. In 1943, Herbert Seddon proposed that further attention needed to be placed on classifications of nerve injuries. Seddon therefore established a classification of three types of nerve injuries that lead to loss of function: neurapraxia (stretch), axonotmesis (partial tearing), and neurotmesis (rupture); listed in order of increasing severity. Later in 1951, Sydney Sunderland further expanded these classifications to include 5 degrees of nerve injury: Sunderland I (neurapraxia), Sunderland II–IV (axonotmesis), and Sunderland V (neurotmesis).[26] These classifications are still utilized today. It is important to note that an avulsion injury can also occur, in which the nerve root is pulled out of the spinal cord.

Although each category of nerve injury carries its unique complications and clinical presentation, as the degree/classification of the injury increases in severity, the probability of recovery decreases proportionately. Sunderland I/Seddon neurapraxia is a stretch without disrupting nerve continuity. This type of injury may present clinically with decreased strength and sensation; however, autonomic function typically remains intact. As there is not permanent damage to the axons, recovery typically occurs spontaneously within 3 months. Sunderland II–IV/Seddon axonotmesis is characterized by a partial tearing of the nerve in which the axon is affected; however, the Schwann cell basal lamina and endoneurium remain intact, as well as the epineurium and nerve trunk itself. Although spontaneous recovery is possible at this level of injury, recovery time is longer due to Wallerian degeneration, followed by axon regeneration, which occurs at a rate of 1–8 mm/day.[27] In Sunderland III injuries, axonal regeneration can occur; however, it is complicated by scarring to the endoneurium, thereby slowing the recovery process. Conversely, in Sunderland IV injuries, the scarring to the endoneurium is severe to the point where it obstructs axon regeneration. In this instance, recovery is not anticipated without surgical intervention to remove the scar tissue and a reanastomosis of the nerve segments. Sunderland V/Seddon neurotmesis results in complete postganglionic transection of the nerve. Lastly, one can sustain a preganglionic avulsion of the nerve root from the spinal cord. This level of injury carries the poorest prognosis with the likelihood that muscle function and/or sensation will not be restored without surgical intervention. Although surgical techniques may be employed in attempts to graft across a postganglionic tear, direct surgical repair of a preganglionic avulsion injury is not possible. In 1989, Mackinnon and Dellon described a sixth degree of injury, the neuroma incontinuity.[28] This type of injury is characterized by varying degrees and patterns of injury to the fascicles, with a resultant mixed pattern of recovery.[1,17,18,25,27,29,30]

Due to the initial similarity in clinical presentation of differing nerve lesions, recovery and extent of the injury cannot be determined immediately following birth. It is reasoned that should an infant not regain near complete recovery within the first weeks of life, anticipated recovery time ranges from several months to absence of full recovery, as more than a neurapraxia injury has occurred.[17,25]

Clinical examination can provide insight into the level(s) of nerve root injury by looking at muscle function. Such identification will aid in predicting recovery and consideration of treatment options. In 1987, Narakas developed a classification tool that groups BPBP into four separate categories (I–IV), based upon the location of muscle weakness/paralysis, with the corresponding nerve roots, and likely outcome.[31] (Tables 11.2 and 11.3)

TABLE 11.2
Narakas Classification of Obstetric Palsy.

Group	Name	Roots Injured	Affected Motion
I	Erb's palsy	C5, C6	Shoulder abduction Shoulder external rotation Elbow flexion Supination
II	Extended Erb's palsy	C5, C6, C7	Shoulder motion Elbow motion Forearm rotation Drop wrist Finger extension (MP joints)
III	Global palsy with no Horner syndrome	C5, C6, C7, C8, T1	Complete flaccid paralysis
IV	Global palsy with Horner syndrome	C5, C6, C7, C8, T1	Complete flaccid paralysis with Horner syndrome

MP, Metacarpophalangeal.
Data from: Al-Qattan MM, El-Sayed AAF, Al-Zahrani AY, Al-Mutairi SA, Al-Harbi MS, Al-Mutairi AM, Al-Kahtani FS. Narakas classification of obstetric brachial plexus palsy revisited. J Hand Surg Eur 2009; 34(6):788–791.

TABLE 11.3
Functional Anatomy of the Brachial Plexus.

Upper Extremity Movement	Primary Nerve Roots Affected
SHOULDER	
Abduction-external rotation	C5, C6
Adduction-internal rotation	C5-T1
ELBOW	
Flexion	C5, C6
Extension	C7
FOREARM	
Supination	C5, C6
Pronation	C7
WRIST	
Extension	C5, C6
Flexion	C6, C7, C8
HAND	
Extrinsic muscles	C7, C8, T1
Intrinsic muscles	C8, T1

Data from: Abid A. Brachial plexus birth palsy: management during the first year of life. Orthop Traumatol Surg Res 2016; 102(1 Suppl): S125–S132.

ASSESSMENT

The therapist's first contact with the patient and their family is ideally during the hospital admission at the time of birth, with a referral made to a brachial plexus injury clinic or specialist following discharge. When consulted to evaluate an infant with recorded shoulder dystocia or possible BPBP as an inpatient therapist, before the evaluation being initiated, radiographs need to be obtained to assess for the presence of a clavicle or humerus fracture if there is any tenderness to palpation or crepitus present. A fracture may be present on the ipsilateral or contralateral side of a BPBP. Additionally, a chest radiograph to assess for a raised hemidiaphragm may also be warranted. Should the imaging be positive for any of these three items, the treatment and caregiver education will differ from when these associated findings are not present. Regardless of the patient's point of entry into therapy, the therapist should be familiar with the brachial plexus injury providers within the immediate geographical area as these infants and children will require specialized assessment and follow-up. Multidisciplinary

teams involved in the care of this population typically include a compliment of pediatric neurologists, neurosurgeons, orthopedic surgeons, physical medicine and rehabilitation physicians, physical and occupational therapists, social workers, or any combination of these providers.[32,33]

Although there exist different developmental milestones to consider when evaluating a newborn with a BPBP versus an older child, the basic tenets of the evaluation remain the same. The skilled therapists' evaluation will assist in classifying the injury and determining the extent of the injury. The evaluation should begin with an in-depth history. Pertinent information to obtain includes the mother's pregnancy and labor course, the infant's hospital course, the initial presentation of the involved upper extremity, the history of any recovery in the upper extremity to date (if any), and any involvement from rehabilitation services (occupational therapy/physical therapy). Specific to the mother's pregnancy and labor, attention is paid to the mother's age, weight gain during pregnancy, presence of maternal or gestational diabetes and whether or not the labor and delivery was complicated in any way, more specifically, if instrumentation was utilized (i.e., forceps or vacuum) or if the patient had shoulder dystocia. Ideally, one would note what if any maneuvers were utilized to relieve the shoulder dystocia. The infants' hospital course should include the infant's birth weight, APGAR scores, whether the normal hospital stay was prolonged for any particular medical reason, as well as any documented or noted impairments in vision, hearing, feeding, or respiration.[27] Additional components of the evaluation include observation of the resting posture (Fig. 11.2) and active movements of the infant (Video 1), skin integrity, passive range of motion, muscle tone, presence or absence of age-appropriate reflexes and protective reactions, sensation, palpation for pain, deformity or muscle tightness, postural control, differential diagnoses/associated findings, and the patient's overall disposition and its impact on the assessment.

Resting posture is examined to identify any asymmetries throughout the cervical spine, trunk, and extremities. Active movements are observed both against gravity, as well as in gravity-eliminated planes where the focus is on identifying unilateral weakness (Video 2) (Fig. 11.3). Passive range is completed bilaterally, with the focus on identifying any unilateral limitations. It is important to describe the end-feels, whether the joint is hypermobile or hypomobile. Range should be assessed at the cervical spine, shoulder, elbow, wrist, and digits, inclusive of assessment of scapulohumeral rhythm.

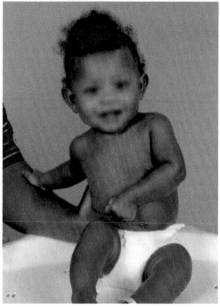

FIG. 11.2 Presentation of a BPBP patient with a resting posture of shoulder internal rotation. (Courtesy of Shriner's Children's Hospital, Philadelphia, PA.)

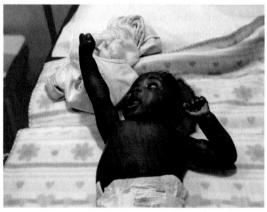

FIG. 11.3 Clinical photograph of a child with BPBP on the right demonstrating active elbow extension against gravity, but no elbow flexion against gravity. (Courtesy of Joshua M. Abzug, MD.)

Upon initial assessment of an infant with a BPBP, if a passive range of motion limitation exists, a differential diagnosis must be considered. Muscle tone should be assessed for normalcy, hypertonicity, hypotonicity, or flaccidity throughout the body. For the infant population, the Moro, Asymmetrical Tonic Neck, Palmar Grasp, Placing, Arm Recoil, and Placing reflexes can be utilized

to elicit active movement and observe for symmetry.[2] In addition, tactile stimulation may elicit active movements in a newborn child (Videos 1 and 2).

Palpation during the clinical examination can be utilized to assess for clinical signs of pain that may be associated with an undiagnosed clavicle and/or humerus fracture, or it can identify muscle tightness. For example, the extremity can be passively placed into abduction and external rotation while assessing for tightness at the pectoralis major, latissimus dorsi, and teres major muscle groups. A significant portion of the population with upper trunk lesions will present at a few months of age with tightness of the internal rotators, often with limited active and passive external rotation (Fig. 11.2). Palpation is also critical in assessing for posterior shoulder subluxation. Clinical indicators for the presence of posterior shoulder subluxation are either the lack of passive external rotation (estimated at −30 degrees to 5 degrees) on initial evaluation, or a loss of passive range at subsequent assessments. In conjunction with the assessment of external rotation for limited range, the posterior aspect of the shoulder should be palpated for what has been described as fullness, which is a result of humeral head displacement. Other clinical factors that raise concern for the potential of a posterior subluxation are asymmetrical soft tissue folds of the proximal aspect of the extremity and asymmetry at the axilla with a deep/concave presentation in the presence of subluxation.[34]

At approximately 4 months old, assessment of the patient's postural control can be conducted (Video 3). For postural control, the therapist is assessing the patient's ability to interact with the environment, moving against gravity while maintaining the position of the cervical spine, trunk, and limbs. Deficits in posture are seen with asymmetry at rest, and atypical movement patterns. As shoulder flexion is limited in many children with BPBP, they utilize postural compensations to achieve their desired movement pattern. A classic compensation is extension or hyper extension of the trunk, with concurrent posterior pelvic tilt and ribcage elevation. Postural control develops in the first months of life in a cephalocaudal fashion. The initial experience of infant's weight bearing from the prone position affects postural control in the shoulder, trunk, pelvis, and lower extremities. Infants with BPBP often are unable to bear weight symmetrically in the prone position, if at all. Missing this key developmental milestone will likely lead to postural control deficits in sitting and standing.[15]

In older children, deep tendon reflexes for the biceps (C5, C6), triceps (C7), and brachioradialis (C6) are assessed. When considering sensation, the Narakas

Sensory Grading System can be utilized. In this system, a rating of S0 is given when there is no reaction to painful stimuli; S1 when there is reaction to painful stimuli, but no reaction to touch; S2 when there is reaction to touch, but not light tough; and S3 when sensation appears to be normal.[33] It is important to remember, however, that sensory feedback is not going to directly correlate to motor function.

Differential diagnoses for BPBP include clavicle and humeral fractures, spinal cord injury, and cerebral anoxia, and therefore assessment for each of these items is warranted.[2] If there is a clavicle or humerus fracture, the upper extremity should be immobilized via a swathe or by pinning the infant's sleeve to the chest of their shirt for a period of 2−3 weeks. It is important to note that clavicle and/or humerus fractures can mimic a BPBP (a pseudopalsy) or can coexist with a BPBP. Due to the nature of the BPBP injury, there may be associated findings outside of the upper extremity. As such, neck positioning should be assessed for the presence of torticollis or muscle imbalance resulting in head rotation preferences with or without lateral tilt. Additionally, the lower extremities should be assessed for atypical muscle tone due to the risk of fetal asphyxia or hypoxia in the presence of a difficult delivery. If the phrenic nerve is involved in the injury, the patient will present with a raised hemidiaphragm and potential feeding difficulties. Horner's syndrome (ptosis, miosis, and anhydrosis) and facial palsies may be seen with lower trunk involvement. Both Horner's syndrome and a hemidiaphragm paralysis have a higher association with preganglionic injuries.

There are several assessment tools that have been developed specifically for the BPBP population for assessing muscle function and ultimately nerve regeneration. These assessment tools are the Toronto Test Score, the Active Movement Scale (AMS), the modified Mallet Classification, Gilbert and Tassin Muscle Grading System, and the Medical Research Council Scale (MRC). The Toronto Test Score, AMS, and modified Mallet Classification have been proven reliable.[2,27] In addition to using these tools, a baseline Narakas level should be recorded during the initial evaluation and each subsequent reevaluation.

The Toronto Test Score, developed by Michelow et al., scores abduction, elbow flexion, wrist extension, digit extension, and thumb extension, each on a scale of 0−2, with zero signifying no function, one equating to partial function and two as normal function, for a total possible score of 10.[35] If by 3 months of life, the patient does not score greater than 3.5 on this tool,

TABLE 11.4
Toronto Test Score.

Score	Movement Against Gravity
0	No joint movement
0.3	Flicker of movement
0.6	Less than 50% range of motion
1.0	50% range of motion
1.3	Greater than 50% range of motion
1.6	Good but not full range of motion
2.0	Full range of motion

Data from: Michelow BJ, Clarke HM, Curtis CG et al. The natural history of obstetrical brachial plexus palsy. Plast Reconstr Surg. 1994; 93:675−680.

surgeons may deem this as an indication for primary nerve surgery.[3] (Table 11.4)

The AMS assesses 15 separate movement patterns, with a seven-point scale for each, that includes both gravity eliminated and against gravity function (Table 11.5). It is important for the therapist to review scoring methodologies for this tool before implementation, due to specific scoring criteria. For example, while a score of zero represents no contraction in a gravity-eliminated plane, a four represents full motion with gravity eliminated and a seven equates to full movement against gravity. A patient must score a four, thus have full motion with gravity eliminated, on a specific

TABLE 11.5
Active Movement Scale.

Active Movement	Score
GRAVITY-ELIMINATED PLANE	
No contraction	0
Contraction, no motion	1
Motion < half range	2
Motion ≥ half range	3
Full motion	4
AGAINST GRAVITY	
Motion < half range	5
Motion ≥ half range	6
Full motion	7

Data from: Ho ES, Curtis CG, Clarke HM. The brachial plexus outcome measure: developmental, internal consistency, and construct validity. J Hand Ther 2012; 25:406−417.

movement pattern before being tested and scored against gravity. In this instance, a patient may score a three for having greater than ½ the available range in the gravity-eliminated plane, even if they have partial against gravity movement, but not full gravity-eliminated movement. It should also be noted that all scores are based upon the patient's available range, such that if there are contractures present or bony deformities that limit achievement of full passive range, active range is assessed within those specific parameters[9,13]

The Modified Mallet classification assesses shoulder function by examining global abduction, global external rotation, and the patient's ability to place their hand on the back of their neck, bring their hand to their mouth, and place their hand on their back. Each of these movement patterns is given a rating of 0–5, with 0 signifying no muscle contraction and five representing normalized movement. However, this assessment is not sensitive enough to ascertain specific motor strength and does not account for forearm, wrist, and digit function.[3] These measures can be used not only at an initial evaluation, but also throughout care. Notably, Abzug and Kozin (2010) proposed a modification to assess improvements in midline function by incorporating a sixth subscale, termed internal rotation, which assesses the patient's ability to move their hand to their belly.[2] This additional assessment focuses on quantifying a patient's midline function and balances out the discrepancy of primarily external rotation measures in the traditional classification.[2] Internal rotation measure to the modified Mallet score aids in assessing midline function in BPBP patients that is vital to evaluating functional independence.[36] (Figs. 11.4 and 11.5)

Gilbert and Tassin's Muscle grading system rates muscle movements from M0, which is no contraction; to M1 where a contraction is present without overt movement; M2 is partial movement against gravity; and M3 is complete movement against gravity.[9] The MRC is a common tool utilized for manual muscle

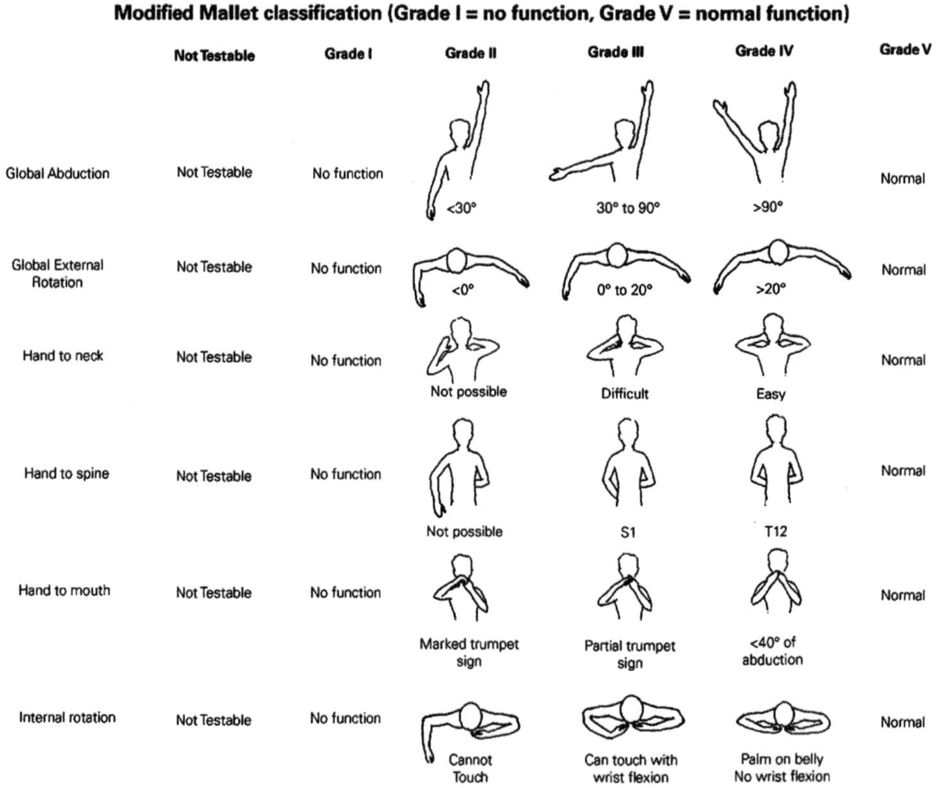

Modified Mallet classification (Grade I = no function, Grade V = normal function)

FIG. 11.4 Modified Mallet classification with additional internal rotational score. Note: Following interventions to improve external rotation and/or shoulder elevation often produce limitations with midline function. The addition measure of hand to trunk allows for greater appreciation of internal rotation changes.

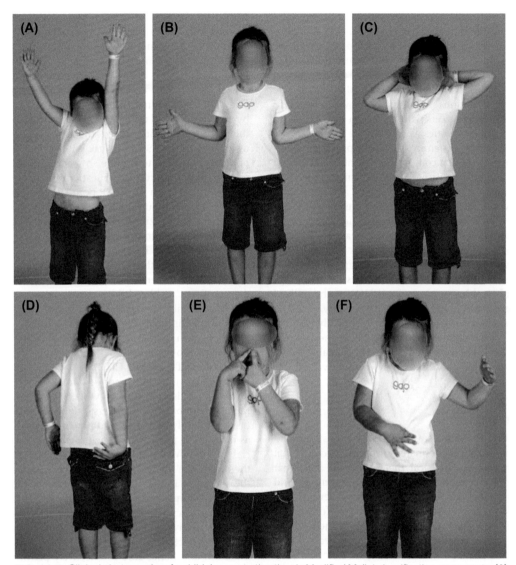

FIG. 11.5 Clinical photographs of a child demonstrating the six Modified Mallet classification movements. **(A)** Global abduction (grade IV) **(B)** Global external rotation (grade IV) **(C)** Hand to neck (grade IV) **(D)** Hand to spine (grade II) **(E)** Hand to mouth (grade IV) **(F)** Internal rotation (grade III). (Courtesy of Shriners Hospital for Children, Philadelphia, PA.)

testing, where specific muscles are assessed against resistance from the therapist and strength of the specific muscle is then graded on a scale of 0–5 with zero equating to no strength/movement and five equating to normal strength. For this scale to be utilized, patients have to be old enough or have the cognitive ability to follow the instructions for the examination. A primary limitation of this exam is that strength is not assessed throughout a movement pattern, but rather at a finite point in the muscle's range.

Regardless of the tool utilized for muscle assessment, the therapist should look to discriminate whether there is weakness, imbalance, or endurance issue present. There also needs to be a focus on muscle function directly related to functional movements such as those required to perform activities of daily living (ADLs). Two additional areas to continuously assess are upper extremity endurance and hand dexterity. Although patients may begin to regain functional movement of the involved upper extremity, endurance is typically limited. A baseline level of endurance should be recorded at the time of the initial evaluation. Although many children are said to have had complete neurologic recovery, there may be long-term sequelae including fine motor dexterity impairments and developmental apraxia. Additionally, children with BPBP may have decreased function because of low self-esteem compared to their peers with respect to their ability to perform motor activities as well as due to the appearance of the upper extremity. Therefore, psychosocial assessments need to be completed. Available assessment tools include the Assisting Hand Assessment, the Pediatric Evaluation of Disability Inventory, and the Pediatric Outcomes Data Collection Instrument. Although BPBP can be classified as a chronic injury for some infants and children, the impact stretches far beyond functional movements and directly impacts quality of life; not only for the patient, but for their family/caregivers as well. For children between the ages of 5 and 18, the Child Health Questionnaire (CHQ) can be utilized to assess general health status. Most recently, in 2012, an assessment tool was created specifically for the brachial plexus injury population, called the Brachial Plexus Outcomes Measure by Ho et al.[13] (Table 11.6). This assessment addressed functional movement of the upper extremity.

TREATMENT

After completing the assessment, the therapist needs to determine what can be managed by the occupational therapist (OT) or physical therapist (PT), and what may require surgical intervention. Treatment should be started immediately after the initial evaluation. When addressing BPBP injuries, therapy is focused on addressing the sequelae of the nerve injury and promoting the optimum environment for nerve healing. The goal is to assist the patient in recovery of motor and sensory input to allow for maximum functional use of the involved upper extremity. This is achieved by initially maintaining passive range of motion (PROM) to permit optimal joint growth and development and prevent contractures. In the shoulder region, it is vital for the therapist to focus on true glenohumeral motion by stabilizing the scapula when performing passive range of motion exercises (Fig. 11.6). As the nerve injury heals and formerly noninnervated muscles regain function, strengthening is performed in conjunction with addressing upper extremity fatigue and, if necessary, sensation.[27] Additionally, as the patient ages, the goal of therapy should be to improve bimanual skills for age-appropriate performance in home, school, and leisure activities. Muscle strength and active range of motion can be addressed by engagement in age-appropriate play and/or functional activities. Stickers can be utilized to encourage a child to perform certain movements as the child will commonly remove the sticker from the location the practitioner places it (Fig. 11.7). Attention is focused on the muscles affected by the injury, and midrange strengthening is recommended. Constraint-induced therapy (CIT) was first developed in the 1980s for use with the stroke injury population. This technique of addressing learned nonuse of an injured upper extremity by forced use can be utilized with the BPBP population; however we do not do this in our practice. Consideration needs to be taken when utilizing this technique regarding the patient's and family's tolerance.[8] The therapist must recognize the extent of the injury far beyond the physical limitations; thus, the impact this potential lifelong injury has on the emotional state of the patients and the caregivers. As the child increases in age, both the parent and child may have concerns about the appearance of the injured extremity (e.g., resting posture, length, or girth) and these should be addressed.[7,18,37,38] There are no long-term studies documenting the success or lack thereof regarding CIT.

Parent/caregiver education is one of the main goals of therapy. It is important to work to establish a solid rapport with parents/caregivers, taking the time to understand family dynamics and parent/caregiver's needs as it relates to providing home programs as well as social support. When initially educating parents about the injury, the therapist should give a full overview of the suspected injury and possible outcomes from full recovery to surgical repair and permanent deficits. Treatment frequency will depend on the parent/caregiver's ability to safely and effectively perform the home program. Research has demonstrated that parents are more apt and better able to effectively perform home programs when video is utilized as a modality instead of written handouts.[1,39] As treatment goals will continuously be adjusted in response to the patient's outcomes, parent education should also be continuously updated. Parents need to be educated on handling, positioning, ADLs, how to maintain and/or assist the patient in improving passive range of motion, strength, and endurance, therapeutic play techniques to address appropriate developmental milestones, sensory reeducation, and why and how to assist in preventing joint contractures (Fig. 11.8). Parents also need to be educated on the risks of subluxation and dislocation. Subsequently, the caregivers must be taught how to perform PROM exercises and how to protect the

TABLE 11.6
The Brachial Plexus Outcomes Measure.

Activity Assessment	Functional Movement Score
SHOULDER	
Head to back of head	
Forward overhead reaching Ex. Uses two hand to place a container directly above child's head	
Midline activity Ex. Undo button or snap at naval level	
Hand to ipsilateral back pant pocket	
ELBOW AND FOREARM	
Hand to mouth	
Uses computer mouse Ex. Uses affected hand with individual finger isolation on mouse	
Playing drums	
Holds plate with palm up	
WRIST, FINGER, AND THUMB	
Opening large container	
Pulls apart medium resistance theraputty Ex. Uses power grasp to pull apart theraputty with active wrist extension	
Stings bead Ex. Holds either bead or string with precision grasp (pinch) with affected hand	

Functional Movement Scale Scoring
1. Cannot complete task
2. Completes task using only unaffected arm
3. Completes task Absent active movement in primary mover(s) May use passive range of motion to complete movement pattern
4. Completes task Initiates all movement actively or position of primary mover(s) is sufficient for function. Compensatory techniques used to complete movement pattern
5. Completes task with normal movement pattern

Self-Evaluation Sliding Scale
My arm works: Very poorly _____ Very well
My hand works: Very poorly _____ Very well
My arm and hand looks: Very bad _____ Very good

Data from: Ho ES, Curtis CG, Clarke HM. The brachial plexus outcome measure: developmental, internal consistency, and construct validity. J Hand Ther 2012; 25:406–417.

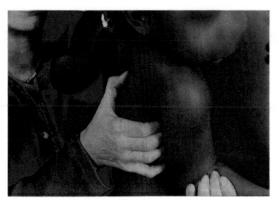

FIG. 11.6 Clinical photograph of a therapist working on true glenohumeral motion. Note the stabilization of the scapula. (Courtesy of Joshua M. Abzug, MD.)

shoulder joint during positioning and play. PROM exercises should always be slow and gentle. During each treatment session with the patient, parents should be asked to demonstrate their technique with passive or active-assisted range of motion with the patient, so that the therapist can ensure proper technique is being utilized. The eventual goal is for the patient to achieve full upper extremity, particularly glenohumeral range with scapular stabilization, to prevent contractures and secondary deformities of the glenohumeral joint. Elbow and forearm range of motion should also be focused on.

When working with the infant population, it is important to remind the parents/caregivers to focus on the entire child, and not just the injured upper extremity to ensure appropriate overall development and bonding between the parent/caregiver and child. For handling and positioning, parents/caregivers should be instructed to protect the injured upper extremity by not allowing it to fall behind the infant when picking them up and when there is a C5-6 nerve root injury, parents should be taught to place a wash cloth roll at the axilla when the patient is at rest to decrease the resting position of adduction and internal rotation. It is important for the parents to complete thorough skin checks, specifically in the area of the axilla and palmar wrist crease, as moisture can get trapped in these locations leading to yeast formation and/or skin breakdown. During ADLs, the injured extremity should be dressed first, followed by the noninjured extremity. Reciprocally, when undressing the infant, the uninjured extremity should be undressed first, followed by the injured upper extremity. This will help to protect the shoulder joint from excessive external rotation and abduction without scapular support. A point of controversy in the literature is whether or not therapists should assist in developing the developmental milestone of crawling with weight bearing over the injured upper extremity, due to the potential for posterior humeral head subluxation. A study conducted by Justice et al., with references made to additional scholarly reviews, noted that weight bearing in the crawling position is not likely to be associated with the incidence of posterior shoulder subluxation.[40] As such, the therapist should use their discretion based upon clinical examination of overall glenohumeral stability to

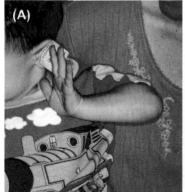
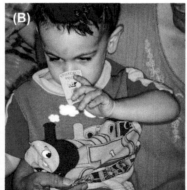
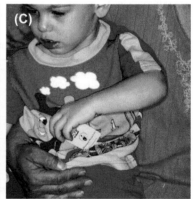

FIG. 11.7 Clinical photographs of a patient with left BPBP. Note the use of a sticker to assess active movement of the child's left upper extremity. (A) The child is removing the sticker from their left ear demonstrating external rotation. (B) The child is removing the sticker from the nose to assess for the presence or absence of a trumpeteer sign. (C) The child is removing the sticker from their abdomen to assess their midline function. (Courtesy of Joshua M. Abzug, MD.)

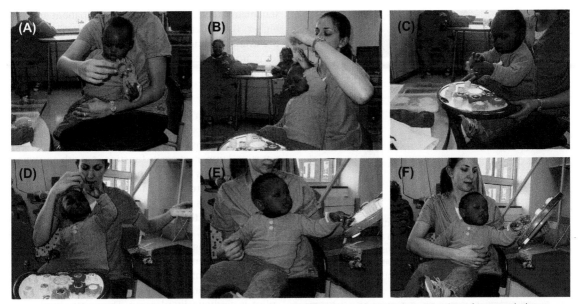

FIG. 11.8 Clinical photographs of a therapist with a BPBP patient. Note the incorporation of toys and play activities to encourage active movement in the injured left upper extremity. (Courtesy of Joshua M. Abzug, MD.)

determine whether or not a patient should be permitted to crawl over the affected extremity. Justice et al. noted that with respect to the arc of range of motion provided during passive range of motion, early full motion with attention to scapular stabilization is beneficial.[40] As active range of motion (AROM) is limited by PROM, and decreased AROM has been noted to be most closely related to the degree of glenohumeral deformation, the thought is that a full arc of PROM with scapular stabilization is warranted. Should a patient plateau or regress in passive external rotation and abduction, the surgeon should be notified, and an MRI or ultrasound may be obtained to determine if substantial dysplasia is present at the glenohumeral joint.[17]

It is important to address fine motor skills during therapy sessions as the child ages. To have solid distal strength and dexterity, proximal stability is required. This includes stability at the pelvis, trunk, and shoulder girdle. When addressing upper extremity functional movements, it is important for the therapist to be aware of age-appropriate norms. Additionally, asymmetry of the injured extremity can lead to postural changes, which can, in turn, impact gait and running patterns. Clinical experience has proven that when children with BPBP begin to learn how to run, falls are often encountered. Parents' concerns related to the patient's limited ability for protective reactions, as well as limited arm swing during running should be addressed.

Although some brachial plexus injury clinics/programs may only have either an OT or a PT, when available, the therapist should consider including the other discipline if the patient continues with deficits after 4 months old. Although similar interventions may be employed, the respective disciplines will be looking at the same movement patterns for different reasons. For example, while the OT may utilize weight-bearing strategies to address strengthening of the intrinsic muscles of the hand, the PT may utilize weight bearing in preparation for crawling.

Children with BPBP are at risk of developing elbow flexion contractures, limiting passive elbow extension. If heterotrophic ossification has not occurred, moist heat, stretching and nighttime splinting should be implemented. When considering the use of Botox, patients and families should be educated to the fact that most functional activities take place with 20 degrees or more of elbow flexion. Therefore, should there be less than a 20 degrees loss in passive range, conservative measures may be most optimal. Older children that have limitations in elbow extension of 40 degrees or greater may be considered for Botox with or without serial casting.[41]

The therapist should also be aware of developmental apraxia with the BPBP population. Specifically, therapists need to decipher if there is a bony deformity limiting movement patterns, or if the atypical movement being observed is a learned pattern with respect

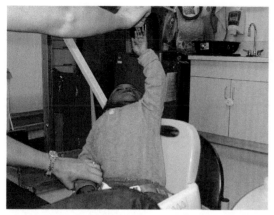

FIG. 11.9 Clinical photograph of a patient with a left BPBP who is utilizing postural compensations in an attempt to obtain additional motion. Postural compensations should be avoided, and rather movement patterns within an active range should be elicited. (Courtesy of Joshua M. Abzug, MD.)

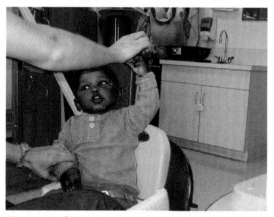

FIG. 11.10 Clinical photograph of the patient in Fig. 11.9 working on active motion within his available range of motion. (Courtesy of Joshua M. Abzug, MD.)

to neuroplasticity and brain mapping. Therapists should only encourage movement patterns that are typical in nature and should avoid eliciting postural compensations (Fig. 11.9). This typically occurs when patients attempt to reach outside of their maximal end range with smooth, isolated upper extremity movement. For example, the child with full passive shoulder flexion may move into a scapular retraction, elbow flexion, and trunk extension position when attempting to actively flex at the shoulder above 90 degrees. This is likely due to the brain map that has been created and repeatedly used while the upper extremity strength was imbalanced. When a patient presents with such patterns of movement, therapists should avoid instruction

statements that are encouraging the patient to reach higher. The upper extremity should be exercised within the available range where normalized movement patterns are observed.[32] (Fig. 11.10)

MODALITIES

Splinting is often utilized for patients with BPBP. When considering the splinting approach and design, therapists need to consider physicians' orders, patients' diagnoses, and upper extremity function. As with any type of splint, therapists need to monitor the patient's status and make adjustments as needed, most often by serial splinting. Splints should be brought into treatment sessions so that the therapists can evaluate fit and function, and if necessary, make adjustments to ensure that the goals of splinting are being maintained. Although it is of great importance to maintain biomechanical principles while splinting, to encourage compliance with splint wear, efforts should be made to ensure that the splint is aesthetically pleasing. Therapists should individualize wearing schedules to meet the goals of the splint, also taking into account relevant information such as contraindications/precautions, patient's tolerance, need of caregivers to assist with donning and doffing (depending on the age of the child), anticipatory compliance, and whether the splint should be donned or doffed for specific ADLs. Considerations should be made when sensory loss is involved because of the BPBP injury. When working with infants or children where the level of potential sensory loss is unknown, thought should be given to increase the surface area of the splint as able, without interfering with the biomechanical design. This modification may decrease the risk of pressure areas. When splinting is being used to address upper extremity function in the presence of BPBP injuries, goals include protecting joints, improving function, and preventing further impairment. When determining if splinting is warranted and if so, which type of splint to employ, the therapist should consider the following: range of motion, muscle tone, presence of contractures, functional use of the upper extremity, developmental norms as it relates to the use of the extremity for fine and gross motor skill function, skin integrity, sensation, and environmental support (i.e., caregivers, home situation, school, etc.).

Bracing about the shoulder can be used to minimize contractures and passively lengthen tight muscles in infants and toddlers during growth. A shoulder abduction orthosis is often warranted for children after undergoing a procedure to address glenohumeral dysplasia such as an open reduction and tendon transfer

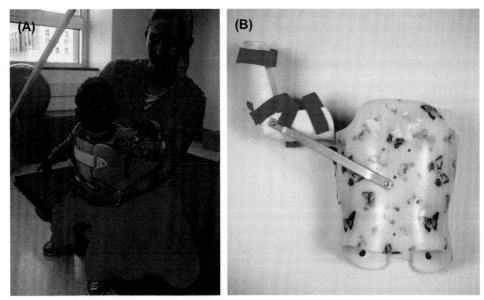

FIG. 11.11 Examples of shoulder abduction orthoses. (Courtesy of Joshua M. Abzug, MD.)

(Fig. 11.11). For infants between four and 8 weeks old presenting with major shoulder external rotation tightness, the Sup-ER (supinator-external rotation) orthosis was created by Durlacher et al. to maintain the affected shoulder in external rotation and the forearm in supination.[42] The design of the brace is made to passively lengthen tight shoulder external rotators and the supination musculature by placing the arm in a soft, long-arm immobilizer and a waistband that keeps the limb in external rotation against the body.[42] For optimal orthotic benefit, it is recommended that the Sup-ER brace is worn for most the day based on the patient's age and clinical assessment, and be removed at least twice a day for parents and/or therapists to perform PROM/AROM exercises.[42] This schedule is gradually tapered as the patient becomes accepting of the brace and improvements are seen.

Three commonly used upper extremity splints for the brachial plexus injury population include wrist cock-up splints, resting hand splints and thumb splints. The wrist cock-up splint provides stabilization at the wrist, while permitting full motion at the metacarpophalangeal, proximal interphalangeal, and distal interphalangeal joints and can be fabricated with either a volar or a dorsal approach, depending on the patient's specific needs. The therapist can utilize either static or dynamic techniques to achieve the desired outcome. The resting hand splint supports the volar surface of a patient's upper extremity, placing the wrist and digits in a static position. A resting hand splint is used to immobilize the wrist and digits to prevent contracture,

or to prevent further impairment such as loss of PROM due to increased muscle tone. Due to the nature of these two types of splints, wrist cock-up splints are usually prescribed for daytime use, as these allow for functional use of the upper extremity with proper positioning of the wrist, while the resting hand splint is often prescribed for nighttime/naptime as it does not allow for functional use of the hand while donned. To address palmar adduction of the thumb because of increased muscle tone or decreased active abduction, thumb splints may be utilized. This is particularly true when there is active movement at the wrist and digits, and therefore, resting hand and wrist cock-up splints are not warranted. For infants and children, soft prefabricated thumb splints can be utilized; however, if needed, custom thermoplastic splints may also be fabricated. For patients with limited supination, supination straps may be added to both custom and prefabricated neoprene and thermoplastic splints.[16,42–44]

A commonly used treatment modality for infants and children with brachial plexus injuries is therapeutic taping, of which the most commonly used product is Kinesio tape. Therapists should explore the various commercially available tapes, as each has different properties or attributes that may best meet a particular patient's needs. The elastic properties of this tape are likened to human skin and were designed to maximize the benefits of taping without limiting joint motion.[16,45] Taping can be utilized to inhibit or facilitate muscle function in addition to providing support regarding joint stabilization. When addressing brachial plexus injuries, this is beneficial to inhibit the strong, unopposed muscles that are not affected by the injury, and to facilitate the weak muscles affected by the injury. As with any treatment intervention, it is important to educate parents on the proper use and wearing schedule. To maximize the elastic properties of the tape, it should remain in place for three to 5 days. Therapists should allow the patient's skin time to recover for 24 hours before reapplying the tape to the same area.[16,46,47]

SUMMARY

BPBP injuries continue to occur in roughly 1 in 1000 live births. Early assessment and intervention from a therapist will aid in the recovery process by limiting contracture development and improving sensory reeducation. Surgical intervention is still needed at times to restore continuity of the nerves. Therapists should focus on maintaining range of motion in the upper extremity, while promoting growth and development. Custom orthoses are commonly utilized to help prevent contracture formation.

SUPPLEMENTARY MATERIALS

Supplementary data related to this article can be found online at doi:10.1016/B978-0-323-53091-0.00011-7.

REFERENCES

1. Abid A. Brachial plexus birth palsy: management during the first year of life. *Orthop Traumatol Surg Res.* 2015; 102:5125–5132. https://doi.org/10.1016/j.otsr.2015.05.008.
2. Abzug JM, Kozin SH. Current concepts: neonatal brachial plexus palsy. *Orthopedics.* 2010;33:430–435. https://doi.org/10.3928/01477447-20100429-25.
3. Waters PM. Obstetric brachial plexus injuries: evaluation and management. *J Am Acad Orthop.* 1997;5(4):205–214.
4. Smith K, Patel V. Congenital brachial plexus palsy. *Paediatr Child Health.* 2016;26(4):152–156.
5. O'Brien DF, Park TS, Noetzel MJ, Weatherly T. Management of birth brachial plexus palsy. *Child's Nerv Syst.* 2005;22(2):103–112. https://doi.org/10.1007/s00381-005-1261-y.
6. Pondaag W, Malessy MJ, van Dijk JG, Thomeer RT. Natural history of obstetric brachial plexus palsy: a systematic review. *Dev Med Child Neurol.* 2004;46(2):138–144.
7. Akel BS, Öksuz C, Oskay D, Firat T, Tarakci E, Leblebicioğlu G. Health-related quality of life in children with obstetrical brachial plexus palsy. *Qual Life Res.* 2013;22(9):2617–2624. https://doi.org/10.1007/s11136-013-0369-x.
8. Buesch FE, Schlaepfer B, de Bruin ED, Wohlrab G, Ammann-Reiffer C, Meyer-Heim A. *Int J Rehabil Res.*
2010;33(2):187–192. https://doi.org/10.1097/MRR.0b013e3283310d6e.
9. Curtis C, Stephens D, Clarke HM, Andrews D. The active movement scale: an evaluative tool for infants with obstetrical brachial plexus palsy. *J Hand Surg.* 2002;27(3): 470–479. https://doi.org/10.1053/jhsu.2002.32965.
10. Fitoussi F, Maurel N, Diop A, et al. Upper extremity kinematics analysis in obstetrical brachial plexus palsy. *Orthop Traumatol Surg Res.* 2009;95(5):336–342. https://doi.org/10.1016/j.otsr.2009.04.012.
11. Foad SL, Mehlman CT, Ying J. The epidemiology of neonatal brachial plexus palsy in the United States. *J Bone Joint Surg Am.* 2008;90(6):1258–1264. https://doi.org/10.2016/jbjs.g.00853.
12. Haerle M, Gilbert A. Management of complete obstetric brachial plexus lesions. *J Pediatr Orthop.* 2004;24(2): 194–200.
13. Ho ES, Curtis CG, Clarke HM. The brachial plexus outcome measure: development, internal consistency, and construct validity. *J Hand Ther.* 2012;25(4):406–417.
14. Hogendoorn S, van Overvest KL, Watt I, Duijsens AH, Nelissen RG. Structural changes in muscle and glenohumeral joint deformity in neonatal brachial plexus palsy. *J Bone Joint Surg Am.* 2010;92(4):935–942. https://doi.org/10.2106/jbjs.i.00193.
15. Ridgway E, Valicenti-McDermott M, Kornhaber L, Kathirirhamby DR, Wieder H. *J Pediatr.* 2013;162(5), 1065-7.
16. Russo SA, Rodriguez LM, Kozin SH, et al. Therapeutic taping for scapular stabilization in children with brachial plexus birth palsy. *Am J Occup Ther.* 2016;70(5):1–11.
17. Waters PM. Update on management of pediatric brachial plexus palsy. *J Pediatr Orthop.* 2005;25(1):116–126.
18. Hale HP, Bae DS, Waters PM. Current concepts in the management of brachial plexus birth palsy. *J Hand Surg Am.* 2010;35(2):322–331. https://doi.org/10.1016/j.jhsa.2009.11.026.
19. Zafeiriou D, Psychogiou K. Obstetrical brachial plexus palsy. *Pediatr Neurol.* 2008;38(4):235–242.
20. Lindqvist PG, Erichs K, Molnar C, Gudmundsson S, Dahlin LB. Characteristics and outcome of brachial plexus birth palsy in neonates. *Acta Paediatr.* 2012;101(6): 579–582.
21. Abzug JM, Mehlman CT, Ying J. Assessment of current epidemiology and risk factors surrounding brachial plexus birth palsy. *J Hand Surg Am.* 2018;(17):S0363–S5023, 31908-1.
22. Foad SL, Mehlman CT, Foad MB, Lippert WC. Prognosis following neonatal brachial plexus palsy: an evidence-based review. *J Child Orthop.* 2009;3(6):459–463. https://doi.org/10.1007/s11832-009-0208-3.
23. Rasmussen L, Justice D, Chang KW, Nelson VS, Yang LJ. Home exercise DVD promotes exercise accuracy by caregivers of children and adolescents with brachial plexus palsy. *PM R.* 2013;5(11):924–930.
24. Russo SA, Loeffler BJ, Zlotolow DA, Kozin SH, Richards JG, Ashworth S. Limited glenohumeral cross-body adduction in children with brachial plexus birth palsy: a contributor

to scapular winging. *J Pediatr Orthop.* 2015;35(3): 240–245.

25. Hoeksma AF, ter Steeg AM, Nelissen RG, van Ouwerkerk WJ, Lankhorst GJ, de Jong BA. Neurological recovery in obstetric brachial plexus injuries: an historical cohort study. *Dev Med Child Neurol.* 2004;46(2):76–83.

26. Sunderland S. A classification of peripheral nerve injuries producing loss of function. *Brain.* 1951;74(4):491–516.

27. Artice MB, Morrison SA, McDowell SL, Ackerman PM, Foy TA, Tefertiller C. Traumatic spinal cord injury. In: Umphred DA, ed. *Neurological Rehabilitation.* 3rd ed. St. Louis: Mosby-Year Book; 1995:459–520.

28. Mackinnon SE, Dellon AL, O'Brien JP, et al. Selection of optimal axon ratio for nerve regeneration. *Ann Plast Surg.* 1989;23(2):129–134.

29. Evans GR. Peripheral nerve injury: a review and approach to tissue engineered constructs. *Anat Rec.* 2001;263(4): 396–404.

30. Nath RK. *Obstetric Brachial Plexus Injuries-Erb's Palsy: The Nath Method of Diagnosis and Treatment.* College Station: VirtualBookworm.com Publishing; 2007.

31. Al-Qattan MM, El-Sayed AA, Al-Zahrani AY, et al. Narakas classification of obstetric brachial plexus palsy revisited. *J Hand Surg Eur.* 2009;34(6):788–791.

32. Brown T, Cupido C, Scarfone H, Pape K, Galea V, McComas A. Developmental apraxia arising from neonatal brachial plexus palsy. *Neurology.* 2000;55(1):24–30.

33. Vander Linden DW. Brachial plexus injury. In: Campbell SK, Palisano RJ, eds. *Physical Therapy for Children.* 3rd ed. St. Louis: Saunders Elsevier; 2006:628–643.

34. Moukoko D, Ezaki M, Wilkes D, Carter P. Posterior shoulder dislocation in infants with neonatal brachial plexus palsy. *J Bone Joint Surg Am.* 2004;86-A(4):787–793.

35. Michelow BJ, Clarke HM, Curtis CG, Zuker RM, Seifu Y, Andrews DF. The natural history of obstetrical brachial plexus palsy. *Plast Reconstr Surg.* 1994;93:675–680.

36. Abzug JM, Wyrick-Glover TO, Case AL, Zlotolow DA, Kozin SH. Loss of midline function in brachial plexus birth palsy patients. *J Pediatr Orthop.* 2019;39(3):e232–e235.

37. Oskay D, Oksüz C, Akel S, Firat T, Leblebicioğlu G. Quality of life in mothers of children with obstetrical brachial plexus palsy. *Pediatr Int.* 2012;54(1):117–122. https://doi.org/10.1111/j.1442-200x.2011.03455.x.

38. Spaargaren E, Ahmed J, van Ouwerkerk WJ, de Groot V, Beckerman H. Aspects of activities and participation of

7–8 year-old children with an obstetric brachial plexus injury. *Eur J Paediatr Neurol.* 2011;15(4):345–352. https://doi.org/10.1016/j.ejpn.2011.03.008.

39. Brown SH, Napier R, Nelson VS, Yang LJ. Home-based movement therapy in neonatal brachial plexus palsy: a case study. *J Hand Ther.* 2015;28(3):307–312.

40. Justice D, Rasmussen L, Di Pietro M, et al. Prevalence of posterior shoulder subluxation in children with neonatal brachial plexus palsy after early full passive range of motion exercises. *PM R.* 2015;7(12):1235–1242.

41. Ho ES, Roy T, Stephens D, Clarke HM. Serial casting and splinting of elbow contractures in children with obstetric brachial plexus palsy. *J Hand Surg Am.* 2010;35(1): 84–91. https://doi.org/10.1016/j.jhsa.2009.09.014.

42. Durlacher KM, Bellows D, Verchere C. Sup-ER orthosis: an innovative treatment for infants with birth related brachial plexus injury. *J Hand Ther.* 2014;27(4):335–339.

43. Chan RK. Splinting for peripheral nerve injury in upper limb. *Hand Surg.* 2002;7(2):251–259.

44. Schwartz DA, McKie A, Gabriel LS. Orthoses for the pediatric population In: Coppard BM, Lohman, H, editors. Introduction to Splinting: A Critical-Thinking & Problem-Solving Approach. St. Louis: Mosby-Year Book, Inc.p.365-392.

45. Russo SA, Zlotolow DA, Chafetz RS, et al. Efficacy of 3 therapeutic taping configurations for children with brachial plexus birth palsy. *J Hand Ther.* 2018;31(3):357–370.

46. Kase K, Martin P, Yasukawa A. *Kinesio® Taping in Pediatrics: Fundamental and Whole Body Taping.* Kinesio® USA, LLC; 2006.

47. Walsh SF. Treatment of a brachial plexus injury using kinesiotape and exercise. *Physiother Theory Pract.* 2010;26(7): 490–496. https://doi.org/10.3109/09593980903578872.

FURTHER READING

1. Hoeksma AF, Wolf H, Oei SL. Obstetrical brachial plexus injuries: incidence, natural course and shoulder contracture. *Clin Rehabil.* 2000;14(5):523–526.

2. Kozin SH. The evaluation and treatment of children with brachial plexus birth palsy. *J Hand Surg Am.* 2011;36(8): 1360–1369. https://doi.org/10.1016/j.jhsa.2011.05.018.

CHAPTER 12

Brachial Plexus: Primary Surgery

SCOTT H. KOZIN, MD

INTRODUCTION

The anatomy, incidence, etiology, demographics, and initial management of a child with brachial plexus palsy have been discussed in this chapter. Timely referral to a brachial center is recommended to allow for obtaining accurate baseline data, to perform serial examinations, and to determine the necessity of surgical intervention. These visits also allow time for the family to understand their child's injury, ask appropriate questions, develop a rapport with the brachial plexus team, and gain confidence in the decision-making process.

The family must be comfortable with the brachial plexus team, as many of these surgeries are lengthy, tedious, difficult, and not without complications. In addition, secondary procedures may be necessary, and long-term follow-up is required. This chapter will discuss the initial referral of the child and the subsequent decision-making process regarding primary nerve surgery. The indications, timing, techniques, and rehabilitation of nerve surgery will be discussed.

INITIAL REFERRAL

Upon referral, the initial evaluation reviews the birth history including prenatal, birth, and postnatal phases. The prenatal period focuses on the mom's health with respect to gestational diabetes and weight gain. The number of previous pregnancies and birth histories are required information. Principal risk factors for shoulder dystocia are fetal macrosomia, gestational diabetes, and history of previous shoulder dystocia. The birth period focuses on the delivery with specific questions concerning the use of instruments (forceps or vacuum), the difficulty of the delivery, and any maneuver necessary to effect delivery. Parents are often unfamiliar with the term shoulder dystocia. We ask if their child was "stuck," that infer dystocia. In addition, the maneuvers performed are unfamiliar terms. We ask were your legs bent to your chest (McRobert's maneuver), did someone push of your belly (suprapubic pressure), and was the bay rotated during the delivery (Corkscrew

or Rubin's maneuver). The postnatal period focuses on the child's health including APGAR scores, birth weight, need for resuscitation, necessity of intubation, results of X-rays, and requirement of neonatal intensive care admission. The initial movement in the affected arm is critical historical information as most parents simple state that their child "could not move their arm." The presence or absence of shoulder, elbow, wrist, and hand (finger opening or closing) movement requires delineation. The goal of the postnatal questioning is to determine the extent of the initial brachial plexus injury and any interim improvement to date. In our clinic, the therapists play an integral role in the examination process and family education. They also guide and oversea any postoperative therapy.

The physical examination of the infant focuses on active and passive movement. Passive motion should be full and painless unless some muscle tightness has occurred following birth. The stretching of tight muscles will yield pain; however, passive motion is necessary to maintain supple joints. Painful passive motion not attributed to muscle tightness warrants further evaluation. X-rays may reveal an undetected fracture of the clavicle, humerus, or elbow. Active motion measurements require patience and experience. Infants are most comfortable resting on the laps of their parents versus stranded on an examination table. The mom or dad can rotate and position the child to allow examination of both limbs and to permit the assessment of gravity eliminated and against gravity movement. Infants respond to tactile stimulation and noise. Stroking the limb will induce movement as will sound, such as a rattle. Patience is truly a virtue during the examination. An uncooperative infant may be tired, poopy, or just irritable. A poopy child is better evaluated after a diaper change. A hungry infant may require feeding before examination; however, a completely satiated child will be somnolent.

The passive examination determines the suppleness of the joints while the active evaluation ascertains the presence or absence of nerve innervation and muscle

TABLE 12.1
Practical Anatomy for Brachial Plexus Injury Pattern.

Trunk (Roots)	Muscles	Sensation
Upper trunk (C5 and C6)	Shoulder (rotator cuff and deltoid) Forearm supination (biceps and supinator) Elbow flexion (biceps and brachialis) Wrist extension (extensor carpi radialis longus)	Median nerve sensibility thumb and index finger
Middle trunk (C7)	Elbow extension (triceps) Latissimus dorsi Forearm pronation (pronator teres) Wrist extension (extensor carpi radialis longus) Digital extension (MCP joints) Wrist flexion (flexor carpi radialis)	Median nerve sensibility long finger
Lower trunk (C8 and T1)	Forearm pronation (pronator quadratus) Extrinsic finger and thumb flexors (flexor digitorum profundus and flexor pollicis longus) Wrist flexion (flexor carpi ulnaris) Digital extension (IP joints) Intrinsic muscles	Ulnar nerve sensibility (ring and small fingers)

IP, interphalangeal; *MCP*, metacarpophalangeal.

activation. Passive motion is simply documented in degrees using a goniometer. In infants, the goniometer can be a protractor or a visual estimate ("ocular goniometer") depending upon the child's cooperation. Active motion utilizes the practical anatomy of the brachial plexus to determine the injury pattern and root involvement (Table 12.1).

Active motion is graded according to the Active Movement Scale (AMS) developed at the Hospital for Sick Children in Toronto, Canada (Table 12.2).[1] A key grading rule during the scoring of the AMS is that a motion cannot be graded as 5 or higher unless the movement is full against gravity (grade 4). For example, elbow flexion must be full with against gravity before achieving a grade of 5, 6, or 7. We have applied a similar concept to our grading during manual muscle testing in older children. In other words, a patient must achieve full motion against gravity (grade 3) before being granted a grade 4 or 5. The AMS is an invaluable tool to assess infants before and after surgery. The AMS been shown to be a reliable measurement between observers.[2]

Sensibility cannot be assessed in an infant. Clinical clues are finger moistness and withdraw from a gentle pinch. Pruning in the tub is another indication of intact nerve supply.

CLASSIFICATION

The classic disease severity measure is the Narakas classification that divides brachial plexus birth palsies into

TABLE 12.2
Active Movement Scale.

Shoulder adduction	Gravity eliminated	Score[a]
Shoulder flexion	No contraction	0
Shoulder external rotation	Contraction, no motion	1
Shoulder internal rotation	<50% motion	2
Elbow flexion	>50% motion	3
Elbow extension	Full motion	4
Forearm supination	Against gravity	
Forearm pronation	<50% motion	5
Wrist flexion	>50% motion	6
Wrist extension	Full motion	7
Finger flexion		
Finger extension		
Thumb flexion		
Thumb extension		
	Total	

[a] A score of 4 must be achieved before a higher score can be assigned. Movement grades are within available range of motion. Adapted from Clarke HM, Curtis CG. An approach to obstetrical brachial plexus injuries. *Hand Clin.* 1995;11:563–580.

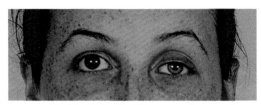

FIG. 12.1 Residual left-sided Horner syndrome with ptosis (drooped eyelid) and miosis (constricted pupil). In addition, Horner's syndrome can lead to different eye colors (heterochromia). (Courtesy of Shriners Hospital for Children, Philadelphia.)

four groups.[3] Group 1 is the classic Erb-Duchenne palsy (C5 and C6) injury. Group 2 is the extended Erb-Duchenne (C5, C6, and C7) injury. Groups 3 and 4 are total plexus palsies separated by the absence (group 3) or presence of Horner syndrome (group 4). The very presence of Horner syndrome (drooped eyelid, constricted pupil, sunken globe, and sweating deficiency along the affected side of the face), usually implies an avulsion injury at C8 and T1 (Fig. 12.1). Horner syndrome has been shown to have independent unfavorable prognostic value.[4] These Narakas groupings have been shown to have prognostic power, with dramatically lower full chances of recovery rates for Narakas 3 and 4 patients.[5,6]

NERVE INJURY

Brachial plexus birth palsy injuries are the result of traction across the brachial plexus. The traction induces strain (change in length) across the nerve roots and trunks. The amount of ultimate strain has several components that affect the degree of nerve damage including the magnitude of the force and the vector along the nerve. The injury represents a continuum with progressive injury to the nerve.[7] Mild stretch disrupts the myelin sheath and interrupts nerve conduction without loss of continuity of the axon (neurapraxia). Recovery takes place via remyelination without Wallerian degeneration. Ongoing stretch exceeds the elastic limit of the nerve, damages the myelin sheath, and the underlying axons with loss of axon continuity (axonotmesis). The connective tissue of the nerve is preserved (epineurium, perineurium, and endoneurium). The entire nerve distal to the injury undergoes Wallerian degeneration that usually begins within 24–36 hours after injury and is complete 1–4 weeks later. The axonal degeneration is followed by degradation of the myelin sheath and infiltration by macrophages. The debris within the distal stump is

removed to allow for regeneration. The motor and sensory cell bodies transition from their normal role as signaling center to a nerve cell growth-promoting center with upregulation and a surge in cellular activity. The cell body synthesizes the structural proteins essential for axonal repair and regeneration. Axonal sprouts emerge just proximal to the injury (first node of Ranvier) and project into the distal nerve stump. Many axon collateral sprouts enter the distal stump with expectations of regeneration. Those sprouts that land into incorrect target contact are pruned. Eventually, accurate motor neurons project their axons into muscle and accurate sensory neurons reach their sensory receptors. Axonal regeneration occurs at a rate of 1–3 mm per day. The extent of recovery is related to the response of the axonal sprouting and the distance to the motor end plate. Longer distances prognosticate lesser recovery as the motor end plates within the muscle undergo irreversible end plate demise between 18 and 24 months. Subsequent to this demise, additional nerve regeneration will be ineffective in reinnervating the muscle.

Continual stretch leads to complete disruption of the nerve including the sheath, axon, and encapsulating connective tissue (epineurium, perineurium, and endoneurium). This injury is called as a neurotmesis and results in irreversible intraneural scarring. The prognosis for recovery is bleak without surgical reconstruction. The intervening scar forms a neuroma that must be resected to allow for nerve reconstruction to allow regeneration across the defect. Another surgical option is nerve transfers distal to the injury that bypass the injury completely.

Neurapraxia is an entity separate and distinct from the more severe injuries of axonotmesis and neurotmesis. Traction axonotmesis and neurotmesis lesions, however, are a continuum with an overlap similar to a Venn diagram (Fig. 12.2). Brachial plexus injuries often have features of neurapraxia, axonotmesis and neurotmesis and even within the same trunk different degrees of nerve injuries can coexist. This combination complicates terminology and the decision-making process for surgery.

Brachial plexus birth injuries are supraclavicular (above the clavicle), although the injury can extend below infraclavicular. Axonotmesis typically occurs at the level of the trunk. Neurotmesis injury can occur at the level of the trunk (a.k.a. rupture). Neurotmesis can also occur when the nerve root is pulled from the spinal cord (a.k.a. avulsion). Currently, there is no reliable technique to restore continuity between an avulsed nerve root and the spinal cord. Surgery can bypass the injury as discussed later.

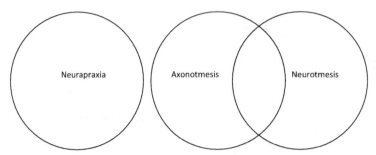

FIG. 12.2 Neurapraxia is a separate entity, but traction axonometesis and neurotmesis can overlap.

ANCILLARY TESTING

Electrodiagnostic testing has a minimal role on brachial plexus birth palsies. The uncooperative infant is unable to tolerate the examination, requires sedation, and cannot follow instructions. Electrodiagnostic studies, including nerve conduction velocity and needle electromyography, overestimates clinical recovery in the proximal muscles of the shoulder and arm.[8] This incorrect prediction provides false hope to the parents and delays referral for surgical intervention.

Radiologic studies can provide usually information by identifying nerve root avulsion injuries. The presence of a pseudomeningocele, a meningeal pouch filled with cerebrospinal fluid that extends through the intervertebral foramen into the paraspinal area infers a nerve root avulsion (Fig. 12.3). This pouch represents an extraction of the dural and arachnoidal sleeve through the intervertebral foramen that often occurs during a root avulsion injury. CT myelography and magnetic resonance imaging have greater than 90% true positive rates for determining avulsion injuries correlated at surgery when pseudomeningoceles are seen.[9,10] Smaller pseudomeningoceles may represent a false positive with preservation of nerve root integrity.[9] Unfortunately, current imaging studies are unable to assess whether the neuroma has axons incontinuity or there has been complete axonal disruption.

TIMING OF SURGERY

The timing of surgery is dependent upon the degree and extent of injury. Mild plexus injuries (neurapraxias) recover quickly via remyelination without Wallerian degeneration. This process occurs in the first 6–8 weeks of life and does not require surgery. Moderate injuries (axonotmesis) recover more slowly following Wallerian degeneration and axonal regeneration. This process occurs at a rate of 1–3 mm per day and results in signs of clinical recovery between 3 and 6 months. The proximal muscles will recover first followed by the more distal

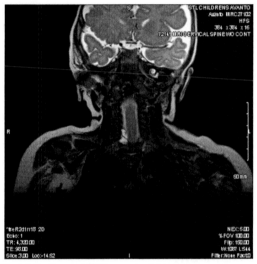

FIG. 12.3 Coronal MRI reveals right-sided pseudomeningoceles that have formed outside the intervertebral foramen indicative of root avulsion injury. (Courtesy of Shriners Hospital for Children, Philadelphia.)

muscles. Neurotmesis (rupture or avulsion) will not recover and requires surgical intervention.

The quandary in brachial plexus birth palsies is determining when to intervene. Surgery must have a positive effect compared to the natural history of recover. Global injuries with a Horner's syndrome (Narakas 4) require early surgery within the first 3–4 months of life.[11] The injury pattern is a combination of ruptures and avulsions that requires surgical reconstruction with nerve grafting and nerve transfers.

The Narakas 1 (C5 and C6) and 2 (C5, C6, and C7) injury patterns are more controversial regarding timing and technique of nerve surgery. There is no universal consensus regarding indications and timing of surgical intervention. Ancillary testing is unreliable in determining the exact extent of injury. We prefer serial examinations every 4–6 weeks to assess recovery.[12] The active movement scale is measured and documented. Failure to demonstrate noteworthy signs of recovery by 5–8 months is an indication for surgeries.[13] Injuries with no recovery or minimal recovery require surgery. In addition, injuries that demonstrate some early recovery but the process subsequently stagnates require surgery.

SURGICAL TECHNIQUES

Nerve Graft

The principle surgical techniques are nerve grafting and nerve transfers. Nerve grafting requires neuroma excision back to proximal and distal viable fascicles.[7] The defect is bridged with nerve grafts harvested from the legs (sural nerves). Additional potential donor nerves include the medial antebrachial cutaneous nerve and the radial sensory nerve. Currently, autograft is preferred over allograft.

Nerve grafting that interposes multiple strands of donor nerve to bride the defect is called as cable grafting. The goal is to place enough cables to satisfy the caliper of the proximal (root) and distal (trunk, division, or branch) recipients. The cable can be secured with microsuture or fibrin glue. The grafts are placed slightly loose without any tension across the coaptation sites. This tension will lessen the chances of the awake child tearing the repair apart.

Nerve Transfer

Selection of the donor nerve

The donor nerve has to be available and expendable.[14] Available implies a functioning and normal nerve that can sustain loss of a portion of its axons. Fortunately, many nerves have built in redundancy in their proximal aspect within the arm. Expendable means that if there is some loss of function from donor harvest, the effect is minimal. For example, harvesting the intercostal nerves has negligible effect on pulmonary function as long as the phrenic nerve is working.[15] Similarly, selection of a radial nerve to a single head of the triceps has miniscule effect on elbow extension as long as the other two heads are preserved.[16]

An additional consideration during nerve transfer is synergism. Logically, using a donor nerve that provides synergistic function with the intended action would facilitate relearning after reinnervation. For example, when selecting an ulnar nerve fascicle for elbow flexion, selecting the fascicle that innervates the flexor carpi ulnaris would ease relearning.

Selection of the recipient nerve

The recipient nerve should be selectively chosen to achieve the desired function. The motor nerve recipient should be close to the endplate to minimize reinnervation time. When selecting recipient motor nerves, there

is a trend to provide dual reinnervation to achieve a desired function. For example, nerve transfers for elbow flexion attempt to reinnervate both the biceps and brachialis muscles. Similarly, nerve transfers for shoulder motion try to reinnervate both deltoid and rotator cuff function.

PRIORITIES OF SURGICAL RECONSTRUCTION

The priorities of brachial plexus reconstruction are different in children compared to adults. In adults, repairing injuries to the lower trunk (avulsions or ruptures) is futile. The distance from the injury and the slow nerve regeneration preclude useful hand recovery. In children, the distance is less and the regeneration is quicker. Hence, useful hand function is obtainable and is the primary goal.[17] The secondary goal is elbow motion, especially flexion for hand-to-mouth activity. The third goal is shoulder stability and motion. The surgical plan should consider this hierarchy during the decision-making process. The next section will detail the potential methods to achieve the hierarchical goals via nerve grafting and/or nerve transfer.

Hand

Nerve grafting

Nerve grafting to the C8 and/or T1 nerve roots is critical to reanimate the hand. The best available nerve root with the greatest number of fascicles is grafted to the lower trunk.[17] A cable graft is placed between the root and the lower trunk (C8, T1 nerve roots). The lower trunk can be mobilized in a cephalad direction to lessen the graft distance.

Nerve transfer

Nerve transfer to the C8 and/or T1 nerve roots is performed in dire straits (Fig. 12.4). In cases with only one or two nerve roots available, nerve transfer can be considered. The primary donor nerve is the contralateral C7 (CC7) nerve root. In the past, the CC7 nerve root was tunneled subcutaneous across the neck to the injured plexus.[18] Long nerve grafts were placed between CC7 and the intended recipients (e.g., lower trunk) with disappointing results. More recently, a passage behind the esophagus has been utilized to shorten the distance and lessen the graft length.[19] This approach requires surgical expertise as the vertebral artery and carotid sheath are in harm's way. We utilize the assistance of our cervical spine surgeons who are comfortable with the exposure for anterior cervical spine procedures. The procedure requires proficiency and meticulous technique to avoid mishaps.

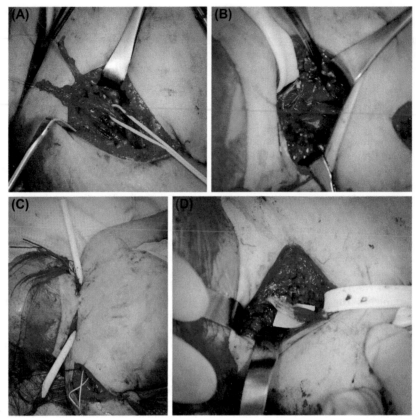

FIG. 12.4 Three-month-old child with right global brachial plexus palsy, Horner's syndrome, and pseudomeningoceles at C8 and T1. **(A)** Exploration revealed frank ruptures of C5 and C6 without continuity. **(B)** Examination of the lower trunk (C8 and T1) beneath the subclavian artery revealed intraforaminal avulsions. **(C)** Passage developed behind the esophagus from the normal left brachial plexus to the injured right brachial plexus. **(D)** Contralateral left C7 nerve trunk grafted to right C8 and T1 nerve roots using 2.5 cm sural nerve grafts. (Courtesy of Shriners Hospital for Children, Philadelphia.)

Elbow

Nerve grafting

Nerve grafting to the anterior division of the upper trunk is a method to restore elbow flexion via reinnervation of the biceps and brachialis muscles (Fig. 12.5). The preferred donor nerve root is C6 to restore the normal anatomy. However, a C6 avulsion precludes this technique and requires an alternative nerve root donor or consideration of nerve transfer.

Nerve transfer

Standard nerve transfers for elbow flexion require an intact lower trunk with preserved ulnar and/or median nerve function. The nerve transfer can reanimate the biceps and/or the brachialis muscles. The single fascicle transfer typically utilizes a group fascicle of the ulnar nerve transferred to the bicep's motor nerve emanating from the musculocutaneous nerve (Fig. 12.6).[20] The double fascicle transfer typically utilizes a group fascicle of the ulnar nerve transferred to the biceps motor nerve and a group fascicle from the median nerve to brachialis motor nerve stemming from the musculocutaneous nerve.[21]

If the lower trunk is injured and abnormal, alternative donors may be necessary. The intercostal nerves are the preferred source of axons. The phrenic nerve should be working and is a prerequisite for intercostal nerve transfer.[15]

Shoulder

Nerve grafting

Nerve grafting to the suprascapular nerve and the posterior division of the upper trunk is a method to restore shoulder abduction. This technique will reinnervate

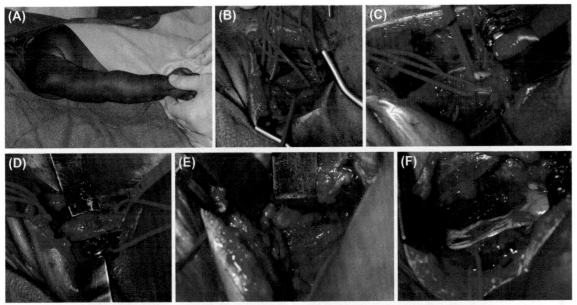

FIG. 12.5 Six-month-old child with right C5/C6 brachial plexus birth palsy and no return of elbow flexion. **(A)** Operative positioning on operating room table. **(B)** Supraclavicular exposure with retraction of omohyoid. **(C)** Isolation of suprascapular nerve, posterior division of upper trunk, and anterior division of upper trunk distal to neuroma. **(D)** Large neuroma of upper trunk. **(E)** C5 nerve root after neuroma resection. **(F)** Sural nerve grafting from C5 and C6 to suprascapular nerve, posterior division of upper trunk, and anterior division of upper trunk. (Courtesy of Shriners Hospital for Children, Philadelphia.)

the supraspinatus, infraspinatus, deltoid, and teres minor muscles. The preferred donor nerve root is C5 to restore the normal anatomy. However, a C5 avulsion precludes this technique and requires an alternative nerve root donor or consideration of nerve transfer.

Nerve transfer
The standard nerve transfer for rotator cuff reanimation requires an intact trapezius muscle (cranial nerve XI). The distal portion of the spinal accessory nerve is transferred to the suprascapular nerve to reinnervate the supraspinatus and infraspinatus.[22] The proximal spinal accessory nerve is retained for maintenance of upper trapezius function. This transfer can be performed from an anterior or posterior approach (Fig. 12.7). A double fascicle transfer can also be used for shoulder motion.[23] A second donor can be transferred to the axillary nerve for deltoid and teres minor function. The donor nerve depends upon the injury pattern. In an upper brachial plexus injury (C5, C6), the triceps muscle (C7) is preserved. A branch from one of its three heads (medial, lateral, or long) can be transferred to the anterior branch of the axillary nerve to reinnervate the deltoid muscle. If the middle trunk (C7) is injured and

abnormal, alternative donors may be necessary. If the lower trunk is normal, a group fascicle of the ulnar nerve can be transferred to the anterior branch of the axillary nerve. Another potential donor is the intercostal nerves as long as the phrenic nerve is working.

Rehabilitation
Nerve grafting
Nerve rehabilitation following nerve grafting is divided into an immobilization phase followed by a mobilization phase awaiting nerve regeneration (Protocol 1). The immobilization position varies with the tightness of any joints. Supple joints allow immobilization in a swathe wrapping the arm against the body. A tight joint, such as a shoulder internal rotation contracture, requires immobilization in a shoulder spica cast stretching the glenohumeral joint.

The mobilization phase is accomplished in therapy and via a home exercise program. The joints are stretched to maintain suppleness awaiting nerve regeneration. Incisional care is also instructed. The therapist must educate the parents on nerve regeneration as months will pass before active motion is seen. In addition, sensory recovery can result in hyperesthesia in

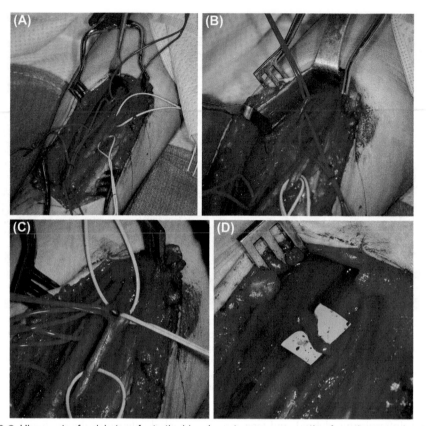

FIG. 12.6 Ulnar motor fascicle transfer to the bicep's motor nerve emanating from the musculocutaneous nerve. **(A)** Medial arm exposure. Yellow loops around ulnar nerve and red loops around musculocutaneous nerve. **(B)** Bicep's motor nerve isolated from musculocutaneous nerve. **(C)** Isolation of a group fascicle from the ulnar nerve. **(D)** Transfer of the group fascicle from the ulnar nerve to the bicep's motor nerve. (Courtesy of Shriners Hospital for Children, Philadelphia.)

infants that manifests as scratching or biting (Fig. 12.8). The biting can be severe and can result in infection and even nibbling away of the affected fingertips. Regrettably, there is no intellectual reasoning with infants and the parents feel horrible about the biting. Numerous medical and home remedies have been tried to no avail as the infants continue to gnaw at their digits. Fortunately, as the sensory recovery progresses and the tactile hyperesthesia lessen, the biting diminishes. The result is often physical scarring to the child and emotional scarring to the parents.

Nerve transfer

Nerve rehabilitation following nerve transfer is straightforward. Following a brief period of immobilization to allow for wound healing, the arm is mobilized. Certain nerve transfers allow unrestricted motion while other nerve transfers have postoperative

limitations (e.g., intercostal nerve transfer—Protocol 2). Nerve regeneration occurs at a rate of 1 mm/day. The patients are instructed to link their donor and recipient nerve function (e.g., flexor carpi ulnaris wrist flexion and elbow flexion following ulnar to bicep's motor nerve transfer) to promote cortical learning. This combined movement pattern is performed numerous times per day awaiting nerve regeneration. When the donor nerve regenerates to the recipient muscle, the patient will "learn" to fire his or her recipient movement independent of donor function (Protocols 12.1 and 12.2).

Outcomes
Nerve grafts

Reported outcomes following nerve grafting are difficult to decipher. There are variable injury patterns, varying surgical approaches, and different methods of assessing

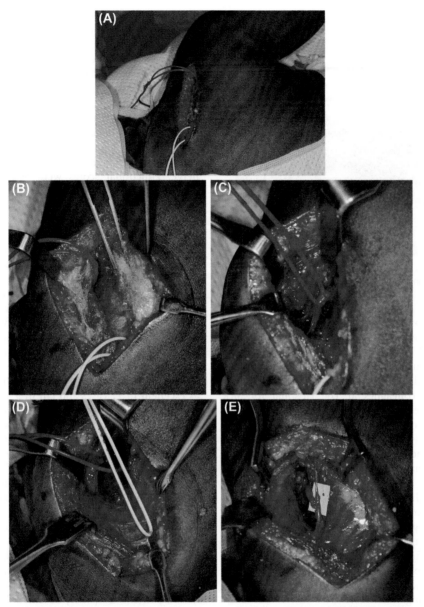

FIG. 12.7 Spinal accessory to suprascapular nerve transfer via posterior surgical approach. **(A)** Infant positioned in the lateral decubitus position. **(B)** Trapezius muscle elevated from scapular spine (forceps). **(C)** Suprascapular nerve identified and traced through the scapular notch with release of the superior transverse scapular ligament. **(D)** Spinal accessory nerve isolated deep to the trapezius muscle. **(E)** Spinal accessory transferred to suprascapular nerve with excessive length to allow for nerve trimming and tension free coaptation. (Courtesy of Shriners Hospital for Children, Philadelphia.)

outcome. The shared theme is that the outcome varies directly with the number of nerve roots ruptured and avulsed. In addition, avulsion of the lower roots portends the worst functional outcome.

Gilbert reported on 436 patients who underwent surgical reconstruction.[24,25] Follow-up was a minimum of 4 years and included those patients who had undergone secondary reconstructive procedure.

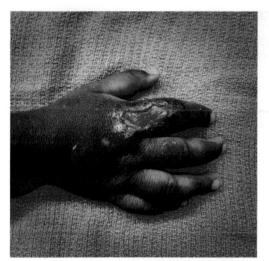

FIG. 12.8 Infant biting her right index finger after brachial plexus exploration attributed to hyperesthesia.

Assessment of outcome and function utilized the Mallet scale. For children with C5–C6 lesions, 80% of patients achieved good or excellent shoulder function. In C5–C7 lesions, 61% attained good or excellent shoulder function. For C5-T1 lesions, only 25% recovered useful hand function.

Clarke and colleagues at The Hospital for Sick Children reported important regarding the role of neurolysis.[26] The cohort consisted of 108 patients with long-term follow-up (minimum of 4 years). Among them, 16 underwent neurolysis of conducting neuromas-in-continuity compared to 92 (48 with C5–C6 lesions and 44 with total plexus palsy) that were treated with neuroma resection and nerve grafting. The authors concluded that early functional improvements following neurolysis were not sustained over time. In contrast, neuroma resection and nerve grafting produced significant functional improvement for both C5–C6 and total plexus palsy. Hence, neurolysis should be abandoned in favor of neuroma resection and nerve grafting.

Nerve transfers

The published reports for nerve transfer in brachial plexus birth palsy have focused on the shoulder and elbow. Many series include variable injury patterns, concomitant nerve grafting, and secondary procedures that confound the results. The spinal accessory to suprascapular nerve transfer has discrepancies in the published outcome, especially concerning external rotation.[27,28] Malessy and colleagues[27] rigorously assessed the results following nerve grafting of C5 to the suprascapular nerve ($n = 65$) or nerve transfer of the accessory nerve to the suprascapular nerve ($n = 21$) in a retrospective analysis 3 years after surgery. Outcome was expressed in degrees of true glenohumeral external rotation, which can be executed only by infraspinatus muscle contraction. Only 17 (20%) of the 86 patients reached more than 20 degrees of external rotation, whereas 35 (41%) were unable to perform true external rotation. There was no statistically significant difference between nerve grafting from C5 and nerve transfer using the accessory nerve. Functional scores were better with 88% of children able to reach their mouth and 75% could touch their head. The authors concluded that restoration of true glenohumeral external rotation after nerve transfer of the suprascapular nerve in infants with brachial plexus birth palsies. However, compensatory techniques allow a considerable range of motion.

Nerve transfers for elbow flexion for elbow in children brachial plexus birth palsy have outcomes that are more positive. Nerve donors have included the medial pectoral nerve, ulnar nerve, and median nerve. Blaauw and Slooff[29] published a large series of 25 children that underwent transfer of the pectoral nerves to the musculocutaneous nerve. Results were reported as excellent in 17 cases and fair in 5 with 2 failures. A small series by Noaman and a larger series by Little and colleagues have reported excellent results with the ulnar and/or median nerve.[30–32] Noaman[30] reported a series of seven children that underwent ulnar nerve transfer to the biceps at an average of 16 months old. Five children recovered M3 or greater elbow flexion while two children recovered less than M3 strength. Little and colleagues[31] reviewed 31 patients that underwent nerve transfer for elbow flexion using the ulnar and/or median nerve fascicle transfer to the biceps and/or brachialis branches of the musculocutaneous nerve. The primary outcome measure was elbow flexion and supination as measured on the AMS. Of the 31 patients, 27 (87%) obtained functional elbow flexion (AMS $\geq$6) and 24 (77%) had full flexion recovery (AMS = 7). Of the 24 patients for whom supination recovery was recorded, only 5 (21%) obtained functional recovery (AM S $\geq$ 6). Single fascicle transfer resulted in functional flexion (AMS $\geq$ 6) in 85% (22/26) and functional supination (AMS $\geq$ 6) in only 15% (3/20). Combined ulnar and median nerve fascicle transfers were performed in five patients. This combination resulted in full elbow flexion (AMS = 7) and supination (AMS $\geq$ 5) in all patients.

PROTOCOL 12.1
Procedure: Primary Nerve Grafting for BPBP

CLINICAL GUIDELINES	
Time Period	**Description**
Preoperative phase	Complete preoperative BPBP evaluation Initiate patient/family education on postoperative immobilization and precautions.
Immobilization phase 0–4 weeks postoperatively *Period of immobilization may be increased if clavicular osteotomy performed	Soft cast applied by surgeon as follows: Position: shoulder adduction, internal rotation, elbow flexion, wrist/hand in resting position (exception will be made if patient has internal rotation tightness—may cast in external rotation)
Mobilization phase 4–6 weeks postoperatively *Guidelines for mobilization may vary if clavicular osteotomy performed	**Precautions:** • Avoid shoulder flexion/abduction PROM of affected extremity above 90 degrees • When completing PROM of affected extremity, avoid lateral neck flexion and head rotation toward unaffected side • Avoid weight-bearing activities • Avoid resistive activities **AROM:** • Shoulder ER/IR • Shoulder abduction/adduction • Shoulder forward flexion • Elbow, forearm, wrist, and digit motion in all planes **PROM:** • Shoulder ER • Shoulder FF to 90 degrees • Shoulder abduction to 90 degrees • Elbow, forearm, wrist, and digit motion in all planes *Stabilize scapula with shoulder PROM exercises to facilitate glenohumeral motion versus scapulothoracic motion **Scar management:** Initiate scar massage 3×/day **Patient education:** Educate patient/family on (1) home program of A/PROM and scar management; (2) postoperative precautions
Mobilization phase 6–12 weeks postoperatively	**Precautions:** None **AROM:** • Same as mentioned earlier **PROM:** • Shoulder ER, full ROM • Shoulder FF, full ROM • Shoulder abduction, full ROM • Elbow, forearm, wrist, and digit motion in all planes *Continue to perform PROM exercises with scapular stabilization *Stabilize trunk to prevent compensatory movement with AROM. **Scar management:** Continue scar massage 3×/day Use of silicone gel sheet or elastomere as indicated **Patient education:** Educate patient/family on changes in home program and precautions

PROTOCOL 12.2
Procedure: BPBP Intercostal Nerve Transfers (to Radial Nerve or Musculocutaneous Nerve)

CLINICAL GUIDELINES	
Time Period	**Description**
Preoperative phase	Complete preoperative BPBP evaluation Initiate patient/family education on postoperative immobilization and precautions
Immobilization phase 0–4 weeks postoperatively	Soft cast applied by surgeon as follows: Position: shoulder adduction, internal rotation, elbow flexion, wrist/hand in resting position (exception will be made if patient has internal rotation tightness—may cast in external rotation)
Mobilization phase 4–6 weeks postoperatively	**Precautions:** • Avoid ROM of affected extremity above 90 degrees shoulder flexion and abduction • Avoid weight-bearing activities • Avoid resistive activities • Avoid passive elbow extension until 6 weeks post-op OR until cleared by surgeon **AROM:** • Shoulder ER/IR • Shoulder abduction to 90 degrees/adduction • Shoulder forward flexion to 90 degrees • Elbow flexion/extension • Forearm pronation/supination • Wrist and digit motion in all planes **PROM:** • Gentle shoulder ER • Shoulder FF to 90 degrees • Shoulder abduction to 90 degrees • Wrist and digit motion in all planes *Stabilize scapula with shoulder PROM exercises to facilitate glenohumeral motion versus scapulothoracic motion *Stabilize trunk to prevent compensatory movement **Scar management:** Initiate scar massage 3×/day **Patient education:** Educate patient/family on (1) home program of A/PROM and scar management and (2) postoperative precautions
Mobilization phase 6–12 weeks	**Precautions:** No shoulder motion beyond 90 degrees until 3 months post-op (or once cleared by MD) **AROM:** Continue as mentioned earlier **PROM:** • Shoulder ER • Shoulder FF to 90 degrees • Shoulder abduction to 90 degrees • Initiate gentle passive elbow flexion/extension • Initiate gentle passive forearm pronation/supination • Wrist and digit motion in all planes *Continue to perform exercises with scapular stabilization *Stabilize trunk to prevent compensatory movement **Scar management:** Continue scar massage 3×/day **Patient education:** Educate patient/family on (1) changes in home program and precautions

REFERENCES

1. Clarke HM, Curtis CG. An approach to obstetrical brachial plexus injuries. *Hand Clin.* 1995;11:563–581.
2. Bae DS, Waters PM, Zurakowski D. Reliability of three classification systems measuring active motion in brachial plexus birth palsy. *J Bone Joint Surg Am.* 2003;85:1733–1738.
3. Narakas AO. Obstetric brachial plexus injuries [Chapter 9]. In: Lamb DW, ed. *The Paralyzed Hand.* Edinburgh: Churchill Livingstone; 1987:117–122.
4. Al-Qattan MM, El-Sayed AAF, Al-Zahrani AY, et al. Narakas classification of obstetric brachial plexus palsy revisited. *J Hand Surg.* 2009;34E:788–791.
5. Sibinski M, Synder M. Obstetric brachial plexus palsy-risk factors and predictors. *Orthop Traumatol Rehabil.* 2007;9: 569–576.
6. Foad SL, Mehlman CT, Foad MB, Lippert WC. Prognosis following neonatal brachial plexus palsy: an evidence-based review. *J Child Orthop.* 2009;3:459–463.
7. Kozin SH. *Nerve Repair Manual.* Beachwood, Ohio: Checkpoint Surgical; 2016.
8. Heise CO, Siqueira MG, Martins RS, et al. Clinical electromyography correlation in infants with obstetric brachial plexopathy. *J Hand Surg.* 2007;32:999–1004.
9. Steens SCA, Pondaag W, Malessy MJA, Verbist BM. Obstetric brachial plexus lesions CT myelography. *Radiology.* 2011;259:508–515.
10. Kawai H, Tsuyuguchi Y, Masada K, Heise CO, Siqueira MG, Martins RS. Identification of the lesion in brachial plexus injuries with root avulsion: a comprehensive assessment by means of preoperative findings, myelography, surgical exploration and intraoperative diagnosis. *Neuro Orthop.* 1989;7:15–23.
11. Al-Qattan MM, Clarke HM, Curtis CG. The prognostic value of concurrent Horner's syndrome in total obstetric brachial plexus injury. *J Hand Surg Br.* 2000;25:166–167.
12. Curtis C, Stephens D, Clarke HM, Andrews D. The active movement scale: an evaluative tool for infants with obstetrical brachial plexus palsy. *J Hand Surg Am.* 2002;27: 470–478.
13. Waters PM. Comparison of the natural history, the outcome of microsurgical repair, and the outcome of operative reconstruction in brachial plexus birth palsy. *J Bone Joint Surg Am.* 1999;85:649–659.
14. Kozin SH. Nerve transfers in brachial plexus birth palsies: indications, techniques, and outcome. *Hand Clin.* 2008; 24:363–376.
15. Malessy MJ, Thomeer RT. Evaluation of intercostal to musculocutaneous nerve transfer in reconstructive brachial plexus surgery. *J Neurosurg.* 1998;88:266–271.
16. Leechavengvongs S, Witoonchart K, Uerpairojkit C, Thuvasethakul P, Malungpaishrope K. Combined nerve transfers for C5 and C6 brachial plexus avulsion injury. *J Hand Surg Am.* 2006;31:183–189.
17. Pondaag W, Malessy MJA. Recovery of hand function following nerve grafting and transfer in obstetric brachial plexus lesions. *J Neurosurg.* 2006;105:33–40.
18. Gu YD, Zhang GM, Chen DS, Yan JG, Cheng XM, Chen L. Seventh cervical nerve root transfer from the contralateral healthy side for treatment of brachial plexus root avulsion. *J Hand Surg Br.* 1992;17:518–521.
19. Wang SF, Li PC, Xue YH, Yiu HW, Li YC, Wang HH. Contralateral C7 nerve transfer with direct coaptation to restore lower trunk function after traumatic brachial plexus avulsion. *J Bone Joint Surg Am.* 2013;95:821–827.
20. Oberlin C, Béal D, Leechavengvongs S, Salon A, Dauge MC, Sarcy JJ. Nerve transfer to biceps muscle using a part of ulnar nerve for C5-C6 avulsion of the brachial plexus: anatomical study and report of four cases. *J Hand Surg Am.* 1994;19:232–237.
21. Mackinnon SE, Novak CB, Myckatyn TM, Tung TH. Results of reinnervation of the biceps and brachialis muscles with a double fascicular transfer for elbow flexion. *J Hand Surg Am.* 2005;30A:978–985.
22. Bertelli JA, Ghizoni MF. Reconstruction of C5 and C6 brachial plexus avulsion injury by multiple nerve transfers: spinal accessory to suprascapular, ulnar fascicles to biceps branch and triceps long or lateral head branch to axillary nerve. *J Hand Surg Am.* 2004;29:131–139.
23. Leechavengvongs S, Witoonchart K, Uerpairojkit C, Thuvasethakul P. Nerve transfer to deltoid muscle using the nerve to the long head of the triceps, part II: a report of 7 cases. *J Hand Surg Am.* 2003;28A:633–638.
24. Gilbert A. Long-term evaluation of brachial plexus surgery in obstetrical palsy. *Hand Clin.* 1995;11:583–594.
25. Gilbert A, Pivata G, Kheiralla T. Long-term results of primary repair of brachial plexus lesions in children. *Microsurgery.* 2006;26:334–342.
26. Lin J, Schwentker-Colizza A, Curtis CG, Clarke HM. *Plast Reconstr Surg.* 2009;123:939–948.
27. Kawabata H, Kawai H, Masatomi T, Yasui N. Accessory nerve neurotization in infants with brachial plexus birth palsy. *Microsurgery.* 1994;15:768–772.
28. Pondaag W, de Boer R, van Wijlen-Hempel MS, Hofstede-Buitenhuis SM, Malessy MJ. External rotation as a result of suprascapular nerve neurotization in obstetric brachial plexus lesions. *Neurosurgery.* 2005;57:530–537.
29. Blaauw G, Slooff AC. Transfer of pectoral nerves to the musculocutaneous nerve in obstetric upper brachial plexus palsy. *Neurosurgery.* 2003;53:338–341.
30. Noaman HH, Shiha AE, Bahm J. Oberlin's ulnar nerve transfer to the biceps motor nerve in obstetric brachial plexus palsy: indications, and good and bad results. *Microsurgery.* 2004;24:182–187.
31. Little KJ, Zlotolow DA, Soldado F, Cornwall R, Kozin SH. Early functional recovery of elbow flexion and supination following median and/or ulnar nerve fascicle transfer in upper neonatal brachial plexus palsy. *J Bone Joint Surg Am.* 2014;96:215–221.
32. Clarke H, Tse R, Malessy M, Kozin S. The role of nerve transfers in the treatment of neonatal brachial plexus palsy, International Federation of Societies for Surgery of the Hand (IFSSH) Scientific Committee on neonatal brachial plexus palsy. *IFSSH Ezine.* 2015;5:17–25.

CHAPTER 13

Brachial Plexus Pre- and Post-Op Management: Secondary

ALLISON ALLGIER, OTD, OTR/L • ROGER CORNWALL, MD

INTRODUCTION

Brachial plexus birth injuries (BPBI) not resolving through natural recovery often result in various sequelae associated with the shoulder, elbow, wrist, and/or hand. These impairments often include decreased range of motion, strength, coordination, and sensation, although functional limitations associated with BPBI can vary substantially in extent and severity.[1] Serial physical examination of children with BPBI is recommended to follow recovery patterns and to determine the need for appropriate therapeutic and/or surgical intervention.[2] Over half of those with BPBI resolve spontaneously while the remaining children may require surgical or nonsurgical intervention to maximize functioning.[3]

SHOULDER

Regardless of the need for primary nerve repair, infants may demonstrate a substantial shoulder contracture as early as a few months of age. Most children with BPBI sustain an injury to the upper plexus (C5, C6) with or without C7.[4] Children with functional impairments at the shoulder often exhibit weakness in abduction, external rotation, and terminal internal rotation due to decreased function of the deltoid and rotator cuff muscles. Unless nerve recovery is early and complete, the denervated muscles fail to grow normally, leading to relative shortening and contractures circumferentially about the glenohumeral joint.[5] The most notable component of the global shoulder contracture is the lack of passive external rotation in adduction, as this motion is the only glenohumeral motion for which scapulothoracic motion cannot compensate.[6,7] In addition, the persistent function of internal rotators, such as the pectoralis major, can create a functional imbalance of the muscles about the shoulder girdle, potentially exacerbating the contracture and leading to glenohumeral deformity.[4] Up to 35% of infants and children with BPBI experience some degree of shoulder weakness, contracture, or joint deformity.[2] Establishing shoulder alignment and stability is important due to the distal aspects of the upper extremity relying on the shoulder to function successfully.

Evaluation

Assessment of the shoulder may begin with active and passive range of motion at the very first session, captured through universal goniometry. Passive internal/external rotation is measured both in adduction and at 90 degrees of abduction. It is important to evaluate shoulder external rotation by passively manipulating bilateral upper extremities simultaneously to prevent natural trunk compensation if an internal rotation contracture is present. Muscle tightness of the pectoralis major is evaluated with direct palpation during passive external rotation in both adduction and abduction. Glenohumeral joint subluxation or dislocation may be determined by posterior palpation of the humeral head, asymmetry of axillary skin folds, and/or an apparently shortened humeral length.[2] Dynamic instability of the joint and degree of scapular winging are assessed when the shoulder is adducted and internally rotated.[2]

The Active Movement Scale and Modified Mallet Scale are both validated instruments utilized consistently with BPBI patients.[8] The Active Movement Scale may be utilized at any age to capture active motion throughout the involved upper extremity, first with gravity eliminated, then against gravity. The original Mallet Scale has been modified to include six components of active motion focusing on shoulder motion:

Pediatric Hand Therapy. https://doi.org/10.1016/B978-0-323-53091-0.00013-0

shoulder abduction, shoulder external rotation, hand to neck, hand to mouth, hand to back, and hand to stomach.[9] As children age, it is important to take precaution to block trunk compensation and ensure slow motions are utilized to not allow momentum to impact demonstrated active motion. Imaging may provide additional information if an internal rotation contracture is noted. For those under 12 months of age, a shoulder ultrasound provides visual confirmation of shoulder alignment, while a shoulder MRI remains the standard of care for full assessment of glenohumeral dysplasia.

Therapy

Therapy is vital to children with BPBI regardless of whether surgery is indicated, although rehabilitative therapy can also preserve and build on gains made possible by surgical interventions.[10] Therapeutic management addressing shoulder imbalance may include active and passive range of motion, use of taping to facilitate positional awareness and give feedback to relevant muscle groups, and use of neuromuscular electrical stimulation (NMES) for strengthening and biofeedback. When a muscle contraction is noted in a weak muscle, NMES can be utilized to facilitate muscle recruitment, provided the practitioner is skilled in its use.[11] Knowledge of the physical and electrical components of this treatment modality is crucial.[10]

Use of splints should be considered in cases where there is weakness, contracture, or to assist in preventing further deformity. Preemptive use of shoulder external rotation splinting may be worthwhile in helping to keep the shoulder developing well through early growth (Fig. 13.1). Proper splinting and casting requires a strong collaboration between the physician and the therapist.[10]

As children grow, the relationship between the shoulder and scapula becomes an area of focus as the scapula is noted to wing and/or tilt. Winging of

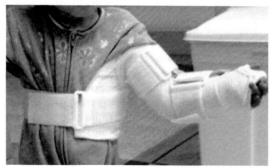

FIG. 13.1 Custom external rotation splint to be worn at night.

the scapula is a common occurrence seen with children with contractures at the glenohumeral joint, as scapular winging compensates for limited glenohumeral motion.[6,7] Joint mobilization and stretching may be utilized to address this limitation.

Botulinum Toxin

Children with incomplete recovery often demonstrate limitations due to cocontraction of agonist and antagonist muscles related to abnormal reinnervation patterns.[12] Management of cocontraction can include temporary weakening of the more powerful muscle with botulinum toxin injection to allow a period of motor learning for the weaker muscle. In addition, the often powerful pectoralis muscle can be used to resist the necessary stretching of the subscapularis muscle, so temporary weakening of the pectoralis with botulinum toxin injection can facilitate appropriate passive range of motion. However, the use of botulinum toxin to directly treat contractures has fallen out of favor, as mounting evidence argues against muscle overactivity as the cause of the contractures.

Surgical Intervention

If active external rotation is absent but full passive range of motion is demonstrated, surgical intervention to restore active motion can consist of nerve reconstruction or tendon transfers. Nerve reconstruction can take the form of excision and grafting of the injured nerves of the brachial plexus or transfer of functioning nerves to paralyzed muscles (e.g., spinal accessory to suprascapular nerve transfer). The relative indications for these nerve reconstruction strategies are covered in a previous chapter. If active external rotation is absent and a persistent internal rotation contracture is noted upon exam, or if poor glenohumeral alignment is noted on imaging studies, surgical intervention may include a contracture release and tendon transfers. The first such procedure was described over a century ago.[13] Since then, many techniques have been described, but most techniques include releasing a portion of the subscapularis muscle, with or without release of the joint capsule or other structures, and transferring the latissimus dorsi and/or teres major tendons to the posterior-superior rotator cuff, where they become active abductors and external rotators of the shoulder.[1] These are the most common procedures utilized to address shoulder imbalance for those with BPBI. A surgical overview has been provided in Appendix A.

A general postoperative guideline for releasing the subscapularis includes having young patients be casted for 4 weeks to hold the shoulder in external rotation.

Subsequently, the child returns to therapy without restriction once the cast is removed. If an orthosis is utilized instead of casting, patients are able to come out of the orthosis daily for bathing and active range of motion. Those not casted may begin therapy immediately after surgery without restriction. A general guideline following the subscapularis release and transfer of the latissimus/teres major includes the patient being casted or in an orthosis full time for 4 weeks. Therapy is then initiated with restrictions associated with protecting the transferred muscle(s) until 3 months after surgery. Restrictions typically include no passive range of motion into internal rotation or shoulder extension as well as no resistive activities. The shoulder and surrounding muscles need appropriate postoperative therapy to adapt to the new configuration, as well as to increase muscle function and strength.[4] Often surgeons differ slightly in their surgical technique and postoperative protocol. If a patient is having surgery, the therapist should reach out to the surgeon to learn more about the procedure and the postoperative therapeutic plan.

A humeral osteotomy may be recommended for patients with long-term internal rotation contractures with substantial glenohumeral deformity or if the internal rotation contracture exists despite prior surgical attempts to improve alignment.[9] An osteotomy is performed in the shaft of the humerus with internal fixation utilized to hold the new position. This new bony alignment creates a new set point for the available active rotation of the shoulder. Following the surgery, a sling is used for comfort only. Therapy may be initiated soon after surgery to facilitate active range of motion and functional use with the new positioning. Resistive activities and passive range of motion are prohibited until radiographic confirmation of bone healing has been completed.

ELBOW

The natural resting position for many children with BPBI is an internal rotation position at the shoulder with a slight bend at the elbow. The reason for development of elbow flexion contractures has historically been unknown, although it has been thought to be due to residual muscle weakness.[1] However, recent basic science data has shown that the elbow flexion contracture actually develops due to impaired growth and thus relative shortening of the biceps muscle, which may also be very weak.[14] This shortening of the biceps may lead to loss of passive range of motion, which often worsens during periods of growth.[15]

Evaluation

Assessment includes active and passive range of motion with use of goniometry. Radiographs may also be valuable in determining bony alignment and growth changes impacting an inability to fully extend the elbow, although bony deformity is a much less common limiting factor than it is at the shoulder. Anterior radial head dislocation is common, but does not in and of itself lead to increased functional difficulties, as it typically occurs in children with severe global brachial plexus involvement with limited functional recovery. Nonetheless, palpable radial head instability can be a concern to the family and can be noticed by the therapist.

Therapy

Because of the limited results of surgical correction of an elbow flexion contracture, splinting and casting are frequently used to maximize elbow extension.[16] If an elbow flexion contracture of less than 20 degrees is noted, splinting may be utilized to maintain the position so it does not worsen. If an initial contracture of 20–40 degrees is noted, serial casting may be first utilized to improve elbow range of motion.[16] This would then be followed by nighttime splinting to maintain gains made through the serial casting. Serial casting has been proven effective in addressing elbow flexion contractures in children with BPBI (Fig. 13.2).[17]

Surgical Intervention

The most common surgery performed at the elbow is a release of the flexion contracture through lengthening of the biceps and brachialis muscles, with or without joint capsule release. Although surgical results may show initial improvements greater than that obtained by serial casting, deterioration of passive elbow extension occurs over time.[18] Overall, surgical treatments

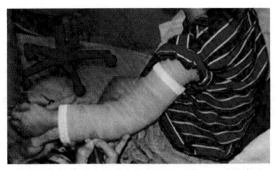

FIG. 13.2 Serial casting to improve elbow extension.

are only able to correct approximately half the passive extension deficit. Postoperatively, patients are casted for 4 weeks followed by splint fabrication. The splint is worn full time for an additional 2 weeks before restarting therapy 6 weeks after surgery. Use of the protective splint continues at this point although it may be removed for light functional use and active range of motion. Gentle passive range of motion may also be started at this time.

FOREARM

Patients with C5, C6, and C7 involvement may demonstrate mild deficits in functional forearm supination due to delayed innervation of the supinator muscle and its biceps support. This often improves with time to a functional level of range of motion. Children with a global BPBI involving C8 and T1 have additional limitations throughout the forearm, wrist, and hand. Those with global injuries appear most prone to developing a supination contracture that limits functional use of the hand. Most daily needs are met through distal upper extremity functioning with the forearm in a pronated position. Forearm rotation can be best assessed using goniometry to capture active and passive range of motion.

Therapy/Surgery

Early therapeutic intervention may include the use of taping, splinting with a rotary strap, and/or serial casting to promote forearm rotation. If active rotation does not recover, or once a rotational contracture has developed, substantial improvement is only seen with surgical intervention. If the forearm remains supple through a full range of rotation, but the patient lacks active protonation, the distal biceps tendon can be rerouted from an active supinator to a pronator function.[19] Following this procedure, patients are casted for 4 weeks and then are able to start therapy. A splint is fabricated for intermittent wearing for an additional 2−4 weeks. Restrictions include no passive or resistive activities until 3 months following surgery. For a fixed contracture, a derotational osteotomy of the radius and/or ulna is the most common surgical procedure performed to improve forearm positioning[1] Postoperative care includes casting for 4 weeks and then therapy is initiated to facilitate active range of motion and functional use with new positioning. Resistive activities and passive range of motion are prohibited until radiographic confirmation of bone healing has been completed.

WRIST

Patients with C6, C7, and C8 involvement may demonstrate decreased active wrist extension. This function is essential in the development of fine motor skills in young children. Adequate wrist extension improves the ability to grip, as a slightly extended wrist results in stronger finger flexion. Wrist function can be best assessed using goniometry to capture active and passive range of motion.

Therapy/Surgery

Therapeutic intervention may include the use of tape and/or NMES to address weak wrist extensors. In those with a more involved injury, wrist support is required for extension and to prevent deviation. Depending on the type of splint used, a rotation strap can be added to support forearm rotation, which may be lacking. Surgical interventions to improve wrist extension include transfer of the flexor carpi ulnaris or flexor carpi radialis to the extensor carpi radialis brevis and/or longus. Studies have shown an average gain in wrist extension of 46.6 degrees and a good result of a four using the modified Medical Research Council muscle grading system.[20,21] Following these procedures, patients are splinted or casted for 4 weeks. Therapy is initiated and a new splint is then fabricated for use during activity and at night.

HAND

Patients with C6, C7, C8 and T1 involvement may lack sensation and active motion in their hand. Hand sensation is essential as awareness and use are both strongly tied to having feeling throughout the volar aspect of the hand. Hand function can be best assessed using goniometry to capture active and passive range of motion of the individual joints of the digits, and sensation is assessed following the sensory dermatomes associated with each involved nerve.

Therapy/Surgery

Early therapeutic intervention may include splinting to maintain and support the anatomical structures of the hand during nonuse. Stimulation along the involved dermatome using a variety of textures promotes awareness given there is noted nerve innervation. NMES may be used to address innervated but weak muscles. Surgical intervention most often includes tendon transfers to provide active extension of the involved digits. Postoperative care follows the same guidelines as provided for intervention at the wrist.

GOAL-DRIVEN THERAPY

Brachial plexus birth injuries have lifelong considerations that may warrant the need for outpatient occupational or physical therapy. It is important to establish a therapeutic relationship locally to access therapy services when needed. Skilled intervention is typically required upon the initial diagnosis, during the postoperative stages, and to address specific functional goals identified by patients and families. These are individualized, goal-driven episodes of care.[22] The ultimate goal of therapy is for the patient and family to have the ability to independently manage their lifelong injury process.[23]

A BPBI evaluation includes an occupational profile with information gathered through an interview with the patient and/or caregiver. Patient's life experiences, daily life roles, meaningful occupations, and caregiver concerns from the profile help to shape the patient's goals. Completion of the Canadian Occupational Performance Measure (COPM) is recommended, as it is an evidence-based outcome measure used to capture a patient or caregiver's perception of performance in daily occupations.[24] This information will assist in prioritizing functional goals and will help to determine the foundational motor skills required to promote participation.

The interventions noted in previous sections of this chapter provide foundational motor and sensory function, the skills needed to achieve goals, and participation. Based on the occupational priorities identified in the patient's profile and COPM, functional activities can be identified and incorporated into intervention with the therapist and in the home program. The therapist is then able to promote engagement through activity modifications or use of adapted equipment in order for the patient to be most successful in their chosen occupations.

Symmetry of Motion

Postural education is an integral part of rehabilitation in children with BPBI. As these children get older, they use specific compensation patterns to be able to perform a given movement. Kinematic findings confirm that children with BPBI display more atypical kinematic patterns in their involved upper extremity than in their uninvolved upper extremity.[25] These atypical patterns may be the result of both the initial injury as well as secondary musculoskeletal deformities. Muscle imbalance at the shoulder may lead to altered resting postures and habitual use patterns that may contribute to the progression of skeletal deformities.[25] A thorough rehabilitation program should introduce the correct movement pattern to recruit the specific muscle groups for a given movement.[10]

Constraint-Induced Movement Therapy

Limitations associated with BPBI often impact the ability to complete activities requiring the use of two hands and may result in participation limitations across many areas of occupation.[26] Constant-induced movement therapy (CIMT) is an intervention in which a constraint is utilized to limit use of the unaffected upper extremity to improve functional use of the involved upper extremity (Fig. 13.3). Bilateral intensive training is an intervention utilized with patients to improve spontaneous performance of tasks that require two hands. Intensive training is completed both in therapy and at home followed by intensive bimanual training. The home program includes a range of functional daily living and play activities of interest to the child to maintain the child's attention.[27] Intensive and repetitive training of the affected limb or a combination of restraint and training have demonstrated improvements in upper extremity function, as practice and repetition are both important components of motor learning.[27] The effectiveness of pediatric CIMT and bimanual training is clearly supported by current evidence.[26]

Aquatic Therapy

Patients lacking engagement in land-based therapy or who have reached a plateau may benefit from incorporating aquatic therapy in their treatment plan. Motion in water eliminates gravity but also provides resistance.[28] The patient may experience improved range of motion and strengthening in water that will then translate to land-based function. Moving from aquatic therapy to community-based swimming can provide a nice transition from structured therapy to age appropriate environments and occupations.

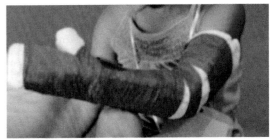

FIG. 13.3 Constraint-induced Movement Therapy (CIMT) device.

Self-Management

As previously noted, outpatient therapy is effective when utilized in an episodic nature with a focus on active engagement in activities of interest to the individual child. Community-based activities such as tumbling, gymnastics, martial arts, certain dance classes, specific sports, and most importantly, swimming, provide a fun and engaging environment promoting functional use and strengthening of the upper extremities. Independent participation in the patient's established home program is strongly encouraged.

Therapeutic management often focuses on minimizing limitations and maximizing the individual's participation at home and in the community. Facilitating a supportive and encouraging environment, with a focus on what the patient is able to do, helps to promote a healthy sense of self-esteem and attitude of independence.

CONCLUSION

BPBI results in mixed residual deficits in strength, range of motion, and coordination throughout the involved upper extremity based on the level of nerve involvement. Appropriately timed initiation of therapy is essential to maximize function as well as capitalize on the gains made available through surgical intervention. Skilled therapists incorporate evidence-based intervention to best address functional deficits and promote participation. Educating the patient and their family regarding home programming and appropriate community-based activities is critical to independent self-management of this lifelong condition.

APPENDIX A

Surgery	Goal	Technique	Post-op Therapy
Release of the subscapularis with or without release of the joint capsule	Release of an internal rotation contracture allowing improved alignment of the glenohumeral joint	Arthroscopic or open release	Cast: • 4 weeks held in shoulder external rotation. • initiate therapy 4 weeks after surgery without restriction. Orthosis: • come out of the orthosis daily for bathing and active range of motion • initiate therapy immediately after surgery without restriction
Release of the subscapularis and transfer of the latissimus with or without the teres major	Release of an internal rotation contracture allowing improved alignment of the glenohumeral joint and providing active muscle(s) to move the shoulder into external rotation	Arthroscopic release of the subscapularis and open transfer of the latissimus and teres major	Cast or orthosis: • 4 weeks held full time in shoulder external rotation • initiate therapy 4 weeks after surgery with restrictions associated with protecting the transferred muscle(s) until 3 months after surgery • restrictions typically include no passive range of motion into internal rotation or shoulder extension as well as no resistive activities.
Humeral osteotomy	Address long-term internal rotation contracture with considerable glenohumeral deformity	Osteotomy of the shaft of the humerus with internal fixation	• sling for comfort only. • initiate therapy soon after surgery to facilitate active range of motion and functional use with new positioning. • resistive activities and passive range of motion are prohibited until radiographic confirmation of bone healing has been completed.

Surgery	Goal	Technique	Post-op Therapy
Biceps and brachialis lengthening with or without joint capsule release	Address elbow flexion contracture	Open release	• cast in extension x 4 weeks. • splint fabricated to wear full time x 2 additional weeks • initiate therapy 6 weeks after surgery. • continue the protective splint, although it may be removed for light functional use and active range of motion. • gentle passive range of motion may also be started at this time.
Biceps rerouting transfer	Provide active motor function for forearm pronation	Rerouting of the biceps around the radius	• casted x 4 weeks • a splint is fabricated for intermittent wearing for an additional 2–4 weeks. • initiate therapy 4 weeks after surgery. • restrictions include no passive or resistive activities until 3 months after surgery.
Forearm osteotomy	Improve positioning of hand for functional use	Radius and/or ulna osteotomy with internal fixation	• casted x 4 weeks • initiate therapy 4 weeks after surgery to facilitate active range of motion and functional use with new positioning. • resistive activities and passive range of motion are prohibited until radiographic confirmation of bone healing has been completed.
Tendon transfers at the wrist	Improve wrist extension	Transfer of the flexor carpi ulnaris or flexor carpi radialis to the extensor carpi radialis brevis and/or longus	• splint/cast x 4 weeks. • new splint is then fabricated for use during activity and at night. • initiate therapy 6 weeks after surgery. • restrictions include no passive or resistive activities until 3 months after surgery.

REFERENCES

1. Price AE, Grossman JA. A management approach for secondary shoulder and forearm deformities following obstetrical brachial plexus injury. *Hand Clin.* 1995;11(4):607–617.
2. Hale HB, Bae DS, Waters PM. Current concepts in the management of brachial plexus birth palsy. *J Hand Surg Am.* 2010;35(2):322–331.
3. Foad SL, Mehlman CT, Foad MB, Lippert WC. Prognosis following neonatal brachial plexus palsy: an evidence-based review. *J Child Orthop.* 2009;3(6):459–463.
4. Safoury YA, Eldesoky MT, Abutaleb EE, Atteya MR, Gabr AM. Postoperative physical therapy program for latissimus dorsi and teres major tendons transfer to rotator cuff in children with obstetrical brachial plexus injury. *Eur J Phys Rehabil Med.* 2017;53(2):277–285.
5. Nikolaou S, Peterson E, Kim A, Wylie C, Cornwall R. Impaired growth of denervated muscle contributes to contracture formation following neonatal brachial plexus injury. *J Bone Joint Surg Am.* 2011;93(5):461–470.
6. Russo SA, Kozin SH, Zlotolow DA, et al. Scapulothoracic and glenohumeral contributions to motion in children with brachial plexus birth palsy. *J Shoulder Elb Surg.* 2014;23(3):327–338.
7. Russo SA, Loeffler BJ, Zlotolow DA, Kozin SH, Richards JG, Ashworth S. Limited glenohumeral cross-body adduction in children with brachial plexus birth palsy: a contributor to scapular winging. *J Pediatr Orthop.* 2015;35(3):240–245.
8. Bae DS, Waters PM, Zurakowski D. Reliability of three classification systems measuring active motion in brachial plexus birth palsy. *J Bone Joint Surg Am.* 2003;85-A(9):1733–1738.

9. Abzug JM, Chafetz RS, Gaughan JP, Ashworth S, Kozin SH. Shoulder function after medial approach and derotational humeral osteotomy in patients with brachial plexus birth palsy. *J Pediatr Orthop.* 2010;30(5):469–474.

10. Ramos LE, Zell JP. Rehabilitation program for children with brachial plexus and peripheral nerve injury. *Semin Pediatr Neurol.* 2000;7(1):52–57.

11. McGillicuddy JE, Yang LJS, Chung KC. *Practical Management of Pediatric and Adult Brachial Plexus Palsies.* Edinburgh: Saunders; 2012.

12. Santamato A, Panza F, Ranieri M, Fiore P. Effect of botulinum toxin type A and modified constraint-induced movement therapy on motor function of upper limb in children with obstetrical brachial plexus palsy. *Childs Nerv Syst.* 2011;27(12):2187–2192.

13. Mehlman CT, DeVoe WB, Lippert WC, Michaud LJ, Allgier AJ, Foad SL. Arthroscopically assisted Sever-L'Episcopo procedure improves clinical and radiographic outcomes in neonatal brachial plexus palsy patients. *J Pediatr Orthop.* 2011;31(3):341–351.

14. Weekley H, Nikolaou S, Hu L, Eismann E, Wylie C, Cornwall R. The effects of denervation, reinnervation, and muscle imbalance on functional muscle length and elbow flexion contracture following neonatal brachial plexus injury. *J Orthop Res.* 2012;30(8):1335–1342.

15. Sheffler LC, Lattanza L, Hagar Y, Bagley A, James MA. The prevalence, rate of progression, and treatment of elbow flexion contracture in children with brachial plexus birth palsy. *J Bone Joint Surg Am.* 2012;94(5):403–409.

16. Ho ES, Roy T, Stephens D, Clarke HM. Serial casting and splinting of elbow contractures in children with obstetric brachial plexus palsy. *J Hand Surg Am.* 2010;35(1):84–91.

17. Duijnisveld BJ, Steenbeek D, Nelissen RGHH. Serial casting for elbow flexion contractures in neonatal brachial plexus palsy. *J Pediatr Rehabil Med.* 2016;9(3):207–214.

18. Strombeck C, Krumlinde-Sundholm L, Remahl S, Sejersen T. Long-term follow-up of children with obstetric brachial plexus palsy I: functional aspects. *Dev Med Child Neurol.* 2007;49(3):198–203.

19. Zancolli EA, Zancolli Jr ER. Palliative surgical procedures in sequelae of obstetric palsy. *Hand Clin.* 1988;4(4):643–669.

20. van Alphen NA, van Doorn-Loogman MH, Maas H, van der Sluijs JA, Ritt MJPF. Restoring wrist extension in obstetric palsy of the brachial plexus by transferring wrist flexors to wrist extensors. *J Pediatr Rehabil Med.* 2013;6(1):53–57.

21. Al-Qattan MM. Tendon transfer to reconstruct wrist extension in children with obstetric brachial plexus palsy. *J Hand Surg Br.* 2003;28(2):153–157.

22. Bailes AF, Reder R, Burch C. Development of guidelines for determining frequency of therapy services in a pediatric medical setting. *Pediatr Phys Ther.* 2008;20(2):194–198.

23. Janssen RMJ, Satink T, Ijspeert J, et al. Reflections of patients and therapists on a multidisciplinary rehabilitation programme for persons with brachial plexus injuries. *Disabil Rehabil.* 2018:1–8.

24. Law M. *Canadian Occupational Performance Measure.* 3rd ed. Toronto: CAOT = ACE; 1998, 1998.

25. Mayfield CH, Kukke SN, Brochard S, Stanley CJ, Alter KE, Damiano DL. Inter-joint coordination analysis of reach-to-grasp kinematics in children and adolescents with obstetrical brachial plexus palsy. *Clin Biomech.* 2017;46:15–22.

26. Pediatric modified Constraint Induced Movement Therapy (mCIMT/BIT) Team CCsHMC. *Evidence-based Clinical Care Guideline Pediatric Modified Constraint Induced Movement Therapy (mCIMT) Plus Bimanual Training (BIT)* (Guideline 34). 2014:1–21.

27. Abdel-Kafy EM, Kamal HM, Elshemy SA. Effect of modified constrained induced movement therapy on improving arm function in children with obstetric brachial plexus injury. *Egypt J Med Hum Genet.* 2013;14(3):299–305.

28. Lai CJ, Liu WY, Yang TF, Chen CL, Wu CY, Chan RC. Pediatric aquatic therapy on motor function and enjoyment in children diagnosed with cerebral palsy of various motor severities. *J Child Neurol.* 2015;30(2):200–208.

CHAPTER 14

Cerebral Palsy

SCOTT H. KOZIN, MD • RICHARD GARDNER, FRCS

INTRODUCTION

Cerebral palsy is often related to hypoxic ischemic encephalopathy (HIE) when the infant's brain is deprived of adequate blood flow secondary to a hypoxic-ischemic event during the prenatal, intrapartum, or postnatal period.[1] HIE requires immediate intervention and affects 20 out of every 1000 full term births. The incidence rate in premature babies is 60% of all live births. HIE caused by asphyxia is the leading cause of infant fatalities in the United States, as well as the primary source of severe impairments. Effects of HIE may include developmental delays, epilepsy, cognitive issues, motor skill delays, and neurodevelopment delays. The true severity of HIE generally cannot be determined until the baby reaches 3–4 years old. The end-result is cerebral palsy with varying signs and symptoms.

There are a number of different causes of HIE that can occur before, during, or after the baby is born.[1] HIE pregnancy risks included maternal diabetes with vascular disease, decreased placental circulation, preeclampsia, cardiac disease, infections of the fetus, drug and alcohol abuse, severe fetal anemia, and lung malformations. HIE birth risks include excessive bleeding from the placenta, low maternal blood pressure, umbilical cord rupture, prolonged late stages of labor, abnormal fetal position, and rupture of the placenta or the uterus. Postpartum period risks include premature babies, severe cardiac or pulmonary disease, infections (sepsis and meningitis), low neonatal blood pressure, brain or skull trauma, and congenital brain malformations.

The orthopedic team is usually consulted when the child fails to reach certain developmental milestones, such as sitting, crawling, or walking. At our center, a team approach is utilized with input from the surgeons and therapists that care for the upper and lower extremities. In addition, a physiatrist with exceptional knowledge is an integral part of our team. Neurologists are relegated to consultants on difficult cases with questionable signs and symptoms or progressive neurologic changes.

CLASSIFICATION

The classification of cerebral palsy denotes the number of limbs involved and the type of spasticity. The classic hemiplegic cerebral palsy child has involvement of one side (arm and leg) with sparing of the other side. The quadriplegic cerebral palsy child has involvement of all four limbs, although the severity may vary. The type of spasticity is either spastic, athetoid, or a combination of spastic and athetoid. Spasticity results from dysregulated reflex arc messaging from the damaged upper motor neurons. We explain this phenomenon to families as the muscles always want to "run" and the intact brain dampens this response. A damaged brain loses this ability and cannot suppress the muscles from moving. Concomitant extrapyramidal involvement causing additional movement disorders, primarily athetosis, which is a rhythmic uncontrollable twisting movement pattern. In addition, to these spastic movement patterns, the limb or portions of the limb may be flaccid without any volitional movement. Various tones results in muscle imbalance across limb segments, which leads to abnormal upper limb position, contracture formation, and hampered function.

ASSESSMENT

The assessment of the child requires input from all team members. In our clinic, the physiatrist manages the spasticity with medications, pumps, and/or botulinum toxin injections. The upper extremity surgeons and occupational therapists treat the arms. The lower extremity surgeons and physical therapists manage the legs. The spine surgeons monitor for spinal deformities, such as scoliosis. The spine surgeons also perform procedures directed at decreasing spasticity, such as the DREZ (human dorsal root entry zone) procedure.[2] This team approach provides optimum case as long as there is communication among the teams to avoid fragmentation of care.

Pediatric Hand Therapy. https://doi.org/10.1016/B978-0-323-53091-0.00014-2

The upper extremity evaluation varies with the patient's age, developmental stage, and cognitive function. Early therapy is the mainstay of treatment in infants. Establishing access for the child and family to therapy and support resources is mandatory. The parents require time, patience, and support to comprehend their child's diagnosis. This process takes time and early surgical intervention is avoided and rarely necessary. Over time, the upper extremity team develops a rapport with the child and family that will ease subsequent decision-making. There is no "quick fix" for cerebral palsy and the family will endure lifelong trials and tribulations. Understanding this monumental effect on the family will enhance the doctor–therapist–family relationship. The physicians and therapist must express the necessary amount of empathy and compassion while avoiding overt expressions of sympathy.

The assessment should include the legacy measures of range of motion and strength. Any joint contracture should be documented. Sensibility tools vary with the age of the child and are discussed in Chapter 3. In addition to legacy measures, a patient reported outcome (PRO) measure (patient and/or parent) should also be performed. The various PROs are covered in Chapter 4 and often shed light into the expectations of the parent and/or child. A set of documented individualized treatment goals is invaluable to prevent unrealistic exceptions from surgery.

Videotape or functional evaluation of the patient performing routine activities or scored functional tests (Jebsen-Taylor, Box and Blocks, Pegboard) can mimic functional loss compared to a clinical visit. Validated evaluation tools, such as the Shriners Hospital for Children Upper Extremity Evaluation, upper extremity cerebral palsy, and Assisting Hand Assessment, can help define upper extremity disability and deformity and guide treatment.[3] In reality, we rarely use videotaping in our clinical practice, but rather rely on clinical acumen and repeated examinations.

SURGICAL INDICATIONS/METHODS

Surgery of the upper extremity in cerebral palsy is reparative and often palliative, but not curative. Surgery can improve the functional limb; however, no operation will not restore normal function to the impaired limb. We discriminate between functional and nonfunctional limbs that have overwhelming spasticity and minimal volitional movement. Hence, there are different indications and procedures based upon the baseline function of the limb. In general, tendon lengthenings and tendon transfers are performed on functional limbs. Tenotomies, myotomies, and fusions are performed on nonfunctional limbs to improve their position and allow hygiene. However, tenotomies, myotomies, and fusions may also be applicable to functional limbs. In addition, nerve surgery for spasticity treatment via nerve stripping or isolated motor neurectomy can be performed.

A muscle–tendon unit can be lengthened using one of three methods (Fig. 14.1). The first method is a Z-plasty of the tendon and suturing the cut ends together in an elongated state. A second method is fractional lengthening whereby the muscle–tendon junction is identified. The tendon is isolated along its origin from the muscle. A tendinous segment is identified that has muscle on both sides of the tendon. The tendon is incised leaving the muscle intact on both sides of the

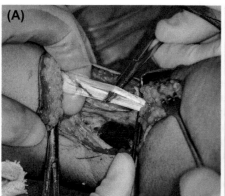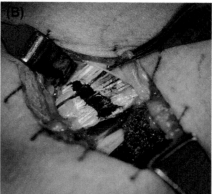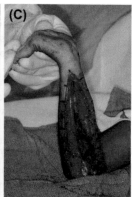

FIG. 14.1 A muscle–tendon unit can be lengthened using one of three methods. **(A)** Z-plasty lengthening of biceps' tendon. **(B)** Fractional lengthening of the brachialis muscle–tendon junction. **(C)** Muscle slide of the flexor pronator origin. (Courtesy of Shriners Hospital for Children, Philadelphia.)

cut. The respective part (e.g., elbow or wrist) is stretched elongating the cut ends of the tendon within the substance of the muscle. No suturing is required. The third method involves releasing the origin of the muscle and allowing it to slide in a distal direction during stretching of the limb.

The particular lengthening technique utilized depends on numerous factors including the anatomy of the muscle–tendon unit, the length required, and the surgeon preference. For example, there are certain muscles that have short muscle–tendon units (e.g., biceps muscle) and are not amenable to fractional lengthening. In addition, if substantial lengthening is required, fractional lengthening would exceed the length of the muscle–tendon junction resulting is discontinuity between the muscle and tendon. Lastly, certain muscles are amendable to release of the origin and allowing the muscles to slide in a distal direction (e.g., flexor pronator mass and thenar muscles).

Release of a muscle or tendon can be performed via tenotomy or myotomy. The method selected also varies with the muscle–tendon anatomy and the surgeon preference. For example, the brachioradialis originates from the supracondylar ridge of the humerus and inserts along the forearm fascia culminating in its attachment to the radial styloid. Simply cutting the tendon at the radial styloid will not negate its ability to flexion the elbow. Hence, myotomy is necessary to eliminate its effect on elbow flexion. In contrast, the flexor carpi radialis has a long tendon that is receptive to tenotomy.

HIERARCHY OF UPPER LIMB FUNCTION

Proximal muscle stability and control is mandatory for hand function. The shoulder must be stable allowing the arm and forearm to function. Surgery to enhance shoulder motion for cerebral palsy has been disappointing. In contrast to brachial plexus injuries, the muscles are spastic and poor candidates for transfer. Surgery is directed toward lessening the myostatic contracture to allow more supple movement. With reference to the elbow, flexor spasticity is commonplace. In mild hemiparesis, this yields elbow flexion posturing during walking and times of excitement. In more severe cases, a myostatic contracture develops that limits elbow extension. Lengthening and myotomies can lessen the elbow flexion tone. The forearm should not be forgotten and is a frequent source of discontentment. The common forearm position is spastic protonation that is initially supple (dynamic) and develops a myostatic contracture over time. Excessive protonation impedes supinations activities, such as

Priority	Function	Task
	TABLE 14.1 Reconstructive Ladder for Hand Function.	
1	Wrist extension	Tenodesis grasp and pinch
2	Lateral pinch	Activities of daily living
3	Grasp	Holding
4	Opening	Object acquisition
5	Coordinated hand function	Dexterity

feeding, carrying a tray, obtaining soap from a dispenser, catching a ball, and wiping one's buttocks.

The management of the wrist and hand in cerebral palsy follows the concepts of "hierarchy of hand function" or the "reconstruction ladder" (Table 14.1).[4] The primary fundamental movement is wrist extension, which yields tenodesis for grip as the fingers flex into the palm and tenodesis for lateral pinch as the thumb adducts against the index finger. Wrist extension also aligns the finger flexors along Blix's length–tension curve for maximum active grip. The second most essential movement is lateral pinch, which is necessary to perform numerous activities of daily living. Most daily activities are accomplished with lateral pinch, such as holding an object, turning a key, or using a fork. The third essential motion is grasp, which allows the holding of objects. The fourth and last movement is digital opening for object acquisition. The reason to place this function lowest on the ladder is that wrist flexion yields passive digital opening, which is often adequate for object procurement. In addition, synchronous digital opening is difficult to achieve via surgery as metacarpophalangeal joint extension is mainly an extrinsic function (extensor digitorum communis, extensor indicis proprius, and extensor digiti quinti) and interphalangeal joint extension is primarily an intrinsic function (interossei and lumbricals).

SHOULDER RECONSTRUCTION
Functional

The functional spastic shoulder is usually positioned in internal rotation. Often the degree of internal rotation has negligible effect on function and treatment is unnecessary. However, the child may be bothered by the posture and their inability to access his or her axilla. The potential culprit spastic muscles include the pectoralis major, subscapularis, latissimus dorsi, and teres major. Clinical examination can often discern the most spastic muscles. These muscles can be treated by lengthening or release depending upon their anatomy. For example, a tight spastic pectoralis major can be addressed by fractional lengthening as there is ample muscle–tendon junction that is assessable via a small anterior axially incision. In contrast, the subscapularis requires a more extensive deltopectoral approach with release of the upper tendinous portion. The goal is to provide ample access to the axilla.

Nonfunctional

The nonfunctional spastic shoulder can be positioned in internal rotation as described earlier. The axilla can be very inaccessible leading to stench and intertriginous infections. Treatment requires release of the offending spastic muscles based upon the clinical examination. The shoulder can also be positioned in excessive external rotation. This awkward position can negate the wheel-chaired child from entering thru a doorway. The offending muscle(s) are usually the infraspinatous, teres minor, and/or posterior deltoid. These muscles can be released form their insertions to lessen the shoulder external rotation. The muscles can also be denervated by isolated neurectomy of their motor nerve. In particular, the posterior branch of the axially nerve and the branch to the teres minor are readily accessible via an axially incision described by Bertelli (see Chapter 15—Tetraplegia).[5]

ELBOW RECONSTRUCTION

Functional

The patient with hemiparesis is frequently bothered by the elbow flexion posture. This posture is evident during running and amplified with stress. Usually, there is full passive elbow extension without a myostatic contracture. Botulinum toxin can provide temporary relief, but the posture uniformly reverts over time. Surgery can resolve this posturing as long as the patient is willing to accept the low risks of undergoing a surgical procedure (Fig. 14.2). The procedure is performed via a transverse incision across the antecubital fossa. The nerve lateral antebrachial cutaneous and radial nerves are mobilized out of harm's way. The brachioradialis muscle is isolated and the muscle cut with an electrocautery (a.k.a. myotomy). The biceps tendon is mobilized, and the underlying brachialis muscle–tendon junction is identified. A fractional lengthening is

performed by cutting the tendon at the muscle–tendon junction. The skin is closed with absorbable suture and dressing applied. A long arm cast is applied for 4 weeks. Following cast removal, therapy is instituted and the arm is mobilized. A nighttime splint is worn for at least 3 months.

Nonfunctional

The nonfunctional elbow is typically more severely flexed with a myostatic contracture. Passive elbow extension is incomplete. Splinting and botulinum toxin are ineffective treatment modalities. Surgery is the only effective treatment (Fig. 14.3). The offending components include the skin, brachioradialis, biceps, and the brachialis. The joint capsule is usually secondarily involved; however, capsular release may jeopardize elbow flexion for any hand to mouth activity. The skin is addressed by a long Z-plasty that allows wide access to the underlying structures. The longitudinal limb is directly down the center of the elbow. The Z-limbs are at the ends of the longitudinal incision and angled approximately 45 degrees. The longitudinal and Z-limbs must be equal lengths. Once the skin is incised, the biceps is lengthened by Z-plasty, the brachialis by fractional lengthening, and the brachioradialis by myotomy. The Z-plasty is closed with absorbable suture and dressing applied. A long arm cast is applied for 4 weeks. Following cast removal, therapy is instituted and the arm is mobilized. A nighttime splint is worn for at least 3 months.

FOREARM RECONSTRUCTION

Functional

The patient with hemiparesis is frequently bothered by the forearm protonation position. This position impedes supinations activities, such as feeding, carrying a tray, obtaining soap from a dispenser, catching a ball, and wiping one's buttocks. However, the surgeon must avoid losing protonation in nondominant hands as table top activities predominate modern day culture, such as typing, cutting food, holding papers, and turning pages in a book. The pronator teres is usually the culprit that impedes forearm supination. The pronator quadratus can also be spastic and the biceps/supinator can be weak. In the past, we have rerouted the pronator teres into a supinator. However, we were unsatisfied with our results, and excessive supination was occasionally seen. Hence, we no longer transfer a spastic pronator teres but favor simple release avoiding the spastic pronator rotating the forearm into too much supination.

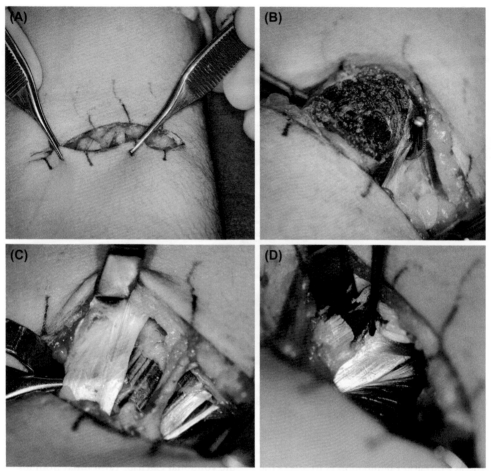

FIG. 14.2 A 16-year-old male with left-sided spastic hemiparesis and excessive elbow flexion posturing. **(A)** Transverse antecubital incision. **(B)** Brachioradialis muscle is isolated and the muscle is cut with an electrocautery. **(C)** Biceps tendon is mobilized. **(D)** The brachialis muscle–tendon junction is identified and a fractional lengthening is performed. (Courtesy of Shriners Hospital for Children, Philadelphia.)

Surgery is performed via a radial incision along the midportion of the radius (Fig. 14.4). The radial sensory nerve is identified emanating from beneath the brachioradialis. Just proximal to this exit point and beneath the brachioradialis, the pronator tendon is identified and released from the radius.

A long arm cast is applied for 4 weeks in supination. The elbow, wrist, and hand position depends on the concomitant procedures performed. Following cast removal, therapy is instituted and the arm is mobilized. A nighttime splint is worn for at least 3 months.

Nonfunctional

The nonfunctional arm is usually fixed in excessive pronation. This position can lead to radial head dislocation. Simple release of the pronator teres will not resolve the underlying contracture. Treatment options include concomitant interosseous membrane release with or without osteotomy of the radius and/or ulna. We have found this combination of procedures to be unreliable in determining the ultimate forearm position. Hence, we prefer a one bone with transposition of the radius on to the ulna when forearm repositioning is necessary.

WRIST RECONSTRUCTION
Functional

The wrist often lacks active extension, which is the fundamental motion for finger tenodesis and grip

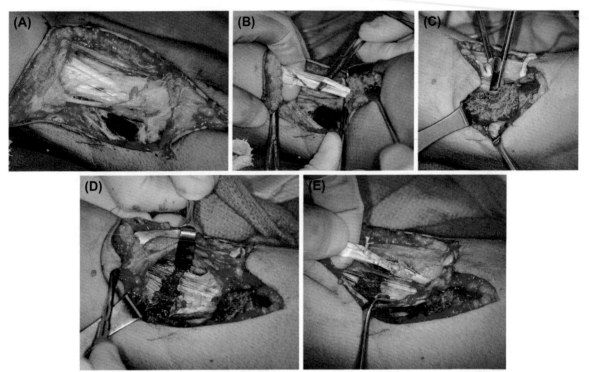

FIG. 14.3 An 18-year-old with spastic quadriplegic cerebral palsy and malpositioned contracted right elbow. **(A)** Z-plasty of the skin across antecubital fossa. **(B)** Z lengthening of the biceps tendon. **(C)** Brachioradialis myotomy. **(D)** Brachialis fractional lengthening. **(E)** Biceps repaired in elongated configuration. (Courtesy of Shriners Hospital for Children, Philadelphia.)

strength. The key physical examination is to assess the ability to open and close the fingers with the wrist positioned in extension. The patient must be able to open their fingers when the wrist is placed into extension to consider augmenting wrist extension. If the patient requires wrist flexion for finger opening, then surgery to enhance wrist extension is contraindicated. The surgeon should also evaluate to integrity and spasticity of the flexor carpi ulnaris and the extensor carpi ulnaris. In the patient with hemiparesis, the flexor carpi ulnaris is usually spastic and the extensor carpi ulnaris is not spastic. This finding forms the basis of our preferred operative strategy.

In the past, we performed a flexor carpi ulnaris to extensor carpi radialis brevis tendon transfer. However, the spastic flexor carpi ulnaris resulting in unintended consequences, mainly excessive wrist extension and/or unwanted forearm supination. We currently prefer transferring the extensor carpi ulnaris to the extensor carpi radialis brevis and a fractional lengthening of the flexor carpi ulnaris (Fig. 14.5). The procedure shifts

the volitional extensor carpi ulnar from an ulnar deviator into a wrist extension and lessens the spasticity of the flexor carpi ulnaris. In addition, the extensor pollicis longus tendon can be removed from the third compartment and transferred in a radial direction to lessen its thumb adduction moment.

A short or long arm cast is applied depending upon the age and compliance of the child. After 3 weeks, the cast is removed, a splint is fabricated, and therapy is instituted (Protocol 14.1). Tendon rehabilitation following extensor carpi ulnaris to the extensor carpi radialis brevis tendon transfer is divided into three phases: early mobilization, mobilization, and strengthening/functional retraining.

Nonfunctional

The nonfunctional wrist usually fixed in flexion. There is marked spasticity of the flexor carpi radialis, flexor carpi ulnaris, and palmaris longus (if present). The status of the thumb and fingers must be considered during the surgical planning. The fingers are often flexed and any

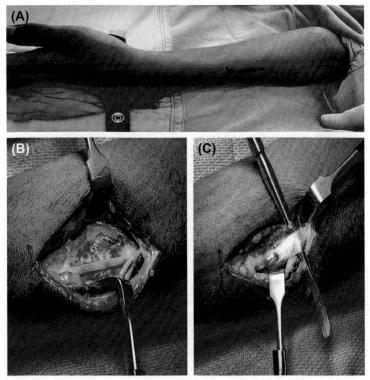

FIG. 14.4 Technique of pronator teres release. **(A)** Longitudinal radial incision. **(B)** Mobilization of cephalic vein and radial sensory nerve. **(C)** Pronator teres tendon isolated beneath brachioradialis and tenotomy performed. (Courtesy of Rick Gardner, FRCS.)

surgical straightening of the wrist will exacerbate thumb and finger flexion. Hence, the digits will likely require surgery and the same time. These finding forms the foundation of our preferred operative strategy. Concerning timing, we prefer to wait until skeletal maturity to allow plate and screw fixation across the wrist arthrodesis. Attempts at wrist arthrodesis using longitudinal wires to preserve growth (a.k.a. chondrodesis) have been uniformly unsuccessful.

The primary procedure to treat the spastic wrist requires tenotomies of the spastic wrist flexors, proximal row carpectomy, and wrist arthrodesis (Fig. 14.6). The wrist flexor tendons are released via an oblique volar incision across the distal forearm. The proximal row carpectomy and wrist fusion are performed via a longitudinal incision. All cartilage must be removed from the distal radius, capitate, and hamate. The wrist is fused in neutral position with an appropriately sized plate and screw construct (usually 2.7 mm). The arm is immobilized in a long arm splint for 4 weeks. Subsequently, a splint is fabricated and therapy initiated. The splint is worn at night for 3 months to ensure healing.

Following wrist fusion, the finger flexor tightness is addressed by lengthening. Surgical options included Z-plasty, fractional lengthening, and flexor pronator slide as discussed later.

HAND RECONSTRUCTION
Functional
The functional hand often has abundant finger flexion and lacks finger dexterity. Unfortunately, there is no surgical remedy for restoration of dexterity. The inability to cross one's fingers, button a shirt, and zipper a jacket is not surgically correctable. The surgical goal is to restore better gross grasp and release. Improving wrist extension will improve grip strength and may be ample treatment. Additional finger flexor tightness can be managed by lengthening of the finger flexors. The surgeon must be careful to avoid over lengthening, especially the flexor digitorum superficialis that could lead to swan neck deformity of the fingers.

Fractional lengthening best elongates the slightly tight finger flexors. The muscle–tendon junction is

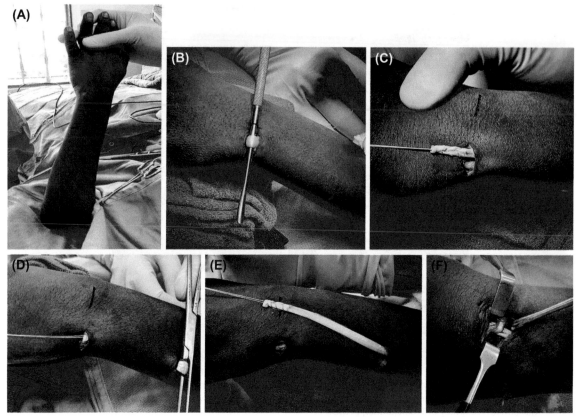

FIG. 14.5 Technique of extensor carpi ulnaris to extensor carpi radialis brevis tendon transfer. **(A)** Skin incisions. **(B)** Extensor carpi ulnaris isolated after opening sixth retinaculum compartment. **(C)** Extensor carpi ulnaris cut and tagged with suture. **(D)** Extensor carpi ulnaris withdrawn into proximal transverse incision. **(E)** Extensor carpi ulnaris passes through subcutaneous tunnel toward extensor carpi radialis brevis tendon. **(F)** Extensor carpi ulnaris woven through extensor carpi radialis brevis tendon. (Courtesy of Rick Gardner, FRCS.)

identified. A tendinous segment that has muscle on both sides of the tendon is identified. The tendon is incised leaving the muscle intact on both sides of the cut. The fingers are gentle straightened and the tendon is elongating between the cut ends within the substance of the muscle. No suturing is required.

A short or long arm cast is applied depending upon the age and compliance of the child. The fingers are gently extended using a webril cotton cast padding roll placed in the palm. The fingers can be mobilized in a few days with removal of the cotton roll and initiating active finger flexion. The webril cotton roll is repositioned between exercise sessions. The cotton roll is discontinued after 3 weeks and a night splint is fabricated stretching the fingers into extension. The nighttime splint is discontinued after 3 months.

Nonfunctional

The nonfunctional hand often has overpowering finger flexion. Improving wrist extension via wrist arthrodesis will exacerbate this problem. The finger flexors require substantial lengthening to allow access to the palm. Fractional lengthening and Z-plasty lengthening do not prove adequate length. Surgical options included a superficialis-to-profundus tendon transfer or flexor pronator slide. Both techniques are affective in resolving the overriding finger flexion. The superficialis-to-profundus tendon transfer is considered a "tendon transfer," also provides little active motion but rather acts as a positioning tenodesis to the fingers. This procedure is performed via longitudinal or curvilinear incision across the forearm. The superficialis tendons are cut as distal as possible and the profundus tendon as proximal as possible. The fingers are

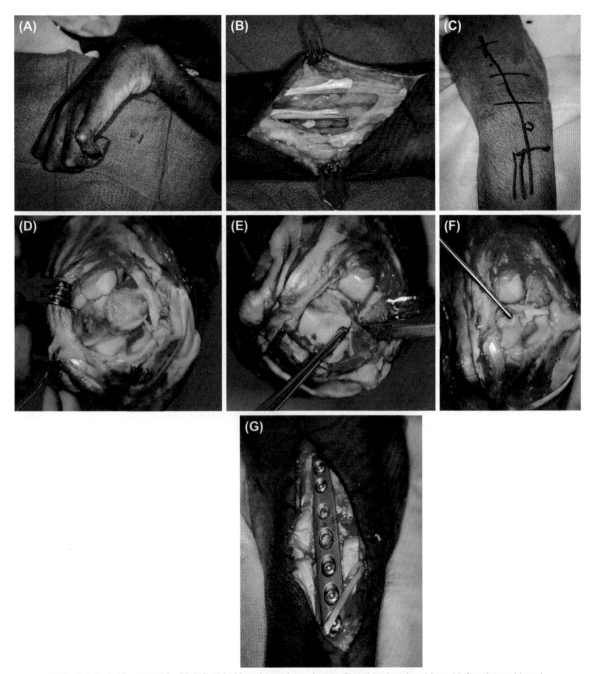

FIG. 14.6 A 19-year-old with left-sided hemiparesis and a nonfunctional malpositioned left wrist and hand. **(A)** Clinical picture. **(B)** Wrist flexor tenotomies. **(C)** Longitudinal dorsal wrist incision. **(D)** Arthrotomy with exposure of the radiocarpal and midcarpal articulations. **(E)** Proximal row carpectomy. **(F)** Removal of articular cartilage. **(G)** Plate and screw fixation in neutral wrist position. (Courtesy of Shriners Hospital for Children, Philadelphia.)

straightened (leaving slight flexion) and the distal superficialis tendons are sutured to the proximal profundus tendons. Theoretically, the superficialis muscle is the motor to the profundus tendons, although this procedure is rarely an active transfer. A short or long arm cast is applied depending upon the age and compliance of the child. The fingers are gently extended using a webril cotton cast padding roll placed in the palm. As there is little active motion, passive mobilization should be initiated in a few days with removal of the cotton roll and passive finger extension. The webril cotton roll is repositioned between exercise sessions. The cotton roll is discontinued after 3 weeks, and a night splint is fabricated stretching the fingers into extension. The nighttime splint is discontinued after 3 months.

The forearm flexor pronator slide is performed via a long medial incision from above the elbow to the ulnar styloid (Fig. 14.7).[6] The ulnar nerve is released enough and transposed in an anterior direction. The flexor pronator mass is incised directly off the ulnar down to the medial collateral ligament of the elbow. The forearm muscle is sequentially released from the ulnar all the way to the wrist. The release continues in an ulnar to radial direction. Any taught muscle is released until the wrist and fingers can be extended completely. Closure is straightforward leaving the ulnar nerve in an anterior position. A long arm cast is applied with the wrist and digits in extension. The forearm is positioned into midsupination. The arm is immobilized in a cast for 4 weeks with the elbow extended to 45 degrees, the forearm supinated, and the wrist/digits in extension. A removable splint is continued for four additional weeks, allowing removal for range of motion and therapy. After 2 months, splinting is converted for night use and discontinued month later unless there is a tendency for recurrence of deformity.

THUMB RECONSTRUCTION

Functional

The thumb is positioned in the palm (thumb-in-palm deformity). This position truly impedes hand function. The thumb blocks finger flexion for grasp and impedes object acquisition. Alleviating the thumb-in-palm deformity would enhance hand function; however, accomplishing this task is difficult. The underlying etiology is intrinsic spasticity (adductor pollicis and thenar muscles) coupled with weakness of thumb retropulsion and extension (abductor pollicis brevis, extensor pollicis brevis, and extensor pollicis longus). The goal is to lessen the intrinsic spasticity and to augment thumb retropulsion and extension. Regrettably, this balance is difficult to achieve.

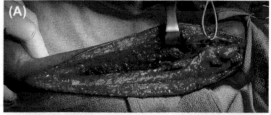
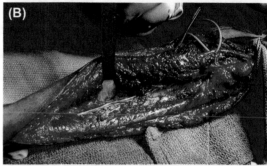
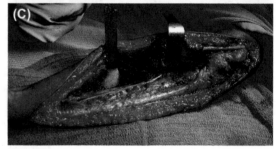

FIG. 14.7 Technique of flexor slide. **(A)** Long ulnar incision and transposition of ulnar nerve. **(B)** Muscles released form ulna and radius. **(C)** Preservation of anterior interosseous neurovascular structure and distal sliding of flexor-pronator musculature. (Courtesy of Rick Gardner, FRCS.)

In the functional thumb, the examination attempts to define spastic agonists from weak antagonist. Typically, the thenar muscles are spastic and the thumb extensor are overwhelmed. The surgical approach involves lengthening the thenar muscles by sliding their origin in a distal direction (Fig. 14.8). Similarly, the adductor muscle is released from its origin (long finger metacarpal) and allowed to slide in a distal direction. Augmentation of the thumb extension is performed by releasing the extensor pollicis longus from the third compartment and transposing the tendon in a radial direction. This transposition augments thumb extension in a radial direction and lessens its unwanted thumb adduction. In addition to thenar slide and extensor pollicis longus transposition, the metacarpophalangeal joint or carpometacarpal joint can be stabilized by

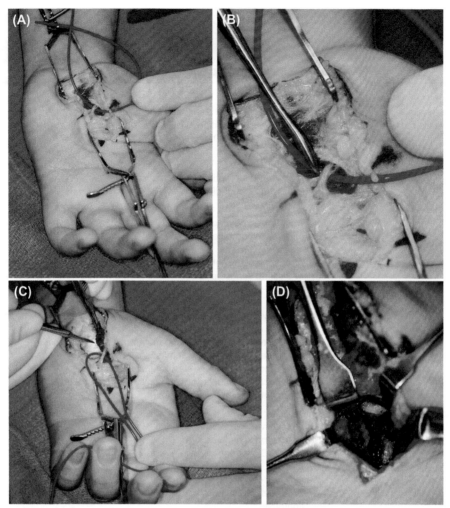

FIG. 14.8 A 12-year-old with left-sided hemiparesis and thumb in palm deformity. **(A)** Skin incision and approach to address the spastic thenar and adductor muscles. **(B)** Recurrent branch of the median nerve isolated and protected. **(C)** Thenar muscles sharply elevated from the transverse carpal ligament and slid in a distal direction. **(D)** Adductor muscle origin released from the long finger metacarpal. (Courtesy of Shriners Hospital for Children, Philadelphia.)

chondrodesis or arthrodesis. This stabilization simplifies the equation by eliminating one of the problematic thumb joints (metacarpophalangeal or carpometacarpal joint).

Nonfunctional

The nonfunctional thumb is also positioned in the palm (thumb-in-palm deformity). This positioning is more dramatic compared to the functional thumb. The underlying etiology is the same with the goal to alleviate the thumb-in-palm deformity. The treatment paradigm is similar with a more extensive approach necessary. A chondrodesis or fusion is always part of the surgical plan. On occasion, the metacarpophalangeal or carpometacarpal joints are both fused to alleviate the thumb-in-palm deformity.

PROTOCOL 14.1
Procedure: ECU (extensor carpi ulnaris) to ECRB (extensor carpi radialis brevis), EPL (extensor pollicis longus) Transposition

CLINICAL GUIDELINES	
Time Period	**Goal**
Immobilization phase 1 week to 3 weeks post-op	Tendon immobilized in a shortened position to protect transfer. UE immobilization position in cast: Wrist: extended 20–30 degrees Thumb: Abducted Treatment: • ROM (range of motion) of uninvolved joints • Edema control of digits
Mobilization phase 3–6 weeks post-op	*Precautions:* No wrist flexion beyond neutral No excessive thumb flexion (into palm) No resistive exercises *Splint:* Volar wrist splint with wrist in 20–30 degrees extension, thumb abducted *Splint wearing schedule:* Off for home program, light functional activities, bathing and therapy sessions, on for sleep and rough activities *Treatment:* *AROM (active range of motion):* *Active wrist extension/thumb abduction through exercise or activities to facilitate tendon recruitment *Stabilize forearm to assure that patient does not rotate forearm *Scar management:* Initiate scar massage 3×/day Use of silicone gel sheet or elastomer as indicated *Patient education:* Educate patient/family on (1) postoperative precautions, (2) scar management, and (3) splint wear/care.
Strengthening **and** functional retraining phase 6–12 weeks post-op	*Precautions:* • no passive wrist flexion *Splint wearing schedule:* week 6–8: Off for nonresistive functional tasks On at night week 8–12: Off all day; on all night week 12: Discontinue use of splint for protection, may use if needed to prevent tightness *Treatment:* *AROM:* *Lateral pinch *Wrist flex and extension Elbow flexion and extension Digit flexion and extension *Stabilize forearm to assure that patient does not rotate. This will promote excursion for wrist extension versus forearm rotation. *Strengthening:* Initiate light resistive exercises at week 8 *Scar management:* Continue scar massage 3×/day Use of silicone gel sheet or elastomer as indicated *Patient education:* Educate patient/family on changes with (1) postoperative precautions, (2) splint wear/care, and (3) incorporate strengthening into home program.

REFERENCES

1. Allen KA, Brandon DH. Hypoxic ischemic encephalopathy: pathophysiology and experimental treatments. *Nborn Infant Nurs Rev.* 2011 1;11(3):125–133.
2. Sindou M, Jeanmonod D. Microsurgical DREZ-ectomy for treatment of spasticity and pain in the lower limbs. *Neurosurgery.* 1989;24:655–670.
3. James MA, Bagley A, Vogler JB, Davids JR, Van Heest AE. Correlation between standard upper extremity impairment measures and activity-based function testing in upper extremity cerebral palsy. *J Pediatr Orthop.* 2017;37:102–106.
4. Kozin SH, Zlotolow DA, Abzug JM. Upper extremity reconstruction in persons with tetraplegia. In: Abzug JM, Kozin SH, Zlotolow DA, eds. *The Pediatric Upper Extremity.* New York: Springer; 2015:735–765.
5. Bertelli JA, Ghizoni MF. Nerve transfers for elbow and finger extension reconstruction in midcervical spinal cord injuries. *J Neurosurg.* 2015;122(1):121–127.
6. Stevanovic M, Sharpe F. Management of established Volkmann's contracture of the forearm in children. *Hand Clin.* 2006;22:99–111.

CHAPTER 15

Tetraplegia: Nerve and Tendon Transfers

SCOTT H. KOZIN, MD

INTRODUCTION

Spinal cord injury is devastating to the patient, the family, and his or her friends. In an instance, life has downgraded dramatically with respect to ambulation, limb usage, bladder/bowel function, and independence. Spinal cord injury has substantial physical, emotional, and psychosocial ramifications. Approximately 54 people per million sustain injuries to the spinal cord each year (17,000 new cases per year), with about half occurring at the cervical spine and 14% resulting in ventilator dependence.[1] Currently, over 300,000 Americans live with some residual paralysis from a spinal cord injury. Most of the persons are young men when the spinal injury occurred, and many require lifelong care to complete their activities of daily living (ADLs) such as feeding, dressing, bathing, bladder/bowel care, and mobility. Maintenance cost estimates for care range from $40,000 to $185,000 per year per patient, depending on the severity and level of the injury.[1] This expensive care places substantial physical and financial stressors on the patient and family.

Spinal cord injuries can be complete or incomplete. In complete injuries, the spinal cord is interrupted blocking any efferent or afferent pathways. In incomplete injuries, the spinal cord maintains some continuity allowing some signal across the injured segment. There are numerous incomplete injury patterns dependent upon the extent and location of the injured and preserved pathways. Hence, the prognosis for spontaneous recovery following incomplete spinal cord injury is more optimistic and varies with the degree of damage.

Since the end of the Second World War, the care for persons with spinal cord injury has considerably improved. There have been advances in numerous aspects of care including the acute management immediately following the injury, the initial rehabilitation to minimize the immediate sequelae of the injury, and

the reconstructive surgical options to improve upper limb usage along with crucial bladder/bowel function. Tendon and nerve transfer surgery are the mainstay procedures to enhance upper limb function. The algorithm for incomplete spinal cord injury follows the same principles as complete spinal cord injury although the variability in presentation negates the establishment of a defined paradigm.

CLASSIFICATION

The American Spinal Injury Association Impairment Scale is most commonly used to classify the level and severity of the injury. This classification documents motor and sensory findings and provides a scoring system. With reference to the upper extremity, the International Classification of Surgery of the Hand in Tetraplegia (ICSHT) is more relevant for planning upper limb reconstruction (Table 15.1).[2] The objective is to identify those muscles distal to the elbow that are potentially transferrable. The classification follows the American Society for Spinal Cord Injury cataloging, but emphasizes muscle strength. Therefore, each muscle below the elbow that is a Grade 4 or greater muscle strength adds an additional grade. The muscle strength and gradation is based upon the muscle's primary nerve innervation. For example, the brachioradialis is mainly innervated by C5. When the brachioradialis muscle is present and strong, but no other muscles are of similar strength, the ICSHT is Grade 1. The subsequent ICSHT grades are also based upon the succeeding muscle principal nerve innervation. In other words, the extensor carpi radialis longus is mainly a C6 muscle. The extensor carpi radialis brevis is principally a C7 muscle as are the pronator teres, flexor carpi radialis, extensor digitorum communis, extensor pollicis longus, and flexor digitorum superficialis. The flexor digitorum profundus and intrinsic muscles are mainly innervated by

Pediatric Hand Therapy. https://doi.org/10.1016/B978-0-323-53091-0.00015-4

TABLE 15.1
International Classification for Surgery of the Hand in Tetraplegia (ICSHT).

Grade	Spinal Cord Segment	Muscle Below the Elbow Function	Motor Description
0	≥C5	None	Elbow flexion and forearm supination
1	C5	+ Brachioradialis	Elbow flexion with some supination/pronation[a]
2	C6	+ Extensor carpi radialis longus	Wrist extension
3	C7	+ Extensor carpi radialis brevis	Strong wrist extension
4	C7	+ Pronator teres	Forearm pronation
5	C7	+ Flexor carpi radialis	Wrist flexion
6	C7	+ Extensor digitorum communis	Finger extension (metacarpophalangeal joints)
7	C7	+ Extensor pollicis longus	Thumb extension
8	C7	+ Flexor digitorum superficialis	Incomplete finger flexion
9	C8	+ Flexor digitorum profundus	Complete digital roll-up
X		Exceptions	Variable

[a] The brachioradialis muscle can supinate and pronate to the neutral position.

C8 and T1 nerve roots. The addition of another strong muscle continually adds a grade to the classification and expands the potential surgical options for upper extremity reconstruction.

REFERRAL FOR UPPER LIMB RECONSTRUCTION

The referral process for persons with spinal cord injury remains disorganized and underutilized. Chung and colleagues[3] have shown that approximately 65% of the 5000 cervical spine injures per year would benefit from upper limb reconstruction by improving function and increasing independence. Despite the potential benefits, less than 500 surgeries are performed annually to improve upper limb function.[3] This disconnect is multifactorial with responsibility levied on physiatrists, surgeons, and institutions.

Published reports of tendon transfers for person with spinal cord injury have shown improvement in quality of life and overall function.[2,3] Despite this evidence, many physicians and even spinal cord rehabilitation facilities remain wary or are unaware of the potential benefits. Many patients that would benefit from surgical reconstruction are never referred for surgical evaluation. With the advent of nerve transfers, this problem will escalate unless knowledge dispersion increases across all subspecialties that manage persons with spinal cord injury. A person with spinal cord injury can typically gain one cervical spinal level of function through

tendon transfers.[2] Augmenting the current tendon transfer paradigm with nerve transfers can restore two cervical spinal cord levels of function.[4–6] However, nerve transfers require a viable muscle target for reinnervation, and irreversible motor endplate demise occurs as early as 18 months from injury. Therefore, most nerve transfers have limited success after 12 months from injury.[7] This window of opportunity highlights the time sensitivity and necessity of prompt referral for upper limb reconstruction.

TENDON VERSUS NERVE TRANSFER

Tendon transfers for upper limb reconstruction have been the gold standard for improving function. Pioneers in tetraplegic surgery, such as Moberg, Zancolli, House, and others, have established the basic tenets of tendon donor and recipient selection.[8] Innovators in nerve surgery, such as Oberlin, MacKinnon, and Bertelli, have introduced nerve transfers into the treatment paradigm. The common prerequisite for tendon and nerve donor selection remains availability and expendability.[4–6,9] In other words, the donor must be available (i.e., strong) and expendable (i.e., the limb can function without the donor nerve or tendon). An expendable donor usually has another muscle that performs the same task. For example, if the patient has an intact extensor carpi radialis longus and brevis tendons, the extensor carpi radialis longus can be transferred without jeopardizing wrist extension.

Nerve transfers warrant further discussion regarding an upper versus lower motor neuron injury. Above the level of injury, the nerve and spinal cord are normal. The afferent and efferent signals are received and transmitted to and from the central nervous system (brain and spinal cord). At the level of injury, there is direct damage to the cord and anterior horn cells. This lower motor neuron injury leads to Wallerian degeneration and secondary muscle changes over time, such as atrophy and fibrosis. This process can be reversed by transferring a donor nerve downstream into a terminal branch of the damaged spinal cord. For example, a lower motor neuron injury to the spinal cord at C7 can be circumvented by transferring a C6 nerve (e.g., supinator nerve) to a C7 motor nerve (e.g., extensor digitorum communis) to regain digital extension. However, nerve transfer procedures for a lower motor neuron injury are time dependent. The surgery must be performed with ample time for nerve regeneration (1 mm/day) to reach the muscle end plate before prevent permanent atrophy and fibrosis (18 months after lower motor neuron injury). Therefore, nerve transfers for lower motor neuron injury are preferably performed within 1 year from injury.

Below the level of injury, the nerve and spinal cord are also normal. However, the afferent and efferent signals are not received by the central nervous system that resides above the damaged cord (brain and spinal cord). This injury is called as an upper motor neuron injury. This situation prohibits volitional activation of these muscles, but promotes involuntary movement, as the dampening effect of the brain is absent. These muscles remain innervated and become spastic, a process that maintains muscle viability. Hence, nerve transfers for an upper motor neuron injury can be performed years after injury as permanent muscle atrophy and fibrosis do not occur. However, some central nervous system pruning may have a negative effect on restoring active movement.

HIERARCHY OF UPPER LIMB FUNCTION

The most common level of cervical spine injury is C5–C6, which leads to ICSHT Grades 1–3. Triceps function is absent, and restoration of elbow extension carries a high priority. The lack of elbow extension hinders function. Deficient elbow extension has multiple negative consequences. Workable reach space is drastically decreased, as the arm is unable to reach out into space. Daily activities for persons with spinal cord injury are compromised such as pushing a wheelchair, transferring in and out of a bed or a chair, and weight

shifting for avoiding decubitus. Reestablishment of elbow extension can have a dramatic increase in reachable workspace, facilitate wheelchair propulsion (uphill and on carpeted surfaces), and facilitate transfers in and out of bed or chair.

The management of the wrist and hand in tetraplegia follows the concepts of "hierarchy of hand function" or the "reconstruction ladder" (Table 15.2). The primary fundamental movement is wrist extension, which yields tenodesis for grip as the fingers flex into the palm and tenodesis for lateral pinch as the thumb adducts against the index finger. Wrist extension also aligns the finger flexors along Blix's length–tension curve for maximum active grip. The second most essential movement is lateral pinch, which is necessary to perform numerous ADLs. Most daily activities are accomplished with lateral pinch, such as holding an object, turning a key, or using a fork (Fig. 15.1). The third essential motion is grasp, which allows the holding of objects (Fig. 15.2). The fourth and last movement is digital opening for object acquisition. The reason to place this function lowest on the ladder is that wrist flexion yields passive digital opening, which is often adequate for object procurement. In addition, synchronous digital opening is difficult to achieve via surgery as metacarpophalangeal joint extension is mainly an extrinsic function (extensor digitorum communis, extensor indicis proprius, and extensor digiti quinti) and interphalangeal joint extension is primarily an intrinsic function (interossei and lumbricals). The only way the extrinsic system can elicit interphalangeal joint extension is by limiting metacarpophalangeal joint extension (e.g., Zancolli tenodesis of the flexor digitorum superficialis).[8] This procedure can cause problems such as limiting flexor digitorum profundus excursion and/or

TABLE 15.2
Spinal Cord Injury Reconstructive Ladder for Hand Function.

Priority	Function	Task
1	Wrist extension	Tenodesis grasp and pinch
2	Lateral pinch	Activities of daily living
3	Grasp	Holding
4	Opening	Object acquisition
5	Coordinated hand function	Dexterity

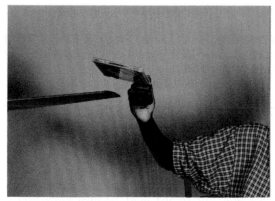

FIG. 15.1 Lateral pinch is the prehension used for most activities of daily living. (Courtesy of Shriners Hospital for Children, Philadelphia.)

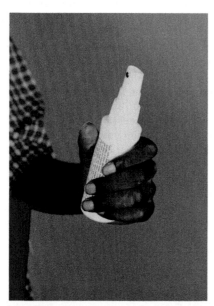

FIG. 15.2 Grasp is imperative for holding and retaining objects within the hand. (Courtesy of Shriners Hospital for Children, Philadelphia.)

attenuating over time. Restoring both metacarpophalangeal and interphalangeal movements by tendon transfer(s) remains a daunting task replete with complications.

ELBOW RECONSTRUCTION

Most persons with cervical spine injury lack triceps function and elbow extension.[2,8,10,11] Restoration of elbow extension carries a high priority. The lack of elbow extension truly hinders function and workable reach space. Elbow extension is a high surgical priority and can be accomplished by nerve or tendon transfer.

Nerve

The principal donor nerve is the posterior branch of the axillary nerve.[12] The axillary nerve has three terminal branches (larger anterior deltoid, smaller posterior deltoid, and teres minor branch). Before surgery, the strength of the posterior deltoid must be strong to ensure an adequate donor nerve. The transfer is completed via an axillary approach (Fig. 15.3A–C). The axillary nerve is identified just proximal to the latissimus dorsi tendon. The three branches are isolated and verified by electrical stimulation. The posterior axially nerve is selected as the donor nerve. The radial nerve is isolated just anterior to the axillary nerve in the arm. Electrical stimulation is helpful as long as the nerve is stimulatable. The triceps motor nerve is isolated. There can be a common branch to all three heads of the triceps muscle, or separate nerve branches can be found. The donor axillary nerve is cut as distal as possible (donor distal) and the recipient triceps motor nerve as proximal (recipient proximal) to negate any tension across the repair. The coaptation between the posterior branch of the axillary nerve and the motor branch to the triceps is secured with microsuture and/or fibrin glue.

Tendon

The two main donors are the biceps and the posterior deltoid muscles.[10,11,13] Each procedure has its own nuances, positives, and negatives. The biceps to triceps is easier and has a less rigid postoperative rehabilitation.[10,13] The posterior deltoid transfer requires an intervening graft that complicates the technique and adds greater postoperative restrictions.[11] We prefer the biceps over the triceps transfer to the deltoid to triceps transfer.

The biceps-to-triceps tendon transfer requires the biceps to be expendable. Therefore, active brachialis and supinator muscles are prerequisites to maintain elbow flexion and forearm supination.[13] The evaluation of their presence requires an attentive physical examination of elbow flexion and forearm supination strength. Effortless forearm supination without resistance will cause supinator function that is palpable along the proximal radius. Similarly, powerless elbow flexion will result in a palpable brachialis contraction along the anterior humerus deep to the biceps muscle. Equivocal cases require additional measures to assure adequate supinator and brachialis muscle activity.

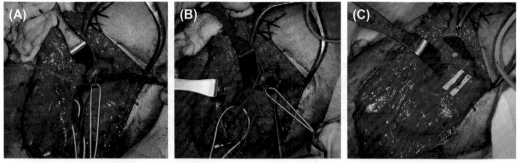

FIG. 15.3 A 16-year-old male 6 months following cervical spine injury. He is ICSHT Grade 1 on both arms and is undergoing nerve transfer of the posterior axillary branch to the triceps motor nerve. **(A)** Axillary nerve and branches isolated. *Red loop* around axillary nerve and larger anterior branch. *Yellow loop* around posterior branch and scissors behind teres minor branch. **(B)** Axillary nerve and motor branch to the triceps isolated (loose yellow loop). **(C)** Coaptation between posterior axillary branch and motor nerve to the triceps muscle. (Courtesy of Shriners Hospital for Children, Philadelphia.)

Injection of the biceps muscle with a local anesthetic induces temporary paralysis of the biceps muscle and allows independent assessment of brachialis and supinator muscle function.

A supple elbow with near complete range of motion is also necessary. Otherwise, the biceps tendon will not reach the olecranon during surgery. Therapy and/or serial casting can decrease the contracture. Surgery is delayed until the contracture is less than 20 degrees.

The surgery is performed via an S-shaped incision along the medial arm, across the antecubital fossa, and over the brachioradialis muscle belly (Fig. 15.4A–F). The biceps tendon is traced to its insertion into the radial tuberosity. The tendon is released at its insertion into the radial tuberosity to maximize length. The tendon and muscle belly are mobilized in a proximal direction to maximize excursion and to improve line of pull. Along the medial side of the arm, the median nerve, brachial artery, and ulnar nerves are isolated.

A separate posterior incision is performed around the olecranon and extended in a proximal direction along the triceps tendon. A subcutaneous tunnel is created between the medial arm and posterior olecranon incision for tendon passage. The tendon is passed over the median nerve and under the ulnar nerve to avoid any ulnar nerve compression. The triceps tendon is split and the tip of the olecranon is exposed. A large bore blind bone tunnel is drilled in the olecranon for acceptance of the biceps tendon. The tendon is passed through the medial leaflet of the triceps tendon and docked into the bone tunnel using suture within the tendon and posterior unicortical holes.[10] The sutures are tied over the posterior olecranon cortex. Additional suturing is performed during closure of the triceps split with incorporation of the biceps tendon. Following closure, a well-padded long arm cast or splint is applied with the elbow in extension. The wrist is included within the cast and the hand position depends upon concomitant procedures performed for hand function.

Rehabilitation

Nerve rehabilitation is much less arduous than tendon rehabilitation. Following a brief period of immobilization to allow for wound healing, the arm allowed normal usage. Nerve regeneration from the axillary to the motor branch of the triceps muscle occurs at a rate of 1 mm/day. The patients are instructed to link shoulder extension (posterior deltoid function) with elbow extension to promote cortical learning. This combined movement pattern is performed numerous times per day awaiting nerve regeneration. When the posterior branch of the axillary nerve regenerates to the triceps activity, the patient will "learn" to fire his or her triceps independent of shoulder extension.

Tendon rehabilitation requires supervised therapy for months. The biceps to triceps can be mobilized early (7–10 days) or delayed (3 weeks) depending upon the patient's age, patient's compliance, and the strength of the tendon transfer repair (Protocols 15.1 and 15.2). The rehabilitation is divided into three phases: early mobilization,

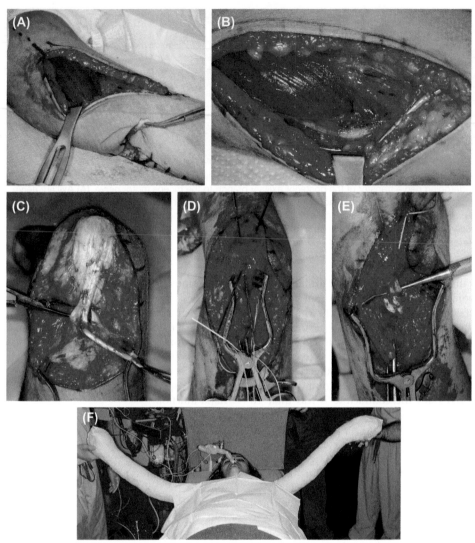

FIG. 15.4 A 16-year-old female 2 years following cervical spinal cord injury. She is ICSHT Grade 2 on both arms and is undergoing biceps-to-triceps tendon transfer. **(A)** Biceps passed along the medial side of the arm to the posterior incision beneath the ulnar nerve. **(B)** Biceps passed beneath the ulnar nerve. **(C)** Biceps tendon passed though triceps tendon before docking into olecranon. **(D)** Suture retrievers to facilitate docking biceps tendon into osseous tunnel. **(E)** Biceps tendon docked into olecranon. **(F)** Postoperative immobilization. (Courtesy of Shriners Hospital for Children, Philadelphia.)

mobilization, and strengthening/functional retraining. Mobilization is initiated in gravity-eliminated plane within a limited arc of flexion. Flexion is progressively increased 15 degrees per week as long as no extension lag develops. Strengthening and wheelchair propulsion are prohibited until 12 weeks from surgery. Transfers and weight shifts are initiated 16 weeks from surgery. Antigravity elbow extension is obtainable in the vast majority of cases (Fig. 15.5).[10,13]

PROTOCOL 15.1
Biceps-to-Triceps Transfer Early Mobilization.

Early mobilization phase 1–5 weeks post-op	Patient is immobilized in bivalved long arm cast or in fabricated splint with elbow in full extension, except during therapy session ***Precautions:*** • Avoid shoulder flexion/abduction above 90 degrees and extension of shoulder beyond 0 degrees • No active elbow flexion until 4 weeks post-op ***Therapeutic intervention*** • Begin early mobilization—passive elbow flexion to 30 degrees, active elbow extension to 0 degrees • Initiate exercises in gravity-eliminated plane, blocking compensatory external rotation and supination • ROM (Range of Motion) of uninvolved joints • Edema management • Week 4: add active elbow flexion in therapy only to 30 degrees
Mobilization phase 5–8 weeks post-op	Cast removed ***Precautions:*** • Avoid shoulder flexion/abduction above 90 degrees and extension of shoulder beyond 0 degrees until 6 weeks post-op • Active elbow flexion and extension is progressed in increments of 15 degrees elbow flexion each week • No elbow flexion beyond allowed elbow range of motion • Do not progress elbow flexion if extension lag is present • No resistive exercises/weight bearing ***Splint*** • Weeks 5–8: • Bledsoe to be worn during the day. At week 5, elbow flexion block at 45 degrees. • Adjust Bledsoe in increments of 15 degrees of flexion per week as patient progresses. Do not increase range in brace if extension lag is present. ***Therapeutic intervention*** • Active elbow flexion to 45 degrees, active extension full. Progress in increments of 15 degrees of flexion per week as patient progresses. Do not increase range if extension lag is present. • Initiate exercises in gravity-eliminated plane, blocking compensatory external rotation and supination • Decrease amount of flexion if extension lag is present. If lag is present focus on end range extension • Edema control and scar management ***Functional Training*** With Bledsoe on, light functional training or activities may begin in allowed elbow ranges (pending time frame and assessment of allowed amount of elbow flexion) only after the therapist is sure, the transfer is firing with the activity.
Strengthening and functional retraining phase 9–12 weeks post-op	***Splint*** • Discontinue Bledsoe splint after 1 week at 90 degrees flexion block (as long as no extension lag present) • Static extension splint at night ***Precautions*** • No resistive exercises or weight bearing • No passive elbow flexion ***Therapeutic interventions*** • Same as described earlier, add against gravity elbow extension as tolerated ***Functional training*** • Same as described earlier
Strengthening/resistive activities	• May begin light progressive resistive exercises at 12 weeks post-op • May begin manual wheelchair propulsion when cleared by surgeon (12–16 weeks post-op) • No restrictions (may resume transfers/weight shifts) at 16 weeks post-op

PROTOCOL 15.2
Biceps-to-Triceps Transfer.

Immobilization phase 1–3 weeks post-op	Patient is immobilized in long arm cast with elbow in full extension. ***Precautions:*** • Avoid shoulder flexion above 90 degrees and extension of shoulder beyond 0 degrees ***Therapeutic intervention*** • ROM of uninvolved joints, edema control

Mobilization phase
3–12 weeks post-op
	Cast removed
	Precautions:
	• Avoid shoulder flexion above 90 degrees and extension of shoulder beyond 0 degrees
	• No passive elbow flexion
	• Active elbow flexion and extension is progressed in increments of 15 degrees elbow flexion each week
	• Do not progress elbow flexion if extension lag is present
	• No resistive exercises
	Splint
	• Fabricate and provide elbow extension splint for night
	  • Continue night time extension splint until postoperative week 12
	• Fit with Bledsoe. To be worn during the day. Set elbow flexion block at 15 degrees.
	  • Adjust Bledsoe in increments of 15 degrees of flexion weekly, as patient progresses. Do not increase range in brace if extension lag is present.
	  • Continue Bledsoe until the patient has achieved 90 degrees elbow flexion and this range has been maintained for 1 week
	Therapeutic intervention
	• Active elbow flexion to 15 degrees, active extension to full
	  • Initiate exercises in a gravity-eliminated plane, blocking external rotation
	  • Progress active elbow flexion in increments of 15 degrees week
	  • Assess for extension lag
	  • Decrease amount of flexion if extension lag is present. If lag is present focus on end range extension
	• Edema control and scar management
	• No passive elbow flexion before 3 months
	Functional training
	Light functional training or activities may begin in allowed elbow ranges (pending time frame and assessment of allowed amount of elbow flexion) only after the therapist is sure the transfer is firing with the activity.

Strengthening/resistive activities	• Initiate light elbow extension strengthening at week 12 as tolerated • May begin manual wheelchair propulsion when cleared by surgeon (12–16 weeks post-op) • No restrictions (may resume transfers/weight shifts) at 16 weeks post-op

ICSHT GRADE 1

Persons with spinal cord injury ICSHT 1 have a strong brachioradialis muscle that is available for transfer. There are no other muscles that are strong and available. According to the reconstruction ladder, the primary fundamental movement to achieve is wrist extension.

Wrist extension can be achieved via tendon and nerve transfer depending upon the donor availability.

Nerve

The potential nerve donor option is the supinator nerves as long as the supinator is working and the

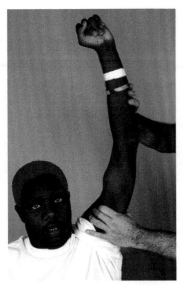

FIG. 15.5 Restoration of strong elbow extension via biceps-to-triceps transfer increases workable reach space, independence, and function use of upper extremity. (Courtesy of Shriners Hospitals for Children, Philadelphia.)

biceps is functioning.[12] Contraction of the supinator muscle can be palpated along the proximal radius, especially as the wrist extensors are atrophic. The biceps is easily accessed during elbow flexion and forearm supination.

If the supinator nerves are deemed available and expendable, we prefer an anterior surgical approach to the posterior interosseous nerve (Fig. 15.6A–C). The radial nerve proper and the posterior interosseous nerve are identified proximal to the supinator muscle and Arcade of Frohse. The posterior interosseous nerve is traced through the arcade and supinator muscle. There are usually two branches to the supinator that can be verified by electrical stimulation. These branches are traced in a distal direction and cut (donor distal). The posterior interosseous nerve is isolated and there is often has a separate branch that innervates the extensor carpi radialis brevis. This branch is traced in a proximal direction and cut (recipient proximal). The coaptation between the supinator branches and the extensor carpi radialis brevis motor branch is secured with microsuture and/or fibrin glue.

Tendon

The brachioradialis can be transferred to the extensor carpi radialis brevis (Fig. 15.7).[8] A longitudinal radial incision is made from the styloid to the proximal third of the forearm. The lateral antebrachial cutaneous and radial sensory nerves are protected. The brachioradialis insertion into the radial styloid is isolated. The tendon is released and the brachioradialis dissected from its investing fascia. The dissection proceeds into the proximal 1/3 of the forearm. The brachioradialis tendon is then woven through the extensor carpi brevis tendon. Tension is adjusted until there is resting tenodesis that maintains the wrist in 30 degrees of extension. Passive lateral pinch can be augmented by performing a tenodesis of the flexor pollicis longus tendon to the volar radius using a bone tunnel (Fig. 15.8). This increases the tension in the flexor pollicis longus during active wrist extension. This maneuver also yields thumb interphalangeal joint flexion that impedes firm lateral pinch. Arthrodesis or a splint flexor pollicis longus tendon transfer can stabilize unwanted interphalangeal joint flexion.

The split flexor pollicis longus transfer is performed via a midaxial incision along the radial side of the thumb (Fig. 15.9A–D). The extensor pollicis longus and the flexor pollicis longus tendons are identified. The radial half of the flexor pollicis longus is traced to its insertion into the distal phalanx and cut. This radial half is passed in a dorsal direction over the interphalangeal joint axis. The tendon is then passed through the extensor pollicis longus and back to itself. Tension is set so that the interphalangeal joint rests in slight flexion. A small nonabsorbable suture is used to secure the transfer. A 0.45 Kirschner is driven from the thumb tip across the interphalangeal joint for stabilization. The pin is cut short and a pin cap applied.

The subcutaneous tissue and skin are closed. A long arm thumb spica cast is applied with the wrist is in extension and the elbow flexed to 90 degrees. The thumb rests along the index finger, and the thumb tip is covered.

Rehabilitation

Nerve rehabilitation is much less arduous than tendon rehabilitation. Following a brief period of immobilization to allow for wound healing, the arm is allowed for

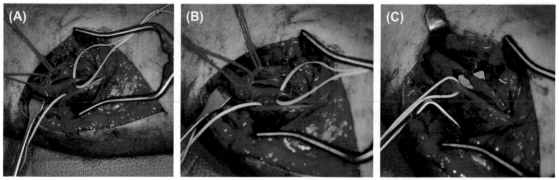

FIG. 15.6 A 22-year-old male 11 months following cervical spine injury. His right side is ICSHT Grade III (absent triceps) and left side ICSHT Grade (I) On the right side, the posterior branch of the axially nerve is transferred to the triceps' motor nerve and the supinator branches are transferred to the posterior interosseous nerve. **(A)** Anterior approach with isolation of the radial sensory nerve (*yellow loop*), posterior interosseous nerve (*blue loop*), and supinator braches (*red loops*). **(B)** Close-up view of nerve branches. **(C)** Supinator branches transferred to the posterior interosseous nerve. (Courtesy of Shriners Hospital for Children, Philadelphia.)

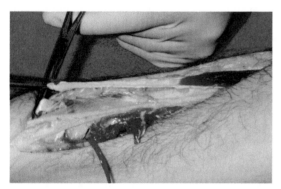

FIG. 15.7 Active wrist extension is restored via transfer of the brachioradialis to the extensor carpi radialis tendon. (Courtesy of Shriners Hospitals for Children, Philadelphia.)

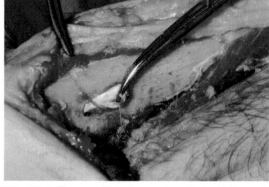

FIG. 15.8 Flexor pollicis longus tenodesis to the volar radius via a bony tunnel. (Courtesy of Shriners Hospitals for Children, Philadelphia.)

normal usage. Nerve regeneration from the supinator to the extensor carpi radialis brevis occurs at a rate of 1 mm/day. The patients are instructed to link forearm supination with wrist extension to promote cortical learning. This combined movement pattern is performed numerous times per day anticipating nerve regeneration. When the supinator branches regenerate to the extensor carpi radialis brevis muscle, the patient will "learn" to fire his or her wrist extension independent of forearm supination.

Tendon rehabilitation following brachioradialis to extensor carpi radialis brevis transfer can be mobilized early (7—10 days) or delayed (3 weeks) depending upon the patient's age and cooperation along with the strength of the tendon transfer repair (Protocol 15.3). The rehabilitation is divided into three phases: early mobilization, mobilization, and strengthening/functional retraining. Regarding the split flexor pollicis longus transfer, the Kirschner wire is removed 3—4 weeks after surgery.

PROTOCOL 15.3
Procedure: Brachioradialis to ECRB/L (Extensor Carpi Radialis Brevis and Longus) with FPL (Flexor Pollicis Longus) Tenodesis (Moberg Procedure).

CLINICAL GUIDELINES

Time Period	Goal
Immobilization phase 1–3 weeks post-op	Tendon immobilized in a shortened position to protect transfer. ***Therapeutic exercise:*** • ROM of uninvolved joints • Edema control of uninvolved digits
Mobilization phase 3–6 weeks post-op	***Precautions:*** • No passive or active wrist flexion beyond neutral • No passive thumb extension/abduction beyond resting • No resistive exercises until 8 weeks post-op • No thumb IP (Interphalangeal joint) flexion ***Splint:*** Volar wrist splint with wrist in 20–30 degrees extension, thumb in adduction ***Splint wearing schedule:*** On at all times; off for home program, bathing, and therapy sessions until consistent recruitment of tendon transfer ***Therapeutic exercise:*** *Muscle reeducation*: Cue simultaneous elbow flexion and wrist extension and passive pinch • Stabilize forearm to assure that patient does not rotate. This will promote excursion for wrist extension versus forearm rotation/gravity assisted extension *Scar management*: Initiate scar massage 3×/day *Patient education*: Educate patient/family on (1) postoperative precautions, (2) scar management, and (3) splint wear/care.

Strengthening and functional retraining phase
6–12 weeks post-op
	Precautions:
	• No passive wrist flexion
	• No passive thumb extension/abduction beyond resting
	• No resistive activities until 8 weeks post-op
	• No thumb IP flexion
	Splint wearing schedule:
	Week 6–8: Off for nonresistive functional tasks; on all night
	Week 8–12: Off all day; on all night
	Week 12: Discontinue use of splint
	Treatment:
	AROM (Active Range of Motion):
	  • Continue recruitment exercises as needed
	  • Active wrist flex and extension (which will promote thumb tenodesis release/pinch)
	*Stabilize forearm to assure that patient does not rotate.
	Strengthening: Initiate light resistive exercises at week 8
	Scar management: Continue scar massage 3×/day
	Patient education: Educate patient/family on changes with (1) postoperative precautions, (2) splint wear/care, and (3) incorporate strengthening into home program.

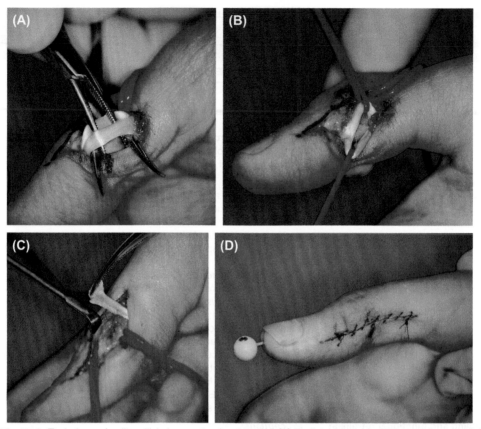

FIG. 15.9 Technique of split pollicis longus tendon transfer. **(A)** Radial midaxial incision and flexor pollicis longus split in the midline. **(B)** Radial half of flexor pollicis longus cut at its insertion. **(C)** Radial half of flexor pollicis longus in a dorsal direction toward the extensor pollicis longus. **(D)** Following split flexor pollicis longus to extensor pollicis longus tendon transfer, a 0.45 Kirschner is driven across the thumb interphalangeal joint. (Courtesy of Shriners Hospitals for Children, Philadelphia.)

ICSHT GRADE 2

Persons with spinal cord injury ICSHT 2 have a strong extensor carpi radialis longus and brachioradialis muscles. According to the reconstruction ladder, the primary fundamental movement of wrist extension is present. The next priority is lateral pinch, which can be obtained by tendon or nerve transfer.

Nerve

The likely nerve donor option is the supinator nerves as they are uniformly working when wrist extension is present.[5,12] The recipient nerve is the anterior interosseous nerve. We prefer an anterior approach to both the posterior interosseous nerve and the anterior interosseous nerve. The incision is longitudinal between the posterior and anterior interosseous nerves. Skin flaps are elevated to gain exposure to both nerves.

The radial nerve proper and the posterior interosseous nerve are identified proximal to the supinator muscle and Arcade of Frohse. The posterior interosseous nerve is traced through the arcade and supinator muscle. There are usually two branches to the supinator that can be verified by electrical stimulation. These branches are traced in a distal direction and cut (donor distal). The median nerve is identified as it enter the pronator teres muscle. The deep head of the pronator teres is released to improve exposure. The anterior interosseous nerve is isolated as it branches from the median nerve. Stimulation is used to identify contraction of the flexor pollicis longus and index flexor digitorum profundus (anterior interosseous nerve). The anterior interosseous nerve is traced in a proximal direction and cut (recipient proximal). The coaptation between the supinator nerves and the anterior interosseous nerve is secured with microsuture and/or fibrin glue.

Tendon

The brachioradialis can be transferred to the flexor pollicis longus for active pinch (Fig. 15.10A–D).[8] A longitudinal radial incision is made from the styloid to the proximal third of the forearm. The lateral antebrachial cutaneous and radial sensory nerves are protected. The brachioradialis insertion into the radial styloid is isolated. The tendon is released, and the brachioradialis is dissected from its investing fascia. The dissection proceeds into the proximal 1/3 of the forearm. The brachioradialis tendon is passed deep to the radial artery and is woven through the flexor pollicis longus. Tension is adjusted until there is resting tenodesis that maintains the thumb against the index finger with the wrist in 30 degrees of extension. Active lateral pinch yields unwanted thumb interphalangeal joint flexion that hinders firm lateral pinch. Arthrodesis or a splint flexor pollicis longus tendon transfer can stabilize the interphalangeal joint as described earlier under ICSHT Grade 1 reconstruction.

The subcutaneous tissue and skin are closed. A long arm thumb spica cast is applied with the elbow at 90 degrees and the wrist positioned in extension. The thumb rests along the index finger and the thumb tip is covered.

Rehabilitation

Nerve rehabilitation is straightforward. Following a brief period of immobilization to allow for wound healing, the arm is permitted normal usage. Nerve regeneration from the supinator to the anterior interosseous nerve occurs at a rate of 1 mm/day. The patients are instructed to link forearm supination with lateral pinch to promote cortical learning. This combined movement pattern is performed numerous times per day anticipating nerve regeneration. When the supinator branches regenerate to the flexor pollicis longus muscle and index flexor digitorum profundus muscles the patient will "learn" to fire his or her thumb and index independent of forearm supination.

The brachioradialis to flexor pollicis longus transfer can be mobilized early (7–10 days) or delayed (3 weeks) depending upon the patient's age and cooperation along with the strength of the

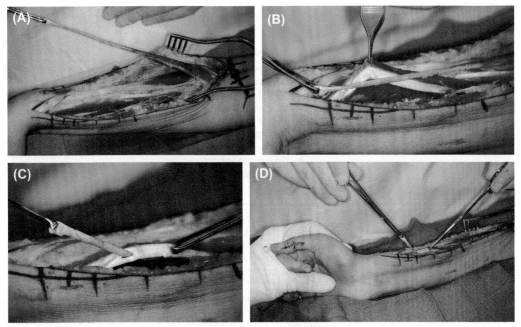

FIG. 15.10 Technique of extensor carpi radialis longus to flexor pollicis longus transfer. **(A)** Brachioradialis tendon released and mobilized into the proximal 1/3 of the forearm. **(B)** Flexor pollicis longus tendon isolated in volar compartment. **(C)** Brachioradialis tendon woven through the flexor pollicis longus tendon. **(D)** Tendon transfer tension is adjusted until there is lateral pinch during wrist extension. (Courtesy of Shriners Hospitals for Children, Philadelphia.)

tendon transfer repair (Protocols 15.4 and 15.5). The rehabilitation is divided into three phases: early mobilization, mobilization, and strengthening/functional retraining. Regarding the split flexor pollicis longus transfer, the Kirschner wire is removed 3−4 weeks after surgery.

PROTOCOL 15.4
Procedure: Brachioradialis into FPL (With Immobilization).

CLINICAL GUIDELINES	
Time Period	**Goal**
Immobilization phase: 1−3 weeks	Tendon immobilized in a shortened position to protect transfer.
Mobilization phase 3−6 weeks post-op	**Precautions:** • Avoid overextension of thumb • No passive wrist extension • Avoid resistive exercises • No passive elbow extension, unless cleared by MD • No IP flexion with FPL split procedure **Splint:** Dorsal forearm based splint with thumb adducted; thumb MP (Metacarpophalangeal) and IP included, wrist in neutral; elbow free **Splint wearing schedule:** On at all times; off for home program, bathing, and therapy sessions. **Treatment:** *Muscle reeducation:* • Cue previous muscle action • Biofeedback as needed *AROM:* • Lateral pinch • Wrist flexion • Wrist extension to 20 degrees−30 degrees (unless cleared by MD for more) • Elbow flexion and extension • Digit flexion and extension *Stabilize forearm to assure that patient is able to pinch in various forearm and elbow positions. *Begin light, functional pinch activities with consistent recruitment *Scar management:* • Initiate scar massage 3×/day *Patient education:* • Postoperative precautions • Scar management • Splint wear/care
Strengthening and functional retraining phase 6−12 weeks post-op	**Precautions:** • Avoid overextension of thumb • Avoid resistive exercises • No IP flexion • No passive elbow extension, unless cleared by MD **Splint wearing schedule:** Week 6−8: Off for nonresistive functional tasks on at night Week 8−12: Off all day; on all night Week 12: Discontinue use of splint **Treatment:** *AROM:* • Lateral pinch • Wrist flex and extension • Elbow flexion and extension • Digit flexion and extension

*Stabilize forearm to assure that patient is able to pinch in various forearm and elbow positions.
Strengthening: Initiate light resistive pinch exercises at week 8
Scar management:
  • Continue scar massage 3×/day
Patient education: Educate patient/family on changes with (1) *postoperative* precautions, (2) splint wear/care, and (3) incorporate strengthening into home program.

PROTOCOL 15.5
Procedure: Brachioradialis into FPL (Early Mobilization).

CLINICAL GUIDELINES	
Time Period	**Goal**
Early mobilization phase: Postop day 3 through 6 weeks	*Precautions:* • Avoid overextension of thumb • No passive wrist extension • Avoid resistive exercises • No passive elbow extension, unless cleared by MD • No IP flexion with FPL split procedure *Splint:* Dorsal forearm based splint with thumb adducted; thumb MP and IP included, wrist in neutral; elbow free *Splint wearing schedule:* On at all times; off for home program, bathing, and therapy sessions. *Treatment:* *Muscle reeducation:* • Cue previous muscle action • Biofeedback as needed *AROM:* • Lateral pinch • Wrist flexion • Wrist extension to 20 degrees–30 degrees (unless cleared by MD for more) • Elbow flexion and extension • Digit flexion and extension *Stabilize forearm to assure that patient is able to pinch in various forearm and elbow positions. *Begin light, functional pinch activities with consistent recruitment after 2.5–3 weeks *Scar management*: • Initiate scar massage 3×/day once incision is completely healed *Patient education*: • Postoperative precautions • Scar management • Splint wear/care

Continued

PROTOCOL 15.5
Procedure: Brachioradialis into FPL (Early Mobilization).—cont'd

CLINICAL GUIDELINES	
Time Period	**Goal**
Mobilization phase 6–12 weeks post-op	**Precautions:** • Avoid overextension of thumb/IP flexion if contraindicated • Avoid resistive exercises (may begin light strengthening at week 8) • No passive elbow extension, unless cleared by MD • Check with MD for return to manual w/c propulsion **Splint wearing schedule:** Week 6–8: Off for nonresistive functional tasks, on at night Week 8–12: Off all day; on all night Week 12: Discontinue use of splint **Treatment:** Same as described earlier, introduce light strengthening at week 8 with consistent recruitment **Scar management:** • Continue scar massage 3×/day

ICSHT GRADE 3

Persons with spinal cord injury ICSHT 3 have a strong extensor carpi radialis brevis, extensor carpi radialis longus, and brachioradialis muscles. According to the reconstruction ladder, the primary fundamental movement of wrist extension is present. The next priorities are lateral pinch and grasp, which can be obtained by tendon or nerve transfer. Digital extension can also be obtained by combining nerve and tendon transfers.

Nerve

The nerve donor options often increase in persons with spinal cord injury ICSHT 3. The supinator nerves are uniformly intact and available. If elbow extension is present, then the motor nerve to the brachialis muscle becomes available, as biceps to triceps transfer is unnecessary.[4,6] Either one of the donor nerves can be transferred to the anterior interosseous nerve or a portion of the median nerve to obtain lateral pinch or grasp, respectively. The motor nerve to the brachialis muscle is transferred via an anterior approach that begins above the elbow and extends into the forearm while the supinator braches are transferred below the elbow as described under ICSHT 2 nerve reconstruction.

Tendon

The brachioradialis can be transferred to the flexor pollicis longus for active pinch, and the extensor carpi radialis longus can be transferred to the flexor digitorum profundus for active grasp (Fig. 15.10A–D).[8] A longitudinal radial incision is made from the styloid to the proximal third of the forearm. The lateral antebrachial cutaneous and radial sensory nerves are protected. The brachioradialis insertion into the radial styloid is isolated. The tendon is released, and the brachioradialis is dissected from its investing fascia. The dissection proceeds into the proximal 1/3 of the forearm. The brachioradialis tendon passed deep to the radial artery and is woven through the flexor pollicis longus. Tension is adjusted until there is resting tenodesis that maintains the thumb against the index finger with the wrist in 30 degrees of extension. Active lateral pinch yields unwanted thumb interphalangeal joint flexion that hinders firm lateral pinch. Arthrodesis or a splint flexor pollicis longus tendon transfer can stabilize the interphalangeal joint as described earlier under ICSHT Grade 1 reconstruction.

Through the same incision, the extensor carpi radialis longus tendon transfer can be performed (Fig. 15.11A and B). The extensor carpi radialis longus and extensor carpi radialis brevis tendons are identified distal to the first compartment. In the proximal part of the incisions, the extensor carpi radialis longus and extensor carpi radialis brevis tendons are also isolated. The extensor carpi radialis longus tendon is then cut as distal as possible and is pulled under the first dorsal compartment. The extensor carpi radialis longus tendon is passed deep to the radial artery and woven through the flexor digitorum profundus tendons using a Pulvertaft weave. Tension is adjusted until there is finger

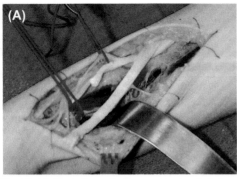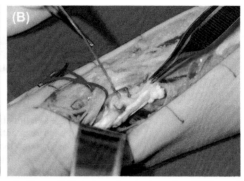

FIG. 15.11 Technique of extensor carpi radialis longus to flexor digitorum profundus transfer. **(A)** Harvest of the extensor carpi radialis longus (and brachioradialis) via longitudinal radial incision. **(B)** Extensor carpi radialis longus tendon woven through the flexor digitorum profundus tendons. (Courtesy of Shriners Hospitals for Children, Philadelphia.)

flexion during wrist extension and tenodesis opening during wrist flexion.

The subcutaneous tissue and skin are closed. A long arm cast is applied with the wrist is in slight extension and the elbow flexed to 90 degrees. The fingers are slightly flexed, and this positioned is maintained with a small roll of webril cotton cast padding.

Nerve and Tendon Transfer

The surgeon can integrate nerve and tendon transfers to gain additional function. The tendon transfers described earlier are used for active lateral pinch and grasp. The supinator nerves can be transferred to the posterior interosseous nerve to achieve finger extension. An anterior surgical approach is used to assess both the supinator nerve braches and the posterior interosseous nerves. The posterior interosseous nerve is traced in a proximal direction (recipient proximal). The supinator braches are traced in a distal direction (donor distal).

The nerves are cut through and the transfer repaired with microsuture and/or fibrin glue.

Rehabilitation

Nerve rehabilitation is similar ICSHT 1 and 2, although the donor and recipient may be different. Nerve regeneration occurs at a rate of 1 mm/day. The patients are instructed to link their donor and recipient functions to promote cortical learning. Once nerve regeneration occurs, therapy is helpful to isolate recipient function.

The brachioradialis to flexor pollicis longus transfer and/or the extensor carpi radialis longus to the flexor digitorum profundus transfer can be mobilized early (7–10 days) or delayed (3 weeks) depending upon the patient's age and cooperation along with strength of the tendon transfer repair (Protocols 15.4–15.6). Early mobilization of the extensor carpi radialis longus transfer can be started on postoperative day 1 by

---

PROTOCOL 15.6
Procedure: Active Grasp: ECRL (Extensor Carpi Radialis Longus) to FDP (Flexor Digitorum Profundus); Early Mobilization.

CLINICAL GUIDELINES	
Time Period	**Goal**
Early mobilization phase Post-op day 1–3 weeks post-op	Tendon immobilized in a shortened position to protect transfer. UE (Upper Extremity) immobilization position in a dorsal blocking cast: Elbow: 90 degrees wrist: Neutral MCPs (Metacarpophalangeal): Flexed to 70 degrees IP's: Extended strap to dorsum of cast, or roll of webril, may be used when not performing exercises to position IP joints in extension to prevent flexion contractures
	Therapeutic exercise: AROM: • Active composite digit flexion • Place/hold digit extension

Continued

PROTOCOL 15.6
Procedure: Active Grasp: ECRL (Extensor Carpi Radialis Longus) to FDP (Flexor Digitorum Profundus); Early Mobilization.—cont'd

CLINICAL GUIDELINES	
Time Period	**Goal**

Mobilization phase
3–6 weeks post-op
	Precautions:
	• No passive or active MCP extension past position of resting tension of transfer
	• No passive or active wrist extension past position of resting tension of transfer unless cleared by MD
	• No passive or active composite extension
	• No resistive exercises
	Splint: Dorsal block splint with wrist in neutral, MPs flexed 70 degrees and IPs extended
	Splint wearing schedule:
	On at all times, off for home program, bathing, and therapy sessions
	Treatment:
	Muscle reeducation:
	  • Cue previous muscle action while manually blocking wrist extension to avoid tenodesis effect digit flexion
	  • Composite flexion place and hold
	AROM:
	  • Protected AROM
	  • Composite digit flexion
	  - When performing this exercise, stabilize the wrist in 30 degrees extension and work on active digit flexion
	  • Active digit IP extension to protected position only
	  • Wrist flexion and extension to resting position—tendon placed in shortened position (i.e., digits fully flexed manually) during this exercise
	  • Passive digit flexion: cComposite flexion and individual joints as indicated
	Scar management: Initiate scar massage 3×/day
	Patient education:
	  • Postoperative precautions
	  • Scar management
	  • Splint wear/care
	  • HEP (Home Exercise Program)

Strengthening and functional retraining phase
6–12 weeks post-op
	Precautions:
	• No composite extension stretching
	• No resistive exercises until postoperative week 8
	Splint wearing schedule:
	Week 6–8: Off for nonresistive functional tasks on at night
	Week 8–12: Off all day; on all night
	Week 12: Discontinue use of splint
	Treatment:
	AROM:
	  • Composite flexion
	  • Composite digit extension to end range (avoid extrinsic flexor stretch)
	Functional retraining:
	  • Patient may remove splint for light ADLs at 6 weeks
	  • At 8 weeks, the patient may begin using extremity to perform transfers with digits in a fisted position (not with composite wrist and digit extension).
	Strengthening: May initiate light strengthening at 8 weeks
	Scar management: Continue as described earlier
	Patient education: Educate patient/*family* on therapy and home program changes

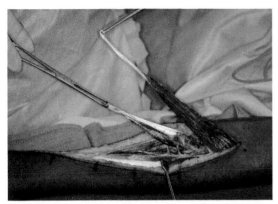

FIG. 15.12 Harvest of the brachioradialis and pronator teres tendons via a radial longitudinal incision. (Courtesy of Shriners Hospital for Children, Philadelphia.)

removing the webril roll and asking the patient to bend his or her fingers. As wrist extension and finger flexion is synergistic, finger flexion is often immediate. The rehabilitation phases of early mobilization, mobilization, and strengthening/functional retraining are detailed on the protocols. Regarding the split flexor pollicis longus transfer, the Kirschner wire is removed 3—4 weeks after surgery.

ICSHT GRADES 4 AND 5

Persons with spinal cord injury ICSHT 4 and 5 have additional strong pronator teres and flexor carpi radialis longus muscles. These muscles are potentially available; however, their function is critical. Forearm pronation is mandatory for daily function and counteracts any supination moment. Similarly, active wrist flexion promotes digital extension and object acquisition. These benefits often disqualify the pronator teres and flexor carpi radialis from being "expendable" for tendon transfer. Hence, the algorithm is similar to that described for person with ICSHT 3. If the pronator and/or flexor carpi radialis are utilized, a similar longitudinal radial incision is made from the styloid to the proximal third of the forearm as described earlier (Fig. 15.12).

ICSHT GRADES 6 AND 7

Persons with spinal cord injury ICSHT 6 and 7 have the ability to extend their fingers and thumb, respectively. This further enhances hand function, especially as grasp and pinch are easily obtained with nerve or tendon transfer. Donor nerves include the supinator branches, brachialis motor nerve, and pronator teres motor

nerve.[4–6] Recipient nerves are the braches from the median nerve for finger and thumb flexion.

ICSHT GRADES 8 AND 9

Persons with spinal cord injury ICSHT 8 and 9 have the ability to flex their fingers and sometimes their thumb. These patients have some ability to grasp and hold items. The surgeon has the option(s) of enhancing grasp and/or attempting intrinsic reconstruction. These patients are treated with similar tenets as combined low median/low ulnar nerve injuries. Tendon transfers are still the mainstays of surgical reconstruction in this group of patients. The objectives of tendon transfers are to restore thumb opposition (opponensplasty), thumb adduction for lateral pinch (adductorplasty), and coordinated grasp (metacarpophalangeal and interphalangeal flexion).

REFERENCES

1. National Spinal Cord Injury Statistical Center, Facts and Figures at a Glance. Birmingham, AL: University of Alabama at Birmingham; 2018. https://www.nscisc.uab.edu/Public/Facts%20and%20Figures%20-%202018.pdf.
2. Zlotolow DA. The role of the upper extremity surgeon in the management of tetraplegia. *J Hand Surg Am.* 2011; 36A:929—935.
3. Curtin CM, Gater DR, Chung KC. Upper extremity reconstruction in the tetraplegic population, a national epidemiologic study. *J Hand Surg Am.* 2005;30(1):94—99.
4. Bertelli JA, Ghizoni MF. Nerve transfers for restoration of finger flexion in patients with tetraplegia. *J Neurosurg Spine.* 2017;26(1):55—61.
5. Bertelli JA, Tacca CP, Ghizoni MF, Kechele PR, Santos MA. Transfer of supinator motor branches to the posterior interosseous nerve to reconstruct thumb and finger extension in tetraplegia: case report. *J Hand Surg Am.* 2010; 35(10):1647—1651.
6. Fox IK, Davidge KM, Novak CB, et al. Nerve transfers to restore upper extremity function in cervical spinal cord injury: update and preliminary outcomes. *Plast Reconstr Surg.* 2015;136(4):780—792.
7. Little KJ, Zlotolow DA, Soldado F, Cornwall R, Kozin SH. Early functional recovery of elbow flexion and supination following median and/or ulnar nerve fascicle transfer in upper neonatal brachial plexus palsy. *J Bone Joint Surg Am.* 2014;96(3):215—221.
8. Kozin SH, Zlotolow DA, Abzug JM. Upper extremity reconstruction in persons with tetraplegia. In: Abzug JM, Kozin SH, Zlotolow DA, eds. *The Pediatric Upper Extremity.* New York: Springer; 2015:735—765.
9. Oberlin C, Béal D, Leechavengvongs S, Salon A, Dauge MC, Sarcy JJ. Nerve transfer to biceps muscle using a part of ulnar nerve for C5-C6 avulsion of the brachial

plexus: anatomical study and report of four cases. *J Hand Surg Am.* 1994;19(2):232–237.

10. Kozin SH, D'Addesi L, Chafetz RS, Ashworth S, Mulcahey MJ. Biceps-to-Triceps transfer for elbow extension in persons with tetraplegia. *J Hand Surg Am.* 2010;35:968–975.

11. LeClerq C, Hentx VR, Kozin SH, Mulcahey MJ. Reconstruction of elbow extension. *Hand Clin.* 2008;24:185–201.

12. Bertelli JA, Ghizoni MF. Nerve transfers fo5r elbow and finger extension reconstruction in midcervical spinal cord injuries. *J Neurosurg.* 2015;122(1):121–127.

13. Kuz J, Van Heest AE, House JH. Biceps-to-triceps transfer in tetraplegic patients: report of the medial routing technique and follow-up of three cases. *J Hand Surg Am.* 1999;24:161–172.

CHAPTER 16

Multiligamentous Laxity

JENNY M. DORICH, MBA, OTR/L, CHT • KEVIN J. LITTLE, MD

INTRODUCTION

Multiligament laxity in children and adolescents results from underlying joint hypermobility.[1,2] Joint hypermobility (JH) is defined as the "capability that a joint (or a group of joints) has to move, passively and/or actively, beyond normal limits along physiological axes."[3] Joint hypermobility that is localized to a less than five joints is called as localized joint hypermobility (LJH). Whereas joint laxity at five or more joints is called generalized joint hypermobility (GJH) and typically genetic in nature, but may be acquired secondary to other conditions such as endocrine disorders, widespread inflammation, or malnutrition. The most common form of inherited GJH is Ehlers–Danlos syndrome (EDS).[3] Throughout this chapter, we will refer to the phenomenon of multiligament laxity as JH.

The prevalence of JH among school-aged children has been reported to range from 16% to 35%[4,5] when diagnosed using the Beighton scale (Table 16.1).[6] Although the prevalence of joint hypermobility is similar between prepubescent females and males, following puberty females demonstrate increased joint laxity while the prevalence is unchanged in males.[2] Joint hypermobility may be present, but unrecognized until the time of injury or onset of joint pain.[7]

TABLE 16.1 Components of the Beighton Scale.		
	Left	Right
1. Passive dorsiflexion and hyperextension of the fifth MCP joint beyond 90 degrees	1	1
2. Passive apposition of the thumb to the flexor aspect of the forearm	1	1
3. Passive hyperextension of the elbow beyond 10 degrees	1	1
4. Passive hyperextension of the knee beyond 10 degrees	1	1
5. Active forward flexion of the trunk with the knees fully extended so that the palms of the hands rest flat on the floor	1	1
TOTAL		/9

The first four elements can be given a maximum score of 2, because these are performed bilateral. The last element is scored with 0 or 1. The maximum score for ligament laxity is 9. A score of 9 means hyperlax. A score of zero is tight.
Adapted from Beighton P, et al. Ehlers-Danlos syndromes: revised nosology. *Am J Med Genet.* 1998;77(1):31–37.

Pediatric Hand Therapy. https://doi.org/10.1016/B978-0-323-53091-0.00016-6

Nine Point Beighton Scale (Beighton et al. 1973)
Nine Point Beighton hypermobility score

Individuals are scored on their ability to	Right	Left
Passively dorsiflex the 5th metacarpophalangeal joint to ≥90°	1	1
Oppose the thumb to the volar aspect of the ipsilateral forearm	1	1
Hyperextend the elbow to ≥10°	1	1
Hyperextend the knee to ≥10°	1	1
Place hands flat on the floor without bending the knees		1
Total		9

One point is gained for each side for each maneuver 1–4, with a total possible score of 9 points.

GJH in children is associated with symptoms of joint pain and fatigue, and GJH in children is associated with a greater risk of joint pain in adolescence.[8] The symptoms of joint pain, fatigue, and stress incontinence have been found to negatively impact quality of life in children with JH.[9] Poor activity tolerance is common,[10] as is exercise tolerance. Eighty-one percent of children receiving care in a rheumatology practice report pain exacerbation with exercise participation.[11] Recurrent joint dislocations and soft tissue injury can lead to chronic joint pain and instability.[12,13] Additionally, children may demonstrate altered proprioception[14] and impaired coordination.[15]

Children/adolescents with JH may present with comorbidities including functional gastrointestinal disorders,[16] neurogenic bladder sphincter dysfunction (more frequently manifested as constipation in males and urinary incontinence in females),[17] headaches,[18] sleep disturbance,[19] and/or postural orthostatic tachycardia syndrome.[20] Children and adults with joint hypermobility exhibit a low pain pressure threshold and increased incidence of hyperalgesia as compared to healthy controls.[21] Adults with joint hypermobility have a higher incidence of anxiety and depression as compared to individuals without joint hypermobility.[22] Kinesiophobia (irrational and debilitating fear of physical movement and activity resulting from a feeling of vulnerability to painful injury or reinjury) is also common in adults with JH.[23] Psychological comorbidities have not been studied in children and adolescents, but have been noted to be a common finding in our clinical experience.

In a 3-year longitudinal cohort study evaluating the natural history of hypermobility and JH in children, those children who presented with more multisystemic comorbidities, poor postural control, and higher levels of pain and fatigue at baseline were most likely to have progressive worsening of symptoms and disability.[13] In children who present with multisystemic comorbidities, coordinated multidisciplinary care is recommended.[24]

When individuals with multiligamentous laxity have underlying JH, the diagnosis of the JH is often delayed. With delayed diagnosis, the child/adolescent may have developed chronic pain, making treatment of the condition more complex.[7] Additionally, children and adolescents may have experienced prior unsuccessful attempts of therapy.[25] Yet, physical therapy is considered the standard treatment for JH.[26,27] Occupational therapy and physical therapy that is holistic in addressing JH is the most effective technique. This allows the therapeutic exercises to be focused on addressing the patient's goals and aimed at addressing the condition's chronicity rather than only the acute symptoms.[7]

CLASSIFICATION

Initial classification of JH was based on phenotypical variants noted to have characteristic physical examination findings. Advancements in genetic testing, combined with the clinical recognition of additional subtypes, have refined and expanded the classification into 13 separate subtypes (Table 16.2).[3] The hypermobile subtype of EDS does not have an associated gene defect and is thought to be genetically heterogenous. This subtype is inherited in an autosomal dominant fashion, and the diagnosis is made on the basis of rigidly applied physical examination findings including a Beighton score ≥ 5.[3]

INITIAL REFERRAL

Children and adolescents who have multiligament laxity may present to a hand and upper extremity specialists with complaints of chronic joint pain or recurrent joint subluxation or episodes of instability. The primary reason for referral may be specific to a particular joint such as the shoulder or wrist. An inciting event may be mild or unknown for the reported level of pain and disability. The presence of an underlying joint hypermobility may or may not be already known.[7]

The initial assessment of the patient should include a thorough history of the current complaint, including any known injuries to the area. Additionally, a thorough history will identify all previous treatment modalities, including casting, splinting, rest, therapy, and/or medications. Finally, the history should elicit any other joints with a history of pain requiring treatment, including multiple sprains, strains, or dislocations.[18]

TABLE 16.2
Clinical Classification of the Ehlers-Danlos Syndromes, Inheritance Pattern, and Genetic Basis.

	Clinical EDS Subtype	Abbreviation	IP	Genetic Basis	Protein
1	Classical EDS	cEDS	AD	Major: *COL5A1, COL5A1* Rare: *COL1A1* c.934C>T, p.(Arg312Cys)	Type V collagen Type I collagen
2	Classical-like EDS	clEDS	AR	*TNXB*	Tenascin XB
3	Cardiac-valvular	cvEDS	AR	*COL1A2 (biallelic mutations that lead to COL1A2 NMD and absence of pro α2(I) collagen chains)*	Type I collagen
4	Vascular EDS	vEDS	AD	Major: *COL3A1* Rare: *COL1A1* c.934C>T, p.(Arg312Cys) c.1720C>T, p.(Arg574Cys) c.3227C>T, p.(Arg1093Cys)	Type III collagen Type I collagen
5	Hypermobile EDS	hEDS	AD	Unknown	Unknown
6	Arthrochalasia EDS	aEDS	AD	*COL1A1, COL1A2*	Type I collagen
7	Dermatosparaxis EDS	dEDS	AR	*ADAMTS2*	ADAMTS-2
8	Kyphoscoliotic EDS	kEDS	AR	*PLOD1* *FKBP14*	LH1 FKBP22
9	Brittle cornea syndrome	BCS	AR	*ZNF469* *PRDM5*	ZNF469 PRDM5
10	Spondylodysplastic EDS	spEDS	AR	*B4GALT7* *B3GALT6* *SLC39A13*	β4GalT7 β3GalT6 ZIP13
11	Musculocontractural EDS	mcEDS	AR	*CHST14* *DSE*	D4ST1 DSE
12	Myopathic EDS	mEDS	AD or AR	*COL12A1*	Type XII collagen
13	Periodontal EDS	pEDS	AD	*C1R* *C1S*	C1r C1s

AD, autosomal dominant; *AR*, autosomal recessive; *IP*, inheritance pattern; *NMD*, nonsense-mediated mRNA decay.
Reproduced with permission from Malfait F, Francomano C, Byers P, et al. The 2017 international classification of the Ehlers–Danlos syndromes. *Am J Med Genet Part C Semin Med Genet.* 2017;175C:8–26) .

A generalized physical examination focusing on hypermobility is useful for these patients when coupled with a more focused physical examination of the affected area. The generalized physical examination should include the Beighton score, as well as signs of skin hypermobility, such as skin striae or widened or atrophic scars. In addition to assessing the affected joint, the examiner should assess the contralateral joint for signs of symmetric hypermobility to better understand the patient's tendencies toward specific joint hypermobility, and to assess if superimposed ligamentous injury is also present. Joint-specific examination features of pathologic hypermobility or multidirectional instability are beyond the scope of this chapter and are detailed elsewhere.[28]

TREATMENT

Initially, conservative treatment is recommended. This includes referral to occupational therapy to address the chief complaint. Physical therapy may also be warranted if the child is found to have pervasive lower extremity pain or postural concerns, such as core weakness,[29] that are contributing to biomechanics underlying the upper extremity concern. If the child presents with debilitating pain, referral to a multidisciplinary pain clinic also may be indicated.[30]

When the child/adolescent has an acute episode of soft tissue trauma associated with edema or unremitting pain, occupational may begin with a short period of immobilization. Prolonged immobilization can lead to weakness and persistent pain,[31] so the period of immobilization should be brief. Additionally, with the increased incidence of hyperalgesia found within this population,[21] a removable upper extremity orthotic that is doffed for bathing and short periods of active range of motion is advised. The child/adolescent should be monitored closely for the presence of allodynia or hyperalgesia, and desensitization exercises should be incorporated if these symptoms emerge.[32]

When the symptoms are more chronic in nature without acute swelling or after a short period of immobilization as outlined earlier in acute presentations, therapy should transition to interventions to minimize pain and maximize function. Patient education is foundational to pain management and facilitating activity participation.[24] Initially, children and their caregivers may have resistance to therapeutic intervention if they have experienced unfavorable results from previous therapy experiences. Additionally, feelings of mistrust in healthcare providers may be present if the diagnosis of JHS is delayed or the child/family feels that the impact of the child's symptoms on their quality of life has been under appreciated.[7] Consequently, developing therapeutic rapport and understanding of the child and family's primary concerns is paramount to establish receptiveness to patient education.

The Canadian Occupational Performance Measure (COPM) can be useful in identifying client-specific goals for the course of therapy (see Chapter 4).[33] This allows the therapist to identify specific activities that may be most impacted by the child's symptoms. The child/adolescent can then be observed attempting to perform these activities identified through the COPM. This allows therapists to determine what interventions may be most beneficial in minimizing pain and enhancing function.

Patient education often includes activity modifications, joint protection, activity pacing, and energy conservation strategies.[31] Additionally, when the child/adolescent has chronic pain associated with JHS therapists can utilize self-management strategies[34] to facilitate the child/adolescent's acceptance of pain management over resolution.[35]

Activity modifications may include use of alternative tools or postures to minimize joint strain during the child's participation in the specific activities identified through the COPM. For example, children who have pain with writing may benefit from using pencil grips, slant boards, or utilizing technology to complete longer written assignments.

Joint protection strategies are employed to minimize joint straining positions and excessive forces.[30] Proprioceptive retraining exercises may be helpful to improve joint mechanics during activities.[36] For example, if a child uses too much force during activities, such as holding a pencil with increased pressure during writing, proprioceptive retraining exercises may achieve improved mechanics to limit joint strain.[22] Upper extremity Orthotics[18] also may be beneficial in activity specific applications to limit excessive range of motion that can cause joint pain. For example, a ring splint may be worn on the finger interphalangeal joints to limit hyperextension if a child who plays the violin has joint pain when playing.

Education in activity pacing[31] and energy conservation[18] strategies is helpful to prevent exacerbation of pain and fatigue. Finally, education in good sleep hygiene habits is recommended if the child/adolescent reports erratic sleep patterns. Limiting screen time and caffeine before bed as well as having a consistent bedtime and bedtime routine helps to establish improved sleep.[37]

Weakness and decreased endurance may contribute to the child's pain, as muscle weakness and impairments in muscle function have been found in the adults with JH.[38] Isometric strengthening of the muscles that provide joint stability such as the rotator cuff and scapular stabilizers in the shoulder or extrinsic wrist muscles at the wrist may be effective in reducing joint pain.[39] Additionally, poor posture may underlie muscle tightness and pain. Decreased core strength often contributes to a shoulder-rounded posture that places strain in cervical and upper trunk muscles. Posture retraining is beneficial to reduce pain and prevent long-term joint damage.[40]

SURGERY

If the child has persistent joint instability following a 3−6-month course of therapy, then surgical treatment may be indicated. Surgery is also an indication in patients with primary, acute ligamentous or bony injury found in the setting of underlying hypermobility. Diagnostic joint arthroscopy, often combined with a fluoroscopic and/or clinical examination under anesthesia, is the procedure of choice for patients where a definitive diagnosis of injury has not been established. This intervention can assess for joint incongruity or pathologic laxity that is difficult to assess in an awake patient who complains of pain with attempted joint manipulation. In patients where ligament instability is noted, surgical procedures are aimed at augmenting the stability of the pathoanatomical ligament or ligaments.

The shoulder joint has limited inherent stability due to the large size of the humeral head and relatively small size of the glenoid and is thus prone to problems with instability. Patients with shoulder diagnosed multidirectional instability (anterior and posterior subluxations or dislocations) or persistent unidirectional instability often benefit from anterior ligament augmentation using an arthroscopic or open capsular-shift procedure[41−43] to improve shoulder stability. However, in an attempt to prevent recurrent instability, a persistent loss of shoulder motion may result from this procedure.

The bony anatomy of the elbow allows for more intrinsic stability of this joint, and persistent instability is less common. Therapy is the first line treatment for pathologic elbow ligamentous laxity,[44] while arthroscopic-assisted or open ligament repair or reconstruction is typically only warranted for patients with single ligament instability leading to recurrent dislocations. Dislocations of the wrist are relatively infrequent, and most often associated with fractures of the distal radius, or because of substantial trauma. In patients with persistent pain and a history of ligamentous hypermobility, wrist arthroscopy can be performed to assess the joint and debride or repair associated ligament injuries to the scapholunate ligament, lunotriquetral ligament, or triangular fibrocartilage complex.[45,46]

REHABILITATION FOLLOWING SURGERY

Specific postsurgical rehabilitation protocols are beyond the scope of this chapter. However, there are principles of rehabilitation with this patient population that are particularly important to consider in the therapeutic approach with children who are recovering from surgery. In the early stages of post-operative therapy, it is important to recognize that wound healing takes longer in this population. Additionally, scarring may be increased.[47] Therefore, the therapist's active role in postoperative wound care and scar management is essential.

The collagen deficiency in children with EDS may lead to weakened soft tissue that is slower to respond to therapeutic intervention.[48] Often, the therapy course is longer with this population as compared to children without JH. The progression of therapy should begin at a low intensity and gradually progressed over time.[18] Therapy should prioritize stabilization[49] and progress from static exercises to dynamic exercises and finally to resistive training.[31] Compensatory patterns of muscle imbalance for joint stabilization are common making it critical that therapists focus on neuromuscular training to facilitate muscular balance.[18]

When children exhibit signs of kinesiophobia, emphasis should be placed on open communication and sensitive handling skills to achieve optimal outcomes.[50] Cognitive behavioral therapy techniques and collaborative intervention with psychology are also effective in maximizing outcomes when kinesiophobia is persistent.[30]

SUMMARY

In conclusion, children with JH require a thorough medical history and clinical evaluation to fully appreciate their full clinical picture. An extensive course of therapy is recommended as the initial course of treatment in the absence of pathology that requires immediate surgical intervention. When surgical intervention is indicated, the postoperative therapy course should progress slowly and consider the need to focus on establishing stability and muscle balance to achieve pain control and maximize functional outcomes.

REFERENCES
1. Decoster LC, et al. Prevalence and features of joint hypermobility among adolescent athletes. *Arch Pediatr Adolesc Med.* 1997;151(10):989−992.
2. Quatman CE, et al. The effects of gender and pubertal status on generalized joint laxity in young athletes. *J Sci Med Sport.* 2008;11(3):257−263.
3. Malfait F, et al. The 2017 international classification of the Ehlers−Danlos syndromes. *Am J Med Genet Part C: Seminars in Medical Genetics.* 2017. Wiley Online Library.
4. Remvig L, et al. Prevalence of generalized joint hypermobility, arthralgia and motor competence in 10-year-old school children. *Int Musculoskelet Med.* 2011;33(4): 137−145.
5. Junge T, et al. Inter-tester reproducibility and inter-method agreement of two variations of the Beighton test for determining Generalised Joint Hypermobility in primary school children. *BMC Pediatr.* 2013;13:214.
6. Beighton P, et al. Ehlers-Danlos syndromes: revised nosology. *Am J Med Genet.* 1998;77(1):31−37.
7. Palmer S, et al. Physiotherapy management of joint hypermobility syndrome–a focus group study of patient and health professional perspectives. *Physiotherapy.* 2016; 102(1):93−102.
8. Sohrbeck-Nohr O, et al. Generalized joint hypermobility in childhood is a possible risk for the development of joint pain in adolescence: a cohort study. *BMC Pediatr.* 2014;14: 302.
9. Pacey V, et al. Quality of life prediction in children with joint hypermobility syndrome. *J Paediatr Child Health.* 2015;51(7):689−695.
10. Rombaut L, et al. Musculoskeletal complaints, physical activity and health-related quality of life among patients

with the Ehlers–Danlos syndrome hypermobility type. *Disabil Rehabil.* 2010;32(16):1339–1345.

11. Adib N, et al. Joint hypermobility syndrome in childhood. A not so benign multisystem disorder? *Rheumatology (Oxford).* 2005;44(6):744–750.

12. Pacey V, et al. Joint hypermobility syndrome: a review for clinicians. *J Paediatr Child Health.* 2015;51(4):373–380.

13. Scheper MC, et al. The natural history of children with joint hypermobility syndrome and Ehlers-Danlos hypermobility type: a longitudinal cohort study. *Rheumatology.* 2017;56(12):2073–2083.

14. Scheper MC, et al. Chronic pain in hypermobility syndrome and Ehlers–Danlos syndrome (hypermobility type): it is a challenge. *J Pain Res.* 2015;8:591.

15. Schubert-Hjalmarsson E, et al. Pain, balance, activity, and participation in children with hypermobility syndrome. *Pediatr Phys Ther.* 2012;24(4):339–344.

16. Kovacic K, et al. Joint hypermobility: a common association with complex functional gastrointestinal disorders. *J Pediatr.* 2014;165(5):973–978.

17. de KORT LM, et al. Lower urinary tract dysfunction in children with generalized hypermobility of joints. *J Urol.* 2003;170(5):1971–1974.

18. Cincinnati Children's Hospital Medical Center, J.M.A.C.f.H.S.E.E.B.C.G. *Evidence Based Care Guideline for Management of Pediatric Joint Hypermobility Guideline Copyright © 2014: Identification and Management of Pediatric Joint Hypermobility in Children and Adolescents Aged 4 to 21 Years Old.* 2014.

19. Sedky K, Gaisl T, Bennett DS. Prevalence of obstructive sleep apnea in joint hypermobility syndrome: a systematic review and meta-analysis. *J Clin Sleep Med.* 2019;15(2):293–299.

20. Hakim A, Grahame RJR. Non-musculoskeletal symptoms in joint hypermobility syndrome. Indirect evidence for autonomic dysfunction? *Rheumatology (Oxford).* 2004;43(9):1194–1195.

21. Scheper MC, et al. Generalized hyperalgesia in children and adults diagnosed with hypermobility syndrome and ehlers-danlos syndrome hypermobility type: a discriminative analysis. *Arthritis Care Res.* 2017;69(3):421–429.

22. Smith TO, et al. The relationship between benign joint hypermobility syndrome and psychological distress: a systematic review and meta-analysis. *Rheumatology.* 2013;53(1):114–122.

23. Celletti C, et al. Evaluation of kinesiophobia and its correlations with pain and fatigue in joint hypermobility syndrome/Ehlers-Danlos syndrome hypermobility type. *Biomed Res Int.* 2013;2013.

24. Bale P, et al. The effectiveness of a multidisciplinary intervention strategy for the treatment of symptomatic joint hypermobility in childhood: a randomised, single centre parallel group trial (The Bendy Study). *Pediatr Rheumatol Online J.* 2019;17(1):2.

25. Keer R, Grahame R. *Hypermobility Syndrome: Recognition and Management for Physiotherapists.* Elsevier Health Sciences; 2003.

26. Kemp S, et al. A randomized comparative trial of generalized vs targeted physiotherapy in the management of childhood hypermobility. *Rheumatology.* 2009;49(2):315–325.

27. Scheper M, et al. Children with generalised joint hypermobility and musculoskeletal complaints: state of the art on diagnostics, clinical characteristics, and treatment. *BioMed Res Int.* 2013;2013.

28. Little KJJTPUE. *Multi-ligament Laxity.* 2013:1–13.

29. Engelbert RH, et al. The evidence-based rationale for physical therapy treatment of children, adolescents, and adults diagnosed with joint hypermobility syndrome/hypermobile Ehlers Danlos syndrome. *Am J Med Genet C Semin Med Genet.* 2017;175(1):158–167.

30. Bathen T, et al. Multidisciplinary treatment of disability in ehlers–danlos syndrome hypermobility type/hypermobility syndrome: a pilot study using a combination of physical and cognitive – behavioral therapy on 12 women. *Am J Med Genet A.* 2013;161(12):3005–3011.

31. Murray KJ. Hypermobility disorders in children and adolescents. *Best Pract Res Clin Rheumatol.* 2006;20(2):329–351.

32. Rabin J, et al. Update in the treatment of chronic pain within pediatric patients. *Curr Probl Pediatr Adolesc Health Care.* 2017;47(7):167–172.

33. Verkerk GJ, et al. The reproducibility and validity of the Canadian occupational performance measure in parents of children with disabilities. *Clin Rehabil.* 2006;20(11):980–988.

34. Gurley-Green SJR. Living with the hypermobility syndrome. *Rheumatology (Oxford).* 2001;40(5):487–489.

35. Branson JA, et al. Managing chronic pain in a young adolescent girl with Ehlers-Danlos syndrome. *Harv Rev Psychiatry.* 2011;19(5):259–270.

36. Sahin N, et al. Evaluation of knee proprioception and effects of proprioception exercise in patients with benign joint hypermobility syndrome. *Rheumatol Int.* 2008;28(10):995–1000.

37. Brown FC, Buboltz Jr WC, Soper BJBm. Relationship of sleep hygiene awareness, sleep hygiene practices, and sleep quality in university students. *Behav Med.* 2002;28(1):33–38.

38. Rombaut L, et al. Muscle mass, muscle strength, functional performance, and physical impairment in women with the hypermobility type of Ehlers-Danlos syndrome. *Arthritis Care Res (Hoboken).* 2012;64(10):1584–1592.

39. Jensen BR, et al. Effect of generalized joint hypermobility on knee function and muscle activation in children and adults. *Muscle Nerve.* 2013;48(5):762–769.

40. Booshanam DS, et al. Evaluation of posture and pain in persons with benign joint hypermobility syndrome. *Rheumatol Int.* 2011;31(12):1561–1565.

41. Burkhead Jr W, Rockwood Jr CJJ. Treatment of instability of the shoulder with an exercise program. *J Bone Joint Surg Am.* 1992;74(6):890–896.

42. Lenters TR, et al. Arthroscopic compared with open repairs for recurrent anterior shoulder instability: a systematic review and meta-analysis of the literature. *J Bone Joint Surg Am.* 2007;89(2):244−254.

43. Neer 2nd C, Foster CRJJ. Inferior capsular shift for involuntary inferior and multidirectional instability of the shoulder. A preliminary report. *J Bone Joint Surg Am.* 1980; 62(6):897−908.

44. Marquass B, Josten CJZfOuU. Acute and chronic instability of the elbow joint. *Orthopade.* 2010;148(6):725−738. quiz 739−40.

45. Earp BE, Waters PM, Wyzykowski RJJJ. Arthroscopic treatment of partial scapholunate ligament tears in children with chronic wrist pain. *J Bone Joint Surg Am.* 2006; 88(11):2448−2455.

46. Farr S, et al. Pathomorphologic findings of wrist arthroscopy in children and adolescents with chronic wrist pain. *Arthroscopy.* 2012;28(11):1634−1643.

47. Kunt TKJWjos. Disorders of wound healing. *World J Surg.* 1980;4(3):271−277.

48. Briggs J, et al. Injury and joint hypermobility syndrome in ballet dancers—a 5-year follow-up. *Rheumatology.* 2009; 48(12):1613−1614.

49. Shultz SJ, et al. Joint laxity is related to lower extremity energetics during a drop jump landing. *Med Sci Sports Exerc.* 2010;42(4):771.

50. Simmonds JV, et al. Exercise beliefs and behaviours of individuals with Joint Hypermobility syndrome/Ehlers-Danlos syndrome − hypermobility type. *Disabil Rehabil.* 2019;41(4):445−455.

CHAPTER 17

Rheumatologic Disorders

DONALD GOLDSMITH, MD

INTRODUCTION

Juvenile idiopathic arthritis (JIA) is the most common inflammatory joint disorder in childhood and may cause substantial intraarticular damage, long-term joint sequelae, and eventual disability. Arthritis occurring with other inflammatory rheumatic disorders in childhood, such as systemic lupus erythematosus, juvenile dermatomyositis, mixed connective tissue disease, and progressive systemic sclerosis is most often milder and nonprogressive. If joint contractures and deformities develop with these latter disorders, they are most often the result of severe extraarticular, intracutaneous, or subcutaneous fibrosis rather than severe intraarticular disease.

The clinical criteria for a diagnosis of JIA include (1) arthritis for more than 6 weeks, (2) onset below the age of 16 years, and (3) exclusion of other causes for arthritis.[1] The advent of new pharmacotherapeutic agents has decreased the negative effects of persistent inflammation on the cartilage and ligamentous structures making the need for surgical evaluation and management of children with upper extremity inflammatory arthritis less common. The orthopedic or hand surgeon nonetheless will still occasionally be asked to evaluate a child with an undiagnosed inflammatory condition or to assess a patient with recalcitrant disease despite medical therapy.

This chapter will include the diagnostic approach, pharmacological management, and surgical considerations of children with pediatric elbow, hand, and wrist inflammatory arthritis.

PRESENTATION AND DIAGNOSIS

Table 17.1 lists the major categories of JIA along with a description of the likelihood of upper extremity joint involvement. Hand arthritis is uncommonly seen in oligoarticular JIA, but the elbow and wrist are the third and fourth most commonly involved joints in this subgroup. All upper extremity joints are not commonly affected in the enthesitis-related subgroup. In other

JIA subtypes, there is a high frequency of upper extremity joint involvement. In particular, dactylitis is quite pathognomonic of psoriatic arthritis (Fig. 17.1). Shoulder arthritis is uncommon in early polyarticular or systemic disease but sometimes develops in more long-standing disease.

At onset, most children present with morning stiffness and mild-to-moderate pain on motion. Shortly thereafter, the child develops recognizable joint swelling and warmth. Erythema is not usually present. Range of motion can be lost rather quickly, notably in extension about the elbow, wrist, and/or digits. Synovial cysts and small out-pouching of synovium are often seen, particularly over the proximal interphalangeal (PIP) joints and about the wrist joint. Extensor tenosynovitis on the dorsum of the hand is common. Limb or digital growth disturbances may occur, particularly when arthritis is poorly controlled. In contrast to adults with rheumatoid arthritis (RA), children with advanced hand arthritis develop ulnar deviation of the wrist with radial deviation of the fingers. Bone pain or tenderness is not common and should alert the clinician to the possibility of osteomyelitis or a malignancy. Night pain is particularly worrisome for the presence of a malignancy or a benign osteoid osteoma.

The most important responsibility of the surgical consultant is to make the correct diagnosis based upon the historical facts, physical examination, and radiographic changes (Fig. 17.2). Patients often present with a history of recent trauma. Differentiating inflammatory mediated from traumatic articular changes is critical to making the diagnosis. The young skeleton is relatively resistant to trauma with thick peripheral cartilage protecting precious ossification centers and stout ligamentous attachments that shield against ligament injuries. The most typical presentation of JIA, particularly the oligoarticular subtype, is relatively painless restricted range of motion of the affected joint(s) along with radiographic abnormalities. Characteristic radiographic findings in children with inflammatory arthropathy include regional osteoporosis, decreased joint

Pediatric Hand Therapy. https://doi.org/10.1016/B978-0-323-53091-0.00017-8

TABLE 17.1
The International League of Associations for Rheumatology (ILAR) Classification.[1]

Oligoarticular	Onset with four or fewer joints. Most often a younger female with an asymmetric pattern and the most commonly involved joints being the knee, ankle, and elbow.
Oligoarticular onset with polyarticular course	Similar to oligoarticular onset except with involvement of five or more joints 6 months after disease onset.
Polyarticular-rheumatoid factor negative	Onset with five or more joints. Most often a younger female with a symmetric pattern involving the wrists and small joints of the hands.
Polyarticular-rheumatoid factor positive	Onset with five or more joints. Most often a teenage female with a symmetric pattern involving the wrists and small joints of the hands
Psoriatic arthritis	Onset with either an oligo or polyarticular asymmetric pattern. Onset most often from 9 to 11 years old with slight female predominance, both upper and lower extremity involvement, and a propensity for the small joints of the hands (dactylitis)—particularly the DIP joints.
Enthesitis-related arthritis (formerly juvenile spondyloarthropathy)	Onset with oligoarticular arthritis in an asymmetric pattern primarily of the large joints of the lower extremities. Most often a male of age 13 years or older with accompanying lower extremity enthesitis and the possible later evolution of sacroiliitis and lumbosacral spine involvement.
Systemic	Onset with either a polyarticular or oligoarticular pattern with both upper and lower extremity involvement at any age with a slight male predominance. There are accompanying signs of systemic disease such as hectic high fevers, cutaneous eruption, lymphadenopathy, and hepatosplenomegaly.
Other or undifferentiated	A subset that does not meet the criteria for one of the designated categories or meets the criteria for two categories.

space, variation in bone outline because of erosions or bone cysts, carpal malalignment, and advanced skeletal maturity of the affected joint. Advanced skeletal maturity is the hallmark X-ray finding and secondary to the hyperemia and inflammation that results in earlier ossification compared to the unaffected side (Fig. 17.3).

In comparison to adults with rheumatoid arthritis (RA), the rheumatoid factor screening test or anticyclic citrullinated peptide antibody (anti-CCP) is negative in all children with oligoarticular JIA. Similarly, most young polyarticular children (younger than 11 or 12 years old) are also rheumatoid factor or anti-CCP negative. Therefore, the absence of these laboratory markers does not rule out the diagnosis of inflammatory arthropathy. In children with both oligoarticular and polyarticular JIA, the antinuclear antibody is often positive. In children with the enthesitis-related arthritis subtype, the HLA B27 antigen is positive in 85%—90%. Inflammatory markers such as the erythrocyte sedimentation rate and C-reactive protein are slightly elevated in oligoarticular JIA, but may also be normal in many affected children.

A history of "trauma" and negative laboratory studies may result in an unnecessary surgical procedure.

When in doubt, a team approach to diagnosis and management is helpful. Blending the knowledge and perspective of a pediatric rheumatologist, pediatric orthopedist and rehabilitation physician will facilitate appropriate diagnosis and disease specific management. For those colleagues without such resources, do not be afraid to reach out for this expertise. The internet and multiple list serve interfaces have expanded the resources for consultation services. It is imperative to remove all patient identifying information when transmitting data.

TREATMENT OF JIA

The management of JIA has changed considerably within the last 10—15 years, primarily because of the recognition that earlier treatment limits irreversible articular cartilage and promotes better outcomes. The introduction of disease-modifying drugs and biologic agents has altered the clinical and radiographic consequences of the disease. This more focused therapeutic approach requires supervision by a pediatric rheumatologist with the knowledge and experience to plan the

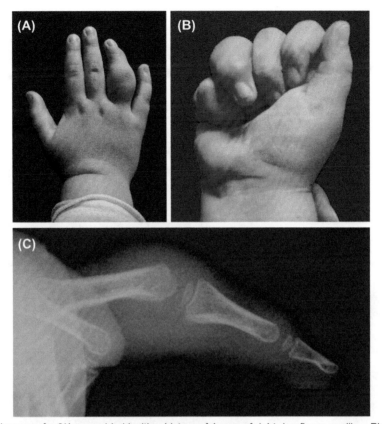

FIG. 17.1 Images of a 3½-year-old girl with a history of 1 year of right ring finger swelling. Rheumatologic work-up was negative. Repeat synovectomy was scheduled, and the patient was seen for a second opinion. The surgery was canceled, and the patient was referred to pediatric rheumatologist and ultimately diagnosed with inflammatory arthritis. Photographs show right ring finger dactylitis **(A)** and decreased flexion **(B)**. **(C)** Lateral radiograph shows fusiform soft-tissue swelling and preservation of the joint structure. (Courtesy of Shriners Hospital for Children, Philadelphia, PA.)

dosage of each medication, assess the risks and benefits of pharmacologic agents, and monitor the necessary parameters to assure safety and efficacy. In addition to the physician team, it is important to provide an occupational therapy program and provide social, psychological, and nutritional support.

The principles of surgical management remain unchanged. A team approach identifies those patients who would benefit from surgical intervention. The child is evaluated by the pediatric hand surgeon as well as the occupational therapist. Function is pivotal with the assessment of independence and ability to perform activities of daily living is pivotal in the decision-making process. Subtle difficulties can often be overcome by utilizing occupational therapy suggestions or simple adaptive equipment (e.g., buttoning and zippering devices).

Children with chronic inflammatory arthritis, systemic lupus erythematosus, and other autoimmune disorders rarely require salvage procedures to treat arthritic changes of their wrists or elbows. Early disease recalcitrant to noninvasive management, however, requires primary surgical treatment in the form of open or arthroscopic synovectomy. Once there is noteworthy loss of articular cartilage and/or the joint architecture is irreversibly altered, the goal is to preserve the unaffected painless portion of the joint for motion or to resurface or eliminate the damaged articular surfaces. Arthroplasty is suitable for the lower extremities of children with inflammatory arthropathies, although the lifelong activity restrictions are stringent and implant longevity remains uncertain. The preservation of lower extremity joint motion is more critical for ambulation and for activities of daily living. In the

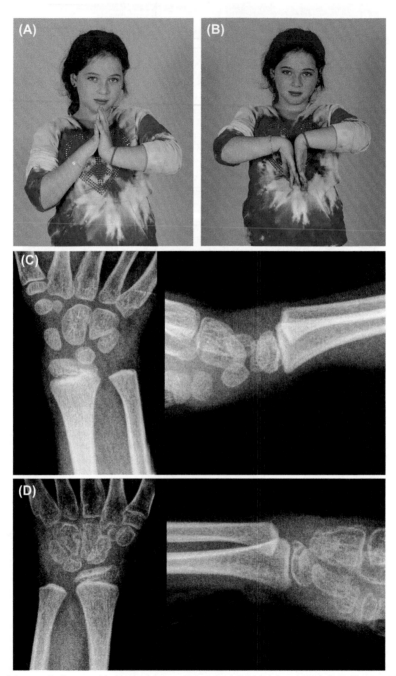

FIG. 17.2 Images of a 5-year-old girl who fell on outstretched right wrist and was placed in a cast for fracture. She presented for a second opinion with surgery scheduled for presumptive diagnosis of perilunate dislocation. Photographs show limited wrist extension **(A)** and symmetric wrist flexion **(B)**. AP and lateral radiographs of a normal left wrist **(C)**. AP and lateral radiographs of a right wrist with advanced skeletal maturity show disruption of the Gilula arcs and dorsal displacement of the capitate relative to the lunate **(D)**. (Courtesy of Shriners Hospital for Children, Philadelphia, PA.)

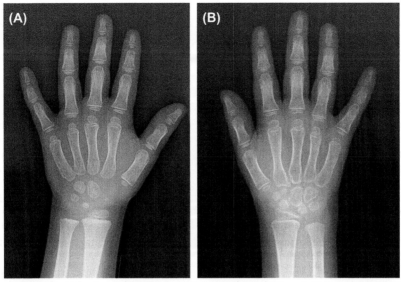

FIG. 17.3 PA radiographs of a 4-year-old girl with juvenile idiopathic arthritis and decreased right wrist motion. **(A)** View of a normal left wrist with four carpal bones ossified. **(B)** View of an affected right wrist with seven carpal bones ossified, consistent with advanced skeletal maturity. (Courtesy of Shriners Hospital for Children, Philadelphia, PA.)

upper extremity (shoulder, elbow, wrist, and hand), biological interposition arthroplasties and limited fusions are more widely accepted, as the durability of upper extremity implant arthroplasty is even more dubious.

EARLY MEDICAL THERAPEUTIC INTERVENTION

Intraarticular Corticosteroid Injections[2]

This therapy is most commonly used for larger joints in oligoarticular JIA, but may also be done for selective joints in other subtypes when these remain active despite more advanced medical intervention. Injections also may be used as bridge management for polyarticular disease as further therapeutic agents are being introduced. Triamcinolone hexacetonide rather than triamcinolone acetonide is favored in children because of its extended therapeutic benefit (at least 6 months in more than 60% of joints treated). Early joint contractures may also respond favorably to intraarticular corticosteroids, and the occurrence of limb length discrepancies is decreased. Complications are limited, most often being mild localized subcutaneous atrophy and hypopigmentation at the injection site. These side effects should be discussed with the patient and family before injection.

Nonsteroidal Antiinflammatory Drugs

Ongoing use of nonsteroidal antiinflammatory drugs (NSAIDs) remains an integral part of medical therapy. If active arthritis persists for more than 2–3 months; however, it is currently recommended that additional medications be included in the regimen. NSAIDs approved for use in juvenile idiopathic arthritis include ibuprofen, naproxen, tolmetin, and celecoxib. Others such as meloxicam, nabumetone, and indomethacin are also regularly used. Serious gastrointestinal side effects in this group of medications remain rare when appropriate dosage is administered in children. During periods of dehydration NSAID's should be stopped to avoid serious adverse renal effects.

FURTHER MEDICAL THERAPEUTIC INTERVENTION

Disease-Modifying Antirheumatic Drugs

Methotrexate was introduced for treatment of JIA approximately 20 years ago and is the foundation of treatment for many children with JIA. The recommended dose is 15 mg/m^2 given orally once weekly.[3] If there is an incomplete response, subcutaneous administration is suggested. Maximum efficacy of methotrexate is seen in patients with extended oligoarthritis, whereas there seems to be little benefit in systemic onset JIA.

Methotrexate limits the rate of progression of radiographic joint damage.[4] The total course of methotrexate is usually from 3 to 5 years depending on the capacity for initial improvement and/or the development of progressive joint disease. Side effects of methotrexate with the suggested dose are minimal, primarily being nausea. Rare hepatic abnormalities are noted with leukopenia and oral ulcerative lesions. Concomitant folic acid is administered to help reduce nausea, limit oral ulcerations, and minimize liver-related abnormalities. Very few serious infections have occurred with the use of methotrexate for JIA.

Although not approved by the food and drug administration (FDA), leflunomide and sulfasalazine are used successfully for both oligoarticular and polyarticular JIA. These agents are considered if there is intolerance to methotrexate.[5] Gold preparations, D-penicillamine, and hydroxychloroquine are no longer used to treat JIA. With the introduction of biologic disease-modifying medications, immunosuppressive drugs such as azathioprine and cyclophosphamide, previously considered for refractory JIA, are rarely needed.

Oral or Intravenous Corticosteroids

Because of their well-recognized and widespread adverse effects, all pediatric rheumatologists attempt to avoid or minimize the use of systemic corticosteroids for JIA. In certain situations, however, bridge therapy is of considerable value while other therapeutic agents (disease-modifying antirheumatic drugs [DMARDs] or biologic agents) are being introduced. Corticosteroids are often needed to control the severe systemic features of systemic onset JIA; however, the recent introduction of anti-interleukin-1 and 6 agents for systemic JIA (see later) has substantially limited the need for corticosteroids.

BIOLOGIC DISEASE-MODIFYING MEDICAL THERAPEUTIC INTERVENTION

Antitumor Necrosis Factor Agents

In children whose arthritis remains considerably active in spite of intraarticular corticosteroid therapy, NSAIDs and DMARDs, biologic drugs are introduced. Two anti-TNF agents, etanercept[6,7] and adalimumab,[8] are approved for the treatment of juvenile idiopathic arthritis. Etanercept is a genetically engineered molecule consisting of a TNF receptor fused with the Fc domain of human IgG1 that binds TNF. Adalimumab is a humanized monoclonal anti-TNF antibody with high binding activity to TNF. Etanercept is administered subcutaneously either once or twice weekly and adalimumab every other week. Etanercept was approved by

the FDA in 2001 for use in children aged 3 years or above with JIA, and adalimumab in 2008 for children age 4 years or above. Both etanercept and adalimumab are also FDA approved for use in adult psoriatic arthritis and ankylosing spondylitis. In 2018, adalimumab was approved for pediatric uveitis associated with JIA.

The safety of TNF inhibitors has been of concern, as there is a slightly increased incidence of infection in patients taking these drugs. However, the rate of serious infections is quite low. All patients must be screened for tuberculosis before starting treatment; however, mycobacterial or fungal infections have rarely been reported in children. The development of overt secondary autoimmune disorders in children with JIA treated with anti-TNF agents is rare. Postmarketing surveillance data on anti-TNF agents collected by the FDA noted 48 malignancies in pediatric patients, 20 of which occurred with treatment of JIA, with most patients taking immunosuppressive agents such as methotrexate, 6-mercaptopurine, azathioprine, and corticosteroids[9a.] Underlying rheumatoid arthritis in adults, however, is known to be associated with an inherent slightly increased risk of malignancy and Beukelman et al.[9b] concluded also that children with JIA had an increased rate of malignancy compared to children without JIA and that treatment of JIA with TNF inhibitors was not significantly associated with the development of malignancy.

Costimulation Modulators

Abatacept is a novel biologic agent that targets the interaction between T cells and antigen-presenting cells and leads to the depletion of T cells. Following a double-blind placebo-controlled trial that showed significant clinical benefit, abatacept was approved for intravenous administration in severe polyarticular JIA in children above 6 years old.[10] Children with systemic JIA were not included in this trial. A subcutaneous preparation is currently also under investigation for use in children, after recently being approved by the FDA for adult RA.

Anti-Interleukin-1 (IL-1) Agents

Systemic onset JIA is less responsive to DMARDs and anti-TNF agents compared to polyarticular and oligoarticular JIA, psoriatic arthritis, and enthesitis-related arthritis. This disease subset is considered by pediatric rheumatologist to be the most recalcitrant to treat, often requiring high doses of corticosteroids. In several recent studies, anakinra, a completely humanized IL-1 receptor antagonist has been shown to be effective for both the systemic and articular manifestations of systemic onset JIA.[11] It has become the preferred initial treatment for children with systemic JIA by many pediatric rheumatologists. Other anti-IL-1 agents such as rilonacept and canakinumab[12] have also been under investigation for systemic onset JIA and in May 2013 the FDA approved canakinumab for the management of systemic onset JIA.

Anti-Interleukin-6 (IL-6) Agents

Interleukin-6 has been considered to be an important mediator of many of the global features of systemic JIA. In a double-blind placebo-controlled study, tocilizumab, a humanized monoclonal antibody that binds to the IL-6 receptor, showed a rapid and positive response in children with systemic JIA,[13] and was subsequently approved for systemic JIA by the FDA in April 2011. In a randomized trial, De Benedetti et al. also recently reported efficacious results with tocilizumab in severe and unresponsive systemic JIA.[14] In May 2013, tocilizumab was also approved by the FDA for polyarticular JIA. The approval of both anti-IL-1 and IL-6 agents represents a recent remarkable achievement in the management of systemic onset JIA.

Other Agents on the Horizon

Janus Kinase (JAK) inhibitors are oral small molecule inhibitors of the janus kinase family of receptors that affect intracellular signaling pathways. *Tofacitinib*, a representative JAK inhibitor, is now approved for use in adult rheumatoid arthritis and psoriatic arthritis. A phase 3 trial is underway to assess its efficacy in polyarticular JIA.

Secukinumab, an anti-interleukin-17 agent, and *ustekinumab* an anti-interleukin 12 and 23 agent are both recently approved for adult psoriatic arthritis. Apremilast, an oral antiphosphodiesterase 4 inhibitor is also approved for adult psoriatic arthritis. Similar efficacy of these three agents for juvenile disease is to be expected.

Interleukin-18 is now considered to be a key mediator of systemic JIA, and several agents with anti-IL-18 properties are currently under initial development.

OCCUPATIONAL THERAPY

Therapy to maintain range of motion and promote limb mobility is likely beneficial, but has not been scientifically demonstrated. The concept of "no pain, no gain" is not applicable to children, particularly in those with underlying active inflammation. These children are not able to tolerate progressive splinting or stretching, which results in guarding and counterproductive muscle cocontraction. A more judicious

approach is necessary, with maintenance of motion followed by small gains in movement once the inflammation subsides. Athletic activities, such as cycling and swimming, are also beneficial. Studies have shown that sporting activities did not negatively influence hand or lower extremity function compared to a nonparticipating control group of patients.[15]

SURGICAL MANAGEMENT

Elbow

Synovectomy is reserved for patients with preservation of articular cartilage and joint congruity but recalcitrant synovitis despite maximal medical management (Fig. 17.4). Synovectomy may be performed via an open incision or using an arthroscopic technique.[16] The arthroscopic approach should be performed by an experienced surgeon, as joint visualization can be difficult due to exuberant synovium with loss of key anatomic landmarks. For children with limited motion, the synovectomy can be combined with capsulectomy for both control of pain and improved motion. For an

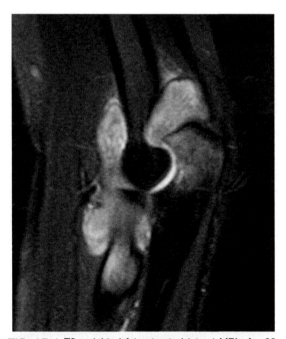

FIG. 17.4 T2-weighted fat-saturated lateral MRI of a 20-year-old woman with juvenile idiopathic arthritis treated with multiple medications including an NSAID, methotrexate, and adalimumab. The right elbow synovitis is persistent despite medical management thus necessitating synovectomy. (Courtesy of Shriners Hospital for Children, Philadelphia.)

open capsulectomy procedure, a utilitarian posterior approach to the elbow is preferred lest subsequent surgical procedures are needed[17.] If there is loss of elbow flexion, it is preferable to begin the synovectomy from the medial side with an ulnar nerve transposition. Transposition of the ulnar nerve eliminates the possibility of a traction neuropathy once elbow flexion is restored. Subsequent elevation the flexor/pronator mass from the medial epicondyle allows access to the joint capsule. The flexor carpi ulnaris and underlying medial collateral ligament are preserved. The median nerve and brachial vessels must be protected before synovectomy/capsulectomy. As the dissection proceeds from medial to lateral, the radial nerve must be protected. The lateral approach is simpler and preferred if adequate elbow flexion is present. The lateral column of the humerus is isolated. The brachioradialis and extensor carpi radialis longus muscle are elevated from the column. The capsule is identified just deep to the brachialis muscle. The anterior neurovascular structures must be protected during the dissection and capsulectomy.

Adolescents with moderate degenerative changes of the elbow can be treated with arthroscopic or open debridement or the Outerbridge—Kashiwagi ulnohumeral arthroplasty.[18] Children with severe elbow arthritis and loss of joint congruity can be managed with distraction interposition arthroplasty.[19—21] As the longevity of any implant in the pediatric elbow is limited, total elbow arthroplasty is contraindicated in the young patient.[22] Interposition arthroplasty is designed to resurface the elbow joint to eliminate pain and enhance motion. Early techniques described removal of a moderate amount of bone, which resulted in instability and interposition wear. Minimal resection of bone, careful repair of the collateral ligaments, and distraction of the articular surfaces (distraction interposition arthroplasty) improves stability, reduces shear forces, and encourages graft healing (Fig. 17.5). The external distractor/fixator device distracts the articulating surfaces that allows for immediate movement. The external fixator also protects the interposed graft material and the soft tissue repairs.[21]

Several interposition materials, including cutis, autologous fascia lata, allograft fascia lata, or allograft Achilles tendon, have been used.[19,21] Fernandez-Palazzi et al.[21] have reported the only cohort of childhood and adolescent elbow interposition arthroplasty. Of the 12 children included, 4 had inflammatory arthropathy as their underlying diagnosis. Follow-up ranged from 25 to 32 years with total range of motion varying from 35 degrees to 150 degrees. Patients were graded according to their amount of elbow flexion. Two patients had an excellent result (elbow flexion > 120 degrees), three patients had a good result (elbow flexion > 90 degrees), four patients had a fair result (elbow flexion > 60 degrees), and three patients had a poor result (elbow flexion < 60 degrees).

Elbow arthrodesis is a viable salvage alternative, but there is not an optimal position that allows performance of all activities of daily living.[22] Children with congenital or acquired fusion across the elbow, however, function at a high level. Children with untreated or unrelenting inflammatory arthritis often present with painless ankylosis of the elbow. The fused elbow is durable for daily function and manual labor. If arthrodesis of both elbows is unavoidable, one should be fused in sufficient flexion to reach the mouth and the other in sufficient extension to reach the other end of the alimentary canal.

Wrist

Radiocarpal and midcarpal synovectomy are reserved for patients with preserved articular cartilage and joint congruity that fails medical management. Synovectomy can be performed via an open incision or an arthroscopic technique. The arthroscopic technique is preferable, as visualization is superior to the open approach, with less potential scarring and less limitation of motion. Partial wrist fusion may be an option when degenerative changes are isolated to the radiocarpal or midcarpal joints (Fig. 17.6). As each joint in the wrist contributes about 50% of the total motion, fusion of a painful radiocarpal or midcarpal joint still allows functional motion. There are several techniques designed to accomplish this task; however, the basic tenets require removal of the remaining cartilage and stabilization across the denuded cartilage until fusion. In children past or near skeletal maturity, adult techniques such as plating and compression screws are viable. In patients with open growth plates, fixation is delegated to Kirschner wires and prolonged casting. X-ray confirmation of fusion is difficult if the carpal bones and distal radial epiphysis have yet to completely ossified. The time interval before wire removal is based on expected time until fusion, which usually requires 6—8 weeks' time.

Extensor tendon synovitis resistant to medical management may benefit from thorough tenosynovectomy. Relentless tenosynovitis may progress to tendon rupture via synovial encroachment and vascular compromise. At the time of surgery, opening the extensor retinaculum provides a more extensile exposure and allows a more thorough debridement compared to working

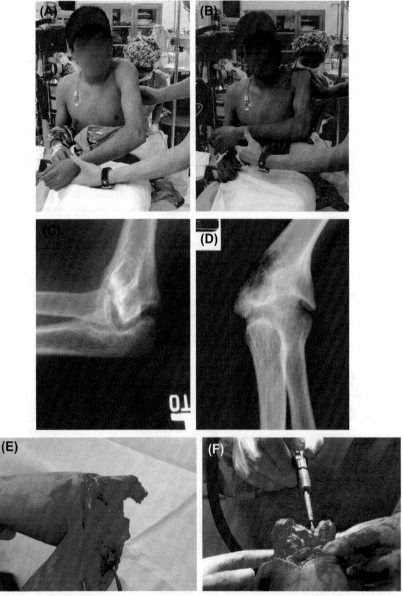

FIG. 17.5 A 16-year-old child from Columbia with painful posttraumatic left elbow arthritis following delayed open reduction of elbow dislocation. **(A)** Limited extension. **(B)** Inadequate flexion. **(C)** AP X-ray with avascular necrosis and loss of joint space. **(D)** Lateral X-ray with loss of joint space but capture of the ulna within distal humerus. **(E)** The joint is dislocated, and the anterior and posterior capsule removed (a straight posterior triceps-splitting approach was used in this case). **(F)** A burr is used to prepare the distal humerus with the goal of producing a rounded cancellous surface for the interposition material and to create an articulation between the distal humerus and ulna. **(G)** Autologous fascia lata harvested from the ipsilateral lateral thigh is used. **(H)** The two-ply fascia lata is draped over the distal humerus and secured to the distal humerus. **(I)** Correct axis wire placement is the critical step to construct the external. **(J)** Adequate elbow extension after closure and external fixator application. **(K)** Excellent elbow flexion after closure. (Courtesy of Shriners Hospital for Children, Philadelphia.)

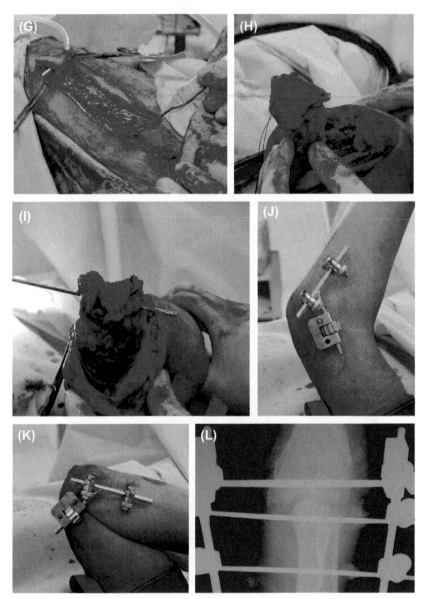

FIG. 17.5 **cont'd.**

around an intact retinaculum and flexing and extending the digits.

Hand

In children with hand involvement, finger deformities are quite variable. Flexion contractures about the involved joints often develop, especially, the PIP joints. Surgical options are limited. Tendon rebalancing procedures in those patients with supple Boutonniere and Swan-neck deformities and preserved articular cartilage may be indicated. In children with pain and loss of articular cartilage, arthrodesis is the principal procedure performed. In the small joints of the hand, there is a minimal role for soft tissue interposition arthroplasty. Implant arthroplasty is contraindicated in children. In those children that have developed

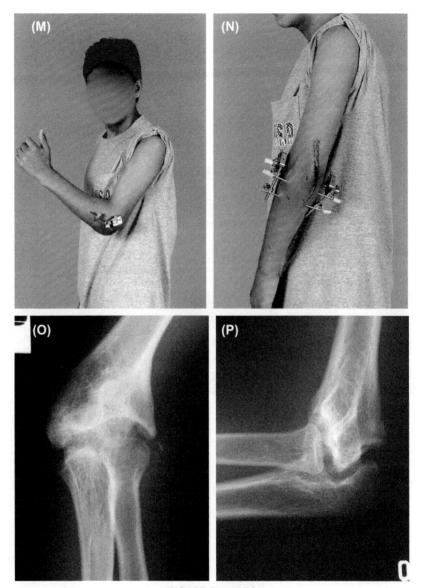

FIG. 17.5 cont'd.

CONCLUSION

JIA and other inflammatory rheumatic disorders in childhood can cause substantial articular damage, loss of joint integrity, and disability. The emergence of new pharmacotherapeutic agents has dramatically lessened the sequelae of childhood inflammatory rheumatic disorders. Hence, the surgical management

spontaneous fusion in a poor position, a repositioning osteotomy can be beneficial.

of children with pediatric hand and wrist inflammatory arthritis is less common. The most important responsibility of the surgeon is to make the correct diagnosis. Children often present with a history of recent or remote trauma that is unrelated, and unremarkable inflammatory markers or negative antibody tests do not rule out the diagnosis of inflammatory joint disease. Surgical management is reserved for recalcitrant synovitis despite optimum medical management with severe joint pain associated with anatomical destructive changes.

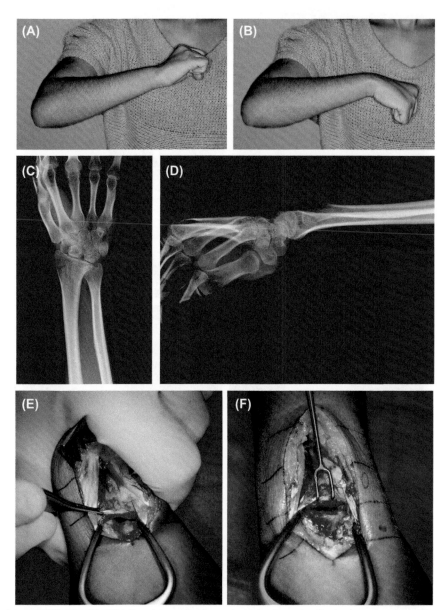

FIG. 17.6 A 20-year-old child (female) architecture student with polyarticular juvenile idiopathic arthritis treated with multiple medications including DMARDs and persistent right wrist pain. **(A)** Limited wrist extension. **(B)** Adequate wrist flexion. **(C)** AP X-ray with radiocarpal arthritis and ulnar translocation. **(D)** Lateral X-ray with loss of radiocarpal joint space. **(E)** Dorsal approach to radiocarpal joint. **(F)** Removal of remaining cartilage. **(G)** Joint reduction of ulnar radiocarpal translation and staple fixation. **(H)** AP X-ray with Kirschner wire and staples. **(I)** Lateral X-ray after fixation. (Courtesy of Shriners Hospital for Children, Philadelphia.)

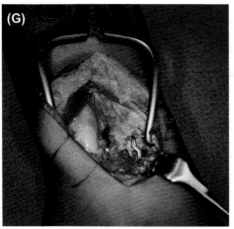

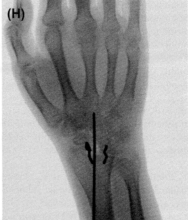

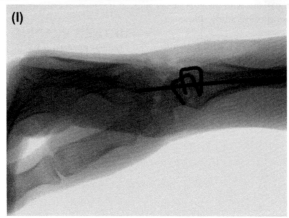

FIG. 17.6 cont'd.

REFERENCES

1. Petty RE, Southwood TR, Manners P, et al. International League of Associations for Rheumatology classification of juvenile idiopathic arthritis; second revision, Edmonton 2001. *J Rheumatol.* 2004;31:390–392.

2. Unsal E, Makay B. Intraarticular triamcinolone in juvenile idiopathic arthritis. *Indian Pediatr.* 2008;45:995–997.

3. Ruperto N, Murray KJ, Gerloni V, et al. A randomized trial of parenteral methotrexate comparing an intermediate dose with a higher dose in children with juvenile diopathic arthritis who failed to respond to standard doses of methotrexate. 2004;50:2191–2201.

4. Ravelli A, Viola S, Ramenghi B, et al. Radiologic progression in patients with juvenile chronic arthritis treated with methotrexate. *J Pediatr.* 1998;133:262–265.

5. Silverman E, Mouy R, Spiegel L, et al. Leflunomide or methotrexate for juvenile rheumatoid arthritis. *N Engl J Med.* 2005;352:1655–1666.

6. Lovell DJ, Giannini GH, Reiff AO, et al. Etanercept in children with polyarticular juvenile rheumatoid arthritis. Pediatric Rheumatology Collaborative Study Group. *N Engl J Med.* 2000;342:763–769.

7. Lovell DJ, Reiff A, Ilowite NT, et al. Safety and efficacy of up to eight years of continuous etanercept therapy in patients with juvenile rheumatoid arthritis. *Arthritis Rheum.* 2008;58:1496–1504.

8. Lovell DJ, Ruperto N, Goodman S, et al. Adalimumab with or without methotrexate in juvenile rheumatoid arthritis. *N Engl J Med.* 2008;359:810–820.

9. a Diak P, Siegel J, La Grenade L, Choi L, et al. Tumor necrosis alpha blockers and malignancy in children: forty-eight cases reported to the Food and Drug Administration. *Arthritis Rheum.* 2010;62:2517–2524.b Beukelman T, Haynes K, Curtis J, et al. Rates of malignancy associated with JIA and its treatment. *Arthritis Rheum.* 2012;64(4): 1263–1271.

10. Ruperto N, Lovell DJ, Quartier P, et al. Abatacept in children with juvenile idiopathic arthritis; a randomized, double-blind, placebo-controlled withdrawal trial. *Lancet.* 2008;372:383–391.

11. Nigrovic PA, Mannion M, Prince FH, et al. Anakinra as first-line disease-modifying therapy in systemic juvenile idiopathic arthritis; report of forty-six patients from an international multicenter series. *Arthritis Rheum.* 2011;63: 545−555.

12. Ruperto N, Brunner HI, Quartier P, et al. Two randomized trials of canakinumab in systemic juvenile idiopathic arthritis. *N Engl J Med.* 2012;367:2396−2406.

13. Yokota S, Imagawa T, Mori M, et al. Efficacy and safety of tocilizumab in patients with systemic-onset juvenile idiopathic arthritis; a randomized, double blind, placebo-controlled, withdrawal phase III trial. *Lancet.* 2008;371: 998−1006.

14. De Benedetti F, Brunner HI, Ruperto N, et al. Randomized trial of tocilizumab in systemic juvenile idiopathic arthritis. *N Engl J Med.* 2012;367:2385−2395.

15. Kirchheimer JC, Wanivenhaus A, Engel A. Does sport negatively influence joint scores in patients with juvenile rheumatoid arthritis. An 8-year prospective study. *Rheumatol Int.* 1993;12:239−242.

16. Tanaka N, Sakahashi H, Hirose K, Ishima T, Ishii S. Arthroscopic and open synovectomy of the elbow in rheumatoid arthritis. *J Bone Jt Surg.* 2006;88A:521−525.

17. Zlotolow DA, Catalano LW, Barron OA, et al. Surgical exposures of the humerus. *J Am Acad Orthop Surg.* 2006;14: 754−765.

18. Kokkalis ZT, Schmidt CC, Sotereanos DG. Elbow arthritis: current concepts. *J Hand Surg.* 2009;34:761−768.

19. Fernandez-Palazzi F, Rodriguez J, Oliver G. Elbow interposition arthroplasty in children and adolescents: long-term follow-up. *Int Orthop.* 2008;32:247−250.

20. Mader K, Koslowsky TC, Gausepohl T, Pennig D. Mechanical distraction for the treatment of post-traumatic stiffness of the elbow in children and adolescents. *J Bone Jt Surg.* 2006;88A:1011−1021.

21. Kozin SH, Zlotolow DA. Distraction interposition arthroplasty: pediatric. In: Glickel SZ, Bernstein RA, eds. *Arthritis of the Hand and Upper Extremity: A Master Skills Publication.* Rosemont, IL: American Society for Surgery of the Hand; 2011:415−428.

22. Morrey BF, Askew LJ, Chao EY. A biomechanical study of normal functional elbow motion. *J Bone Jt Surg.* 1981; 63A:872−877.

FURTHER READING

1. Morrey BF, Adams RA, Bryan RS. Total replacement for post-traumatic arthritis of the elbow. *J Bone Jt Surg.* 1991;73B: 607−612.

CHAPTER 18

Fractures: Hand and Wrist

ALEXANDRIA L. CASE, BSE • HEATHER WEESNER, OT •
DANIELLE A. HOGARTH, BS • JOSHUA M. ABZUG, MD

INTRODUCTION

Most children experience at least one fracture during their childhood and adolescence.[1,2] Pediatric and adolescent fractures are more commonly observed in males than females (65% vs. 50% of children, respectively), with the highest incidences observed at 14 years in males and 11 years in females.[2] Injuries in this population can frequently be attributed to falls and sports participation.[3] Falls between planes cause a large proportion of injuries, while traffic and downhill falls are also frequently reported injury mechanisms.[3] The developing skeleton is more susceptible to injury, particularly about the growth plates (physes), as this is biomechanically the weakest portion of a child's skeleton.[1,4,5]

FOREARM FRACTURES

Approximately 40% of all pediatric fractures are diaphyseal forearm fracture.[6] These fractures are observed primarily between the ages of 8 and 14 years, and are commonly caused from ground level falls, direct trauma, and/or sporting activities.[7,8]

Clinical and Radiographic Examination

If an injury to the forearm is suspected, the entire upper extremity should be assessed. The physical examination should begin with a visual inspection of the extremity to identify any lacerations, ecchymosis, edema, and/or obvious deformities. If possible, gentle active range of motion (AROM) testing should occur, although pain may limit this assessment. Neurovascular injury should then be assessed, considering the associated motor and sensory deficits that would be caused by an injury to the radial, ulnar, or median nerves. When assessing radiographs for a suspected both-bone forearm fracture, it is important to ensure that true orthogonal views are present, as well as radiographs of the elbow and wrist, to ensure the entire scope of the injury is noted.

Treatment

Both-bone fractures of the forearm in the pediatric population are largely treated nonoperatively with cast immobilization. Closed reductions may be required to obtain satisfactory alignment, followed by the application of a well-molded cast[8–10] (Fig. 18.1). Close follow-up with radiographs for the first 2–3 weeks following the injury is recommended to monitor for any loss of reduction. In children under 9 years old, up to 20 degrees of sagittal angulation is considered acceptable and capable of remodeling.[8,11] The allowable angulation gradually decreases for children over the age of 9, as they approach skeletal maturity and the likelihood of remodeling diminishes.[8,11]

In approximately 10% of pediatric both-bone forearm fractures, operative intervention is required.[8] Flexible nailing, with or without open reduction techniques, is performed in younger patients and those with fracture patterns amenable to this technique, such as transverse and short oblique patterns (Fig. 18.2). Open reduction with plate and screw fixation is performed in children/adolescents approaching skeletal maturity and in comminuted and long oblique fracture patterns. Postoperatively, patients are immobilized until definitive fracture healing has occurred. Flexible nails are typically scheduled for removal 3–4 months after the initial procedure, assuming complete healing has occurred, while plate and screw constructs are typically retained unless they are symptomatic.

Outcomes and Therapeutic Management

Potential complications associated with pediatric and adolescent forearm fractures include compartment

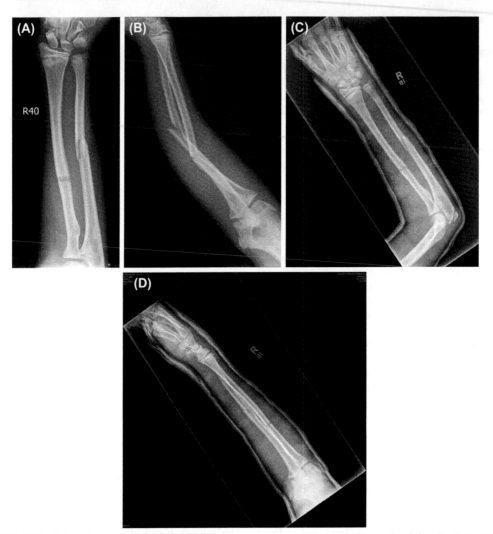

FIG.18.1 Plain radiographs of a child with both-bone forearm fracture with apex volar deformity that was managed with successful closed reduction and long arm casting. **(A)** AP view prereduction. **(B)** Lateral view prereduction. **(C)** AP view postreduction. **(D)** Lateral view postreduction. (Courtesy of Joshua M. Abzug, MD.)

syndrome, decreased range of motion (ROM), particularly forearm rotation, skin breakdown, tendon and/or nerve injury, and refractures up to 6–12 months following the initial injury.[4,7,12] The rotational deficits can lead to a functional impairment in activities of daily living (ADLs) such as self-feeding, washing, and grooming, as well as leisure activities. Although these limitations may be the result of bony malalignment, they may also occur due to soft-tissue contractures. Therefore, therapy may be prescribed to minimize any potential long-term deficits. In the pediatric population, the incorporation of play, along with functional exercises, can assist in regaining strength and mobility of the wrist and forearm and aid in building endurance. Example

exercises that are wellreceived with this population include finger painting using an easel, playing card games that require forearm rotation, sporting activities such as dribbling a basketball, and other play activities such as tossing a beanbag. Throwing a ball overhead, crab walking, and playing the Wii or other computer games are excellent activities to focus on the restoration of forearm and wrist ROM.

Hand therapists are often incorporated in the treatment of patients with both-bone forearm fractures and concomitant nerve injuries. The hand therapists' role is to assist in splinting to prevent joint contractures and to place the affected hand in the most optimal functional position, desensitization, and neuromuscular

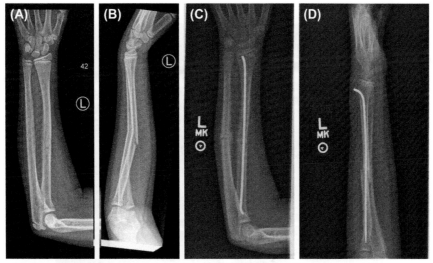

FIG.18.2 Plain radiographs of a 10-year-old female with a both-bone forearm fracture that was treated with flexible nailing. **(A)** AP view preoperatively. **(B)** Lateral view preoperatively. **(C)** Postoperative AP view. **(D)** Postoperative lateral view. (Courtesy of Joshua M. Abzug, MD.)

reeducation. Therapists also provide critical information to the patient and their caregivers about the key safety factors surrounding loss of protective sensation to the hand or affected digits.

FRACTURES OF THE DISTAL RADIUS

Fractures of the distal radius are common in children, accounting for approximately 30% of pediatric fractures.[3,12] These injuries are commonly caused by a fall onto an outstretched hand.[13] Distal radius fractures are often observed in the nondominant limb, most commonly between the ages of 4−15 years.[14] Male children are more prone to fractures of the distal radius and experience a slightly delayed peak incidence (ages 11−14 years) when compared with the peak incidence observed in female children (ages 8−11 years).[15] The overall incidence rates of pediatric distal radius fractures have a trend that is hypothesized to be associated with increased sporting activity participation.[16]

Clinical and Radiographic Examination

The entire extremity should be inspected for wounds, deformity, ecchymosis, and/or edema. Palpation throughout the extremity is necessary to assess the extent of the injury and to identify any associated injuries,[17] such as radial neck fractures, supracondylar humerus fractures, and Monteggia fracturedislocations.[18] Posteroanterior (PA) and lateral plain radiographs are typically sufficient in diagnosing the injury.

Treatment

Fractures of the distal radius can often be treated nonoperatively in the pediatric population. Those fractures that are nondisplaced or have minimal displacement are typically treated with immobilization in a short arm cast or orthosis for 3−4 weeks. Fractures that have the potential for displacement due to their fracture pattern are commonly placed in a long arm cast and radiographs are obtained weekly for at least 2−3 weeks to ensure no loss of alignment. When there is displacement at the fracture site, a closed reduction can be attempted in the emergency department, outpatient office, or operating room before immobilization in a long arm cast (Fig. 18.3). Close follow-up with weekly radiographs for at least 2−3 weeks must be performed. When casting, it is important to utilize optimal casting techniques, with an interosseous or three-point mold, to maximize the success in maintaining the reduction. Molding above the humeral condyles to prevent the cast from sliding down is also recommended when applying long arm casts.[19]

Operative intervention is indicated for irreducible fractures, fractures with intraarticular involvement, open fractures, distal radius fractures with concurrent injuries, and fractures that have lost alignment following an initial reduction[20,21] (Fig. 18.4). The vast majority of pediatric and adolescent distal radius fractures can be treated with a closed reduction with percutaneous pinning. Open reduction with internal fixation (ORIF) is reserved for open fractures, nascent malunions that do not involve the physis, and fractures in

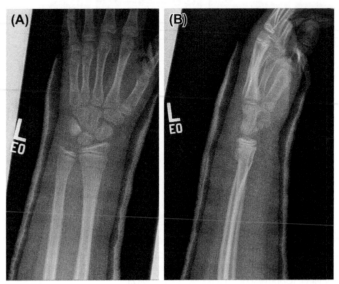

FIG.18.3 Plain radiographs of a minimally displaced distal radius fracture after closed reduction in the emergency department in an 11-year-old female. **(A)** AP view. **(B)** Lateral view. (Courtesy of Joshua M. Abzug, MD.)

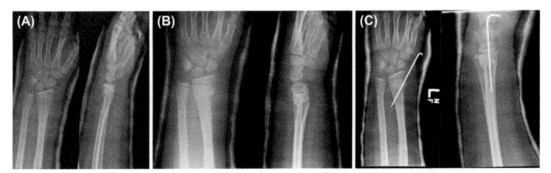

FIG.18.4 PA and lateral radiographs of the wrist demonstrating a worsening displacement of a distal radius fracture: **(A)** Initial injury. **(B)** Worsening displacement 1 week after initial immobilization. **(C)** Final treatment utilizing closed reduction and percutaneous pinning. (Courtesy of Joshua M. Abzug, MD.)

skeletally mature individuals that are amenable to ORIF followed by early ROM[20,21] (Fig. 18.5). Following operative intervention, patients are commonly immobilized for 3–4 weeks and then early AROM is initiated.

Outcomes and Therapeutic Management

Distal radius fractures heal without complications in the vast majority of pediatric patients. Complication rates increase if there are multiple attempts to reduce a physeal fracture, as this has been shown to increase the risk of physeal damage and subsequent physeal arrest. The rate of physeal arrest associated with distal radius fractures is 4%–7%, and is seen more commonly in Salter–Harris III and IV fractures as well as in children approaching skeletal maturity.[11,22] Nonunion, malunion, and radioulnarsynostosis are other potential complications following distal radius fractures in pediatric patients but are quite rare.[11] Specific complications associated with operative intervention include pin tract infections, neurovascular damage, and painful hardware.[11]

Therapy is typically not required for pediatric distal radius fractures whether they are treated with immobilization alone or with closed reduction and

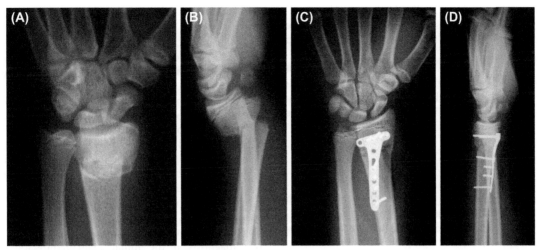

FIG. 18.5 Preoperative **(A)** AP view and **(B)** lateral view and postoperative **(C)** AP view and **(D)** lateral view radiographs of a distal radius fracture treated with open reduction and internal fixation. (Courtesy of Joshua M. Abzug, MD.)

percutaneous pinning (CRPP). Patients that underwent ORIF procedures are typically treated following the same treatment algorithms as adults. These patients are often immobilized in a short arm cast for 3—4 weeks and then transitioned to a circumferential fracture brace for continued protection for a total of 6—8 weeks postoperatively. The goals of initial hand therapy following an ORIF procedure are edema control, orthosis fabrication, ROM of the uninvolved joints, and light activities of daily living within the orthosis[23] (Fig. 18.6) (Fig. 18.7). Patients may experience extensor tendon irritation, swelling along the dorsum of the hand, and pain with composite extension during this phase, and ROM should be altered based on patient's complaints and discomfort level. Caution with early AROM should be considered, as associated extensor tendon rupture has been reported during the early postoperative phase.[23—25]

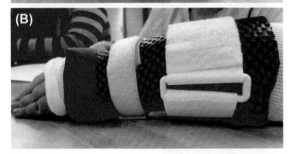

FIG. 18.6 Clinical photograph of a custom-molded removable wrist splint to allow for light, active range of motion. **(A)** Top view. **(B)** Side view. (Courtesy of Joshua M. Abzug, MD.)

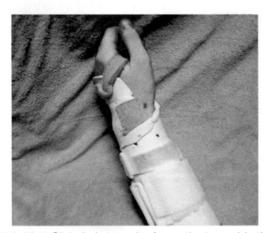

FIG. 18.7 Clinical photograph of an orthosis used in the immobilization of a pediatric distal radius fracture following removal of a pin utilized for stabilization. (Courtesy of Joshua M. Abzug, MD.)

Once adequate bony healing has occurred, the initiation of active, active-assisted, and passive ROM to the wrist may be initiated.[23] Now, the patient is allowed to increase the use of the effected extremity in daily activities and may be able to wean out of the orthosis use for functional tasks. For the athletic patient, return to full contact sports may be allowed 3–6 months postoperatively, once full ROM and strength are regained in the affected extremity.[23]

SCAPHOID FRACTURES

Scaphoid fractures account for nearly 90% of all pediatric carpal fractures[26] and are commonly associated with other injuries such as distal radius fractures, ulnar styloid fractures, or contralateral scaphoid fractures. These injuries are often caused by a ground level fall onto an outstretched hand or sports participation.[26,27]

Clinical and Radiographic Examination

When a patient presents with radial sided hand/wrist pain, the physical examination should cover the entirety of the hand and forearm to rule out any concurrent injuries. Any edema, ecchymosis, and abrasions should be noted. Patients with a scaphoid fracture often present with tenderness over the snuffbox region, or over the distal pole of the scaphoid. Studies have shown that pressure applied to the snuffbox region or scaphoid tubercle or axial pressure applied over the first metacarpal have high sensitivity but lesser specificity depending on the region where pressure is applied.[28] Four radiographic views are recommended to identify a scaphoid fracture: posteroanterior, lateral, pronated oblique, and an ulnar-deviated posteroanterior view[29] (Fig. 18.8). CT and MRI can be used to obtain a definitive diagnosis if the initial plain radiographs are negative.

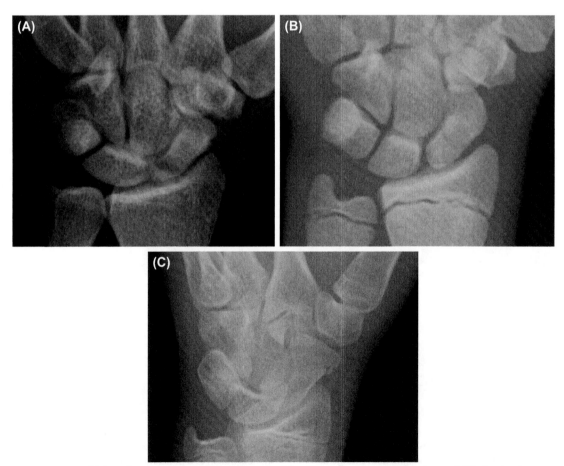

FIG. 18.8 Plain radiographs of scaphoid fractures of the **(A)** proximal pole, **(B)** waist, and **(C)** distal pole. (Courtesy of Joshua M. Abzug, MD.)

Treatment

Nondisplaced scaphoid fractures are typically treated nonoperatively, with 90% of nondisplaced pediatric scaphoid fractures healing successfully without complication.[27] Operative indications include fractures presenting more than 6 weeks postinjury, displaced fractures, and those fractures that were unsuccessfully managed nonoperatively.[27] Nondisplaced fractures are typically treated with percutaneous screw fixation; however, K-wires may be used in young children. ORIF is indicated for displaced fractures[30] (Fig. 18.9).

Outcomes and Therapeutic Management

Patients who present with an acute injury and are treated with appropriate immobilization tend to have more favorable outcomes. Toh et al. reported in a study of 63 pediatric scaphoid fractures, the rate of successful healing upon initial treatment (operative or nonoperative) was 97% ($n = 58$).[31] The cases that did not immediately heal eventually went on to successful bony union after repeated intervention.[31] Most pediatric scaphoid fractures are treated with cast immobilization, with a long arm thumb spica cast initially, transitioned to a short arm thumb spica cast at the 2-week follow-up appointment.[32] Bae et al. reported a 90% rate of healing for acute, nonoperative scaphoid fractures in children, commenting that immobilization of at least 3 months may be required.[33] However, for fractures requiring operative intervention, the same study reported a 97% rate of healing and a shorter time to union.[33]

Pediatric patients typically experience excellent functional outcomes with cast immobilization alone, and most do not require formal hand therapy outside of the fabrication of an appropriate orthosis. Athletes and performing artists are an exception to this generalization, as their performance and return-to-sport may be optimized through the prescription of formal hand therapy given the required ROM, proprioception, and dexterity associated with such activities. In treating these patients, it may be beneficial to use static,

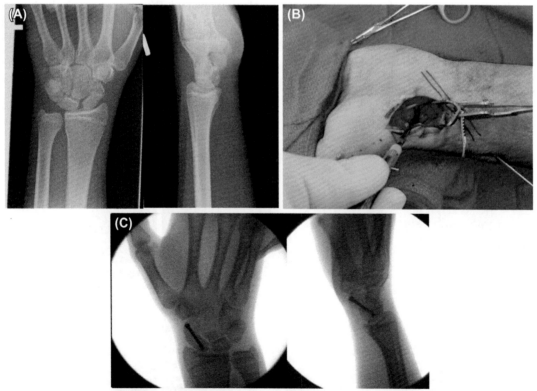

FIG. 18.9 A scaphoid waist fracture nonunion in a skeletally immature child. **(A)** Preoperative AP and lateral radiographs demonstrate a displaced waist fracture with dorsal intercalated segment instability (DISI) deformity of the wrist. **(B)** Intraoperative photograph demonstrating the volar approach for open reduction and internal fixation using iliac crest bone graft and a compression screw. **(C)** Postoperative AP and lateral fluoroscopic images at final follow-up demonstrate restoration of scaphoid alignment with complete bony union. (Courtesy of Shriner's Children Hospital, Philadelphia, PA.)

progressive orthoses to target ROM lost during cast immobilization. Furthermore, the implementation of therapy protocols including exercises that concentrate on wrist/forearm proprioception, strength and endurance, and activity-specific activities is recommended. Exercises such as dart throwers movements and wrist gyroscopes can aid in achieving optimal results for rapid and complete return to the desired activities.[34]

Bae et al. assessed 63 pediatric scaphoid fractures, treated both operatively and nonoperatively.[35] In this study, all fractures were observed to heal successfully and 95% of patients reported Disability of the Arm, Hand, and Shoulder (DASH) scores at, or above, the level of the general pediatric population.[35] Interestingly, when patients were given the sports/performing arts module of the DASH evaluation, 11% of the patients reported persistent functional limitations.[35] This may be due to the more specific nature of recognizable functional limitations in the pediatric population. As a hand therapist, this outcome measure is an important tool in your evaluation that can allow you to tease out the functional limitations for your patient that can be targeted in therapy.

FRACTURES OF THE HAND AND FINGERS

Hand and finger fractures are the most commonly observed fractures in the pediatric population, with 24 of every 100,000 children reporting a hand fracture each year.[36] An increase in incidence is observed toward adolescence, as children begin increasing sports participation, with the peak ages for pediatric hand fractures ranging from 10 to 14 years old.[37–40] Within the hand, metacarpal fractures, and phalanx fractures are the most commonly observed injuries.

Metacarpal fractures account for roughly 35% of hand fractures in the pediatric population.[3,36] The fifth metacarpal is the most commonly fractured metacarpal, with the thumb metacarpal the second most commonly injured.[16,40] Metacarpal fractures typically occur in later childhood and adolescence.[40] Fractures of the metacarpal are described by location: metacarpal base, metacarpal shaft, metacarpal neck, and metacarpal head (Fig. 18.10). Additional descriptions for metacarpal fractures of the thumb include Bennett fractures and Rolando fractures, which are intraarticular fractures of the metacarpal base, with either two or three fragments, respectively.

Phalanx fractures are the most common hand fractures observed in the pediatric population and are classified using the Salter–Harris Classification when the physis is involved. These fractures can be further categorized by location: phalangeal base fractures, phalangeal shaft fractures, phalangeal neck fractures, and phalangeal condyle fractures (Fig. 18.11). Other specific classifications for the distal phalanx include the Seymour fracture, which is an open fracture about the physis of the distal phalanx, crush injuries that have distal tuft fractures, and avulsion fractures at the attachment of the extensor tendon to the epiphysis, described as

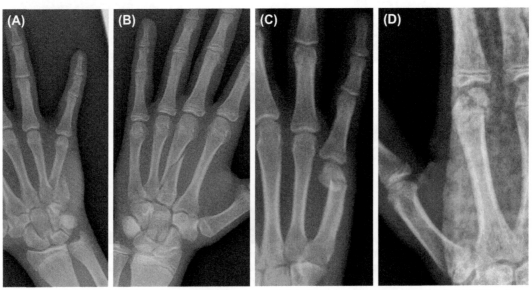

FIG. 18.10 Series of preoperative metacarpal fractures of the **(A)** base, **(B)** shaft, **(C)** neck, and **(D)** head. (Courtesy of Joshua M. Abzug, MD.)

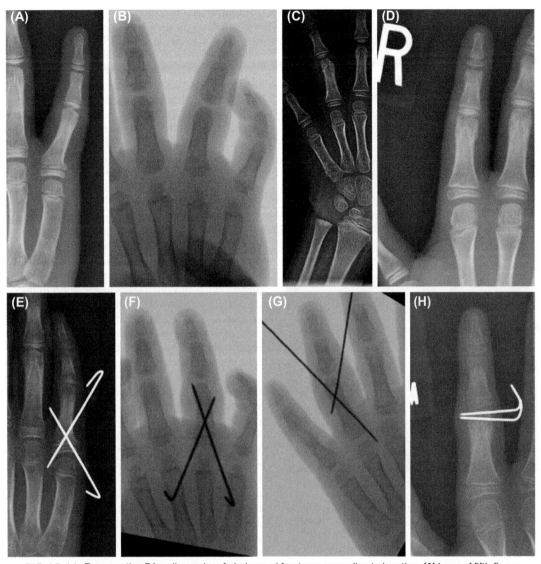

FIG.18.11 Preoperative PA radiographs of phalangeal fractures according to location: **(A)** base of fifth finger proximal phalanx (P1), **(B)** shaft of fourth finger P1, **(C)** neck of fourth finger P1, and **(D)** distal condyle of second finger P1. PA radiographs of postoperative closed reduction percutaneous pinning plain radiographs of phalangeal fractures according to location: **(E)** base of fifth finger P1, **(F)** shaft of fourth finger P1, **(G)** neck of fourth finger P1, and **(H)** distal condyle of second finger P1. (Courtesy of Joshua M. Abzug, MD.)

bony mallet injuries (Fig. 18.12). The thumb phalanges also have unique fracture patterns such as Salter–Harris III avulsion fractures of the first proximal phalanx due to the ulnar collateral ligament (UCL) attachment, which are termed gamekeeper or skier's thumb.[16,30,41–43] The most common pediatric phalanx fracture is a Salter–Harris I fracture of the proximal phalanx.[44,45]

Clinical and Radiographic Examination

When assessing an injury of the hand and/or fingers, a thorough visual inspection looking for abrasions, lacerations, ecchymosis, edema, or deformity should be performed. The entirety of the wrist, hand, and digits should be palpated to identify areas of tenderness and any possible associated injuries. For finger injuries, the nail complex should be thoroughly inspected, as

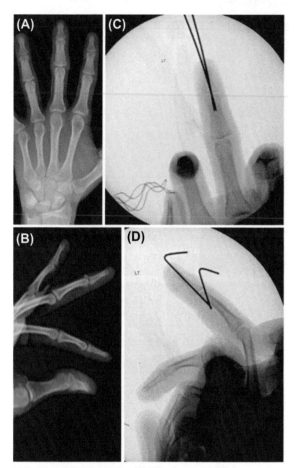

FIG. 18.12 Preoperative **(A)** PA view and **(B)** lateral view and postoperative **(C)** PA view and **(D)** lateral view radiographs of a bony mallet fracture of the distal phalanx of the long finger. (Courtesy of Joshua M. Abzug, MD.)

injuries to the nailbed are common with distal phalanx injuries and may indicate an associated fracture. Malrotation of a metacarpal or phalangeal fracture will cause a change in the digital cascade. Therefore, an assessment of the digital cascade via the tenodesis effect is recommended to identify malrotation.[46] Assessment of the contralateral side is beneficial, as some patients may normally have some overlapping or underlapping of the digits at baseline. Active and passive ROM assessments should be performed if possible to assess an associated tendon injury. An alternative technique is to squeeze the child's volar forearm musculature and observe the fingers flex to ensure tendon integrity. Neurovascular assessment should also be performed for these injuries. Capillary refill testing can assist in

identification of underlying vascular injuries while two-point discrimination is beneficial in determining any sensory impairment associated with the injury in older children and adolescents.[47] Sweat and wrinkle tests may be utilized to assess sensation in younger children (under 6 years old) who lack the ability to accurately communicate sensory responses.[47]

Radiographic imaging is the mainstay modality to evaluate the hand for a fracture. PA and lateral views of a particular finger can be obtained when the injury is isolated to one digit. If the whole hand or multiple digits are involved, then three views of the hand should be obtained, by obtaining an oblique view in addition to the PA and lateral views.[45,48,49]

Treatment

The treatment of metacarpal fractures is largely dependent on the fracture angulation and location. Coronal plane angulation is less tolerated than sagittal plane angulation as this often leads to alteration of the digital cascade. One degree of coronal angulation in the metacarpals equates to 5 degrees at the fingertips.[50] Nonoperative treatment with cast immobilization or an orthosis is performed for nondisplaced and minimally displaced fractures without deviation or malrotation.

Metacarpal base fractures with extraarticular involvement are often displaced and may require operative intervention. In the first ray, fractures with more than 30 degrees of angulation should be treated operatively.[45,51] In the second and third rays, only 5 degrees of angulation is acceptable before operative intervention is indicated.[45,51] Moreover, 15 degrees of angulation is tolerated in the fourth and fifth rays.[45,51] Bennett fractures with greater than 30 degrees of angulation should be treated operatively,[45,52] and Rolando fractures with substantial angulation and/or displacement of more than 1 mm should be treated operatively.[53] Fractures that have less than 3 mm of displacement may be successfully managed with CRPP if the fragment is large enough and an anatomic reduction can be obtained, while greater displacements and/or small fragments will likely require ORIF.[53]

The amount of acceptable angulation associated with metacarpal neck fractures is based on the digit injured. In the first and second digits, operative intervention is indicated if more than 10–20 degrees of angulation is present.[30,54] In the third and fourth digits, slightly more angulation is acceptable, with 30–40 degrees of angulation of the neck being well tolerated.[30,54] In the fifth digit, up to 70 degrees of angulation at the neck can be treated successfully without operative intervention.[17,55] Fractures of the

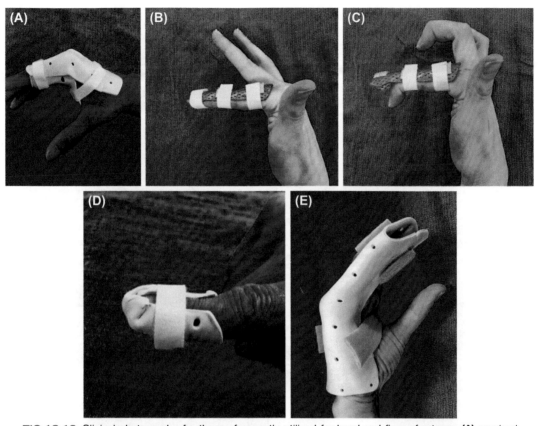

FIG.18.13 Clinical photograph of orthoses frequently utilized for hand and finger fractures: **(A)** proximal phalanx orthosis with free flexion of the distal interphalangeal joint. **(B)** A middle phalanx fracture orthosis with DIP held in extension. **(C)** Splint from B with distal strap removed to permit DIP joint active motion. **(D)** Distal phalanx fracture orthosis. **(E)** Metacarpal ulnar gutter orthosis commonly utilized for fourth and fifth metacarpal fractures. (Courtesy of Joshua M. Abzug.)

metacarpal head with more than 20% involvement of the articular surface should be treated operatively if any displacement is present.[56] Metacarpal shaft fractures that have a spiral or long oblique pattern should be treated operatively to correct the rotational deformities typically present with these fracture patterns.[30] Additional indications for operative treatment of metacarpal fractures include those with concurrent puncture wounds, such as those caused during a fight, as these will need to be irrigated and debrided to reduce the risk of infection and an assessment of tendon integrity should be performed.[48,50,51,56]

For most nondisplaced or minimally displaced phalanx fractures, nonoperative treatment in a cast or orthosis is sufficient (Fig. 18.13). When substantial displacement is present, a closed reduction with or without percutaneous pinning should be performed, paying close attention to the digital cascade. Indications

for operative intervention include incongruency at the articular surface, coronal plane angulation, malrotation, and/or substantial displacement.[46,57–61] Additional operative indications include comminuted fractures or those that have a spiral or oblique pattern.[62] Phalangeal neck fractures that have coronal angulation or malalignment, a lack of cortical contact, substantial displacement, or joint incongruency are treated operatively.[46,57–61]

Phalangeal condyle fractures are commonly treated operatively due to their articular surface involvement. Fractures that have more than 5 degrees of angulation or displacement greater than 1.5–2 mm are best treated operatively with closed reduction and percutaneous pinning or ORIF when necessary.[42] Open fractures such as Seymour fractures are often treated operatively to allow for a thorough debridement as well as fracture stabilization[16,37] (Fig. 18.14). Bony mallet injuries with greater than one third of the articular surface involved

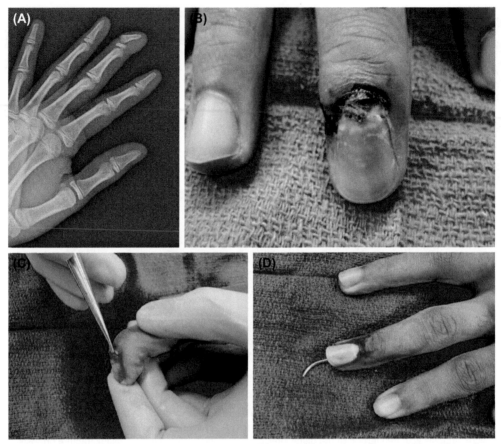

FIG.18.14 Radiograph and clinical photographs of a Seymour fracture in a 12-year-old boy whose finger was caught in the door of a vehicle. **(A)** Oblique radiograph demonstrating displacement through the physis of the long finger distal phalanx. **(B)** Clinical photograph demonstrating the nail plate is located superficial to the eponychial fold. **(C)** Intraoperative photograph demonstrating a gentle debridement of the fracture site by using hyperflexion of the DIP joint. **(D)** Intraoperative photograph after the gentle irrigation and debridement, percutaneous pinning, and replacement of the nail plate for stabilization. (Courtesy of Joshua M. Abzug, MD.)

should be treated operatively, which is commonly done using an extension block pinning technique.[63,64] Thumb phalanx fractures that are displaced and have associated ligamentous injuries, such as a UCL avulsion fracture in a gamekeeper/skier's thumb, should also be treated operatively.[42,65]

Outcomes and Therapeutic Management

Fractures of the hand in children typically heal with minimal complications. Potential complications include malunion, nonunion, stiffness, and/or persistent angulation or malrotation. Extended periods of immobilization due to poor follow-up may result in stiffness. Procedures utilized to treat phalangeal neck and bony mallet fractures may result in stiffness, which

can be addressed with a brief course of therapy focused on regaining ROM.[66]

Therapy can typically be addressed with at-home programs centered around ROM. Reengagement in ADLs is generally sufficient for regaining motion. In fact, patients with thumb injuries can be instructed to use video gaming systems and cell phones to regain ROM.[67] However, if concomitant injuries were present or there are concerns about compliance regarding engagement in home exercises, formal therapy may be pursued. The use of early ROM exercises for metacarpal fractures is controversial, as this requires the use of a removable orthosis for immobilization and the patient must be capable of complying with the immobilization between periods of therapy.

For patients that are capable of complying with orthosis wear, early AROM is beneficial, especially for those patients that have been treated with an ORIF of metacarpal neck and shaft fractures. Adhesions can occur along the extensor digitorumcommunis (EDC) tendon that can result in decreased MCP joint flexion and tightness along the joint capsule and collateral ligaments, leading to decreased functional use of the patient's hand.[68] If the therapist observes a decrease in EDC gliding, with the permission of the surgeon, the patient should be transitioned from an ulnar gutter orthosis to a circumferential hand-based orthosis that allows the patient to perform AROM of the hand.[68] Subsequently, light EDC strengthening to increase distal gliding of the EDC can be initiated.[68]

Proximal phalanx fractures in the pediatric patient treated by ORIF may require formal hand therapy. Once stable, these fractures require initiation of early AROM. The surgical scar can produce adherence of the underlying tendons, joint capsule, or ligaments, resulting in an overall decrease in extensor tendon gliding and subsequent joint stiffness.[69] Hand therapists can provide a functional position orthosis with the wrist in slight flexion to increase the tension in the extensor mechanism with the MCPs blocked to maximize PIP joint active extension, extensor, and flexor tendon gliding exercises to increase total active motion (TAM) of the affected digit and increase functional use of the affected hand.[69]

SUMMARY

Hand, wrist, and forearm fractures are common in the pediatric population. With prompt diagnosis and treatment, most are able to be treated nonoperatively due to the quality and remodeling potential of pediatric bone. Open fractures, substantial angulation, malrotation, and concomitant injuries are some of the operative indications for fractures of the upper extremity. Therapy is often beneficial in regaining ROM for such injuries and is notably most advantageous in cases that have been treated operatively. Splinting can be a helpful means to continue partial immobilization in young patients while working to slowly regain strength and ROM of the upper extremity following traumatic injuries. Therapy protocols are specific to the injury and should be decided upon by a multidisciplinary team of orthopedic physicians and therapists while involving the patient and their family in the decision-making process.

REFERENCES

1. Arora R, Fichadia U, Hartwig E, Kannikeswaran N. Pediatric upper-extremity fractures. *Pediatr Ann.* 2014;43(5):196–204.
2. Cooper C, Dennison EM, Leufkens HG, Bishop N, van Staa TP. Epidemiology of childhood fractures in Britain: a study using the general practice research database. *J Bone Miner Res.* 2004;19(12):1976–1981.
3. Hedström EM, Svensson O, Bergström U, Michno P. Epidemiology of fractures in children and adolescents. *ActaOrthop.* 2010;81(1):148–153.
4. Carson S. Pediatric upper extremity injuries. *Pediatr Clin N Am.* 2006;53(1):41–67.
5. Jacobsen FS. Periosteum: its relation to pediatric fractures. *J Pediatr Orthop B.* 1997;6(2):84–90.
6. Landin LA. Fracture patterns in children: analysis of 8,682 fractures with special reference to incidence, etiology and secular changes in a Swedish urban population, 1950-1979. *Acta Orthop Scand Suppl.* 1983;202:1–109.
7. Sinikumpu JJ, Pokka T, Serlo W. The changing pattern of pediatric both-bone forearm shaft fractures among 86,000 children from 1997 to 2009. *Eur J Pediatr Surg.* 2013;23:289–296.
8. Smith VA, Goodman HJ, Strongwater A, Smith B. Treatment of pediatric both-bone forearm fractures: a comparison of operative techniques. *J Pediatr Orthop.* 2005;25(3):309–313.
9. Reinhardt KR, Feldman DS, Green DW, Sala DA, Widmann RF, Scher DM. Comparison of intramedullary nailing to plating for both-bone forearm fractures in older children. *J Pediatr Orthop.* 2008;28(4):403–409.
10. Zionts LE, Zalavras CG, Gerhardt MB. Closed treatment of displaced diaphyseal both-bone forearm fractures in older children and adolescents. *J Pediatr Orthop.* 2005;25:507–512.
11. Chia B, Kozin SH, Herman MJ, Safier S, Abzug JM. Complications of pediatric distal radius and forearm fractures. *Instr Course Lect.* 2015;64:499–507.
12. Zlotolow DA. Pediatric both bone fractures: spotting and managing the bad actors. *J Hand Surg.* 2012;37(2):363–366.
13. Rodríguez-Merchán EC. Pediatric fractures of the forearm. *Clin Orhtop Relat Res.* 2005;432:65–72.
14. Hassan FOA. Hand dominance and gender in forearm fractures in children. *Strategies Trauma Limb Reconstr.* 2008;3(3):101–103.
15. Khosla S, Melton LJ, Dekutoski MB, Achenbach SJ, Oberg AI, Riggs BL. Incidence of childhood distal forearm fractures over 30 years: a population-based study. *J Am Med Assoc.* 2003;290:1479–1485.
16. Nellans KW, Chung KC. Pediatric hand fractures. *Hand Clin.* 2013;29:569–578.
17. Mercan S, Uzun M, Ertugrul A, Ozturk I, Demir B, Sulun T. Psychopathology and personality features in orthopedic patients with boxer's fractures. *Gen Hosp Psychiatry.* 2005;27(1):13–17.

18. Noonan KJ, Price CT. Forearm and distal radius fractures in children. *J Am Acad Orthop Surg.* 1998;6:146–156.

19. Bae DS, Waters PM. Pediatric distal radius fractures and triangular fibrocartilage complex injuries. *Hand Clin.* 2006;22:43–53.

20. Dua K, Abzug JM, Sesko Bauer A, Cornwall R, Wyrick TO. Pediatric distal radius fractures. *Instr Course Lect.* 2017;66: 447–460.

21. Lee BS, Esterhai Jr JL, Das M. Fracture of the distal radial epiphysis. characteristics and surgical treatment of premature, post-traumatic epiphyseal closure. *Clin Orthop Relat Res.* 1984;185:90–96.

22. Smith DW, Brou KE, Henry MH. Early active rehabilitation for operatively stabilized distal radius fractures. *J Hand Ther.* 2004;17(1):43–49.

23. Schnur DP, Chang B. Extensor tendon rupture after internal fixation of a distal radius fracture using a dorsally placed AO/ASIF titanium pi plate. *Ann Plast Surg.* 2000; 44(5):564–566.

24. Lowry KJ, Gainor BJ, Hoskins JS. Extensor tendon rupture secondary to the AO/ASIF titanium distal radius plate without associated plate failure: a case report. *Am J Orthop.* 2000;29(10):789–791.

25. Brudvik C, Hove LM. Childhood fractures in Bergen, Norway: identifying high-risk groups and activities. *J Pediatr Orthop.* 2003;23(5):629–634.

26. Gholson JJ, Bae DS, Zurakowski D, Waters PM. Scaphoid fractures in children and adolescents: contemporary injury patterns and factors influencing time to union. *J Bone Joint Surg Am.* 2011;93(13):1210–1219.

27. Freeland P. Scaphoid tubercle tenderness: a better indicator of scaphoid fractures? *Arch Emerg Med.* 1989;6(1): 46–50.

28. Cheung GC, Lever CJ, Morris AD. X-ray diagnosis of acute scaphoid fractures. *J Hand Surg Br.* 2006;31(1):104–109.

29. Cornwall R. Finger metacarpal fractures and dislocations in children. *Hand Clin.* 2006;22(1):1–10.

30. Toh S, Miura H, Arai K, Yasumura M, Wada M, Tsubo K. Scaphoid fractures in children: problems and treatment. *J Pediatric Orthop.* 2003;23:216–221.

31. Anz AW, Bushnell BD, Bynum DK, Chloros GD, Wiesler ER. Pediatric scaphoid fractures. *J Am Acad Orthop Surg.* 2009;17(2):77–87.

32. Bae DS, Howard AW. Distal radius fractures: what is the evidence? *J PediatrOrthop.* 2012;32(suppl 2): S128–S130.

33. Hagert E. Proprioception of the wrist joint: a review of current concepts and possible implications on the rehabilitation of the wrist. *J Hand Ther.* 2010;23(1):2–17.

34. Bae DS, Gholso JJ, Zurakowski D, Waters PM. Functional outcomes after treatment of scaphoid fractures in children and adolescents. *J Pediatr Orthop.* 2016;36(1):13–18.

35. Mahabir RC, Kzemi AR, Cannon WG, Courtemanche DJ. Pediatric hand fractures: a review. *Pedaitr Emerg Care.* 2001;17(3):153–156.

36. Young K, Greenwood A, MacQuillan A, Lee S, Wilson S. Paediatric hand fractures. *J Hand Surg Eur.* 2013;38E(8): 898–902.

37. Abzug JM, Kozin SH. Seymour fractures. *J Hand Surg Am.* 2013;38(11):2267–2270.

38. Naranje SM, Erali RA, Warner Jr WC, Sawyer JR, Kelly DM. Epidemiology of pediatric fractures presenting to emergency departments in the United States. *J Pediatr Orthop.* 2016;36(4):e45–e48.

39. Chew EM, Chong AK. Hand fractures in children: epidemiology and misdiagnosis in a tertiary referral hospital. *J Hand Surg Am.* 2012;37:1684–1688.

40. Liu EH, Alqahtani S, Alsaaran RN, Ho ES, Zuker RM, Borschel GH. A prospective study of pediatric hand fractures and review of the literature. *Pediatr Emerg Care.* 2014;30(5):299–304.

41. Abzug JM, Dua K, Bauer AS, Cornwall R, Wyrick TO. Pediatric phalanx fractures. *Instr Course Lect.* 2017;66:417–427.

42. Williams AA, Lochner HV. Pediatric hand and wrist injuries. *Curr Rev Musculoskelet Med.* 2013;6(1):18–25.

43. Al-Qattan MM, Al-Zahrani K, Al-Boukai AA. The relative incidence of fractures at the base of the proximal phalanx of the fingers in children. *J Hand Surg Eur.* 2008;33(4): 465–468.

44. Hastings 2nd H, Simmons BP. Hand fractures in children. A statistical analysis. *Clin Orthop Relat Res.* 1984:120–130.

45. Cornwall R, Waters PM. Remodeling of phalangeal neck fracture malunions in children: case report. *J Hand Surg.* 2004;29(3):485–561.

46. Dua K, Lancaster TP, Abzug JM. Age-dependent reliability of Semmes-Weinstein and 2-point discrimination tests in children. *J Pediatr Orthop.* 2016;39(2):98–103.

47. Capo JT, Hastings H. Metacarpal and phalangeal fractures in athletes. *Clin Sports Med.* 1998;17(3):491–511.

48. Chin SH, Vedder NB. MOC-PS(SM) CME article: metacarpal fractures. *Plast Reconstr Surg.* 2008;121(1 suppl):1–13.

49. Menckhoff C. *Pediatric Hand Injuries, Part I: Fractures and Dislocations.* AHC Media - Continuing Medical Education Publishing; 2009. https://www.ahcmedia.com/articles/ 114255- pediatric-hand-injuries-part-i-fractures-and-dislo cations.

50. McNemar TB, Howell JW, Chang E. Management of metacarpal fractures. *J Hand Ther.* 2003;16(2):143–151.

51. Beatty E, Light TR, Belsole RJ, Ogden JA. Wrist and hand skeletal injuries in children. *Hand Clin.* 1990;6(4): 723–738.

52. Coplin L, Kimball N, eds. *Pediatric Trauma Care II: A Clinical Reference for Physicians and Nurses Caring for the Acutely Injured Child.* Atlanta, GA: AHC Media; 2014.

53. Lindley SG, Rulewicz G. Hand fractures and dislocations in the developing skeleton. *Hand Clin.* 2006;22(1): 253–268.

54. Campbell Jr RM. Operative treatment of fractures and dislocations of the hand and wrist region in children. *Orthop Clin N Am.* 1990;21(2):217–243.

55. Statius Muller MG, Poolman RW, van Hoogstraten MJ, Steller EP. Immediate mobilization gives good results in boxer's fractures with volar angulation up to 70 degrees: a prospective randomized trial comparing immediate mobilization with cast immobilization. *Arch Orthop Trauma Surg.* 2003;123(10):534–537.

56. Yaeger SK, Bhende MS. Pediatric hand injuries. *ClinPediatrEmerg Med*. 2016;17(1):29–37.

57. Jansenn SJ, Molleman J, Guitton TG, Ring D, Science Of Variation Group. What middle phalanx base fracture characteristics are most reliable and useful for surgical decision making? *ClinOrthopRelat Res*. 2015;473(12): 3943–3950.

58. Dean BJF, Little C. Fractures of the metacarpals and phalanges. *Orthop Trauma*. 2011;25(1):43–56.

59. Kang HJ, Sung SY, Ha JW, Yoon HK, Hahn SB. Operative treatment for proximal phalangeal neck fractures of the finger in children. *Yonsei Med J*. 2005;46(4):491–495.

60. Hennrikus WL, Cohen MR. Complete remodelling of displaced fractures of the neck of the phalanx. *J Bone Joint Surg Br*. 2003;85(2):273–274.

61. Tada K, Ikeda K, Tomita K. Malunion of fractures of the proximal phalangeal neck in children. *Scand J Plast Reconstr Surg Hand Surg*. 2010;44(1):69–71.

62. Oetgen ME, Dodds SD. Non-operative treatment of common finger injuries. *Curr Rev Musculoskelt Med*. 2008; 1(2):97–102.

63. Pegoli L, Toh S, Arai K, Fukuda A, Nishikawa S, Vallejo IG. The ishiguro extension block technique for the treatment of mallet finger fracture: indications and clinical results. *J Hand Surg Br*. 2003;28(1):15–17.

64. Ishiguro T, Itoh Y, Yabe Y, Hashizume N. Extension block with Kirschner wire for fracture dislocation of the distal interphalangeal joint. *Tech Hand Up Extrem Surg*. 1997; 1(2):95–102.

65. Al-Qattan MM. Juxta-epiphyseal fractures of the base of the proximal phalanx of the fingers in children and adolescents. *J Hand Surg Br*. 2002;27B(1):24–30.

66. Boyer J, London D, Stephan J, Goldfarb C. Pediatric proximal phalanx fractures: outcomes and complications after the surgical treatment of displaced fractures. *J Pediatr Orthop*. 2015;35(3):219–223.

67. Kozin SH. Fractures and dislocations along the pediatric thumb ray. *Hand Clin*. 2006;22:19–29.

68. Chinchalkar S, Pipicelli J. Addressing extensor digitorum-communis adherence after metacarpal fracture with the use of a circumferential fracture brace. *J Hand Ther*. 2009; 22(4):377–381.

69. Freeland AE, Hardy MA. Rehabilitation for proximal phalangeal fractures. *J Hand Ther*. 2003;16(2):129–142.

FURTHER READING

1. Randsborg PH, Gulbrandsen P, SaltyteBenth J, et al. Fractures in children: epidemiology and activity-specific fracture rates. *J Bone Joint Surg Am*. 2013;95:e42.

2. Alla SR, Deal ND, Dempsey IJ. Current concepts: mallet finger. *Hand (N Y)*. 2014;9(2):138–144.

3. Lane CS. Detecting occult fractures of the metacarpal head: the Brewerton view. *J Hand Surg Am*. 1977;2(2):131–133.

CHAPTER 19

Fractures of the Pediatric Elbow and Shoulder

REETI R. DOUGLAS, OTD, OTR/L • CHRISTINE A. HO, MD

ELBOW FRACTURES

Anatomy and Classification of Elbow Fractures

Fractures about the pediatric elbow are common; they account for 5%−10% of all fractures in children.[1,2] The unique anatomy of the elbow has three articulations; the ulnohumeral joint that allows for flexion−extension, the radiohumeral joint that articulates in both flexion−extension and forearm rotation, and the proximal radioulnar joint that allows for forearm rotation. This bony relationship brings static osseous stability to the joint. Dynamic stabilizers include the medial collateral ligament, the lateral ulnar collateral ligament, and the 23 muscles that are associated with the elbow joint.

In addition, there are six secondary ossification centers in the elbow that often leads to confusion when assessing for and diagnosing pediatric elbow fractures. These centers develop in a predictable progression—capitellum, radius, medial epicondyle, trochlea, olecranon, and then the lateral epicondyle. The capitellum ossification center is first radiographically apparent at around 2 years old, and each subsequent ossification center appears sequentially about every 2 years (Fig. 19.1).

Common fractures in the pediatric elbow include supracondylar humerus fractures, transphyseal distal humerus fractures, lateral condyle humerus fractures, medial epicondyle fractures, radial head and neck fractures, and olecranon fractures. Fortunately, most of these pediatric injuries heal quickly, and patients regain 90% of elbow motion and full function without the need for therapy.[3−6] However, in certain elite-level athletes, early and full return of elbow motion is critical. Such sports include basketball, baseball pitching, gymnastics, and competitive cheerleading. In our experience, the most problematic fractures for this population include supracondylar humerus fractures, medial epicondylar fractures (both with and without a concomitant elbow dislocation), and olecranon stress fractures, although certainly any fracture around the elbow has the potential for causing stiffness.

Supracondylar humerus fractures

Supracondylar humerus fractures account for 50%−70% of pediatric elbow fractures, and most commonly occur between the ages of 3 and 6 years.[7−9] The medial and lateral columns connect the articular surfaces of the trochlea and capitellum to the humeral shaft. The unique anatomy of the distal humerus predisposes fractures to occur in the thin area of bone between the medial and lateral columns where the coronoid fossa anteriorly and the olecranon fossa posteriorly are located. The fracture may occur in hyperextension when the olecranon acts as a fulcrum in the olecranon fossa, or may occur in flexion with an anteriorly directed force. In both cases, supracondylar humerus fractures generally occur at the level of the olecranon and coronoid fossae.

Extension supracondylar humerus fractures make up 95%−98% of supracondylar fractures and are generally classified by the Wilkins' modification of the Gartland classification.[10,11] Gartland type I fractures are nondisplaced or minimally displaced. Gartland type II fractures have posterior angulation with disruption of cortical continuity anteriorly but an intact posterior bony hinge. Type III injuries are completely displaced, with both posterior and anterior cortices fractured (Fig. 19.2). A type IV has been added, which describes a multidirectionally unstable fracture with complete loss of the periosteal hinge; these are diagnosed intraoperatively.[12] Wilkins added subtypes A and B for type II fractures; type IIA fractures purely have extension deformity, while type IIB fractures have coronal and/or rotational malalignment.

Medial epicondyle fractures

Medial epicondyle fractures typically occur between ages 7 and 15 years, and are associated with concomitant elbow dislocations 60% of the time. The medial

Pediatric Hand Therapy. https://doi.org/10.1016/B978-0-323-53091-0.00019-1

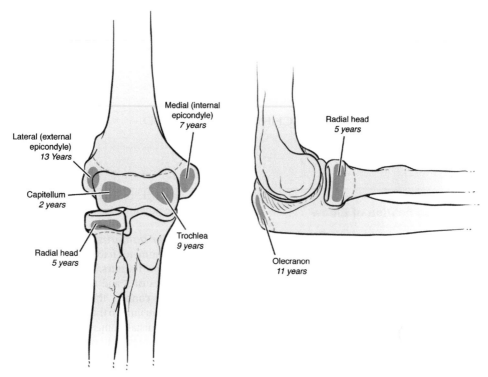

FIG. 19.1 Elbow secondary ossification centers and age of appearance. Although the ossification centers may appear at a younger age in girls and an older age in boys, the sequence remains constant.

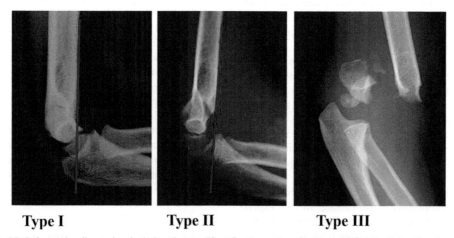

Type I   Type II   Type III

FIG. 19.2 Lateral radiographs depicting the modified Gartland classification of SCH Fx. Type I fractures are nondisplaced. The anterior humeral line (red) intersects the capitellum. Type II fractures have loss of cortical continuity anteriorly with an intact posterior cortex. The anterior humeral line (red) does not intersect the capitellum that is displaced posteriorly. Type III fractures have complete loss of anterior and posterior cortical continuity and are unstable.

epicondyle is significant for the soft tissue stabilizers of the elbow that originate on it; the flexor pronator mass and the medial collateral ligament of the elbow are strong stabilizers that resist valgus instability. In addition, the ulnar nerve runs posteriorly to the medial epicondyle, making the nerve susceptible to injury in medial epicondyle fractures. There is no widely accepted classification system for medial epicondyle fractures; there does not even exist a commonly accepted definition of minimally or maximally displaced fractures, as there is poor accuracy and reliability in measuring displacement of the fragment on plain radiographs.[13]

Olecranon stress fractures

Repeated traction forces across the olecranon physis occur in pediatric overhead throwing athletes and gymnasts. Traction apophysitis may occur, as the physis is weaker than the bone and the triceps tendon-bone insertion. With repeated force of the olecranon in the olecranon fossa during forceful elbow extension, a stress fracture may also develop in children whose olecranon physis has closed or is near closing. There is no classification system for these fractures.

Preoperative Evaluation and Treatment for Elbow Fractures

Although it is tempting to immediately examine the injured elbow, this should be delayed until the end of the examination. Evaluation of any injury in the elbow begins with palpation and inspection of the bones and joints above (humerus and shoulder) and below (forearm, wrist, and hand) the obviously injured area. The "floating elbow" variant (supracondylar humerus fracture with ipsilateral forearm fracture) occurs in approximately 5% of supracondylar humerus fractures and is associated with higher morbidity and complications, such as neuropraxia, pulselessness, and compartment syndrome.[14–17] The skin should always be carefully inspected to rule out the possibility of an open fracture. In addition, signs of severe soft tissue injury such as ecchymoses, substantial swelling, and puckering should be noted as this may aid in determining the timing and urgency of treatment. Substantial global elbow swelling in the setting of a medial epicondyle fracture should alert the clinician to the possibility of a spontaneous relocation of a pediatric elbow dislocation.

A complete and thorough neurovascular exam should be performed. Because of young age and anxiety, some children may be uncooperative with the examination after an acute elbow injury and therefore parents should be warned that there is a possibility of

discovering a neurologic injury later. Examining the contralateral uninjured extremity is helpful to establish baseline cooperation in the young, anxious child. Peripheral nerve injuries occur in 10%–15% of pediatric supracondylar fractures; the anterior interosseous and median nerve are the most commonly injured in extension-type supracondylar humerus fractures although the radial nerve can also be injured. Ulnar nerve injuries occur most commonly with flexion-type supracondylar fractures and medial epicondyle fractures. Elbow dislocations often occur in the setting of medial epicondyle fractures and have had reported iatrogenic injury of the median and ulnar nerves after reduction of the dislocation due to entrapment of the nerve in the joint.

It is always possible to establish the vascular status of an injured limb, even in an uncooperative child. In addition to noting warmth, color, and capillary refill of the ipsilateral hand, the presence of a palpable radial pulse can be ascertained on physical examination. If the presence of a palpable radial pulse is in doubt, use of a doppler ultrasound is helpful in ascertaining the presence of patent arterial flow to the hand. Nonpalpable pulses have been reported in 6% of Gartland type 3 supracondylar humerus fractures and may be due to spasm, extrinsic constriction, incarceration in the fracture site, thrombosis, or laceration. Although vascular injury is uncommon with medial epicondyle fractures and elbow dislocations, careful vascular assessment is mandatory, especially after reduction of an elbow dislocation.

The final step in evaluating the child with an elbow fracture is to carefully and gently palpate the injured elbow; performing this step first will lead to pain and the child's subsequent distrust of the examiner. Supracondylar fractures have tenderness both medially and laterally over the supracondylar ridges. Lateral condyle fractures have tenderness over the lateral ridge, and medial epicondyle fractures have tenderness medially. Careful palpation of both the olecranon and radial neck will also help to assess for a fracture in those areas. Valgus instability that can be seen in the setting of a medial epicondyle fracture is often only possible to elicit when the child is completely anesthetized. Olecranon apophyseal stress fractures have tenderness over the apophysis, but patients have intact active elbow extension; patients with displaced olecranon fractures are unable to extend their elbow.

Good quality radiographs of the injured elbow are essential to diagnosis. True anteroposterior (AP) and lateral orthogonal views must be obtained, with oblique views if a lateral condyle humerus fracture or occult fracture is suspected. Contralateral radiographs of the uninjured elbow can be helpful to differentiate incomplete ossification from a fracture in an unossified elbow. Any forearm or wrist tenderness should alert the clinician to the possibility of an ipsilateral forearm or wrist fracture, and orthogonal forearm or wrist radiographs should be obtained.

Surgical Steps, Indications for Immobilization, and Postoperative Rehabilitation for Elbow Fractures

The surgical technique for elbow fracture varies for each type of fracture.

Supracondylar humerus fractures

Surgical steps. Closed reduction and percutaneous pinning is the mainstay of treatment of displaced pediatric supracondylar humerus fractures. With the child supine under general anesthesia, longitudinal traction is first applied to obtain length. Coronal plane malalignment and displacement is then corrected, then a gentle hyperflexion movement with an anteriorly directed force over the distal fragment reduces the fracture. Two or three percutaneous laterally based entry pins are then placed retrograde, entering the capitellum and exiting the medial cortex of the distal humerus (Fig. 19.3). Occasionally, fracture pattern or fracture instability dictates the need for a medial entry pin, but this pin does endanger the ulnar nerve as it courses posterior to the medial epicondyle (Fig. 19.4). Rarely, an open reduction is performed for an irreducible fracture or for neurovascular exploration. The child is immobilized for 3—4 weeks in a long arm splint or cast, and the pins are then removed in the clinic.

Indications for immobilization. Postoperatively after a supracondylar humerus fracture, children are placed in a long arm splint or cast with their elbow flexed less than 90 degrees, especially if a medial pin was placed that may cause a traction injury to the ulnar nerve. Supracondylar humerus fractures that are treated nonoperatively are generally immobilized in a long arm cast flexed to 90 degrees. Children are immobilized in the long arm splint or cast for 3—4 weeks.

Postoperative rehabilitation. The week the splint or cast is removed, children are given a home exercise program due to frequent elbow stiffness, particularly in elbow extension. The home exercise program consists of early active assistive range of motion (ROM), early active ROM, and early gentle passive ROM focusing on elbow extension but also including elbow flexion, forearm protonation, and forearm supination. Children are to complete the home exercise program three times a day for 1 month. Most children only require a home exercise program for elbow ROM and do not require any further rehabilitation. Goals for the postoperative phase for most children are a pain-free elbow, a functional elbow, and a stable elbow, which are obtained with only a home exercise program.[18]

However, for pediatric athletes, the goals are unique. For pediatric athletes, end ROM in elbow extension is necessary. Basketball players require full elbow extension for success in free throws. Gymnasts need full

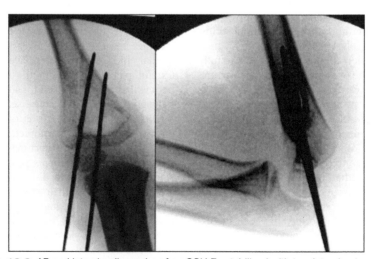

FIG. 19.3 AP and lateral radiographs of an SCH Fx stabilized with two lateral entry pins.

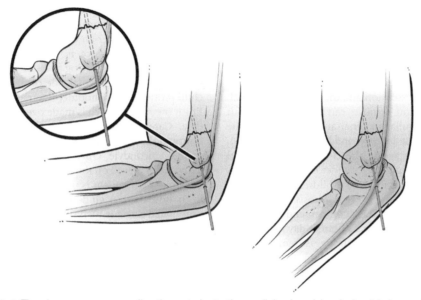

FIG. 19.4 The ulnar nerve courses directly posterior to the medial epicondyle, placing it in jeopardy during medial pin placement.

elbow extension for elbow extension symmetry on rings and symmetrical weight bearing while tumbling. Cheerleaders require full elbow extension to perform stunts where holding a formation safely needs to have full elbow extension. For these athletes, elbow symmetry is also necessary when tumbling safely. These athletes are not able to participate to their full potential in their sports if they do not achieve full extension of their elbow. With an increase in high-level pediatric athletes, the need for full elbow extension is more often seen. For pediatric athletes, their sport is often their most meaningful "occupation" in their life. In these cases, serial

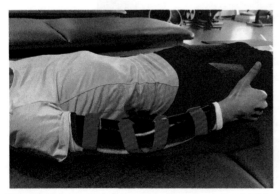

FIG. 19.5 Aquaplast elbow extension orthosis for obtaining end range of elbow extension after supracondylar humerus fracture.

TABLE 19.1 Serial Orthoses Treatment Schedule.	
First treatment session	• PROM to elbow in extension and moist heat to achieve maximum extension • Take elbow ROM measurements • Fabricate elbow extension orthosis
Weekly treatment sessions	• PROM to elbow in extension and moist heat to achieve maximum extension • Take elbow ROM measurements • Remold elbow extension orthosis • Provide new straps, Velcro, and stockinette as needed
Last treatment session	• Take elbow ROM measurements • Check fit of orthosis and transition to nighttime wear schedule • Provide new straps, Velcro, and stockinette as needed

orthoses to obtain end range of elbow extension may be necessary. Serial orthoses are beneficial for improving elbow extension, because it maintains shortened tissue at maximum tolerable length without stress, and adjustments are easily made to the orthoses.[19]

Serial elbow extension orthoses are fabricated with maximum elbow extension and the forearm in neutral. An elbow extension orthosis can be fabricated with Aquaplast or a similar material and is applied to the radial surface of the forearm and humerus (Fig. 19.5). Depending on the age of the child, thicker material such as 1/8 in. is required for older children; whereas, 1/16 in. can be used for younger children with an additional bar for reinforcement. The orthosis should allow for easy movement of the shoulder and wrist. The orthosis should be worn for 23 hours a day for ideal results. Once a week, the orthosis is remolded for increased extension. Before remolding, passive range of motion (PROM) to the elbow in extension and moist heat is recommended to achieve maximum stretch. Four to six weeks of orthosis adjustments are required depending on individual improvements and compliance. Once end ROM is achieved, extension is maintained with a nighttime orthosis for 3 months (Table 19.1).

Medial Epicondyle Fractures

Surgical steps. Medial epicondyle fractures are typically treated with open reduction and internal fixation due to the proximity of the ulnar nerve. In addition,

one common indication for operative fixation of the medial epicondyle fracture is when it is incarcerated in the elbow joint after an elbow dislocation (Fig. 19.6). The author's preference is prone positioning, which avoids the valgus displacing stress of supine positioning when exposing the medial side of the elbow. With the child prone and the shoulder internally rotated, a curvilinear medial approach is made over the medial epicondyle. Careful dissection is used to avoid iatrogenic injury to the ulnar nerve, which may often be near the medial epicondyle. Once the epicondyle is identified, a towel clip placed on the flexor pronator mass to avoid crushing the fragment is used to reduce the epicondyle in its bony bed. A guide wire for a partially threaded cannulated screw is then placed up the medial column with a second guide wire placed as a derotational guide wire. The appropriate length screw is then placed over the guidewire after a cannulated drill opens the cortex. Utilization of a washer allows for greater surface area of distribution of compressive forces over the small fragment. The derotational guidewire is then removed.

Indications for immobilization. For nonathletes, the elbow is immobilized in a long cast for 3–4 weeks postoperatively before they are allowed self-directed elbow ROM at home. In athletes, the long arm posterior splint or cast is removed at 7–10 days after their medial epicondyle fixation. At this time, children are placed in a posterior splint or a hinged elbow brace. A hinged elbow brace allows for early

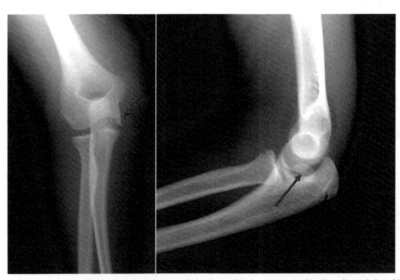

FIG. 19.6 AP and lateral radiographs depict a medial epicondyle incarcerated in the elbow joint. Although the patient did not report a history of elbow dislocation, elbow dislocation with spontaneous immediate relocation is often only diagnosed when the fractured medial epicondyle is visualized intra-articularly.

motion while still protecting the joint and allows for the therapist to control the ROM restrictions. A hinged elbow brace is preferred for pediatric athletes who need to return to their sport early. If there are concerns with healing and compliance, posterior splint is preferred (Fig. 19.7).

Postoperative rehabilitation. Once the athlete is placed in a hinged elbow brace, the child and family are instructed to perform a home exercise program to initiate early gentle passive ROM in elbow flexion and extension within the limitations of the hinged elbow brace. The child should be in the elbow brace at all times except bathing. When the child is pain-free with palpation of the medial epicondyle, a home exercise program consisting of active ROM of the elbow in flexion and extension and the forearm in supination and protonation can be initiated. The child should continue to remain in a hinged brace for 4−6 weeks. If in 6−8 weeks, the child has not regained full ROM, outpatient therapy should be initiated to assist with gaining full ROM for both athletes and nonathletes. At 3 months, the child is normally cleared for all activities and sports.[20] If the child is a baseball player, an interval throwing program is initiated for gradual return to throwing.

Returning gradually to throwing is important for skeletally immature overhead athletes due to the stress applied to the medial epicondylar physis during throwing.[21] An interval throwing program needs to be utilized in conjunction with a comprehensive program including injury-specific treatments as well as total body conditioning and training to address poor form. Soreness dictates the progression of the program that normally takes approximately 6 weeks. Interval throwing programs should be completed according to the child's age level and Little League Pitch Rules (www. littleleague.org).

The following is an example of an interval throwing program for high school level pitchers (Table 19.2).

Olecranon stress fractures

Surgical steps. Initial treatment of olecranon apophysitis and nondisplaced stress fractures consists of nonoperative management with rest, NSAIDs, ice, and physical therapy. If the child continues to be symptomatic after 3−6 months of nonoperative treatment and rest, surgical management is considered. Although many different fixation options have been described, the authors prefer a partially threaded large diameter cannulated screw, placed percutaneously from the tip of the olecranon across the olecranon physis, compressing across the stress fracture (Fig. 19.8). The need for open bone graft is not universally accepted but certainly may be considered if the initial screw fixation fails to relieve symptoms or allow closure of the olecranon physis. Need for future hardware removal is common due to prominent screw head irritation at the olecranon physis.

Indications for immobilization. Postoperatively, the elbow is immobilized in 90 degrees flexion in either a posterior long arm splint or cast.

Postoperative rehabilitation. Immediately postoperatively, ROM of the wrist, hand, and shoulder should be encouraged to decrease the chance of stiffness. It is recommended to provide a handout with exercises and review the exercises preoperatively to ensure the exercises are initiated immediately postoperatively. At 7−10 days postoperatively, unlimited passive ROM of the elbow is allowed; however, no active elbow flexion is allowed beyond 90 degrees. At this time, full active rotation of the forearm is initiated. At 6 weeks postoperatively, full active ROM of the elbow can be initiated. At 8 weeks postoperatively, light strengthening can be initiated.[20] For baseball pitchers, the beginning phase of an interval throwing program and light strengthening can be initiated at this time. At 12 weeks, full strengthening can be allowed and advancement to the final stages of a throwing program is permitted (Fig. 19.9).

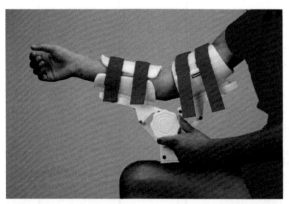
FIG. 19.7 Hinged elbow brace used for athletes after medial epicondyle fixation.

TABLE 19.2
Interval Throwing Program for High School Pitch.

WARM UP AND STRETCHING
Light jogging or arm bike for 5 minutes
Upper extremity and dynamic total body stretches for 10 minutes
SORENESS RULES
If sore during warm-ups: repeat previous workout if soreness is gone after warm-ups.
If warm-up soreness continues through first 15 throws: Stop, take 2 days off, and upon return drop down one step.
If sore only after throwing: Take one day off as you would anyway, and then stay at that same program step on the next day you resume throwing.
SORENESS RULES APPLY FOR ENTIRE PROGRAM

PHASE 1: EARLY THROWING STEPS
- Do not exceed 50% effort
- Stop if there is pain

Step	Distance	Routine
1	45 ft	Warm-up throws
		25 throws
		Rest
		Warm-up throws
		25 throws
2	45 ft	Warm-up throws
		25 throws
		Rest
		Warm-up throws
		25 throws
		Rest
		25 throws
3	60 ft	Warm-up throws
		25 throws
		Rest
		Warm-up throws
		25 throws
4	60 ft	Warm-up throws
		25 throws
		Rest
		Warm-up throws
		25 throws
		Rest
		25 throws
5	90 ft	Warm-up throws
		25 throws
		Rest
		Warm-up throws
		25 throws
6	90 ft	Warm-up throws
		25 throws
		Rest
		Warm-up throws
		25 throws
		Rest
		25 throws
7	120 ft	Warm-up throws
		25 throws
		Rest
		Warm-up throws
		25 throws
8	120 ft	Warm-up throws
		25 throws
		Rest
		Warm-up throws
		25 throws
		Rest
		25 throws

PHASE 2: FLAT-GROUND THROWING FOR PITCHERS STEPS

Step	Routine
1	Warm-up throwing
	Throw 60 ft, 10-15 throws
	Throw 90 ft, 10 throw
	Throw 120 ft, 10 throws
	Throw 60 ft flat ground using pitching mechanics, 20-30 throws
2	Warm-up throwing
	Throw 60 ft, 10-15 throws
	Throw 90 ft, 10 throw
	Throw 120 ft, 10 throws
	Throw 60 ft flat ground using pitching mechanics, 20-30 throws
3	Warm-up throwing
	Throw 60 ft, 10-15 throws
	Throw 90 ft, 10 throw
	Throw 120 ft, 10 throws
	Throw 60 ft flat ground using pitching mechanics, 20-30 throws
	Throw 60-90 ft, 10 throws
	Throw 60 ft flat ground using pitching mechanics, 20-30 throws

PHASE 4 GUIDELINES: SIMULATED GAME
10 minutes warm-up of 50–80 pitches with gradually increasing velocity
5–8 innings for starters, 3–5 innings for relievers, 2–3 innings for closers
15–20 pitches per inning, including 10–15 fastballs
9 Minutes rest between innings

PHASE 3: RETURN TO PITCHING FROM THE MOUND STEPS

Step	Routine:
1	Long toss to 90-120' x 50 throws
	15 fastballs at 50%
2	Long toss to 90-120' x 50 throws
	30 fastballs at 50%
3	Long toss to 90-120' x 25 throws
	45 fastballs at 50%
4	Long toss to 90-120' x 25 throws
	60 fastballs at 50%
5	Long toss to 120' x 25 throws
	30 fastballs at 75%
6	30 fastballs at 75%
	45 fastballs at 50%
7	45 fastballs at 75%
	15 fastballs at 50%
8	45 fastballs at 75%
	15 fastballs at Batting practice
9	45 fastballs at 75%
	30 fastballs at Batting practice
10	30 fastballs at 75%
	15 curve balls at 50%
	40-60 fastballs at BP
11	30 fastballs at 75%
	30 curve balls at 75%
	30 fastballs at BP
12	30 fastballs at 75%
	60-90 pitches at BP (25% curve)

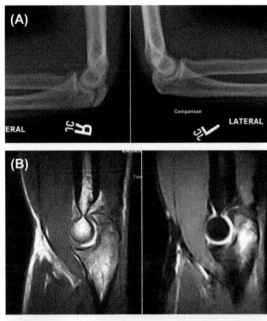

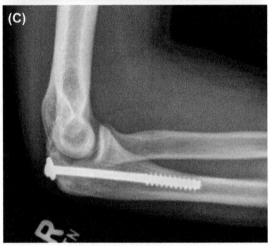

FIG. 19.8 Surgically treated olecranon stress fracture.

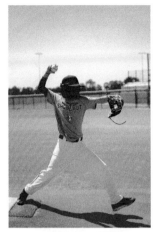

FIG. 19.9 Little League baseball pitcher utilizing interval throwing program to safely return to pitching.

Posttraumatic elbow stiffness

Pediatric elbows are at risk for stiffness after most types of fractures. With children, longer immobilization in often required to ensure proper healing and compliance, but this can lead to increased stiffness. Once elbow motion is allowed, children can be fearful of using the injured elbow and may guard the elbow, increasing the elbow stiffness. Early rehabilitation is recommended when there is a risk of elbow stiffness. Specific treatment of a stiff elbow depends on timing, severity, patient specific factors, and underlying pathology.[18] However, all treatment should include an early mobilization phase, an intermediate phase of recovery, an advance phase of strengthening, and a final phase of returning to meaningful "occupations.."[22] During the early mobilization phase, active ROM exercises should begin gravity-assisted and progress to against gravity using pain as a guide to progress. Exercises should include ROM of the shoulder, elbow, forearm, and wrist in all directions. Low-load prolonged stretching is also beneficial in this early phase for both elbow flexion and extension. In the intermediate phase of recovery, exercises can be progressively completed in traction, compression and suspension, and stretching can be more aggressive to prevent elbow stiffness. Light strengthening can begin in this phase to focus on the elbow flexors and extensors, the forearm supinators and pronators, the wrist flexors and extensors, and the entire shoulder girdle. The advance strengthening phase should begin once the child has gained full painless ROM of the elbow. Advance strengthening can include theraband exercises, exercises with weights, and body-weight exercises with the goal of the child returning to their prior level of strength. During the final phase, the focus is on functional activities that are meaningful and motivating to the child and assists them with returning back to their daily school, home, leisure, job, sport, and community activities. If a child is returning to a sport or job, it is essential that exercises specific to the individual's job or sport are completed.

Therapy treatment for stiff elbows can include static and static progressive elbow orthoses depending on the severity of the stiffness and the individual child's tolerance. Use of orthoses should be considered when exercises

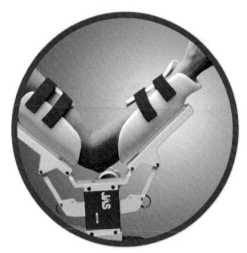

FIG. 19.10 Prefabricated static progressive elbow orthoses used for elbow stiffness with older children.

and outpatient therapy are unsuccessful in improving ROM for the elbow. In the pediatric population, the least aggressive elbow orthoses that are static elbow orthoses for extension or flexion are preferred. Due to the unique size of each child's upper extremity, these orthoses are usually custom fabricated. If the child is not making elbow ROM improvements with static elbow orthoses and is able to tolerate more aggressive orthoses, a static progressive elbow orthosis is recommended. Static progressive elbow orthoses are most successful with compliant older children that are able to tolerate the more aggressive stretch of a static progressive orthosis and are capable of being compliant with a strict orthosis wearing schedule (Fig. 19.10). Dynamic splints are generally not recommended for the pediatric population as they may lead to cocontraction, thus inhibiting any potential gains and actually leading to worsening results.

SHOULDER FRACTURES

Although most fractures in the pediatric shoulder girdle heal uneventfully, three specific fractures more commonly warrant intervention by the occupational therapist: (1) clavicle fractures for recovery of ROM and scar desensitization after open reduction and internal fixation, (2) proximal humerus fractures for recovery of ROM, and (3) humeral shaft fractures treated with a humeral cuff/fracture brace.

Clavicle Fractures
Anatomy and classification of clavicle fractures
The clavicle is the first bone to ossify, and it has the last physis in the body to close, the medial clavicular physis

during the third decade of life. The clavicle is "S-shaped" with the biomechanically weakest point at the joining of the curves of the "S" in its midportion. Inferiorly, the costoclavicular ligaments insert medially while the coracoclavicular ligaments insert laterally. The subclavius muscle and clavipectoral fascia protect the subclavian vessels and brachial plexus that travel beneath the clavicle when there is a middle third clavicle fracture. The medial and lateral physes of the clavicle make true dislocations of the sternoclavicular and acromioclavicular joints rare in children and adolescents; these are typically physeal separations with an intact inferior periosteal sleeve. In medial clavicular physeal injuries, the lateral metaphyseal fragment displaces anteriorly or posteriorly, and the periosteal sleeve with the costoclavicular ligaments, sternoclavicular ligaments, and medial epiphyseal fragment remain intact. In lateral clavicular physeal injuries, the medial clavicle typically displaces superiorly, while the coracoclavicular ligaments remain attached to the periosteal sleeve and lateral epiphyseal fragment. Posterior displacement also occurs laterally, but less frequently. Clavicle fractures are generally classified by location; middle third, medial physeal separation, and lateral physeal separation.

Preoperative evaluation and treatment of clavicle fractures
For displaced clavicle shaft fractures the integrity of the overlying skin must be evaluated; an impending open fracture is a relative indication for open reduction and internal fixation. Clavicle fractures are easily identified on routine AP radiographs. Most pediatric clavicle fractures are treated nonoperatively with symptomatic sling or figure-of-eight harness supports for 1−4 weeks. Indications for operative treatment include neurovascular injury, posterior displacement with impingement of underlying structures, open fractures, and impending open fractures with skin compromise. Open reduction and internal fixation of pediatric clavicle fractures has not demonstrated improved outcomes or return to sports when compared to nonoperative treatment of displaced pediatric clavicle fractures. In addition, complication rates following fixation of pediatric clavicle fractures have been reported to be 21%−86%, including secondary surgery for implant removal, anterior chest wall numbness, wound dehiscence, infection, skin breakdown, peri-implant fracture, refracture after plate removal, flexible nail deformity and breakage, and nonunion.[23−25]

Anteriorly displaced medial clavicular physeal separations have an often palpable medial clavicle end directly beneath the skin. As the sternocleidomastoid muscle is pulled anteriorly, the child's head may be tilted toward the affected side. Posteriorly displaced medial clavicular physeal separations may threaten the posterior visceral structures. Airway, esophageal, and neurovascular injury must be carefully evaluated in these cases. The presence or absence of dyspnea, hoarseness, decreased distal pulses, paresthesias, and motor weakness must be assessed for and documented. Medial physeal injuries are difficult to identify on routine radiographs; often a serendipity view with a 40-degree cephalic tilt to include both clavicles can demonstrate the anatomy, as can a CT scan. A CT scan can also aid in the evaluation of the trachea and other underlying structures that may be injured or compressed in a posteriorly displaced pattern. Due to the substantial remodeling of the medial clavicle physis, symptomatic nonoperative treatment with a sling or figure-of-eight harness is the mainstay for anteriorly displaced injuries. Operative treatment is reserved for the posteriorly displaced fracture with airway, esophageal, or neurovascular impingement.

Lateral clavicle physeal injuries are often mistaken for acromioclavicular separations. On examination, the clavicle may be palpable or even tenting the skin if it is markedly displaced superiorly. The examiner should also view the clavicle from above to look for possible posterior displacement. Lateral physeal injuries often require a radiograph centered on the acromioclavicular joint using a soft tissue technique. An AP radiograph taken with a 20-degree cephalic tilt can also demonstrate the displacement, as can an axillary lateral view for a posteriorly displaced injury. The amount of superior displacement dictates the need for symptomatic treatment with a sling versus operative treatment. Injuries with complete disruption of the lateral physis, whether superiorly or posteriorly displaced, are treated with open reduction and internal fixation.

Surgical Steps, Indications for Immobilization, and Postoperative Rehabilitation for Clavicle Fractures
Clavicle fractures
Surgical steps. Operative midshaft clavicle fractures are typically treated with plate fixation. The approach mirrors that for an adult clavicle shaft fracture, with incision of the platysma and clavipectoral fascia. The cutaneous sensory branches of the supraclavicular nerve are identified and protected if possible to prevent a painful neuroma or postoperative permanent chest wall numbness. After the periosteum is incised, the clavicle can be stabilized with a plate placed either anteriorly or superiorly on the clavicle. Commercially available anatomic clavicle plates rarely fit, even in larger adolescent patients. Fixation options include a straight or recon 3.5 mm or 2.7 mm plate; precontouring of the plate with both a bend and a twist by the surgeon is required to fit the "S" shape of the clavicle. Typically, three screws on either side of the fracture are sufficient for stable fixation. The periosteum is then reapproximated over the clavicle if possible, and the fascia and subcutaneous tissue closed in layers.

For posteriorly displaced medial clavicular physeal fractures with visceral or neurovascular impingement, an attempt at closed reduction under general anesthesia, with thoracic surgery back-up available, is warranted. A bolster is placed between the shoulder blades of the supine patient, and longitudinal traction is applied to the adducted ipsilateral arm. A posteriorly directed force is applied to the shoulder, while a carefully placed towel clip is applied to the medial clavicle to reduce the fragment anteriorly. If closed reduction is successful and stable, Velpeau immobilization is applied for 6 weeks. Open reduction is reserved for failed closed reduction. Suture fixation from the medial clavicle to the sternum and medial epiphysis with periosteal sleeve repair is usually sufficient for fixation. Similarly, lateral clavicular physeal fractures can also often be fixed by simply repairing the ruptured periosteal sleeve.

Indications for immobilization/mobilization. Postoperatively, the child is immobilized in a Velpeau shoulder immobilizer for 4–6 weeks. Nonoperatively treated clavicle fractures are treated symptomatically with a sling and allowed to be out of the sling and start shoulder ROM when their pain has subsided.

Postoperative rehabilitation. Typically children do not require postoperative rehabilitation for clavicle fractures. Pendulum exercises can be initiated immediately after surgery. Before bony union, shoulder movement should be limited to below 90 degrees in all planes. Once bony union is noted, full shoulder ROM is permitted and should be checked to ensure that no stiffness has occurred. If shoulder stiffness occurs, a home exercise program is provided for shoulder ROM. Scar pliability and height should also be assessed. If the child's scar is raised or firm, a scar management home program should be initiated including scar massage and a scar pad.

Proximal Humerus and Humeral Shaft Fractures
Anatomy and classification of humerus fractures
Most proximal humerus fractures in children are physeal injuries. As 80% of the longitudinal growth in the

humerus occurs from the proximal humeral physis and there is universal motion of the glenohumeral joint, there is a tremendous remodeling potential, and nonoperative treatment is the mainstay for proximal humerus fractures in children. The supraspinatus, infraspinatus, and teres minor muscles insert onto the greater tuberosity, and the subscapularis inserts onto the lesser tuberosity. The pectoralis major inserts onto the inferior crest of the greater tuberosity and the teres major inserts onto the inferior crest at the lesser tuberosity, both at the metadiaphysis of the proximal humerus. Proximal humerus fractures are usually classified utilizing the Salter–Harris classification for physeal injuries and the Neer–Horowitz classification to describe the amount of displacement (Table 19.3).

The humeral shaft is cylindrical; the anterior compartment consists of the deltoid, biceps brachii, and brachialis muscles. The posterior surface is covered by the triceps and deltoid. The neurovascular bundle (brachial artery, median nerve, musculocutaneous nerve, ulnar nerve) courses along the anterior compartment along the medial aspect of the humerus, and the radial nerve runs in a shallow spiral groove between the medial and lateral heads of the triceps in the posterior compartment.

Preoperative Evaluation of Humerus Fractures

Pediatric proximal humerus fractures can have minimal clinical findings if minimally displaced or a dramatic clinical presentation when the fracture is displaced. In displaced fractures, the child's arm may be shorted with a puckering in the anterior axillary fold from the distal fragment that is displaced anteriorly and medially. Radiographic views include orthogonal views of the glenohumeral joint to include a true AP of the glenohumeral joint and an axillary lateral as well as a Y-scapular view.

Pediatric humeral shaft fractures are easily diagnosed due to pain, swelling, and deformity. Because of the potential of an associated neurovascular injury, a thorough and complete neurovascular evaluation must be performed and documented. The radial nerve is especially at risk as it runs along the spiral groove about the posterior humerus. The radial nerve can be tested by assessing active wrist extension, thumb interphalangeal joint extension, and finger metacarpophalangeal joint extension as well as sensation in the first dorsal webspace of the hand. AP and lateral orthogonal radiographs are usually sufficient to make the diagnosis of a humeral shaft fracture.

Surgical Steps, Indications for Immobilization, and Postoperative Rehabilitation for Humerus Fractures
Surgical steps

Surgical treatment for pediatric proximal humerus fractures is rare and reserved for patients nearing skeletal maturity with Neer–Horowitz Grades III and IV injuries, polytrauma, open fractures, neurovascular injury, and/or intraarticular fractures. Closed reduction under anesthesia or sedation is first attempted; the reduction maneuver consists of traction, abduction, forward flexion, and external rotation. After reduction, sling and swathe immobilization or a hanging arm cast is applied for 2–3 weeks for those that are stable after reduction. If the reduction is unstable, the fracture can be stabilized with smooth percutaneously placed pins for 3–4 weeks. On occasion, open reduction is required to extricate interposed periosteum, the biceps tendon, deltoid muscle, and/or bony fragments that are preventing an adequate reduction.

Pediatric humeral shaft fractures are generally treated with closed techniques. At initial presentation, a coaptation splint is placed. When the swelling subsides, typically in 2 weeks, the child is transitioned to a sling, hanging arm cast, or a humeral fracture brace for an additional 4–8 weeks, depending on their pain and the radiographic fracture union (Fig. 19.11).

Indications for immobilization

In pediatrics, a custom molded humeral cuff/fracture brace is often recommended for accurate sizing. Humeral cuffs/fracture braces are fabricated circumferentially around the humerus while allowing for both shoulder and elbow ROM.

Postoperative rehabilitation

When beginning early motion of the shoulder, early controlled motion needs to be carefully monitored to adapt for stability of the fracture. Early motion can be initiated at 7–10 days postoperatively depending on

TABLE 19.3	
Neer–Horowitz Classification.	
Grade I	**<5 mm Displacement**
Grade II	Displacement between 5 mm and 1/3 shaft diameter
Grade III	Displacement between 1/3 and 2/3 shaft diameter
Grade IV	Displacement >2/3 shaft diameter

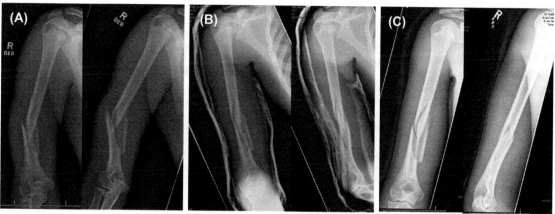

FIG. 19.11 A 14-year-old male with displaced right comminuted humeral shaft fracture after a motor vehicle accident. **(A)** AP and lateral radiographs of the humeral shaft fracture demonstrate shortening and angulation. **(B)** AP and lateral radiographs showing improved alignment in a coaptation splint after sedated closed reduction. **(C)** AP and lateral radiographs after a custom humeral cuff placed by the occupational therapist 10 days after injury; fracture alignment has been maintained.

the child and surgery. Early motion includes pendulum exercises and passive shoulder forward flexion and passive shoulder external rotation. Active assisted motion of the shoulder in forward elevation and external rotation to 40 degrees can be initiated once the child is pain-free for 1 week with passive motion. At 4 weeks postoperatively, isometric exercises can be started with full active motion of shoulder. At 8 weeks postoperatively, light resistive exercises can be initiated. Functional strength for the child related to their recreational activities is the goal during rehabilitation of a humerus fracture. Exercises for children should be tailored to the individual child's interests and "occupations" in their daily life including school and sports activities.[26]

REFERENCES

1. Landin LA, Danielsson LG. Elbow fractures in children. An epidemiological analysis of 589 cases. *Acta Orthop Scand.* 1986;57(4):309–312.
2. Worlock P. Supracondylar fractures of the humerus. Assessment of cubitus varus by the Baumann angle. *J Bone Joint Surg Br.* 1986;68(5):755–757.
3. Zionts LE, et al. Time of return of elbow motion after percutaneous pinning of pediatric supracondylar humerus fractures. *Clin Orthop Relat Res.* 2009;467(8):2007–2010.
4. Wang YL, et al. The recovery of elbow range of motion after treatment of supracondylar and lateral condylar fractures of the distal humerus in children. *J Orthop Trauma.* 2009; 23(2):120–125.
5. Spencer HT, et al. Prospective longitudinal evaluation of elbow motion following pediatric supracondylar humeral fractures. *J Bone Joint Surg Am.* 2010;92(4):904–910.
6. Bernthal NM, et al. Recovery of elbow motion following pediatric lateral condylar fractures of the humerus. *J Bone Joint Surg Am.* 2011;93(9):871–877.
7. Hanlon CR, Estes Jr WL. Fractures in childhood, a statistical analysis. *Am J Surg.* 1954;87(3):312–323.
8. Farnsworth CL, Silva PD, Mubarak SJ. Etiology of supracondylar humerus fractures. *J Pediatr Orthop.* 1998;18(1):38–42.
9. Holt JB, Glass NA, Shah AS. Understanding the epidemiology of pediatric supracondylar humeral fractures in the United States: identifying opportunities for intervention. *J Pediatr Orthop.* 2018;38(5):e245–e251.
10. Gartland JJ. Management of supracondylar fractures of the humerus in children. *Surg Gynecol Obstet.* 1959;109(2): 145–154.
11. Wilkins KE. Fractures and dislocations of the elbow in children. In: *Rockwood and Wilkins' Fractures in Children.* Philadelphia, PA: Lippincott Williams & Wilkins; 1996.
12. Leitch KK, et al. Treatment of multidirectionally unstable supracondylar humeral fractures in children. A modified Gartland type-IV fracture. *J Bone Joint Surg Am.* 2006; 88(5):980–985.
13. Edmonds EW. How displaced are "nondisplaced" fractures of the medial humeral epicondyle in children? Results of a three-dimensional computed tomography analysis. *J Bone Joint Surg Am.* 2010;92(17):2785–2791.
14. Muchow RD, et al. Neurological and vascular injury associated with supracondylar humerus fractures and ipsilateral forearm fractures in children. *J Pediatr Orthop.* 2015; 35(2):121–125.
15. Roposch A, et al. Supracondylar fractures of the humerus associated with ipsilateral forearm fractures in children: a report of forty-seven cases. *J Pediatr Orthop.* 2001;21(3): 307–312.
16. Blakemore LC, et al. Compartment syndrome in ipsilateral humerus and forearm fractures in children. *Clin Orthop Relat Res.* 2000;(376):32–38.

17. Tabak AY, et al. Closed reduction and percutaneous fixation of supracondylar fracture of the humerus and ipsilateral fracture of the forearm in children. *J Bone Joint Surg Br.* 2003;85(8):1169–1172.

18. Nandi S, et al. The stiff elbow. *Hand (N Y).* 2009;4(4): 368–379.

19. Schwartz DA. Static progressive orthoses for the upper extremity: a comprehensive literature review. *Hand (N Y).* 2012;7(1):10–17.

20. Redler LH, Dines JS. Elbow trauma in the athlete. *Hand Clin.* 2015;31(4):663–681.

21. Lawrence JT, et al. Return to competitive sports after medial epicondyle fractures in adolescent athletes: results of operative and nonoperative treatment. *Am J Sports Med.* 2013;41(5):1152–1157.

22. Fusaro I, et al. Elbow rehabilitation in traumatic pathology. *Musculoskelet Surg.* 2014;98(Suppl 1):95–102.

23. Li Y, et al. Complications after plate fixation of displaced pediatric midshaft clavicle fractures. *J Pediatr Orthop.* 2016.

24. Luo TD, et al. Complications in the treatment of adolescent clavicle fractures. *Orthopedics.* 2015;38(4): e287–e291.

25. Rapp M, Prinz K, Kaiser MM. Elastic stable intramedullary nailing for displaced pediatric clavicle midshaft fractures: a prospective study of the results and patient satisfaction in 24 children and adolescents aged 10 to 15 years. *J Pediatr Orthop.* 2013;33(6):608–613.

26. Basti JJ, et al. Management of proximal humeral fractures. *J Hand Ther.* 1994;7(2):111–121.

CHAPTER 20

Tendon Injuries and Trigger Digits

REBECCA NEIDUSKI, PHD, OTR/L, CHT

INTRODUCTION

Flexor tendon injuries in children are less prevalent and have less evidentiary support as compared to the adult population. Most authors agree that immobilization protocols comprise a safe and efficacious choice. This chapter will review rehabilitative regimens and correlated literature regarding the outcomes of immobilization, *early passive flexion*, and *true active flexion* in the pediatric population. Contextual factors influencing adherence and outcomes will also be discussed. Finally, the conservative and surgical management of trigger digits and trigger thumb in children will be summarized.

SECTION I: FLEXOR TENDON INJURY

Background

The literature regarding rehabilitation following flexor tendon injury includes several fundamental concepts that facilitate clinical reasoning and direct efforts in evaluation and intervention. These concepts, studied primarily in the adult population, include both necessary information regarding injury and surgery as well as therapeutic parameters that can be modulated by the treating therapist.

Elapsed time is of particular interest in time between injury and surgery, time between surgery and initiation of therapy, and total time elapsed between injury and initiation of therapy. It is suggested that an increase in any of these timeframes will have a negative impact on outcomes, as a delay in gliding of the healing tendon across adjacent structures allows adhesions to form, limiting both proximal and distal excursion for the production of motion.[1-7] Multiple studies support the concept that early controlled motion is beneficial to both tendon healing and strength, while also decreasing work of flexion and subsequent adhesion formation.[2-9]

Specific information related to surgical procedure, including the number of strands of suture crossing the repair site and any concomitant injuries and/or repairs help guide rehabilitative choices to facilitate gliding of the repaired tendon within and across adjacent structures. Decisions for postoperative rehabilitation are made in conjunction with the surgeon and include type of orthosis, initiation of controlled motion, and progression of exercise. Clear and consistent language has recently been suggested to describe exercise strategies.[10] The term *true active flexion* should be used to describe an arc of volitional motion toward flexion. *Early passive flexion* is recommended for regimens incorporating passive flexion of the digit regardless of extension, and *place and hold* should be for those regimens that incorporate passive digital flexion with an isometric hold at end range. In addition to and as important as any surgical or therapeutic specifics, the ability of the patient to adhere to the suggested regimen and participate in the rehabilitative process is crucial to outcomes.

The first section of this chapter will examine how these fundamental concepts apply to the rehabilitation of children following flexor tendon injury. Previous studies have suggested that recovery is observed more quickly following pediatric flexor tendon repair and with fewer adhesions due to favorable blood supply and remodeling capabilities.[11,12] The flexor tendons of children have been described as smaller and more delicate, requiring a meticulous surgical technique.[13] Age categories of children, including those younger than 5, between 5 and 10, and those 11 or older have been suggested to influence suture technique, size of suture, and rehabilitative approach.[14] These concepts have informed surgical and postoperative decision-making and, in concert with the adult literature, have afforded multiple approaches to rehabilitation that will be reviewed herein.

Rehabilitative Options

The primary controversy with regard to pediatric flexor tendon outcomes is centered on postoperative immobilization. Converse to the adult population, immobilization following pediatric flexor tendon repair continues to be suggested as producing comparable outcomes

Pediatric Hand Therapy. https://doi.org/10.1016/B978-0-323-53091-0.00020-8

with a lessened chance for rupture during the rehabilitative phase.[15-21] Four weeks has been established as the common, agreed upon maximal timeframe for immobilization.[15,16,21] A collection of studies published between 1994 and 2006 compared immobilization protocols with early motion in children without significant differences in outcomes.[16-19] High percentages of good and excellent results using *early passive flexion*[13,22,23] and *true active flexion*[24,25] have also been reported. A summary of these approaches is presented in the following sections.

Immobilization

An example of a specific immobilization protocol has been offered by Amy Lake and her surgeon colleagues at the Texas Scottish Rite Hospital for Children.[15] This protocol delineates children into two age brackets: those 4 years and younger and those 5 years and older. Children in the younger group are immobilized in a long arm "mitten" cast with the wrist positioned in 20–25 degrees of flexion, the metacarpophalangeal (MP) joints in 50–60 degrees of flexion, and the interphalangeal (IP) joints in mild flexion for 4 weeks. The older group is immobilized in the same position for only 3 weeks.

Progression for both age groups is guided by number of weeks following the immobilization phase. During the first week after the cast is removed, children are placed in a dorsal blocking orthosis with the wrist positioned in neutral and distal joints maintained in mild flexion. As rationale for this continued, open-packed position, the authors offer a greater concern with attenuation of the repair and resultant swan neck deformities versus IP extensor lags. During the first postimmobilization week, the children and their caregivers are educated on initiation of passive protected extension (Duran's passive range of motion) in the splint, and wrist active motion with relaxed digits performed out of the splint.

Over the course of the subsequent second through fifth week after immobilization, *true active flexion* is progressed using a percentage approach. During the second week, children are encouraged to create *true active flexion* to 25% of full effort (fifth to sixth postoperative week), the third week 50% (sixth to seventh postoperative week), fourth week 75% (seventh to eighth postoperative week), and during the fifth week (eighth to ninth postoperative week) the child is encouraged to demonstrate *true active flexion* with 100% of their effort. The orthosis is typically weaned during the third week after the cast has been removed (sixth to seventh postoperative week).

Outcomes of immobilization following flexor tendon repair in children have been published by Elhassen et al.[18] The authors employed a retrospective design of children who had been treated with immobilization compared to those progressed through *early passive flexion*. No significant differences were found in total active motion between the two groups. Final outcomes in both groups included good to excellent results; children with zone I injuries and those without concomitant nerve repairs were noted to have better outcomes. The authors reported two complications, both in the immobilization group, including a 2-year-old child who sustained tendon rupture and one 6-year-old who developed joint stiffness requiring tenolysis. Each of these children ultimately achieved good outcomes. This study supports the use of immobilization following flexor tendon repair in children as similar to *early passive flexion*.

Early Passive Flexion

Moehrlen et al.[23] focused solely on the assessment of *early passive flexion* using age groupings: up to 4 years, 4–10 years, and 10–16 years. Forty-nine tendons were repaired in 39 children using a two-strand core suture with a modified Kessler technique. The sample was not limited to zone II injuries. Postoperative orthoses were positioned in 45 degrees of wrist flexion with the MPs and IPs in extension; immobilization was extended proximal to the elbow in children younger than 4. Rationale for wrist positioning was not provided by the authors.

Similar to immobilization protocols, children in this study were progressed through postoperative rehabilitation based on age. *Early passive flexion* and active-assisted extension via Kleinert traction were pursued during the first 3 weeks after surgery in all age groups, and children were immobilized in flexion between exercises. The youngest group of children, less than 4 years old, received assisted finger mobilization during therapy at 3 weeks and returned to activity at week 7. Those children between 4 and 10 years old began *true active flexion* at 4 weeks and were encouraged to discontinue the orthosis and resume full activity after 8 weeks. Children greater than 10 ears old also initiated *true active flexion* at 4 weeks and resistance of the exercise was gradually increased through the eighth postoperative week. The oldest children remained in their orthoses until the 10-week point. Moehrlen et al.[16] reported good or excellent results in 93% of these cases with no subsequent ruptures. The authors found no statistically significant differences in total active motion or Strickland's percentage between age groups; however, children with zone II injuries were noted to have significantly lower Strickland's percentages than children with injuries in other zones.

True Active Flexion

Although cast immobilization through the fourth postoperative week is considered the norm, some international authors have reported successful results in pursuing early mobilization following flexor tendon repair in children. Nietosvaara[24] and colleagues in Finland completed a retrospective review of 45 fingers in 28 children, including two-, four-, and six-strand repairs. Eleven fingers were treated with an immobilization protocol and casted for an average of 27 days, 1 was treated using elastic traction, and 33 fingers were treated with an active motion protocol initiated 1–3 days following repair. The average age of children in this study was 10 years, ranging from 3.2 to 15.9 years and including 21 boys and 7 girls. The active motion protocol included application of a dorsal blocking orthosis with the wrist held in a neutral position, MPs flexed to approximately 60 degrees and IPs held in extension. The orthosis was removed for active exercises four times a day including five repetitions of synergistic exercise: passive wrist flexion with active digital extension followed by wrist extension with *true active flexion*. The exercises were completed by the patient, caregiver, or therapist completing passive digital flexion through the available range.

According to Strickland's original criteria, good and excellent results were noted in 36 fingers in this study. Ninety-four percent of fingers in the mobilization group achieved these results as compared to only 62% in the immobilization group. Three fingers with two-strand repairs sustained tendon rupture; two following cast immobilization and the 1 patient for which elastic traction was used. All cases of rupture were in male patients. The authors in this study concluded that *true active flexion* can be used for children older than 5 years, and delineated age groupings for number of strands as opposed to length of immobilization. Six-strand repairs were suggested for zone I and II injuries in adolescents, while four-strand repairs were advocated for younger children and zone V repairs.

A more recent study completed by Al-Qattan in Saudi Arabia retrospectively reviewed 44 children ranging from 5 to 10 years of age whose tendons were repaired using a six-strand core technique achieved through "figure of eight" sutures and venting of the proximal pulley.[25] The children were placed in a dorsal blocking orthosis with the wrist in 30 degrees of flexion, MPs in 30–40 degrees of flexion, and IPs fully extended. *True active flexion* and extension were initiated immediately following surgery; the orthosis was discontinued after 4 weeks. Excellent results were reported in 85% of cases with the remainder classified as good results; no complications were reported by the authors.

The aforementioned literature, while disparate in both surgical and rehabilitative suggestion, typically employs age as a factor that influences decision-making in the pediatric population. In both immobilization and *early passive flexion* regimens, children under the age of four are immobilized proximal to the elbow postsurgically, and those 5 and older initiate *true active flexion* during the fourth postoperative week.[15,18] One *true active flexion* study, in comparison, focused age-related choices on surgical repair and number of strands.[24] Despite previous research suggesting no difference in rehabilitative outcomes,[16–19] the more recent studies indicating greater than 90% good and excellent results with early passive and active protocols provide promising evidence for consideration[13,22–25] (see Tables 20.1 and 20.2).

Nonoperative and Secondary Procedures

A handful of international studies have been published related to nonoperative and secondary procedures for children with flexor tendon injuries. Stahl[26] and colleagues in Israel retrospectively studied a group of 23 children who had partial lacerations of less than 75% in zones II–III. The first group included 11 children with a mean age of 6.6 years who received surgical procedures based on percent laceration. Tendons with less than 25% laceration were trimmed, those with 25%–50% lacerations were repaired with an epitendinous suture, and those with greater than 50% lacerations were treated with a primary repair and epitendinous suture. The second group included 12 children with a mean age of 7.4 years and less than 75% lacerations; all tendons were trimmed to prevent triggering, but no primary or epitendinous repairs were completed. All children were placed in a postoperative orthosis with the wrist flexed to 40 degrees, MPs flexed to 90 degrees, and the IPs in slight flexion. Children younger than 5 years old were immobilized; those older than 5 completed an *early passive flexion* regimen with Kleinert traction. Excellent results were observed in 11 out of 12 cases that were not repaired, as compared to 8 out of 11 cases that were repaired.

Al-Qattan[27] and Yamazaki et al.[28] reported on secondary procedures for ruptured and neglected tendon injuries in children. In the former study, 10 children sustained ruptures of a primary flexor tendon repair in zone I or II and were treated with a primary rerepair using a six-strand, "figure of eight" method. Children between the ages of 5 and 10 were immobilized for 4 weeks while those older than 10 began *true active flexion* within 2/3 range starting 2–3 days after surgery. Only 1 child had an excellent outcome, with four good

TABLE 20.1
Pediatric Flexor Tendon Protocols.

		Postoperative	Week 3	Week 4	Week 5	Week 6	Week 7	Week 8	Week 9	Week 10
Texas Scottish Rite	<4 years	Long arm mitten cast 20–25 degrees wrist flexion 50–60 degrees MP flexion Mild flexion IP joints			Dorsal block orthosis with wrist neutral Duran's PROM Wrist AROM	25% true active flexion	50% true active flexion Wean orthosis	75% true active flexion	100% true active flexion	
	>5 years	Long arm mitten cast 20–25 degrees wrist flexion 50–60 degrees MP flexion Mild flexion IP joints		Dorsal block orthosis with wrist neutral Duran's PROM Wrist AROM	25% true active flexion	50% true active flexion Wean orthosis	75% true active flexion	100% true active flexion		
Moehrlen et al. (2009)	<4 years	Long arm orthosis 45 degrees wrist flexion MP and IP extension Passive digital flexion and active-assisted extension via Kleinert traction	Assisted finger mobilization		True active flexion		Return to activity			
	4–10 years	Dorsal blocking orthosis 45 degrees wrist flexion MP and IP extension Passive digital flexion and active-assisted extension via Kleinert traction	True active flexion					Discontinue orthosis Return to activity		
	10–16 years	Dorsal blocking orthosis 45 degrees wrist flexion MP and IP extension Passive digital flexion and active-assisted extension via Kleinert traction	True active flexion with increasing resistance							Discontinue orthosis Return to activity
Nietosvaara et al. (2007)	>5 years	Dorsal blocking orthosis: Wrist neutral, 60 degrees MP flexion, IPs extended Synergistic exercise 4×/day, 5 repetitions: Passive wrist flexion with active digital extension, wrist extension with true active flexion Passive digital flexion								

TABLE 20.2
Comparison of Research Outcomes.

	Elhassen et al. (2006)	Moehrlen et al. (2009)	Nietosvaara et al. (2007)
Design	Retrospective comparison of immobilization versus early passive flexion	Retrospective comparison of three age groups using early passive flexion	Retrospective comparison of true active flexion versus immobilization
Subjects	41 fingers (35 patients) Mean age 7 years (range 2–15)	49 fingers (39 children) Mean age 6 years (range 1.2–14.8)	45 fingers (28 children) Mean age 10 years (range 3.2–15.9)
Groups	22 early passive flexion 19 immobilized	<4 years: 8 subjects 4–10 years: 18 subjects 10–16 years: 13 subjects	33 true active flexion 11 cast immobilization 1 elastic bands
Results	• Good to excellent TAM in 100% of cases • Zone I favorable to zone II • Isolated tendon repairs favorable to those with concomitant nerve injuries • No significant difference between rehabilitation strategies or age groups	• Good to excellent results on 93% of cases • No significant differences based on age • Less favorable results in zone II	• Good and excellent results in 94% of fingers in the mobilization group (Strickland's) • Good and excellent results in 62% of fingers in the immobilization group (Strickland's)
Complications	1 rupture, 1 tenolysis Both in immobilization group	1 tenolysis due to surgical error No ruptures	3 ruptures of two-strand repairs: 1 elastic bands, 2 immobilization

and four fair results spread across age groups. Yamazaki et al.[28] achieved more promising outcomes using a one-stage grafting technique in a slightly older group of children. Seven children ranging in age from 7 to 15 years were treated with a tendon graft 3–78 months (mean 25 months) after initial tendon injury. All children were treated with an *early passive flexion* regimen and Kleinert traction, resulting in five excellent, 1 good, and 1 fair result assessed through long-term follow-up.

Contextual Factors

Although research articles and patient outcomes provide interesting academic discourse and potentially useful rehabilitative information, providing intervention for children can also be confounded by contextual factors.

Age has been suggested not only as a means by which to guide surgical and therapeutic parameters, but also as a potential, limiting personal factor as it pertains to comprehension and cooperation.[3] Age and maturity of individual pediatric patients can influence their ability to understand cause and effect, their willingness to follow instructions, and their tenacity in participating in therapy sessions and completing home programs. Careful analysis of the developmental maturity of each child, beyond its simple age, is suggested before initiation of a rehabilitative program following flexor tendon repair.

In addition to the personal factors of each client, the environment in which they live and are cared for can markedly impact their rehabilitative success. Although some adolescents can be instructed in and expected to be responsible for home programs, most pediatric patients have a parent or caregiver who becomes an integral part of the rehabilitative team. Caregiver support and assistance can range dramatically, fundamentally altering all aspects of medical care from simply keeping appointments to monitoring adherence to orthotic and exercise instructions. As per previous, careful analysis of the environmental factors is suggested, especially in cases where *early passive flexion* or *true active flexion* is under consideration.

A recent study by Cole et al.[29] addressed the factors contributing to adherence in children who had sustained a traumatic injury to their hand(s). The authors worked with 47 parents: 21 with 6–11-year-old children and 26 with 12–17-year-old children. Thirty-eight percent of children were reported to be nonadherent to their immobilization regimens; 8 in the younger group and 10 in the older group. The adherence percentage increased to 76% when the subgroup of children who underwent a procedure involving anesthesia was analyzed separately. Of those who were nonadherent to recommendations, 80% reported removing orthoses or dressings for less than an hour, typically to complete hygiene activities. Odor, discomfort, and restriction of activities of daily living were additional reasons for removal. The authors of this study suggest careful attention to choice of materials and feedback regarding comfort to ensure follow-through. The inclusion of activities of daily living as an important component of flexor tendon rehabilitation has been previously published[30] and is reinforced here for the pediatric population.

Recommendations

The provision of rehabilitation for a child with a flexor tendon injury is not without challenge. It is certainly tempting to want to treat the pediatric hand as a tiny, adult version and attempt *true active flexion* regimens based on the results reported herein. However, it is also important to consider the majority of literature that suggests a more rapid recovery, fewer adhesions, and the incorporation of a 4-week immobilization period for children following flexor tendon repair.[11,12,15,16,21] Finally, it is imperative to think about the size of the anatomy and the meticulous surgical skill required to successfully repair the tendons in a child's hand[13,14] (see Fig. 20.1).

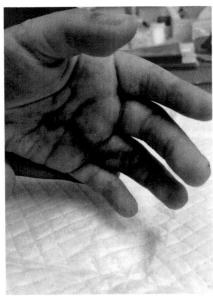

FIG. 20.1 Presentation of the pediatric operative site within the first week postoperatively.

Striking a balance between *true active flexion, early passive flexion,* and immobilization optimally lies in the choice of postoperative dressing and the ability of the surgeon and therapist to monitor wound healing, joint mobility, and tendon glide during the first 4 weeks. The use of web roll covered with 2–3 layers of quick cast is suggested to create this opportunity, providing easy removal during therapy visits.[31] The cast is applied with the wrist in neutral, the MP joints in 60–70 degrees of flexion, and the IP joints in extension. Multiple studies support the positioning of the wrist in a neutral to extended position as a safe and effective choice to decrease passive and resultant active tension on the flexor tendon system.[32–35] In addition to the cast, the provision of an "emergency" orthosis that can be applied by the parents is recommended.[31] This will allow protection for the children who manage to remove their casts or get them wet, and will help the parents avoid an urgent trip to the hospital on a night or weekend.

The patient is scheduled for weekly visits during the first 4 weeks, during which the therapist removes the cast and assesses joint mobility through passive flexion and gentle passive extension of the IP joints with the MP joints blocked in flexion. Tendon gliding can also be safely assessed by positioning the wrist in a neutral to extended position, passively positioning the digits into midrange flexion, and asking the child to very gently hold the position.[34,35] Timing of this assessment should be discussed with the surgeon based on perceived tendon integrity after the repair, and can be deferred to the second or third postoperative week as needed.

Progression of therapy based on physiologic response is recommended with careful attention to both maturity and environmental support. Lack of tendon glide or joint mobility noted in the early stages may be better addressed through supervised therapy visits for the young, less-mature, or less-supported child. Patients with acceptable joint mobility and tendon glide are treated with continued immobilization. In all cases, as careful assessment indicates a need for progression of treatment, exercises and activity should be added in a way that both attends to force production and is logical for the pediatric patient.

When the therapist and surgeon deem progression as a beneficial and safe option, children 4 years or older are moved from a cast to a dorsal blocking orthosis with the same joint positions (see Fig. 20.2). In concert with the Texas Scottish Rite protocol,[15] passive protected extension (Duran's passive range of motion) and wrist active motion with relaxed digits are

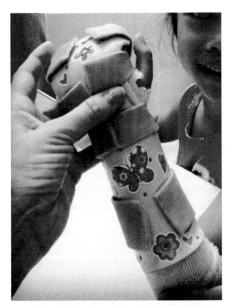

FIG. 20.2 Dorsal blocking orthosis.

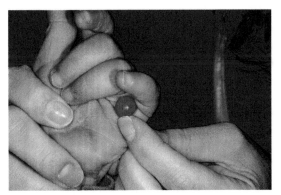

FIG. 20.3 True active flexion using bead to guide to midrange. (Photo courtesy of Shriner's Hospital for Children Philadelphia.)

suggested as an effective way to begin to facilitate tendon glide. Active motion is initiated based on number of strands crossing the repair site; two-strand repairs necessitating deferral until at least 3 weeks postoperative. Rather than asking a child to estimate percentage of force, the use of midrange flexion may be easier to understand and complete. The use of small beads and puzzle pieces can help the child and therapist discern *true active flexion* through play and purposeful activity (see Figs. 20.3–20.5). Picture cards can be used to assess tendon glide and isolate joint motion (see Figs. 20.6–20.7). Discontinuation of the protective orthosis and return to function are based on adherence and response to treatment, but also with great caution in allowing a child full use of their hand again (see Table 20.3 for pediatric flexor tendon regimen).

SECTION II: TRIGGER DIGITS

Trigger thumbs and trigger digits are observed in the pediatric population; however, the incidence of trigger thumb is suggested as 10 times more prevalent.[36] The second section of this chapter will provide a brief review of the evidence guiding conservative and surgical management.

Trigger Digits

Trigger digits are estimated to occur in less than 0.05% of children[37] and, as such, has received limited attention in the surgical and therapeutic literature. Common

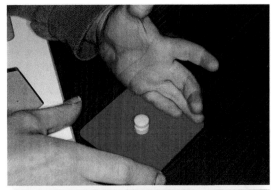

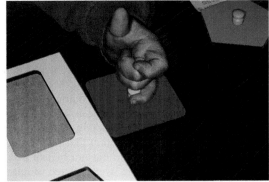

FIGS. 20.4–20.5 The use of a pegged puzzle piece to facilitate motion from extension to flexion. (Photo courtesy of Shriner's Hospital for Children Philadelphia.)

approaches to this uncommon diagnosis include observation for spontaneous recovery, conservative management with orthotic fabrication, and/or surgical release of the A1 pulley with or without flexor digitorum superficialis (FDS) slip separation.[38,39]

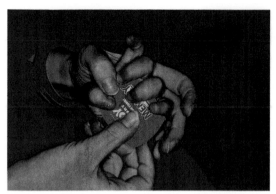

FIG. 20.6 The use of a playing card to facilitate blocked/isolated DIP flexion. (Photo courtesy of Shriner's Hospital for Children Philadelphia.)

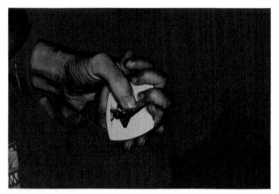

FIG. 20.7 The use of a playing card to facilitate blocked/isolated PIP flexion. (Photo courtesy of Shriner's Hospital for Children Philadelphia.)

Shiozawa et al.[39] reviewed outcomes of children seen over 29 years, initially treated with either observation or an orthosis before surgical intervention. Twenty-four fingers were treated with an orthosis; 67% of these cases resulted in resolution. Comparably, 23 digits were observed for spontaneous resolution that occurred in 30% of cases. The children who did not benefit from these conservative approaches were offered surgical release of the A1 pulley; 92% chose the surgical option and went on to complete resolution of triggering. Orthoses used in this study held the wrist, MP joints, and IP joints in full extension. Single digit orthoses were used for children with 1 affected digit; resting pan splints that incorporated all digits were used for children with multiple trigger digits.

A recent systematic review published by Womack et al.[40] intended to gather the available studies as a means to create an evidence-based treatment algorithm.

Upon review of 7 studies comprising 118 trigger digits, the authors offered the following conclusions. Based on the final resolution rates of conservative management both instead of and as a precursor to A1 pulley release, the authors suggest starting with a trial of nonoperative therapy. Trigger digits in the studies reviewed did not have less favorable results if surgical procedures were delayed as a means to attempt conservative management. In fact, 57.8% of total cases reviewed experienced resolution of triggering with conservative management.

The importance of identifying concomitant diagnoses that could potentially contribute to triggering has also been suggested in the literature, including mucopolysaccharidosis, juvenile rheumatoid arthritis, Ehlers–Danlos syndrome, and Down syndrome.[41] Bauer and Bae also stress the importance of careful anatomical assessment, including location of decussation of the FDS tendon, insertion of lumbricals, and the relationship between FDS and flexor digitorum profundus (FDP) tendons.[41] Procedures added to resolve triggering, such as A2/A3 pulley releases and/or resection of FDS slips, should be communicated to the treating therapist for proper postoperative care.

Trigger Thumb

A more common diagnosis, trigger thumb, is typically observed in children between the ages of 1 and 4 and currently considered to be acquired as opposed to congenital.[41] Sugimoto (as described by Ogino[42]) provided a classification system for trigger thumb, including stage I: palpable "Notta" nodule without observable snapping of IP joint; stage II: triggering with IP extension; stage III: lack of active extension with triggering during passive IP extension; and stage IV: IP cannot be passively extended. The literature provides a consensus that release of the A1 pulley is recommended for children over 1 year and for those in whom triggering persists during a period of conservative management.[43] Although some authors have reported success using orthotic intervention during an observation period, consensus has not been reached with regard to conservative management.[44] Passive range of motion, immobilization using a neoprene or rigid thumb extension splint, and observation for spontaneous recovery are cited methods of conservative management.

A practice pattern survey completed by Marek et al.[44] noted that 85% of respondents would treat a 2-year-old patient with stage IV trigger thumb with surgical release, while 52% would observe the same patient if the triggering was intermittent. These authors also surveyed the caregivers of children who had a locked trigger thumb for greater than 6 months and received surgical

TABLE 20.3
Pediatric Tendon Regimen.

Timeline	Priorities	Orthosis	Exercise	Progression
0–4 weeks	Wound healing Joint mobility Tendon glide	Web roll covered with 2–3 layers of quick cast "Emergency" orthosis for children who remove casts or get them wet Wrist neutral MP joints 60-70 flexion IP joints in extension	Home: Gentle passive flexion and extension of IP joints with MPs held in flexion: 3 × /day, 10 reps Clinic: Assess joint mobility through IP passive range of motion Assess tendon glide with gentle place and hold flexion at midrange **with MD approval*	If joint mobility and tendon glide are consistently progressing: STAY THE COURSE! Increase frequency of passive range of motion if joint mobility issues are noted: 6×/day, 10 reps Add true active flexion to midrange if patient is unable to maintain place and hold in clinic: 3×/day, 10 reps **with MD approval* **Two-strand repairs are not progressed before 3 weeks*
4–6 weeks	Tendon glide Synergistic motion	Removable orthosis Wrist neutral MP joints 60-70 flexion IP joints in extension	Home: Continue gentle passive flexion and Duran's passive motion: as needed Active wrist extension and flexion with relaxed digits; focus on digital extension during wrist flexion and digital flexion during wrist extension (synergistic motion): 3×/day, 10 reps, out of orthosis True active flexion to midrange with active extension to dorsal orthosis: 3×/day, 10 reps, in orthosis **with MD approval*	If joint mobility and tendon glide are consistently progressing: STAY THE COURSE! Progress toward composite, true active flexion between weeks 4 and 6
6 + weeks	Composite flexion and extension Careful progression of ADL tasks	6–8 weeks: Remove orthosis for supervised, light ADLs, and play 8 weeks: Discontinue orthosis **with MD approval*	Home: Continue gentle passive flexion and Duran's passive motion: as needed Composite flexion and extension out of orthosis	Use for supervised, light play out of orthosis between weeks 6 and 8 Progress slowly to full activity starting at week 8; monitor and grade resistive activity (brushing teeth, sustained grasp, turning knobs and handles) Add isolated joint passive and active motion as needed to maximize joint mobility and tendon glide Strengthening is NOT a therapeutic priority; encourage child to resume typical activity to regain strength and dexterity

release of the A1 pulley. The average age at trigger onset was 25 months with a mean timeframe of 11 months between onset and surgery. High levels of satisfaction were reported, and 99% of caregivers recommended the surgery for other children.

In a recent systematic review, Farr et al.[45] analyzed 17 retrospective and 1 prospective study comparing surgery (759 thumbs), orthoses (138 thumbs), and passive exercises (108 thumbs). The mean age of all children in the reviewed studies was 32 months (range 15–90 months). Children who received an A1 pulley release were followed for an average of 59 months, and 95% demonstrated full range of IP joint motion without triggering. Comparably, children who received an orthosis were followed for 23 months and only 67% were noted to achieve full IP motion within that timeframe. Finally, only 55% of those who were treated with passive range of motion, while followed for 76 months, were able to demonstrate full range of IP joint motion. It was noted by the authors that a majority of cases in these studies included stage IV, or fixed flexion deformities, which may not be as amenable to orthoses or passive range of motion. Adherence to orthotic regimens was also identified as an issue with as many as 24% of children dropping out of orthotic groups and electing surgery instead. Future studies that align conservative management with stages of trigger thumb were recommended by the authors; surgical release was favored as a "reliable and rapid outcome" for children with triggering or locked thumb IP joints.

CONCLUSION

Although previous research has suggested no difference between immobilization and early mobilization in the pediatric population,[16–19] more recent studies have provided promising results for both *early passive flexion*[13,22,23] and *true active flexion*[24,25] regimens. Incorporation of these progressive approaches is suggested when modulated by careful analysis of age, developmental maturity, and caregiver support during the postoperative phase. Immobilization for the first 4 weeks following flexor tendon repair in children remains the most clearly articulated and supported rehabilitative option.[11,12,15,16,21] Future research is suggested to increase our collective understanding of repair strength in children, optimal age ranges for early active motion, and cost-effectiveness of rehabilitative strategies based on number of therapy visits.

Trigger digits are rare in children, often treated with a progression from conservative to surgical management with attention to concomitant diagnoses and abnormal anatomy. Acquired trigger thumbs are more common

and potentially less likely to resolve spontaneously. Favorable results of A1 pulley release for children greater than 1 year old have been published, with 99% of caregivers recommending the procedure for other children.[44]

REFERENCES

1. Hitchcock TF, Light TR, Bunch WH, et al. The effect of immediate constrained digital motion on the strength of flexor tendon repairs in chickens. *J Hand Surg.* 1987;12A:590–595.
2. Tanaka T, Amadio PC, Zhao C, et al. Gliding resistance versus work of flexion-two methods to assess flexor tendon repair. *J Orthop Res.* 2003;21:813–818.
3. Zhao C, Amadio PC, Paillard P, et al. Digital resistance and tendon strength during the first week after flexor digitorum profundus tendon repair in a canine model in vivo. *J Bone Jt Surg.* 2004;86:320–327.
4. Zhao C, Amadio PC, Tanaka T, et al. Short-term assessment of optimal timing for postoperative rehabilitation after flexor digitorum profundus tendon repair in a canine model. *J Hand Ther.* 2005;18:322–328.
5. Cao Y, Tang JB. Investigation of resistance of digital subcutaneous edema to gliding of the flexor tendon: an in vitro study. *J Hand Surg.* 2005;30A:1248–1254.
6. Cao Y, Tang JB. Resistance to motion of flexor tendons and digital edema: an in vivo study in a chicken model. *J Hand Surg.* 2006;31A:1645–1651.
7. Cao Y, Chen CH, Wu YF, et al. Digital oedema, adhesion formation and resistance to digital motion after primary flexor tendon repair. *J Hand Surg.* 2008;33E:745–752.
8. Gelberman RH, Botte MJ, Spiegelman JJ, Akeson WH. The excursion and deformation of repaired flexor tendons treated with protected early motion. *J Hand Surg.* 1986;11A:106–110.
9. Gelberman RH, Woo SL-Y. The physiological basis for application of controlled stress in the rehabilitation of flexor tendon injuries. *J Hand Ther.* 1989;2:66–70.
10. Neiduski RL, Powell RK. Flexor tendon rehabilitation in the 21st century: a systematic review. *J Hand Ther.* 2019;32(2):165–174.
11. Al-Qattan M, Posnick J, Lin K, et al. Fetal tendon healing: development of an experimental model. *Plast Reconstr Surg.* 1993;92:1155–1160.
12. Grobbelaar A, Hudson D. Flexor tendon injuries in children. *J Hand Surg.* 1994;19:696–698.
13. Navali AM, Rouhani A. Zone 2 flexor tendon repair in young children: a comparative study of four-strand versus two-strand repair. *J Hand Surg.* 2008;33E(4):424–429.
14. Al-Qattan MM. Flexor tendon injuries in the child. *J Hand Surg.* 2014;39E(1):46–53.
15. Lake A, Oishi SN, Ezaki M. Flexor tendon injuries, repair and rehabilitation in children. In: Skirven T, Osterman AL, Fedorczyk J, Amadio P, eds. *Rehabilitation of the Hand and Upper Extremity.* 6th ed. St. Louis, MO: Mosby; 2011:1647–1650.
16. O'Connell S, Moore M, Strickland J, et al. Results of zone I and zone II flexor tendon repairs in children. *J Hand Surg.* 1994;19:48–52.

17. Berndtsson L, Ejeskär A. Zone II flexor tendon repair in children. A retrospective long term study. *Scand J Plast Reconstr Surg*. 1995;29:59–64.

18. Elhassan B, Moran S, Bravo C, et al. Factors that influence the outcome of zone I and zone II flexor tendon repairs in children. *J Hand Surg*. 2006;31:1661–1666.

19. Fitoussi F, Lebellec Y, Frajman JM, Pennecot GF. Flexor tendon injuries in children: factors influencing prognosis. *J Pediatr Orthop*. 1999;19:818–821.

20. Kato H, Minami A, Suenaga N, Iwasakin N, Kimura T. Long term results after primary repairs of zone 2 flexor tendon lacerations in children younger than age 6 years. *J Pediatr Orthop*. 2002;22:732–735.

21. Sikora S, Lai M, Arneja JS. Pediatric flexor tendon injuries: a 10-year outcome analysis. *Can J Plast Surg*. 2013;21(3): 181–185.

22. Kayali C, Eren A, Agus H, Arslantas M, Ozcalabi IT. The results of primary repair and early passive rehabilitation in zone II flexor tendon injuries in children. *Acta Orthop Traumatol Turcica*. 2003;37:249–253.

23. Moehrlen U, Mazzone L, Bieli C, Weber DM. Early mobilization after flexor tendon repair in children. *Eur J Pediatr Surg*. 2009;19:83–86.

24. Nietosvaara Y, Lindfors NC, Palmu S, Rautakorpi S, Ristaniemi N. Flexor tendon injuries in pediatric patients. *J Hand Surg*. 2007;32:1549–1557.

25. Al Qattan MM. Finger zone II flexor tendon repair in children (5–10 years of age) using three 'figure of eight' sutures followed by immediate active mobilization. *J Hand Surg*. 2011;36E(4):291–296.

26. Stahl S, Kaufman T, Bialik V. Partial lacerations of flexor tendons in children: primary repair versus conservative treatment. *J Hand Surg*. 1997;22B(3):377–380.

27. Al-Qattan MM. Re-repair of ruptured primary flexor tendon repairs in zones I and II of the fingers in children. *J Hand Surg*. 2015;40E(3):271–275.

28. Yamazaki H, Kato H, Uchiyama H, Iwasaki N, Ishikura H, Minami A. *J Hand Surg*. 2011;36E(4):303–307.

29. Cole T, Underhill A, Kennedy S. Adherence behavior in an acute pediatric hand trauma population: a pilot study of parental report of adherence levels and influencing factors. *J Hand Ther*. 2016;29:299–306.

30. Powell RK, von der Heyde RL. The inclusion of activities of daily living in flexor tendon rehabilitation: a survey. *J Hand Ther*. 2014;27(1):23–29.

31. Bassini Lynn. *Personal Communication*. June 22, 2019.

32. Savage R. The influence of wrist position on the minimum force required for active movement of the interphalangeal joints. *J Hand Surg*. 1988;13B:262–268.

33. Lieber RL, Amiel O, Kaufman KR, et al. Relationship between joint motion and flexor tendon force in the canine forelimb. *J Hand Surg*. 1996;21A:957–962.

34. Evans RB, Thompson DE. The application of force to the healing tendon. *J Hand Ther*. 1993;6:266–284.

35. Lieber RL, Silva MJ, Amiel D, Gelberman RH. Wrist and digital joint motion produce unique flexor tendon force and excursion in the canine forelimb. *J Biomech*. 1999; 32:175–181.

36. Cardon LJ, Ezaki M, Carter PR. Trigger finger in children. *J Hand Surg*. 1999;24:1156–1161.

37. Ryzewicz M, Wolf JM. Trigger digits: principles, management, and complications. *J Hand Surg*. 2006;31:135–146.

38. Moon WN, Suh SW, Kim IC. Trigger digits in children. *J Hand Surg*. 2001;26B:11–12.

39. Shiozawa R, Uchiyama S, Sugimoto Y, et al. Comparison of splinting versus nonsplinting in the treatment of pediatric trigger finger. *J Hand Surg*. 2012;37:1211–1216.

40. Womack ME, Ryan JC, Shillingford-Cole V, Speicher S, Hogue GD. Treatment of paediatric trigger finger: a systematic review and treatment algorithm. *J Child Orthop*. 2018; 12:209–217.

41. Bauer AS, Bae DS. Pediatric trigger digits. *J Hand Surg*. 2015;40:2304–2309.

42. Ogino T. Trigger thumb in children: current recommendations for treatment. *J Hand Surg*. 2008;33A:982–984.

43. Bae DS. Pediatric trigger thumb. *J Hand Surg*. 2008;33A: 1189–1191.

44. Marek DJ, Fitoussi F, Bohn DC, Van Heest AE. Surgical release of the pediatric trigger thumb. *J Hand Surg*. 2011; 36A:647–652.

45. Farr S, Grill F, Ganger R, Girsch W. Open surgery versus nonoperative treatments for paediatric trigger thumb: a systematic review. *J Hand Surg*. 2014;39E(7):719–726.

CHAPTER 21

Surgical and Therapeutic Management of Volkmann's Ischemic Contracture and Free Functional Muscle Transfer

JAMIE BERGGREN, OTR/L, BS • GINA KIM, MA OTR/L • ERIN MEISEL, MD • MILAN STEVANOVIC, MD

INTRODUCTION

Volkmann's ischemic contracture is the outcome of prolonged muscle and nerve ischemia resulting most commonly from delayed or untreated acute compartment syndrome. Increased compartment pressures decrease capillary perfusion to the muscle ultimately leading to muscle necrosis and fibrosis, which clinically presents as contracture. Nerve dysfunction may also result from the initial trauma and/or subsequent scar formation as well as impaired nerve perfusion. The deep flexor compartment of the forearm and the median nerve are the most vulnerable (Figs. 21.1 and 21.2).

Mild contractures with deep flexor involvement and no neurologic deficit that have failed nonoperative treatment respond well to soft tissue procedures such as a flexor origin or flexor pronator slide. This procedure relatively lengthens the forearm flexor muscles and is effective when good active finger flexion is present. Moderate contractures that involve both superficial and deep compartments and have neurologic dysfunction may also be treated with a flexor origin slide however its usually paired with complete median and ulnar nerve neurolysis and possible resection and grafting to restore protective sensation. Tendon transfers may be involved in the reconstruction as well, depending on the degree of neurologic injury. Severe contractions are best treated with free functional muscle transfers (Figs. 21.3 and 21.4).[1]

THERAPY CONSIDERATIONS ACCORDING TO TYPE OF SEVERITY

Sustained ischemia results in irreversible changes to muscle whereby the necrotic muscle is replaced with fibrotic tissue. The maturation of fibrotic tissue occurs over 6 months to a year, resulting in progression of contracture severity over time. Nerve impairment occurs as fibrosis compresses the nerve and/or prevents gliding. The most vulnerable muscle group is the deep flexor compartment in the forearm.[1]

Hand rehabilitation is directed toward maintenance of passive joint motion, preservation and strengthening of remaining muscle function, and correction of contracture through static progressive splinting of wrist, fingers, and thumb web space. Splinting is maintained until skeletal maturity (Table 21.1).[1,2]

FREE FUNCTIONAL MUSCLE TRANSFER
Introduction

Functional deficits in the upper extremity that are not amenable to tendon, nerve, or rotational muscle transfers for reconstruction often require the use of a free functional muscle transfer as the most effective means to restore function. Common indications are Volkmann's ischemic contracture, late reconstruction of brachial plexus injuries, traumatic muscle loss, oncologic resection, and congenital absence of motor function such as arthrogryposis. The gracilis has long been used as the workhorse of most upper extremity free muscle transfers due to its favorable neurovascular and musculotendinous anatomy. Other commonly used donor muscles include latissimus dorsi, medial gastrocnemius, pectoralis major, serratus anterior, tensor fascia lata, and rectus femoris.[3]

Success of these procedures requires impeccable surgical technique paired with comprehensive therapy both preoperatively and postoperatively (Figs. 21.5 and 21.6).

Pediatric Hand Therapy. https://doi.org/10.1016/B978-0-323-53091-0.00021-X

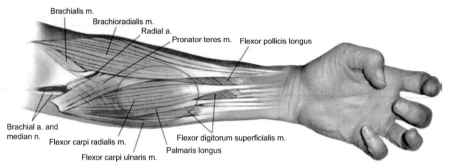

FIG. 21.1   Zone of injury caused in anterior compartment. (Primary authors retain copyrights.)

Before free functional muscle transfer, it is imperative that the patient has passive motion across the affected joint and that the soft tissue envelope is optimized for soft tissue gliding. This may mean that an antecedent surgery be performed for tenolysis, contracture release, and/or soft tissue coverage. At the time of muscle transfer surgical incisions are planned to maximize soft tissue coverage over the planned tenorrhaphy site. The transplanted muscle origin is spread to best match the width of the old origin and is secured to bone or periosteum using bone tunnels or nonabsorbable sutures. Marking and restoring the resting length of the gracilis during its harvest is of critical importance in ensuring its maximal function. Pulvertaft weave is the preferred method of distal tenorrhaphy. Vascular anastomosis should be performed first to minimize ischemic muscle changes, followed by venous anastomosis, and finally neurorrhaphy as close to the transplanted muscle as possible. Wound closure, dressings, and postoperative splinting are critical as to not compress the anastomoses. The operative extremity is immobilized with the elbow in flexion and hand in position of safety to protect the new muscle origin and insertion as well as the neurovascular anastomosis. Viability of the muscle flap is monitored for 48–72 hours via the skin flap using Doppler ultrasound and clinical exam.[3-5]

In this part of the chapter, we will focus on the therapeutic management during the pre- and postoperative periods following free functional gracilis transfers (FFGT) for elbow flexion and digital flexion and extension (Figs. 21.7–21.9).

PREOPERATIVE ASSESSMENT AND THERAPY

When nerve and muscle recovery has plateaued, preoperative assessment is critical to help the surgeon identify donor muscles and nerves, and guide targeted preoperative therapy. (Box 21.1).

Full passive range of motion of the affected joint as well as full passive and active range of motion of neighboring joints is considered crucial for successful surgical outcome. Serial splinting may be effective in resolving joint contractures in addition to an extensive stretching program.

Decreased sensation in the involved upper extremity may lead to poor postoperative functional outcomes. Assessment of protective sensation, light touch, and two-point discrimination provides valuable information of specific areas of nerve injury. However, sensory exams can be difficult to perform and may be unreliable in young children.

Assessing the strength and motor function of antagonistic muscle will predict and prepare for future concerns regarding muscle imbalance between the antagonistic and transplanted muscle.

The child and caregiver's commitment to comply with the preoperative home program (i.e., stretching and splinting) will help to gauge their readiness to commit to the long and complex rehabilitative journey ahead.

POSTOPERATIVE ASSESSMENT AND THERAPY

Therapeutic management following FFGT is limited in the literature and does not exist for children. Some authors have contributed brief guidelines,[5,6] but it is up to the therapist to gather relevant information about the procedure and work together with the surgeon to design a course of postoperative care. Therapists unfamiliar with this procedure would benefit from the mentorship of a colleague who has gained successful experience with these cases (Box 21.2).

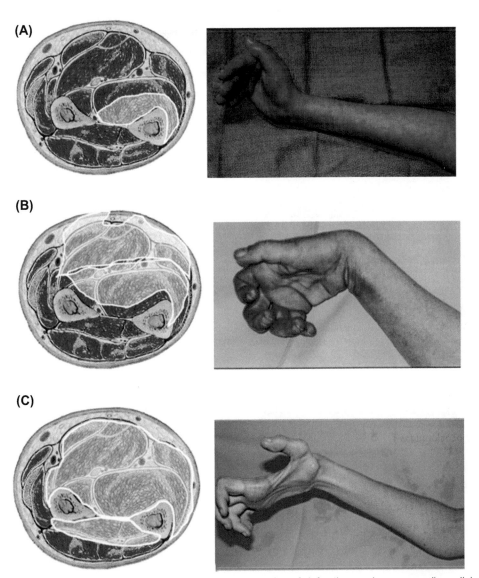

FIG. 21.2 Cross-section of forearm with various severity of infarction and corresponding clinical presentation. **(A)** Mild type involving flexor digitorum profundus and flexor pollicis longus. **(B)** Moderate type involving flexor digitorum superficialis, flexor digitorum profundus, flexor pollicis longus, wrist flexors, and pronator. **(C)** Severe type involving both flexor and extensor compartments. (Primary authors retain copyrights.)

STANDARD ASSESMENT AND OUTCOME MEASURES

The British Medical Research Council (MRC) grading system is a well-accepted scale that is used to grade muscles individually (Box 21.3).[7]

The Active Movement Scale (AMS) designed for infants with brachial plexus birth palsy is an accepted scale to measure motion in infants and younger children (Box 21.4).[8]

Surface electromyography (sEMG) is an effective measure of determining muscle reinnervation.[5,6]

It is also helpful in giving visual or auditory feedback to induce synergist pairing, gain muscle control, and determine when pairing is no longer

(A)

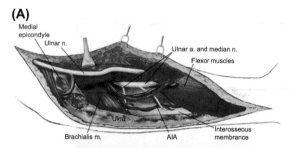

(B)

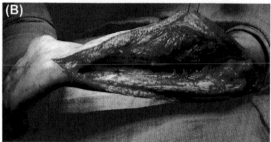

FIG. 21.3 **(A)** Detachment of the origins of PT, FCR, PL, FCU, FDS, FDP, and FPL muscles from the medial epicondyle which slide 2–3 cm distally. **(B)** Intraoperative photograph of the flexor origin slide. (Primary authors retain copyrights.)

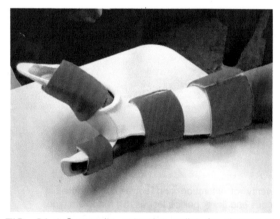

FIG. 21.4 Composite extension splint for therapeutic management of Volkmann's ischemic contracture and postoperative positioning following flexor origin slide.

needed. Placement of sensors should be standardized during each use.

SPLINTING REQUIREMENTS: IMMOBILIZATION PHASE

FFGT to restore elbow flexion: The upper extremity is held in a sling with 90 degrees–100 degrees of elbow flexion. An additional strap may be needed to maintain shoulder

TABLE 21.1
Tsuge Classification for Volkmann's Ischemic Contracture of the Forearm.[2]

Type	Findings	Treatment Option
Mild	Localized Volkmann's contracture Deep flexor compartment FDP of long and ring finger Little or no nerve involvement	Therapy management: Stretching Composite ext. splint/night Surgical management: Selective fractional lengthening Selective flexor origin slide
Moderate	Nearly all FDP, FPL, and partial FDS Median nerve impairment Intrinsic minus posture Poor sensation along ulnar nerve	Therapy management: Stretching Intrinsic/extrinsic muscle balance Support pinch MCP block splint/day Intrinsic plus, composite ext. splint/night Surgical management: Flexor origin slide
Severe	All the flexor compartment Varied extensor compartment No intrinsic muscles Median, ulnar nerve impairment	Therapy management: Stretching Wrist gauntlet, cock up splint/day Composite ext. splint/night Surgical management: Tendon transfer Functional free muscle transfer

adduction, in cases when intercostal or phrenic nerve transfers are used. Great care is taken, as even a brief period of shoulder abduction in the post-op period can lead to rupture of the nerve repair.[5] Postoperative immobilization is 4–8 weeks depending on surgeon's preference.

FFGT to restore finger flexion or extension: Please refer to Table 21.2 for specific postoperative positioning (Fig. 21.10).

SPLINTING REQUIREMENTS: FOLLOWING IMMOBILIZATION PHASE

FFGT to restore elbow flexion: Following immobilization, the sling is lowered 10–20 degrees each week until

(A)   **(B)**

(C)

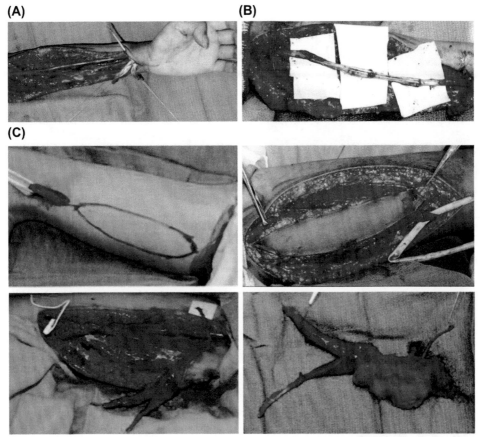

FIG. 21.5 **(A)** Dissection, identification, and tensioning of the distal tendons. **(B)** Cable grafts of the median nerve using sural nerves as donor. **(C)** Various stages of harvesting the gracilis muscle with its tendon, vessels, and obturator nerve in preparation for FFGT.

elbow extension is achieved A gentle serial elbow extension splint at night may be required if elbow flexion contracture develops. Some authors advocate for a slight elbow flexion contracture as it will put tension on the gracilis and help to facilitate the initiation of elbow flexion.[5] Monitor need for night splinting until skeletal maturity is achieved.

FFGT to restore finger flexion or extension: Following immobilization a variety of splints may be required dependent on the presentation of the patient and the aim of reconstruction. Splints are fabricated with the joints affected by the transfer to protect the resting tension of the transfer. Night splinting may involve progressive static splinting toward composite extension or wrist neutral with fingers in intrinsic plus position to preserve intrinsic finger motion. Day splinting may involve a wrist gauntlet for stability in power grip and or, MP block splint to prevent finger extensors from over powering intrinsic muscles. Periodic serial

casting of the wrist into extension may be required. Monitoring is needed for night and day splinting until skeletal maturity is achieved (Fig. 21.11).

EARLY PASSIVE MOBILIZATION VERSUS CONVENTIONAL PROTOCOLS

Successful outcomes following FFGT can be complicated by the muscle length-tension curve. Overstretching or under tensioning the transferred muscle will lead to inefficient muscle output (excursion and strength) and poor active range of motion. Tendon adherence also affects active range of motion. Adhesions of the tendon mostly occur underneath the pulley at the coapted tendon and around the site of tenorrhaphy.[3] In some cases, a secondary surgical procedure of tenolysis may be required to achieve desired outcomes.

Doi and colleagues compared the outcomes between conventional and early mobilization protocols. Active

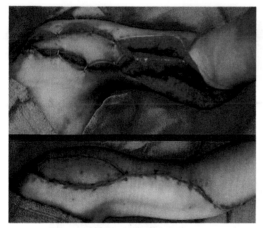

FIG. 21.6 Attention to wound closure is critical to avoid compression of the anastomoses or compartment syndrome.

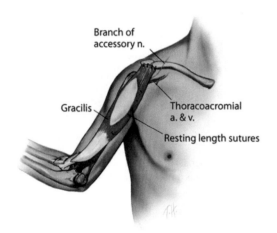

FIG. 21.7 Gracilis muscle used to restore elbow flexion. (Copyright © Timothy C. Hengst, primary authors retains copyright.)

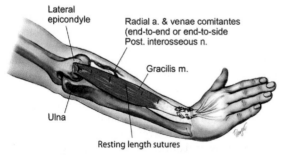

FIG. 21.8 Gracilis muscle used to restore finger extension. (Copyright © Timothy C. Hengst, primary authors retain copyright.)

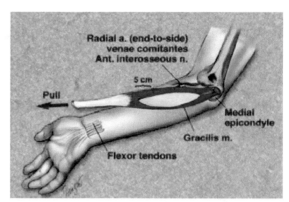

FIG. 21.9 Gracilis muscle used to restore finger flexion. (Copyright © Timothy C. Hengst, primary authors retain copyright.)

range of motion and incidence of tenolysis were reviewed. The early mobilization group did not require tenolysis and had better range of motion outcomes. The conventional group, required tenolysis in 26% of muscle transfers and had poorer range of motion outcomes. After tenolysis, the range of motion outcomes was the same between both groups.[6]

In conventional protocols, the tendon and muscle can start moving after 4−8 weeks of immobilization dependent on surgeon's preference. Early passive mobilization begins at 1 week, consisting of the following tendon compression and tenodesis exercises:

NERVE REINNERVATION PHASE: MRC 1/AMS 1

Reinnervation of the FFGT depends on various factors such as age, vascular complications, and the distance from nerve coaptation to muscle. Most authors suggest muscle contraction can be detected in 3−4 months following the transfer.[3,5] This long period of inactivity in the transferred muscle requires supportive strategies. Passive range of motion of the surrounding joints, scar massage, tendon gliding, and electrical stimulation (ES) help minimize muscle atrophy and improve contractile response after reinnervation.[3,6,9]

If there are concurrent tendon transfers for thumb extension or flexion, splinting and activation will be required during this phase.

Daily PROM of the surrounding joints is essential to prevent stiffness. Check with the surgeon about specific precautions regarding PROM. Shoulder motion may be guarded if phrenic or intercostal nerves were used.

Scar massage is performed daily with special attention to adhesion sites. Tendon adherence interferes with motion and mostly occurs underneath the pulley at the coapted tendon and around the site of tenorrhaphy.[3] In addition, the presence of tendon adhesions in distal forearm, palm, or digits must be monitored when FFGT was used for finger flexion or extension.[10]

Begin or continue the early passive mobilization technique described in Table 21.3 until 50% of the expected motion is achieved.[6]

Several authors advocate the use of ES on the FFGT during the reinnervation phase.[3,6,11] The effect of ES on nerve regrowth is unclear. Direct motor ES has been shown to increase muscle bulk.[12] However, long pulsed (ms) durations can be uncomfortable and are controversial when used during nerve regeneration.[13,14] Some studies using short pulsed (μs) sensory ES after peripheral nerve repair have shown comparatively earlier sensory and functional recovery times.[15–18]

We begin short pulsed sensory ES after the immobilization period and continue until reinnervation can be seen by sEMG. The pulse duration is set at 100 μs with 20 Hz or pulses per second. The program is performed two times a day for 30 minutes. Amplitude is to sensory awareness or trace muscle contraction without inducing muscle or joint movement.[19]

The strategies used during the reinnervation phase are performed in a daily home program. It is important to develop a gentle but firm rapport with the child and caregivers to coach and guide them through this challenging process. First movements and handling of the postsurgical arm can be painful and instill fear among all parties. Engaging the nonsurgical arm in soothing activities such as games, coloring, or listening to music can help to lessen the anxiety and focus on specific procedures.

MUSCLE AND NERVE ACTIVATION PHASE: MRC 1–2/AMS 1–4

The first sign of reinnervation is an exciting time for the child and caregivers, but the activation phase can prove to be frustrating. Early on, there is lack of AROM and scant visible joint motion. Therapist's knowledge of the physiology of muscle recovery following nerve reinnervation is essential for success.

Keep a close watch on muscle recovery by performing outcome measures (MRC, AMS, sEMG) monthly. These measures help guide progression and modification of treatment toward expected outcomes.

Table 21.4 lists the five stages of muscle recovery following nerve reinnervation as published by David Chuang MD.[20] Keep in mind, the timelines are based on adults, and children will often recover sooner.

Authors express preference for certain nerve donors over others to reanimate the FFGT according to the

TABLE 21.2
Technique Summary for Biceps, Finger Extension, and Finger Flexion Reconstruction.

	Elbow Flexion	Finger Extension	Finger Flexion
Donor muscle options	Gracilis[a] Latissimus dorsi Tensor fasciae latae Medial gastrocnemius	Gracilis[a] Latissimus dorsi Tensor fasciae latae	Gracilis[a] Latissimus dorsi Tensor fasciae latae
New origin	Distal half of clavicle (gracilis) Coracoid (latissimus)	Lateral epicondyle, common extensor fascia	Medial epicondyle of humerus, flexor-pronator fascia
New insertion	Distal biceps tendon Bone at radial tuberosity Bone at ulna-level of tuberosity	Tendons of EDC, EPL	Tendons of FDP at distal forearm
Recipient nerve (options)	Musculocutaneous Spinal accessory (terminal branch) Intercostal Medial pectoral (not preferred because of size)	Posterior interosseous Motor branch to pronator teres	Anterior interosseous Median motor fascicles
Position for restoration of resting length	Full elbow extension	Elbow, wrist, and fingers in full extension	Full elbow extension, wrist flexion at 20–30[a], finger MCP 90[a] flex
Postoperative Position	Immobilization at 90[a] elbow flexion for 8 weeks.	Immobilization with elbow at 90[a] flexion, wrist at 30[a] ext., full MCP ext., IP joints left free for 6 weeks.	Immobilization with elbow at 90[a] flex, wrist at 30[a] flex, MCP at 90[a] flex. Thumb in palmar abduction, IP flex.

[a] Preferred muscle.
Compilation of Tables 21.3–21.4, Stevanovic M, Sharpe F. Functional free muscle transfer for upper extremity reconstruction. Plast Reconstr Surg 2014; 134:257e.

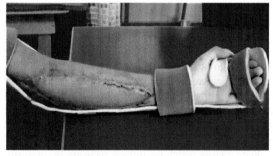

FIG. 21.10 Dorsal-based protective postoperative splint following FFGT to restore finger flexion.

number of functioning axons needed for the specific muscle movement to be achieved. Active elbow flexion requires several hundred axons for activation versus intrinsic hand function that requires several thousand axons. The intercostal nerve has 1300 myelinated axons, spinal accessory 1700, and the ulnar nerve 1600.[11,21,22]

The reinnervated muscle takes on the characteristics of the donor nerve.[11] This prior nerve function needs to be paired with the new muscle movement in a synergistic pattern. The following table lists the nerves and the synergistic pattern required for activation (Table 21.5).

When the phrenic or intercostal nerves are used, it is important to encourage the child to take a daily brisk walk to improve deep inspiration.[23] The child can practice making animal sounds, singing, blowing bubbles, or imitating funny positions to see if they can incite more movement. Use sEMG biofeedback to help the child understand how the synergistic pattern promotes movement. Biofeedback is especially helpful when displayed in a graphic format that the child and family can see. If there is a robotic-assisted arm-hand rehabilitation system such as Tyromotion© in the clinic, introduce it and continue to use it as a motivating activity for task-oriented training (Fig. 21.12).

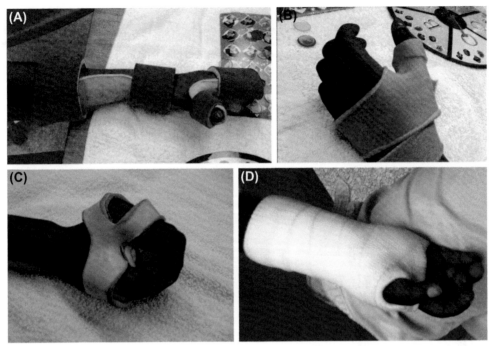

FIG. 21.11 **(A)** Progressive static splint to increase composite extension. **(B)** Short thumb spica to place thumb CMC in position of opposition while IP is allowed to flex and extend. **(C)** MCP block splint with thumb loop to place fingers in intrinsic positive position and thumb in opposition. **(D)** Periodic serial casting of the wrist into extension.

Gaining control to move the FFGT requires learning to activate the muscle and nerve in a new role and then practicing it repeatedly. Practice enough and the motor map is established, don't practice enough and the motor map is not stable. Principles of motor learning apply throughout all phases of rehabilitation. In the activation phase, the child must acquire the ability to move the transfer and retain that ability after long delays between work periods. During the strength and function phase, the child must acquire the flexibility to vary movement according to task and develop motor efficiency to minimize energy expenditure.[24]

Mirroring with the other limb will provide visual and proprioceptive feedback to engage the mirror and activity observation neurons in the contralateral hemisphere. Ultimately, this may aid in initial movement of the involved limb.[9]

Once gravity-eliminated movement is noted, therapist and caregivers create clinic and home activities that are fun, task specific, and encourage repetition. Table top activities with a sling, towel, or skate board will facilitate elbow flexion to bring objects to midline, hug a ball, hit a balloon, or place objects in a container, finger flexion to grasp cylindrical objects from large to small and push around until holding is possible, or finger extension to sweep light objects off table into a container or keep a disk spinning.

Aquatic therapy is especially beneficial during this phase, as it provides a gravity-eliminated environment for practice.

As gravity-eliminated movement improves, begin place and hold. This is best performed in midranges. Play games with elbow held in a gravity-eliminated position, sustain contact with finger flexion on light objects such as cotton balls, or place and hold finger extensors in a cat's paw position. As control increases, incorporate light bimanual activities (Fig. 21.13).

When full active gravity-eliminated movement is achieved, begin motion against gravity and add progressive resistance.

All throughout the activation phase, therapist and caregivers need to watch for signs of fatigue and modify the program accordingly. Engage in motor practice with intervals of rest. Home program: start with 10 reps, 10 times a day to build control and endurance. One author recommends practice intervals of 4 minutes followed by a 5 minutes rest break, working up to a daily full hour of activity.[25]

TABLE 21.3
Early Passive Mobilization of FFGT to Restore Finger Flexion or Extension.[6]

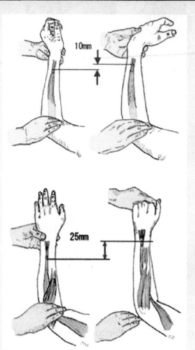

1. Compress and hold tendon at flexed elbow (medial epicondyle). Move the fingers into flexion and extend the wrist. Release fingers and flex wrist (tenodesis).
2. Compress and hold tendon at flexed elbow. Hold wrist in neutral and passively flex and extend the MCPs
   - Perform 10 repetitions, 2 × a day.
   - Take caution to protect tenorrhaphy sites.
   - Continue until 50% of expected motion achieved.

Fig. 4. Tendon compression at the elbow could move the gracilis tendon 5 mm, and the tenodesis technique at the wrist also moved the tendon 10 mm (*above*). However, by adding the assisted movement of the metacarpophalangeal joints and the wrist, the sliding distance of the gracilis tendon by the compression technique increased to 25 mm (*below*).

Fig. 4, license to reuse at RightLinks.com.

TABLE 21.4
Five Stages of Muscle Recovery Following Nerve Graft/Transfer.

Timeline	Intervention	Outcome Measure
0–3 months	Squeezing muscle results in pain in area of coapted nerve function (squeezing FFGT coapted by intercostal nerves results in pain in the chest).	Reinnervation sEMG
3–6 months	Visible muscle contraction without movement during induction of coapted nerve function (see Table 21.5 for synergistic pairing)	MRC 1 AMS 1
6–12 months	Muscle movement with gravity-eliminated support	MRC 2 AMS 2–4
12–18 months	Muscle movement against gravity	MRC 3 AMS 5–7
M3 reached	Strength training with steady increase of 0.5 kg every 6 months	3–6 kg weightlifting maximum

TABLE 21.5
Donor Nerve and Synergistic Activation Pattern.

Donor Nerve	Synergistic Pattern
Spinal accessory	• Shoulder shrug • Scapular adduction
Intercostals	• Deep inspiration/expiration • Coughing, singing
Phrenic	• Deep inspiration • Belly push
Ulnar	• Wrist flexion, ulnar side
Median	• Wrist flexion, radial side • Pronation
Long Thoracic	• Scapular protraction

MUSCLE STRENGTH AND FUNCTION PHASE: MRC 3–4/AMS 5–7

Following reinnervation and activation of muscle transfer the aim of rehabilitation is to integrate the function of the transplanted gracilis in the context of age-appropriate and meaningful bimanual activities. Through practice in multiple settings and activities, motor learning or relearning continues to take place to support cortical remapping.[26]

A child who has experienced a lack of finger flexion, extension, or elbow flexion function in the affected hand/arm for a prolonged period must overcome learned nonuse. If the child continues to ignore the use of the affected hand despite activation of the gracilis and lack of progress is noted, then a short period of

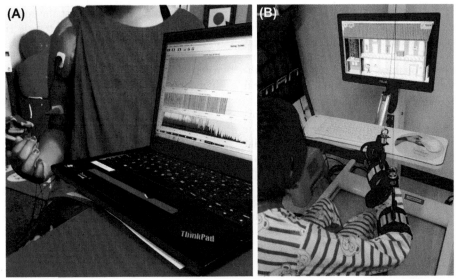

FIG. 21.12 **(A)** Surface EMG displays contraction of the gracilis in a graphic format. **(B)** Tyromotion © - robotics-assisted therapeutic device promotes hand-arm rehabilitation.

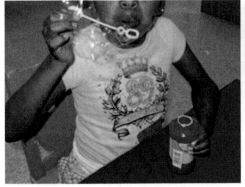
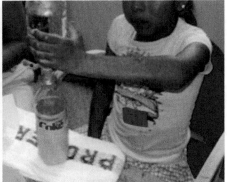

FIG. 21.13 Place and hold activities for finger flexion performed in midranges.

modified constraint induced movement therapy may be beneficial. Through the restraint of the unaffected hand and extensive practice of the affected hand, motor learning takes place with subsequent use-dependent cortical reorganization.[27]

Although this upper extremity intervention was originally developed for patients with hemiparesis cerebral palsy, the concept can also be applied for child with learned nonuse to relearn that the hand or arm powered by the gracilis is a useful hand/arm.

The therapist may observe clinically that midrange isometric contraction is where the transplanted gracilis produces maximal force. The amount of force a skeletal muscle generates during maximal force contraction varies according to its length at the beginning of a contraction.[28] In midrange contraction, the actin and myosin myofilaments that comprise the muscle sarcomere are overlapped optimally and generate its maximal force.[28] The length of the muscle's sarcomeres is at the plateau of the length–tension curve.[28] For example, maximal strength of gracilis may be noted at approximately 70 degrees of elbow flexion and approximately 45 degrees of finger flexion. Gentle strengthening activities are aimed at producing maximal isometric tension at the muscle's optimal length.

Zuker states that the goal of the gracilis muscle transfer is to restore a functional nondominant hand.[10] For transplanted gracilis to restore finger flexion, the child may be prompted to use finger flexion to maintain a static grip around an empty cup. Over time, the child can steadily work to hold items that are smaller in diameter. A child may sustain finger extension to finger paint on a vertical surface. A child may stabilize a lightweight ball or balloon against their trunk using both hands via bilateral elbow flexion. The therapist's ability to assess, grade, and creatively modify objects and activities is critical for the child to be successful during this period of function and gentle strengthening.

As the child integrates the function of gracilis with fewer cues, the therapist can scaffold the goal of building strength and endurance of the gracilis by introducing activities that require work against resistance (MRC 3–4). In his protocol, Chuang (Table 21.4) recommends that once MRC 3 is reached for elbow flexion, resistance training can begin by integrating weightlifting exercises.[20] The aim is to increase 0.5 kg every 6 months up to 3–6 kg maximum.[23]

In the context of motivating activities, the child may be challenged to stabilize cylindrical wooden projects with their finger flexors while sanding with their dominant hand. A child can be prompted to create art on rainbow scratch paper by using finger extension to scrape their fingernails against the resistive paper. A child can propel an arm-driven tricycle (i.e., Ambuks tryke©) or other resistive ride on toys (i.e., power pumper bike) by recruiting their elbow flexion coordinated with their intact triceps. Gentle traditional strengthening activities can also be integrated such as therapy putty and therapy band with an aim for MRC 4–5 (Fig. 21.14).

Optimizing outcome is heavily dependent on caregiver education and home program. The caregivers are supported by the therapist to offer motivating, repetitive, and sustained resistive activities in the child's natural environment. The child continues to build strength and endurance in their FFGT and integrate the function of the muscle transfer in a wider number of everyday, age-appropriate activities (Figs. 21.15 and 21.16).

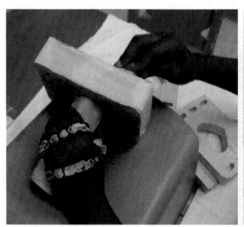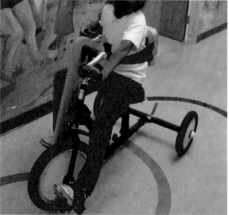

FIG. 21.14 Strengthening of finger flexion through motivating activities to promote resistive grasp.

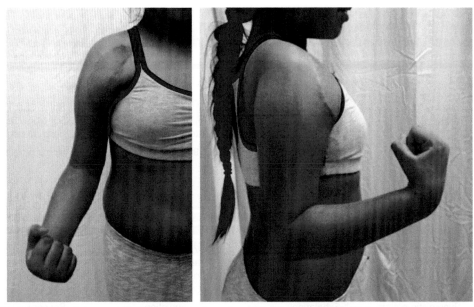

FIG. 21.15 AS status post-FFGT to restore elbow flex. AS achieved AMS 5/MRC 3 elbow flexion at 34 weeks post-FFGT.

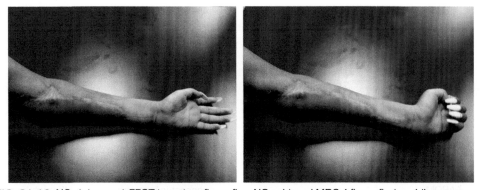

FIG. 21.16 NC status post-FFGT to restore finger flex. NC achieved MRC 4 finger flexion, 1 lb gross grasp, and 0.25 lb lateral pinch at 52 weeks post-FFGT.

CASE STUDY ONE: FFGT FOR ELBOW FLEXION

A.S. is a 9-year-old formerly right-handed girl who sustained a viral illness 3 years prior, and this resulted in acute flaccid myelitis. She was managed conservatively and recovered a modest amount of motion of the right upper extremity with substantially poor elbow flexion. On examination, elbow flexion was AMS 4 with the inability to bring a cup to her mouth. Surgical plan involved transplanting the gracilis muscle from the left medial thigh to the right shoulder region. The transfer was anchored to the clavicle proximally and to the biceps tendon distally. The plan was to power the gracilis muscle with either the spinal accessory or the intercostal nerves. Stimulation of the spinal accessory nerve resulted in no contractions in the trapezius muscle. Stimulation of intercostal nerves 3, 4, 5 showed strong contractions in these and was independently sutured to the obturator nerve for an excellent match. No tension was placed on the nerves and coaptation was performed with the shoulder in 75 degrees of abduction (Table 21.6).

TABLE 21.6
Case Study One: FFGT for Elbow Flexion.

Timeline	Intervention	Measure/Protocol	Outcome	Miscellaneous
10/2014 onset	IVIG × 4		Rehab stay	Outpt. Therapy
7/7/17	Surgery to reconstruct biceps		(a) FFGMT (b) Neurotization intercostal 3,4,5	Spica Cast 75*Sh ab 90* elbow flex Forearm neutral
4 weeks post-op	Sling/elbow flex Sensory estim PROM shoulder Elbow/Hand Tendon compression	−10*/week 20 pps/100pd 30 minutes 2 × /day 45* Full Clavicle/Acromion Gentle elbow flex/ext.	−90*	Home program
8 weeks	Sling PROM shoulder Scar massage Synergistic pattern	−10*/week 90* Exhalation	−70* Pain over 45* Contraction of FFGT	
10 weeks	Synergistic pattern Sling PROM shoulder Gravity eliminated	Exhalation AMS 90* sEMG 5 trials	Reinnervation AMS 1 −50* 70* 83.2 μV 4−9 s	Sensory estim stopped Gracilis innervated HEP include gravity eliminated
13 weeks	Sling Soft elbow ext. Brace Gravity eliminated/ Synergistic pattern	Discontinued	Tightness at biceps insertion 50% movement	Night use Skateboard
16 weeks	Tendon compression Gravity eliminated AAROM	Stopped AMS/MRC Pulley	50% expected movement AMS 3/MRC 2 70% movement 1lb off weight	Towel/table top Home pulley system
18 weeks	Soft elbow ext. Brace Isometric holding	Discontinued	Smooth motion	Games
20 weeks	Robotic program AAROM Against gravity	Tyro motion Diego©	Smooth motion concentric/isometric 10−90* 1lb off weight 90−150*	Excellent follow through home program
25 weeks	Splint Against gravity	Composite ext./elbow/wrist/hand AMS	Full ROM/40 reps AMS 4	Night use
28 weeks	Against gravity Mild resistance Sustained elbow flexion	Elbow flex 0−85* AMS/MRC	30−50 reps Rest break at 10 1# weight full elbow flexion AMS 5/MRC3	Swimming program
34 weeks	sEMG biofeedback	Elbow flex sEMG AMS	0−100* Controlled, isolated elbow flexion 200 μV sustained AMS 6	Fatigues easily Home program No trunk compensation

CASE STUDY TWO: FFGT FOR FINGER FLEXION

N.C. is a 7-year-old girl who fell off the monkey bars and sustained a supracondylar humeral fracture to her nondominant, left upper extremity. Following closed reduction percutaneous pinning and casting of her fracture, N.C. experienced compartment syndrome that was undetected. As a result, N.C. developed severe Volkmann's ischemic contractures to her left upper extremity and presented with severe neurologic and motor deficits. Within a year, N.C.'s forearm was atrophied and the underlying muscles of the volar compartment were firm and fibrotic. N.C. had a significant forearm protonation contracture as well as dorsal subluxation of her radial–ulnar joint. Extensor function was limited. She was able to activate her lumbricals in a limited AROM via ulnar nerve; however, she had no motor function and no sensation in her median nerve. Within a year of injury, she had learned to perform most self-care, school-based, and leisure occupations using just her right upper extremity.

Approximately 1-year postinjury, she underwent a free functional gracilis muscle transfer surgery to restore finger flexion. Necrotic and fibrotic muscles of the volar compartment were resected. Donor vessels, motor nerve, and gracilis muscle were harvested. Neurolysis and repair of the median nerve was performed using four cable grafts from a donor sural nerve. Anastamosis of the nerves and vessels was completed. Skin markings were made to establish the appropriate resting and contractile length of the gracilis. The gracilis was then attached to the medial epicondyle proximally. Distally, the tendons of the flexor digitorum profundus were jointed together as one unit and coapted to the tendon of the gracilis. The surgeon also transferred extensor carpi radialis longus to the flexor pollicis longus for independent thumb flexion. The patient's pronation contracture was released, and the subluxated radioulnar joint was reduced (Table 21.7).

TABLE 21.7
Case Study Two: FFGT for Finger Flexion.

Timeline	Intervention	Measure/Protocol	Outcome	Miscellaneous
11/15/08 onset	CRPP following L humerus Gartland Type III fx.		Compartment syndrome: Volkmann's contracture	Ulnar, median, and radial nerve neuropathies
Time i.e. 4 weeks post-op	Hand rehabilitation Splint: Composite wrist/ finger ext.	Severe Volkmann's contracture		Night splint
11/14/09	Surgery to restore finger/ thumb flex		(a) FFGT (b) Neurotization median nerve (c) Tendon transfer: ECRL to FPL	Complication: Vascular compromise of gracilis/ tissue death
11/23/09	Debridement of prior surgery		(a) Second FFGT (b) Repair of distal neurorrhaphy median nerve	Soft dressing 90* elbow flex 30* wrist flex 90* MCP flex Thumb in palmar ab.
4 weeks post-op	Post-op splint:	30* elbow flex, wrist flex, fingers in natural cascade		Day and night use
5 weeks post-op	Sensory estim	20pps/100pd 30 minutes second 2×/day	0.7–0.8 cm of tendon excursions noted	Home program
	PROM shoulder Elbow/Hand Tendon gliding	Full Early passive mobilization (Table 21.3)		

Continued

TABLE 21.7

Case Study Two: FFGT for Finger Flexion.—cont'd

Timeline	Intervention	Measure/Protocol	Outcome	Miscellaneous
8 weeks	PROM finger flex/ext. Tendon gliding Scar massage ECRL to FPL activation AROM	Full Pair thumb IP flex with radial deviation Finger flex.	Full PROM 15* thumb flex 15* IP flex	Home program Silicone w/splint Tendon transfer active Gracilis innervated, sensory estim stopped
9 weeks	Gravity eliminated AROM sEMG biofeedback	MRC sEMG	MRC 1 via sEMG assessment Cocontraction noted in finger extensors with gracilis	HEP: gravity-eliminated finger flex/ext. Repetition 100x/day
10 weeks	Place and hold AROM finger flex Passive hold objects with wide circumference		20* finger flex Contact pads of fingers on 2.5″ diameter container 25% of the time	HEP: Passive hold of light, wide objects
12 weeks	Splint Gravity eliminated AROM	MP block w/thumb loop MRC	Decreased flex at MPs and thumb CMC in AD 25*IP flex MRC 2	Day use Transition dorsal splint to school and night HEP: Hold lightweight, circumferential containers
16 weeks	Gravity eliminated AAROM Cylindrical grasp and palmar grasps		Decreased flex at MPs, 40* finger flex Grasps 2–3″ objects off tabletop, holds for up to 30 s	Objects are wrapped in dycem or foam built up handle to prevent slippage and increase success
22 weeks	Isometric holds AROM	Bimanual activities	Sustains finger flex around 1.5 diameter object to hold for up to 5 minutes	Lightweight play, games (i.e., holding light bubble/paint container)
24 weeks	Splint Against gravity AROM	Neutral wrist/fingers ext. MRC	Developing wrist ext. Contracture and tightness in finger flex MRC 3	Night use
40 weeks	Incorporate resistive activities Orient objects	Strength training MRC	0–70* MP flex,0–60* PIP flex, 0–40* DIP flex, and 30–80* thumb IP flex MRC 4	Sanding projects, Ambuks© arm tryke, swings, min. Resistive Thera putty
52 weeks	ADLs/leisure activities mCIMT	Dynamometry: 30 minutes, 2×/day using bivalve cast MRC	Gross grasp 1lb Lateral pinch 0.25lb MRC 4	Tying shoelaces, fixing hair, Wii controller, jump roping, power pumper bike

OUTCOMES AND TIMELINES

Progress can be expected up to 2 years following FFGT.[3,10] Continued rehabilitation is essential in maximizing the efficacy of the transfer. Even in patients who achieved an MRC 4 or higher following FFGT, histology revealed only 46% of muscle fibers appeared healthy and only 60% of regenerated nerves had met there receptor targets.[3,29]

FFGT for Elbow Flexion

- Kay et al. compared outcomes in adults and children and found that 64% of all those studied achieved an MRC 4 or higher. In that same group, 92% of children with perinatal brachial plexus achieved an MRC 4 or higher.[5]
- Chuang et al. assessed weight lifting outcomes and determined the ability to lift 0.5–3 kg as good, and 3–8 kg as excellent.[23]

FFGT for Finger Flexion

- Zuker et al. published the following outcomes.[10]
- Average 1.45 cm pulp to proximal palmar crease
- Average total active motion (TAM) = 158 degrees
- 25% of grip strength of contralateral hand
- Functional nondominant hand

REFERENCES

1. Stevanovic M, Sharpe F. Management of established Volkmann's contracture of the forearm in children. *Hand Clin.* 2006;22:99–111.
2. Tsuge K. Treatment of established Volkmann's contracture. *J Bone Joint Surg Am.* 1975;57A(7):925–929.
3. Stevanovic M, Sharpe F. Functional free muscle transfer for upper extremity reconstruction. *Plast Reconstr Surg.* 2014; 134:257e.
4. Oishi SN, Ezaki M. Free gracilis transfer to restore finger flexion in Volkmann ischemic contracture. *Tech Hand Surg.* 2010;14:104–107.
5. Kay S, Pinder R, Wiper J, Hart A, Jones F, Yates A. Microvascular free functioning gracilis transfer with nerve transfer to establish elbow flexion. *J Plast Reconstr Aesthet Surg.* 2010; 63:1142–1149.
6. Doi K, Hattori Y, Yamazaki H, Wahegaonkar A, Addosooki A, Watanave M. Importance of early passive mobilization following double free gracilis muscle transfer. *Plast Reconstr Surg.* 2008;121:2037.
7. Medical Research Council. *Aids to the Investigation of the Peripheral Nervous System.* London: Her Majesty's Stationary Office; 1943 (Medical Research Council).
8. Curtis C, Stephens D, Clarke HM, Andrews D. The active movement scale: an evaluative tool for infants with obstetrical brachial plexus palsy. *J Hand Surg.* 2002; 27(3):470–478, 2002.
9. Campbell MEJ, Cunnington R. More than an imitation game: top-down modulation of the human mirror system. *Neubiorev.* 2017;75:195–202.
10. Zucker RM, Egerszegi EP, Manktelow RI, McLeod A, Candlish S. Volkman's ischemic contracture in children. The results of free vascularized muscle transplantation. *Microsurgery.* 1991;12:341–345.
11. Liu Y, Lao J, Zhao X. Comparative study of phrenic and intercostal nerve transfers for elbow flexion after global brachial plexus injury. *Injury.* 2015;46:671–675.
12. Gordon T, Mao J. Muscle atrophy and procedures for training after spinal cord injury. *Phys Ther.* 1994;74(1): 50–60.
13. Gigo-Benato D, Russo TL, Geuna S, Domingues NR, Salvin TF, Parizo HO. Electrical stimulation impairs early functional recovery and accentuates skeletal muscle atrophy after sciatic crush injury in rats. *Muscle Nerve.* 2010; 41:685–693.
14. Tam SL, Gordon T. Neuromuscular activity impairs axonal sprouting in partially denervated muscles inhibiting bridge formation and Schwann cells. *Dev Neurobiology.* 2003;57(2):221–234.
15. Smania N, Berto G, Marchina E. Rehabilitation of brachial plexus injuries in adults and children. *Eur J Phys Rehabil Med.* 2012;48:483–506.
16. Rosenkranz K, Rothwell JC. Differences between the effects of three plasticity inducing protocols on the organization of the human motor cortex. *Eur J Neurosci.* 2006;23: 822–829.
17. Gordon T, Brushart TM, Amirjan N, Chan M. The potential of electrical stimulation to promote functional recovery after peripheral nerve injury comparisons between rats and humans. *Acta Neurochir Suppl.* 2007;100:3–11.
18. Asensio-Pinilla E, Udina E, Jaramillo J, Navarro X. Electrical stimulation combined with exercise increase axonal regeneration after peripheral nerve injury. *Exp Neurol.* 2009;219:258–265.
19. Berggren J, Baker LL. Therapeutic application of electrical stimulation and constraint induced movement therapy in perinatal brachial plexus injury: a case report. *J Hand Ther.* 2015;28:217–221.
20. Chuang DC. Nerve transfers in adult brachial plexus injuries: my methods. *Hand Clin.* 2005;21:71–82.
21. Hattori Y, Doi k, Fuchigami Y, Abe Y, Kawai S. Experimental study on donor nerves for brachial plexus injury: comparison between the spinal accessory nerve and the intercostal nerve. *Plast Reconstr Surg.* 1997;100(4):900–906.
22. Gutowski KA, Orenstein HH. Restoration of elbow flexion after brachial plexus injury: the role of nerve and muscle transfers. *Plast Reconstr Surg.* 2000;106(6):1348–1357.
23. Chuang DC, Epstein MD, Yeh MC, Wei FC. Functional restoration of elbow flexion in brachial plexus injuries: results in 167 patients. *J Hand Surg.* 1993;18:285–291.

24. Muratori LM, Lamberg EM, Quinn L, Duff SV. Applying principles of motor learning and control to upper extremity rehabilitation. *J Hand Ther.* 2013;26:94–103.

25. Udina E, Puigdemasa A, Navarro X. Passive and active exercise improves regeneration and muscle reinnervation after peripheral nerve injury in the rat. *Muscle Nerve.* 2011; 43:500–509.

26. Novak C, Von der Hedye R. Rehabilitation of the upper extremity following nerve and tendon reconstruction: when and How. *Semin Plast Surg.* 2015;29:73–80.

27. Taub E, Ramey SL, DeLuca S. Efficacy of constraint-induced movement therapy for children with cerebral palsy with asymmetric motor impairment. *Pediatrics.* 2004;113(2):305–312.

28. Gordon A, Huxley A, Julian F. The variation in isometric tension with sarcomere length in vertebrate muscle fibres. *J Physiol.* 1966;184:170–192.

29. Bullinger KL, Nardelli P, Pinter MJ, Alvarez FJ, Cope TC. Permanent central synaptic disconnection of proprioceptors after nerve injury and regeneration. II. Loss of functional connectivity with moto neurons. *J Neurophysiol.* 2011;6:2471–2485.

FURTHER READING

1. Doi K, Kazuhiro S, Kuwata N, Ihara K, Kawai S. Reconstruction of finger and elbow function after complete avulsion of the brachial plexus. *J Hand Surg.* 1991;5(16A):796–803.

CHAPTER 22

Amputations and Replants

RITU GOEL, MS, OTR/L • ALEXANDRIA L. CASE, BSE • DANIELLE A. HOGARTH, BS • JOSHUA M. ABZUG, MD

INTRODUCTION

Traumatic amputations are a challenge at any age, often requiring extensive input from the medical and therapy team to provide the patient with the optimal functional outcome. Therapists are involved in the treatment program to assist the patient in achieving functional independence through improved use of their remaining limb. In the case of a pediatric traumatic amputation, involving the parents and family in the treatment team and explaining the treatment plan and goals are of utmost importance.

Traumatic limb loss in the pediatric population is an emotionally and psychologically stressful occurrence for a child and their family. A knowledgeable healthcare team, including the medical and therapy team, is essential to minimize the stress.[1] Children have a significant advantage in healing as compared to adults in that their bones and soft tissues heal faster, with less scar formation and adhesion, as well as impeccable speed and potential for nerve regeneration and recovery following repair.[1]

This chapter aims to provide the treating therapist with a background of various types of traumatic amputations, medical intervention, and rehabilitation. Upper extremity traumatic amputations proximal to the digits are much less commonly seen in the pediatric population and therefore, this chapter will focus solely on traumatic digital amputation and replantation.

MECHANISM OF INJURY

Various types of traumatic injuries are typically associated with amputations: crush injuries, avulsion-type injuries, abrasions, and lacerations.[2,3] Crush and avulsion-type injuries typically occur in younger children, between 0 and 5 years old, whereas lacerations more common in adolescents and are often caused by a sharp object.[3–6] Crush injuries may be caused by a finger caught in a doorway, bicycle chain or from

interaction with a stationary exercise bicycle[2,3]; whereas, avulsion injuries may result from a forceful traction.[7] (Fig. 22.1). Treadmills are also a common cause of traumatic injury, often leading to abrasions and lacerations occurring when a child places its fingers in the moving parts while the parent is exercising.[2]

Nontraumatic amputations can also occur that are performed for various reasons including infection, tumors, congenital abnormalities, or vascular abnormalities.[2] Typically, nontraumatic amputations are an elective procedure performed to prevent further medical issues related to a problem on a digit.

MEDICAL INTERVENTION

Replantation refers to the reattachment of a completely severed body part; whereas, revascularization refers to the reattachment of a part with an intact bridge of soft tissue that requires vascular repair to prevent necrosis of the partially severed distal part.[8] Not all upper extremity amputations are appropriate for replantation procedures, although the pediatric population has better results than the adult population in terms of replantation success.[8,9]

Following an acute injury, the physician will examine the patient to identify any exposed bone, tissue loss, and nail and/or nail-bed involvement.[10] The injury is typically debrided (cleaned to remove dead tissue and contaminants) at this time to decrease the risk of infection in the wound.[11] Radiographs may be obtained if there is concern for bony involvement.[10] The medical team will also determine if replantation of the severed part is indicated. In pediatrics, replantation is often attempted for optimal functional outcomes and psychological considerations.[12]

Replantations following sharp amputations are typically approached with a direct repair, and are the most favorable instance of traumatic amputation for such procedures. Although all pediatric amputations should be considered for replantation, optimal indications

Pediatric Hand Therapy. https://doi.org/10.1016/B978-0-323-53091-0.00022-1

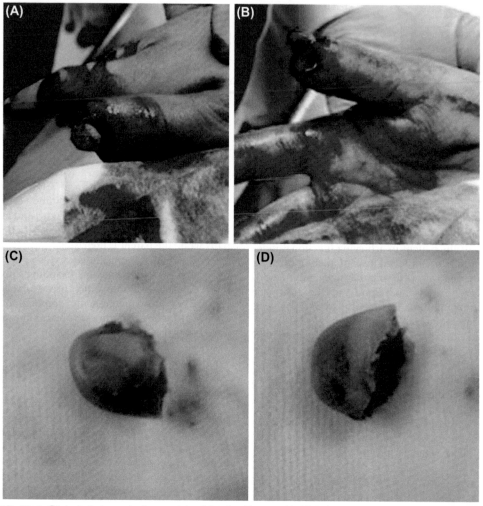

FIG. 22.1 Clinical photograph of an avulsion injury in a 7-year-old child who's thumb was slammed in a door. **(A)** Dorsal view of thumb with exposed distal phalanx. **(B)** Volar view of thumb with exposed distal phalanx. **(C)** Dorsal view of amputated part. **(D)** Volar view of amputated part with visible bruising indicating a crush component to the injury as well. (Courtesy of Joshua M. Abzug, MD.)

include clean, guillotine amputations; thumb amputations; multiple digit amputations; digit amputations distal to the flexor digitorum superficialis (FDS) insertion; and hand level and proximal amputations.[3,10,13] Crush and avulsion amputations are often approached using grafts due to the greater extent of tissue and vascular injuries typically associated with such injury mechanisms. In cases where multiple digits have been amputated, it is recommended that a stepwise approach be performed across all fingers, working through each of the previous described steps for each finger before moving onto the repair of the next structure (Fig. 22.2). Alternatively, surgeons may elect to perform complete

replantations in the order of most functionality to least with the thumb, then middle digit, followed by the index, ring, and small digits. Failed replantation procedures are addressed with revisions, if possible, or ray resections.

For amputated digits, the goal of operative intervention is to preserve as much tissue as possible while repairing existing structures to restore functionality. First, the vessels and nerves are identified and tagged with suture, then both the stump and the detached portion of the digit are thoroughly irrigated and debrided. The next priority is skeletal fixation, followed by repair of the flexor tendon. Then, the surgeon will

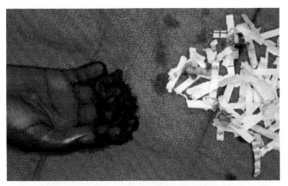

FIG. 22.2 Clinical photograph of a multidigit amputation trauma caused by fingers being trapped in a paper shredder. (Courtesy of Joshua M. Abzug, MD.)

perform anastomoses of the arteries with interpositional vein grafting, as needed. Following the artery anastomosis, the nerves will be repaired, and then venous anastomosis will be performed, with or without interpositional vein grafting. Finally, the skin will be closed if possible (Figs. 22.3 and 22.4). It is also important to note that additional procedures, such as a tenolysis, may be necessary to improve function following a successful replantation.[3,14,15] Postoperatively, the replanted part is placed in a bulky dressing to permit resting of the extremity in an elevated position to assist with venous return (Fig. 22.5).

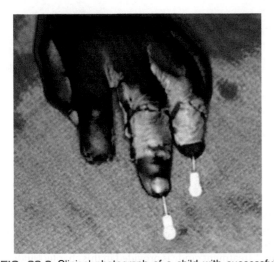

FIG. 22.3 Clinical photograph of a child with successful replantation surgery after fingers were trapped in an exercycle machine. Note that revision amputation of the index finger was necessary because of the severity of the injury caused by the wheel spokes. (Courtesy of Shriners Hospital for Children, Philadelphia, PA.)

FINGERTIP AMPUTATION AND NAIL-BED INJURY

In the case of a nail-bed injury, the nail plate is removed, and the nail-bed laceration is repaired. The nail plate or a substitute is then replaced to act as a protective splint until new nail plate growth occurs. Complete and partial amputations may be treated operatively when it is thought that the remaining piece is viable (Fig. 22.6). Alternatively, these injuries can be allowed to heal by secondary intention via scarring and epithelialization[16] (Fig. 22.7). Most children will not require formal therapy for this type of injury, as they will regain their range of motion and sensation over time. A mitten cast or cap splint may be utilized in the acute phase to limit the sensitivity that can occur when the digit is accidentally touched or banged into.

Composite grafts are another option for surgical repair of a digital fingertip amputation or avulsion injury. The benefit of such procedures is the low disruption in digit integrity, specifically the avoidance of digital shortening and functional ability by utilizing the patient's own skin at the fingertip.[17]

DIGITAL RECONSTRUCTION FOR SKIN LOSS

Surgical intervention options for digital amputation include skin grafts, skin flaps, and ray resection with possible transposition procedures. Skin grafts include composite grafts, full- or split-thickness skin graft, and/or substitute skin graft materials. Skin flaps for partial digital reconstruction include regional or local soft tissue flaps such as the V–Y advancement flap, volar advancement, Moberg flap, and cross-finger flaps.[16] In cases where the amputation occurs more proximally on the digit, near the metacarpophalangeal joint, a ray resection can be performed. A ray resection, which may improve the aesthetics following a digit amputation, can compromise hand width and grip strength.[18]

A skin graft is used when the wound is too large in size and depth for wound closure or local flap reconstruction, thus requiring skin from an alternate donor site to cover the wound. The wound/skin graft and donor site are both closed with absorbable sutures. Following a skin graft, the postoperative management is of utmost importance. Graft survival is improved by a stringent local immobilization protocol, often requiring immobilization of associated joints with a splint or cast for protection and to decrease the risk of shearing the graft.[16] Patients are typically referred to occupational therapy for rehabilitation. Therapy sessions should focus on wound care and scar management, mobility, and

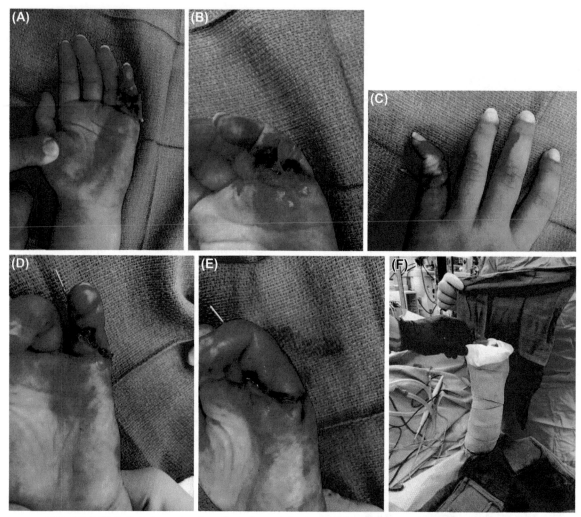

FIG. 22.4 Clinical photographs of a patient who sustained an avulsion partial amputation by getting their finger caught between a boat and a dock with significant vascular and soft tissue damage. Note the lack of perfusion to the distal aspect of the affected digit. **(A)** Volar view, **(B)** ulnar view, **(C)** dorsal view, **(D)** postoperative volar view, **(E)** postoperative ulnar view, and **(F)** postoperative bulky splint Clinical photograph of postoperative fixation. Note the incomplete wound closure due to swelling of the digit. (Courtesy of Joshua M. Abzug, MD.)

desensitization. Therapists should also address the patient's edema, sensory reeducation, range of motion, and fine motor coordination skills, as well as protective and functional splinting (Table 22.1).

THERAPY
Therapists are involved in the treatment program to assist the patient in achieving their functional independence through improved use of their hand/remaining limb. The ultimate goal of treatment is

for a pain-free limb, healthy skin coverage, and normal function of the hand. Although digit length and aesthetics are considered, preserving functional use with decreased pain and concerns of infection are prioritized.

A treatment guide is provided in this chapter for digit amputation and reconstruction as well as digital replantation (Appendix). Therapists are encouraged to review protocols with the referring physician before implementation to ensure agreement and appropriateness for the patient (Table 22.2).

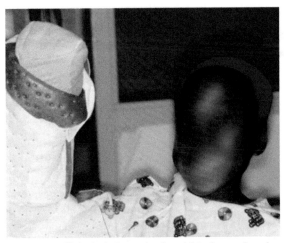

FIG. 22.5 Clinical photograph of a child after undergoing finger replantation. Note upright elevation of fingers and hand to promote venous return for optimal healing. (Courtesy of Shriners Hospital for Children, Philadelphia, PA.)

PEDIATRIC-SPECIFIC CONSIDERATIONS

In all aspects of therapy, patient and family education are a constant. In the case of a pediatric amputation or replantation, involving the parents in the treatment team and explaining the treatment plan and goals are of utmost importance. The necessary education must go a step further to explain the treatment and plan, while including the patient and their parents in the treatment for carryover, and ensuring there is comfort with the intervention. It is sometimes helpful to speak to the parents without the child present to allow time for questions or concerns, and to provide reassurance. When speaking to the patient, it is vital to explain the components of treatment in terms that they understand, keeping in mind their age and grade level. Using familiar analogies and keeping the conversation as comfortable as possible for the child will ease their fear and anxiety toward the injury and treatment. Although some adult patients will embrace an attitude of "do what you have to do," when working with children, it is generally better to explain what you are going to do before you do it to minimize the element of surprise, guarding due to the anticipation of pain, and to decrease overall anxiety. Gaining the trust of pediatric patients will make the therapy experience more positive and successful.

Pediatrics spans a wide age range, including patients from birth to until their 18th birthday. During this time frame, an extensive array of developmental milestones and levels of independence are encountered. It is beneficial to remain mindful of the child's age, stages of development for bone formation and healing time, family/social environment, and vocabulary for communication. Furthermore, having treatment modalities that are age appropriate and engaging for the child may increase the success of a treatment session. For example, toys with music, bright colors, and blinking lights tend to be attention grabbing and intriguing for young children. Colorful stacking blocks, bouncing balls, and even a child-sized table and chair for the child to sit at may promote engagement and comfort in the treatment room for many school age children. Older children and adolescents may benefit from competitive, challenging games and activities such as beanbag toss or cornhole, video games such as Wii sports, and incorporating basic cooking skills.

The healing capacity and healing time are enhanced within the pediatric group, which differs from adult and geriatric groups. Although the injury may be similar to that of an adult, the healing time and treatment protocol varies substantially between the two populations. This is largely due to the accelerated healing time of pediatric patients that results in fewer secondary complications, as compared to adults.[8,9]

GENERAL EVALUATION AND ASSESSMENT CONSIDERATIONS

Careful attention should be given to the referring physician's protocol, clarifying restrictions and precautions the physician may have related to a specific case. The following protocol, evaluation, and treatment specifications are meant to be a guide for treating therapists. Therapists are encouraged to discuss appropriateness of the protocol with the referring physician to ensure agreement.

Upon evaluation of a pediatric patient with a digit, hand, or proximal upper extremity amputation and subsequent surgical repair, it is beneficial to assess the following: medical history, mechanism of injury, wound assessment, objective measures (range of motion and strength), fine motor coordination skills/prehensile patterns, and overall functional use of the upper extremity.

Sensory testing can produce inconsistent results in children, as they may experience a challenge with describing sensory changes or paresthesias in their hands.[20] Dua et al. (2016) established normative values for the pediatric population using the Semmes–Weinstein Monofilament Test and two-point discrimination, static and moving, which should be used for comparison during assessment as well as to determine the level of sensory compromise.[20] Dua et al. (2016) also determined objective testing with monofilaments

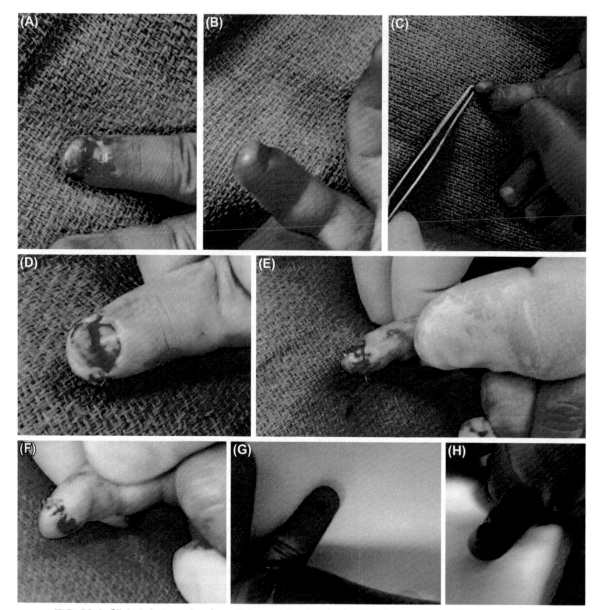

FIG. 22.6 Clinical photographs of a partial amputation in a young child that was bitten by a parrot. **(A)** Dorsal view, **(B)** volar view, **(C)** intraoperative assessment, **(D)** dorsal view postoperatively, **(E)** ulnar view postoperatively, **(F)** radial view postoperatively, **(G)** 1-year follow-up showing near-normal appearance of the digit but persistent nail plate deformity, and **(H)** ulnar aspect of digit at 1 year postoperatively. (Courtesy of Joshua M. Abzug, MD.)

to be reliable in children 4 years old and above, whereas density testing using two-point discrimination is reliable in children age 6 and above.[20] Knowing normative values and age-appropriateness of sensory assessments are two integral pieces of information for clinicians in determining appropriateness of sensory assessments with the pediatric population.

The functional assessment includes observation of fine motor coordination skills, prehensile patterns, as well as use of the involved upper extremity with activity

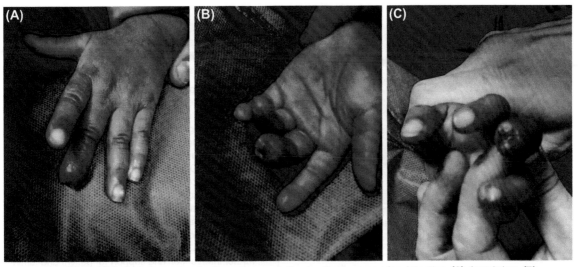

FIG. 22.7 Clinical photographs of a fingertip amputation healing by secondary intention. **(A)** dorsal view, **(B)** volar view, and **(C)** tip view. (Courtesy of Joshua M. Abzug, MD.)

TABLE 22.1
Overview of Treatement Goals After Hand or Finger Amputation Injuries.

Treatment Goals

- Pain management and reduction
- Optimize healing time
- Preserve sensibility and length of limb
- Prevent painful neuromas
- Avoid or limit nail deformity
- Minimize time away from school/play
- Aesthetically pleasing appearance

Data from Peterson SL, Peterson EL, Wheatley MJ. Management of fingertip amputations. *J Hand Surg Am.* 2014; 39(10):2093–2101.

TABLE 22.2
Phases of Rehabilitation Following Hand Replantation.

Initial Phase	• Protecting the repair • Edema management • Wound care • Splinting
Intermediate phase	• Scar management • Scar desensitization • Range of motion • Address emotional/ psychological concerns
Late phase	• Functional retraining • Strengthening skills • Sensory reeducation • Activities of daily living retraining

Data from Bueno E, Benjamin MJ, Sisk G, Sampson CE, Carty M, Pribaz JJ, Pomahac B, Talbot SG. Rehabilitation following hand transplantation. *Hand (N.Y)* 2014; 9(1):9–15.

performance. Standardized assessments typically used to assess fine motor skills and hand function include Functional Dexterity Test,[21–23] Nine Hole Peg Test[24] (Fig. 22.8), Box and Block Test[25] (Fig. 22.9), Purdue Pegboard,[26,27] and Jebsen Taylor Hand Function Test.[28] Reviewing assessment norms for age appropriateness is recommended. Observation is another method of assessing functional use of the hand and upper extremity during play activity, object handling, and manipulation, as well as during activities of daily living tasks such as self-feeding and fastener management skills.

GENERAL TREATMENT CONSIDERATIONS

General treatment considerations to have during the rehabilitation process when caring for pediatric patients

who have sustained partial or complete amputation injuries are the following (Tables 22.3 and 22.4).

WOUND CARE

Patient and family education on signs of infection should be discussed on the first therapy visit in addition to dressing change technique and frequency. Initial wound care will typically consist of a nonadherent (Xeroform or Adaptic) dressing. Specifics regarding

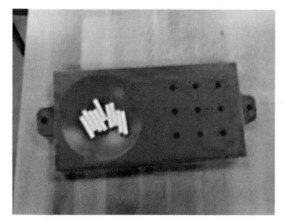

FIG. 22.8 Nine Hole Peg Test. (Courtesy of Ritu Goel, OTR/L.)

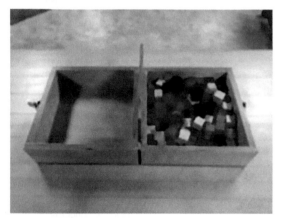

FIG. 22.9 Box and Block Test. (Courtesy of Ritu Goel, OTR/L.)

preferred dressings should be discussed with the physician (Table 22.3).

Following removal of the sutures and wound closure, scar management protocols should include massage, mobility, and desensitization, as needed. Scar massage with cocoa butter after the incision has closed using a cross-friction massage technique may assist with scar tissue breakdown, as well as improve scar and joint/limb mobility. Parents and the patient are educated on performing this technique when outside of therapy as part of a home program to minimize scar tissue development.

Despite steps taken for scar management, hypertrophic or keloid scars can present. This type of abnormal scarring can cause irritation (increased temperature, redness, and pain) around the skin, as well as increase the firmness

---

TABLE 22.3
Treatment Goals for Therapy Following Partial or Full Amputation Injuries.

Treatment Goals

- Protect all repaired structures: nerves, vessels, tendons, bones/fractures
- Promote and monitor wound healing and closure
- Edema management and reduction
- Functional and protective splinting as needed
- Pain management and reduction
- Full active ROM of all involved and uninvolved joints
- Desensitization/sensory reeducation of the amputated digit/part
- Patient and family education
- Prosthetic evaluation and training, as needed
- Return to functional activity and independence
- Psychological evaluation and determination need for further intervention and support for patient and family

Data from Walsh JM, Chee N. Replantation. In: Saunders RJ, Astifidis RP, Burke SL, Higgins JP, McClinton MA, editors. Hand and upper extremity rehabilitation: a practical guide 4th ed. St. Louis: Elsevier; 2016. 431–439.

TABLE 22.4
Potential Complications to be Aware of During Recovery Period.

Potential Complications

- Infection
- Hypersensitivity
- Diminished sensation
- Cold intolerance
- Neuroma formation
- Scar/keloid formation
- Scar immobility
- Stiffness
- Phantom pain

Data from Boulas HJ. Amputations of the fingers and hand: indications for replantation. J Am Acad Orthop Surg 1998; 6(2):100–5; Jaeger SH, Tsai TM, Kleinert HE. Upper extremity replantation in children. Orthop Clin North Am 1981; 12(4):897–907.; Koczan BJ, Ware LC. Digital amputation and ray resection. In: Saunders RJ, Astifidis RP, Burke SL, Higgins JP, McClinton MA, eds. *Hand and upper extremity rehabilitation: a practical guide.* 4th ed. St. Louis: Elsevier; 2016. 441–446; Urgurlar M, Kabakas F, Purisa H, Sezer I, Celikdelen P, Ozcelick IB. Rehabilitation after successful finger replantation. *North Clin Istanb* 2016; 3(1):22–6.

and height of the scar.[31] Silicone gel sheeting is an effective method of topical scar management used to minimize scar volume, tenderness, itching, and redness.[31] Additional topical methods of scar management including elastomer putty and silicone gel digit caps (such as Silopad), can assist with scar desensitization, protection, healing, and patient comfort.[32]

EDEMA MANAGEMENT

Postoperative edema is a common presentation in the hand due to the inflammatory response during tissue healing.[33,34] During the fibroplastic stage of healing, edema is promptly addressed to prevent additional joint stiffness, pain, and delays in healing.[34] Following an amputation, circulatory, venous, and arterial compromise, as well as decreased sensation are common presentations. In such cases, methods of edema management are limited as common techniques are often contraindicated as they may have adverse effects on tissue healing.[33,34] Cryotherapy, retrograde massage, and compression are all commonly employed methods of edema reduction that are too aggressive following an amputation.

Active range of motion (AROM), upon medical clearance, in an elevated position is a beneficial method of edema management, as it uses active movement to pump fluid out of the hand.[34] Furthermore, this method is completely controlled by the patient, with no external pressure involved, and therefore often gives the patient the added comfort of being in control of the movement. In addition, this is also a good exercise for the child to perform for their home exercises, and therefore their parents should also be educated on this exercise to ensure adequate carryover.

SPLINTING

For digital amputations, splinting may include a clamshell tip protector or trough splint to allow the finger time to heal in a protective position. Infants and toddler age children are commonly referred to as "Houdinis," due to their impeccable ability to "escape" out of a cast or splint without undoing straps.[35] Using a hand-based splint, such as a hand-based digit extension splint, is beneficial compared to a tip protector or trough splint for younger children, as it increases the difficulty of splint removal by the patient. However, it is important to note that a hand-based splint may involve more digit inclusion than necessary; therefore, therapists should encourage parents to mobilize the unaffected joints or digits at every diaper and/or dressing change to keep the uninvolved digits supple.

For older children and adolescents, a tip protector, cap splint, or trough splint can be beneficial following a digital amputation (Fig. 22.10). This type of splint would be used for protective purposes as well as to stabilize the involved joint(s). Furthermore, the low profile would allow for proximal joint movement, thereby limiting unnecessary stiffness of uninvolved joints.

DESENSITIZATION AND SENSORY REEDUCATION

Following splint discontinuation, issuing the patient a silicone gel digit cap (such as Silopad) may assist with scar healing, desensitization, and patient comfort.[32] Encouraging use of the hand will expose the digit to various textures through everyday use, allowing the amputated digit to be exposed for desensitization. In therapy, sensory sticks of various textures, rice bins with appropriately sized objects, Fluidotherapy, and shaving cream activities are a few options for desensitization of the affected limb (Fig. 22.11).

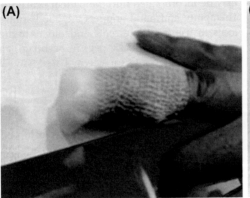
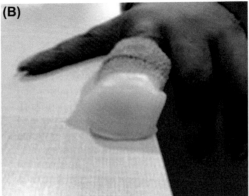

FIG. 22.10 Clinical photograph of a child with a therapist molded tip protector orthosis: **(A)** side view and **(B)** tip view. (Courtesy of Ritu Goel, OTR/L.)

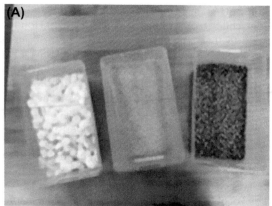 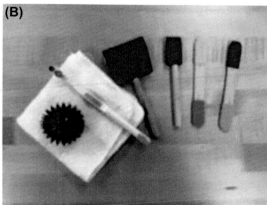

FIG. 22.11 Desensitization therapy modalities including **(A)** rice bins and **(B)** various textured sensory sticks. (Courtesy of Ritu Goel, OTC/L.)

Education of safety concerns with sensory deficits is imperative to review with the patient and parents. For example, a patient with compromised sensation may be unable to decipher if the temperature of an object on the hand is too hot or cold.

Phantom limb pain is another common symptom experienced by patients following an amputation. Phantom limb pain refers to a neuropathic pain of the amputated limb's presence postamputation.[36] Neuropathic pain is typically described with symptoms of numbness, tingling, burning, and/or shocking descriptors. Mirror therapy has been found to be an effective method to decrease phantom limb pain.[36] Mirror therapy is a treatment technique in which the uninvolved extremity performs movements while watching its mirror image on a mirror box laid overtop the unseen impaired extremity, thereby causing a visual illusion of the impaired extremity performing the movements.[37,38]

THERAPEUTIC EXERCISE

Before attending therapy, parents and the patient are educated on AROM exercises for all uninvolved joints, from the shoulder to the hand, which are performed regularly throughout the day to limit guarding and stiffness from disuse. Upon medical clearance, active and passive range of motion (PROM) exercises are initiated to the involved joints. Initial treatment exercises may include a tenodesis pattern to promote passive digit motion with active wrist motion or tendon gliding exercises. Patients and parents should be educated on all exercises performed in therapy to carryover at home as part of their home exercise program.

Blocking exercises are beneficial for isolated FDS and flexor digitorum profundus (FDP) tendon excursion and should be incorporated into the treatment plan. However, therapists should be aware of the surgical procedures performed as this may impact when certain exercises are introduced. Initiating blocking exercises prematurely following an FDS or FDP tendon repair can put too much tension on the repair, which could rupture the repair.

Place-and-hold exercises are also effective digit exercises to increase composite motion. In this exercise, the therapist places the digit in a composite flexion position and has the patient attempt to hold that position for a period of time, typically 5–10 seconds. This is a good exercise for pediatric patients of any age, with an age-appropriate explanation of the exercise for the younger population.

Upon medical clearance, strengthening exercises may be incorporated into the patient's treatment plan. Theraputty and hand grippers are good strengthening tools to use for adolescents and older children. Play toys such as Lego blocks, pegs in pegboard, and Play-doh, are good options for activity-based hand strengthening for younger children.

FUNCTIONAL RETRAINING

Children often need to be restricted from performing too much movement when they sustain an injury; however, depending on the child's personality, he or she may be timid to return to using the affected hand functionally after healing has occurred. The ultimate goal is for the patient to return to functional use of the involved extremity. Therefore, a focus on functional tasks and games should be incorporated into the treatment plan.

Once the hand splint has been discontinued and the incision is healed, play activities to encourage active motion and use of the hand is beneficial to the patient, as well as the family, to see what types of movements the child can perform. For example, to improve digit extension, activities may include clapping hands or playing pat-a-cake, rolling Play-doh, and/or making handprints on the wall with finger paint. To improve digit flexion, activities such as grasping utensils or writing, holding/throwing a ball, and/or holding bike handles may be utilized. Age-appropriate board games, card games, corn hole, or beanbag toss are functional activities that will encourage upper extremity use and engagement in the treatment session. In the case of sensory concerns, finding objects in dry rice, sand, and/or water may be helpful for desensitization.

PROSTHETIC EVALUATION AND TRAINING

Although many options for static and dynamic prostheses are available for pediatric patients, not all patients will be interested in a prosthesis following an amputation. James et al. (2006) explored the quality of life and functional performance in children with unilateral, congenital below elbow deficiency.[39] The results of their study showed that nonprosthesis wearers have the same or better functional performance as compared to prosthesis wearers.[39] The authors concluded that an infant or young child's function and/or quality of life does not seem to be improved with the use of a prosthesis.[39] However, prostheses may assist with aesthetics and social acceptance, as well as, performance in specialized activities.

For those patients interested in pursuing a prosthesis, they can be directed to a prosthetist who will discuss the prosthesis that best suits the patient's and family's interest. These may be designed for aesthetic or functional purposes, or a combination of both. Upon receiving a prosthesis, the patient may return to therapy for training as needed. For additional information and details on prosthetics, please refer to the prosthetics chapter of this book.

EMOTIONAL AND PSYCHOLOGICAL CONSIDERATIONS

Although the protocol for advancement in functional use and performance of the extremity is of priority in therapy, it is also imperative for the therapist to be cautious and conscientious of the patient's emotional and psychological state of mind. Emotional and psychological effects of an amputation, prosthesis, and/or replantation can have immense effects on a child.

School-aged children can experience a myriad of obstacles in school without the addition of physical disfigurement or altered aesthetics. Speaking candidly about school, friends, the home environment, and their siblings can help the child feel comfortable with the therapist and allow the child to discuss frustrations and concerns related to the injury. Furthermore, directing the conversation toward subjects such as games, play, and sports can help the therapist understand what activities the child is interested in returning to, which can then be incorporated into the treatment sessions. The therapist can offer alternative methods of coping such as adaptive techniques or equipment to assist with task performance as well as having the child interact with counselors or support groups.

CONCLUSION

Treating a child following a traumatic amputation is challenging. Being aware of the patient, their family, as well as their social environment are important to consider when developing the treatment plan. Creative fabrication of a variety of orthoses is beneficial to ensure maximal functionality, as well as optimal aesthetics, for children with these injuries. Keeping the parents involved in the treatment plan and sessions is encouraged to ensure adequate carryover in the home environment. Finally, consideration of the patient and their family's goals is of utmost importance to assure full compliance and reach full healing potential. Using adaptive equipment and modified techniques to return the child to the playground or their desired activities will highly improve the child's and their families' overall quality of life.

APPENDIX

POSTOPERATIVE THERAPY PROTOCOLS
Postoperative Therapy Protocol for Nail-Bed Repair Procedures

Time Postoperative	Therapy Type	Instructions
10–14 days, upon cast removal	Splinting	• Tip protector orthosis to protect fingertip • Protective orthosis maintaining digit in extension, keeping next proximal joint free to limit stiffness. • For younger children, it may be beneficial to fabricate a hand-based splint including only the involved digit. A larger splint will be more difficult to doff by the child independently.
	Range of motion	• Range of motion exercises should be immediately initiated to patient tolerance. • Exercises be performed five times per day, for 10-minutes sessions. • Be aware of the above listed precautions before initiating ROM in the event of concurrent injuries.

Data from Cannon NM. Amputation. In: Cannon NM, ed. *Diagnosis and Treatment Manual for Physicians and Therapists: Upper Extremity Rehabilitation. Indianapolis*: The Hand Rehabilitation Center of Indiana PC; 2001. 1.

Postoperative Therapy Protocol for Fingertip Amputation Procedures

Time Postoperative	Therapy Type	Instructions
10–14 days, upon cast removal	Splinting	• A trough splint or a clamshell tip protector orthosis should be fabricated for single-digit amputations. • The protective orthosis should maintain digit extension, keeping the next proximal joint free to limit stiffness of uninvolved joints • For younger children, it may be beneficial to fabricate a hand-based splint including only the involved digit(s). A larger splint will be more difficult to doff by the child independently.
2 weeks	Range of motion	• Initiate active and passive range of motion exercises immediately, to patient tolerance, every 2 hours. • No pressure should be placed on the distal stump. • Be mindful of previously listed precautions before initiating ROM in the event of concurrent injuries.
	Edema management	• Before wound closure: elevation, AROM exercises • Upon wound closure: compression sleeves, retrograde massage
	Phantom pain management	• Mirror therapy, desensitization, active motion, functional use
	Scar management	• Initiated upon wound closure • Scar massage and mobilization • Elastomer™ molds, silicone gel sheets, silicone gel digit cap (such as Silopad), kinesiotape • Initiated upon wound closure
8 weeks	Strengthening	• Strengthening exercises should be initiated when motion is achieved. • Use of products such as TheraPutty, hand gripper, stress balls, and resistive clothespins can be beneficial in gradually regaining strength in affected digit(s).

Data from Cannon, 2001[41] and Koczan BJ, Ware LC. Digital amputation and ray resection. In: Saunders RJ, Astifidis RP, Burke SL, Higgins JP, McClinton MA, eds. *Hand and Upper Extremity Rehabilitation: A Practical Guide*. 4th ed. St. Louis: Elsevier; 2016. 441–446.

Postoperative Therapy Protocol for Composite Grafts

Time Postoperative	Therapy Type	Instructions
10—14 days, upon cast removal	Wound care	• The fingernail of affected digit is removed to perform procedure, then replaced to act as a splint following repair. • Antibiotic ointment with bulky, yet loose postoperative dressing applied for protection. • Postoperative bandages should be left intact until first follow-up visit at approximately 5—8 days after the procedure.
	Range of motion	• Range of motion exercises should be immediately initiated to patient tolerance. • Exercises be performed five times per day, for 10-minutes sessions. • Be aware of the above listed precautions prior to initiating ROM in the event of concurrent injuries.
	Splinting	• Clamshell tip protector orthosis with nonadherent gauze (Xeroform or Adaptic) can be applied over the tip of the amputation. • A nighttime digit extension orthosis with tip protector may be beneficial for the pediatric population to prevent inadvertent orthosis removal.

Data from Heistein JB, Cook PA. Factors affecting composite graft survival in digital tip amputations. *Ann Plast Surg*. 2003;50(3):299—303 and Levin LS. Management of skin grafts and flaps. In: Skirven TM, Osterman AL, Fedorczyk JM, Amadio PC, eds. *Rehabilitation of the Hand and Upper Extremity*, 6th ed. Philadelphia: Elsevier; 2011. 244—254.
Remaining course of care for composite grafts consistent with "fingertip amputation" protocol above.

Postoperative Therapy Protocol for Ray Resections

Time Postoperative	Therapy Type	Instructions
4 weeks, upon cast removal	Range of motion Splinting	• AROM and PROM should be initiated for all digits, five times per day. • Resting hand orthosis for comfort. • Static flexion and/or extension orthosis as needed to regain motion. • Be aware of the previously listed precautions before initiating ROM in the event of concurrent injuries.
6 weeks	Scar management	• Scar massage/mobilization • Elastomer or other silastic material (Rolyan 50/50) • Desensitization with sensory sticks, rice bin, etc. for residual hypersensitivity
8—12 weeks	Progressive Strengthening	• Strengthening exercises should be initiated following wound closure. • Use of products such as Theraputty, hand gripper, stress balls, and resistive clothespins can be beneficial in gradually regaining strength in affected digit(s).

Data from Cannon NM. Amputation. In: Cannon NM, ed. *Diagnosis and Treatment Manual for Physicians and Therapists: Upper Extremity Rehabilitation*. Indianapolis: The Hand Rehabilitation Center of Indiana PC; 2001. 1.

Postoperative Therapy Protocol for Digital Replantation

Time Postoperative	Therapy Type	Instructions
4 weeks, upon cast removal	Splinting	• Dorsal block orthosis in neutral wrist position, 45–50 degrees of metacarpophalangeal (MP) flexion, interphalangeal (IP) joints in extension to 0°.

	Range of motion	• Be mindful of the previously listed precautions before initiating ROM in the event of concurrent injuries.
		  • Active wrist flexion to tension, allowing digit MP and IP extension via tenodesis.
		  • Active wrist extension to neutral with gentle passive MP flexion, where wrist and MP motion are proportional.
		  • AROM/PROM of uninvolved digits that do not have an effect on the repaired digit(s).

	Edema management	• Elevation, AROM exercises.
		• Compression sleeves if cleared by physician.
		  • Light compressive dressing applied for edema control
		  • Compressive dressing should be evenly applied from distal to proximal end of digit and should not be constricting
		  • Retrograde massage

	Scar management	• Initiated upon wound closure • Scar massage and mobilization • Elastomer molds, silicone gel sheets, silicone gel digit cap (such as Silopad), Kinesio Tape
	Sensory reeducation	• Use of various textures to decrease hypersensitivity or encourage sensory return in digit • Rice, corn, sand bins; stereognosis skills
6–8 weeks	Range of motion	• Continue ROM protocol from aforementioned • Hook fist with neutral wrist, MP extension to neutral, proximal interphalangeal (PIP) flexion to 60 degrees, and minimal DIP flexion. • Tabletop position (intrinsic plus position) with neutral wrist MP flexion, IP extension • Place-and-hold exercises initiated • Initiate active/passive wrist extension past neutral to patient tolerance • Initiated active/passive digit composite flexion/extension with neutral wrist
	Splinting	• A nighttime resting hand orthosis including involved and neighboring digits to address flexor tightness can be created at this stage of healing.
8 weeks	Strengthening	• Initiate gentle/light resistive activities, progress as patient tolerates • Use of products such as TheraPutty, hand gripper, stress balls, and resistive clothespins can be beneficial in gradually regaining strength in affected digit(s)

Data from Cannon NM. Replantation. In: Cannon NM, ed. *Diagnosis and Treatment Manual for Physicians and Therapists: Upper Extremity Rehabilitation*. Indianapolis: The Hand Rehabilitation Center of Indiana PC;2001. 1; Silverman PM, Willette-Green V, Petrilli J. Early protective motion in digital revascularization and replantation. *J Hand Ther* 1989;2(2):84–101; Ugurlar et al., 2016; Walsh JM, Chee N. Replantation. In: Saunders RJ, Astifidis RP, Burke SL, Higgins JP, McClinton MA, eds. *Hand and Upper Extremity Rehabilitation: A Practical Guide*. 4th ed. St. Louis: Elsevier; 2016. 431–439.

Postoperative Therapy Protocol for Thumb Replantation

Time Postoperative	Therapy Type	Instructions
4 weeks, upon cast removal	Splinting	• Dorsal block splint in neutral wrist position, thumb in wide palmar abduction, thumb MP and IP joints flexed to 15 degrees, with remaining digits free.
	Range of motion	• Be mindful of previously listed precautions before initiating ROM in the event of concurrent injuries. • Initiate gentle passive thumb carpometacarpal (CMC) ROM • If PROM of the thumb CMC is well tolerated, initiate AROM of the thumb CMC. • Initiate gentle passive wrist flexion to tension and extension to neutral. • AROM/PROM of uninvolved digits that do not have an effect on the repaired digit(s).
	Edema management	• Elevation, AROM exercises • Compression sleeves if cleared by physician 　• Light compressive dressing applied for edema control. 　• Compressive dressing should be evenly applied from distal to proximal end of digit and should not be constricting. 　• Retrograde massage.
	Scar management	• Initiated upon wound closure • Scar massage and mobilization • Elastomer™ molds, silicone gel sheets, silicone gel digit cap (such as Silopad™), Kinesio® Tape
	Sensory reeducation	• Use of various textures to decrease hypersensitivity or encourage sensory return in digit • Rice, corn, sand bins; stereognosis skills
6–8 weeks	Splinting	• Discontinue dorsal block orthosis as permitted by physician. • Thumb in wide palmar abduction and full thumb MP and IP extension orthosis to address extrinsic flexor tightness during daytime. • Nighttime web spacer orthosis to maintain or improve first web space to limit risk of adduction contracture development.
	Range of motion	• Continue ROM protocol • Initiate gentle isolated passive thumb MP and IP ROM, if free from fixation. • AROM initiated to thumb MP and IP joints, within restrictions of dorsal block splint. • Initiate gradual active/passive wrist extension past neutral to patient tolerance. • Initiate passive composite thumb and wrist motion. 　• Active motion to thumb and wrist to tolerance. 　• To maximize tendon excursion: 　　• Active thumb flexion with wrist flexion. 　　• Active thumb extension with wrist extension 　• Initiate blocking exercise: 　　• Blocked thumb IP flexion 　　• Reverse blocking for maximum extensor pollicis longus (EPL) excursion: 　　　• With the wrist in slight flexion and MP joint in 30 degrees of flexion, the patient should attempt IP extension.
8 weeks	Strengthening	• Initiate gentle/light resistive activity, progress as patient tolerates • Use of products such as TheraPutty®, hand gripper, stress balls, and resistive clothespins can be beneficial in gradually regaining strength in affected digit(s).

Data from Cannon NM. Replantation. In: Cannon NM, ed. *Diagnosis and Treatment Manual for Physicians and Therapists: Upper Extremity Rehabilitation*. Indianapolis: The Hand Rehabilitation Center of Indiana PC; 2001. 1; Walsh JM, Chee N. Replantation. In: Saunders RJ, Astifidis RP, Burke SL, Higgins JP, McClinton MA, eds. *Hand and Upper Extremity Rehabilitation: A Practical Guide*. 4th ed. St. Louis: Elsevier; 2016. 431–439.

REFERENCES

1. Abzug JM, Zlotolow DA, Kozin SH. Upper extremity replantation. In: Abzug JM, Herman MJ, eds. *Pediatric Orthopedic Surgical Emergencies.* New York: Springer; 2012: 111−123.
2. Carmen C, Chang B. Treadmill injuries to the upper extremity in pediatric patients. *Ann Plast Surg.* 2001;47(1): 15−19.
3. Jaeger SH, Tsai TM, Kleinert HE. Upper extremity replantation in children. *Orthop Clin N Am.* 1981;12(4):897−907.
4. Borne A, Porter A, Recicar J, Maxson T, Montgomery C. Pediatric traumatic amputations in the United States: a 5-year review. *J Pediatr Orthop.* 2017;37(2):e104−e107.
5. Eberlin KR, Busa K, Bae DS, Waters PM, Labow BI, Taghinia AH. Composite grafting for pediatric fingertip injuries. *Hand (N Y).* 2015;10(1):28−33.
6. Giddins GE, Hill RA. Late diagnosis and treatment of crush injuries of the fingertip in children. *Injury.* 1998;29(6): 447−450.
7. Mohan R, Panthaki Z, Armstrong MB. Replantation in pediatrics. *J Craniofac Surg.* 2009;20(4):996−998.
8. Jones NF, Chang J, Kashani P. The surgical and rehabilitative aspects of replantation and revascularization of the hand. In: Skirven TM, Osterman AL, Fedorczyk JM, Amadio PC, eds. *Rehabilitation of the Hand and Upper Extremity.* 6th ed. Philadelphia: Elsevier; 2011:244−254.
9. Chicarilli ZN. Pediatric microsurgery: revascularization and replantation. *J Pediatr Surg.* 1986;21(8):706−710.
10. Peterson SL, Peterson EL, Wheatley MJ. Management of fingertip amputations. *J Hand Surg Am.* 2014;39(10): 2093−2101.
11. Fassler PR. Fingertip injuries: evaluation and treatment. *J Am Acad Orthop Surg.* 1996;4(2):84−92.
12. Abzug JM, Kozin SH. Pediatric replantation. *J Hand Surg Am.* 2014;39(1):143−145.
13. Boulas HJ. Amputations of the fingers and hand: indications for replantation. *J Am Acad Orthop Surg.* 1998;6(2): 100−105.
14. Kim JY, Brown RJ, Jones NF. Pediatric upper extremity replantation. *Clin Plast Surg.* 2005;32(1):1−10.
15. Urgurlar M, Kabakas F, Purisa H, Sezer I, Celikdelen P, Ozcelick IB. Rehabilitation after successful finger replantation. *North Clin Istanb.* 2016;3(1):22−26.
16. Levin LS. Management of skin grafts and flaps. In: Skirven TM, Osterman AL, Fedorczyk JM, Amadio PC, eds. *Rehabilitation of the Hand and Upper Extremity.* 6th ed. Philadelphia: Elsevier; 2011:244−254.
17. Heistein JB, Cook PA. Factors affecting composite graft survival in digital tip amputations. *Ann Plast Surg.* 2003; 50(3):299−303.
18. Marchessault JA, McKay PL, Hammert WC. Management of upper limb amputations. *J Hand Surg Am.* 2011; 36(10):1718−1726.
19. Bueno E, Benjamin MJ, Sisk G, et al. Rehabilitation following hand transplantation. *Hand (N.Y).* 2014;9(1): 9−15.
20. Dua K, Lancaster TP, Abzug JM. Age-dependent reliability of Semmes-Weinstein and 2-point discrimination tests in children. *J Pediatr Orthop.* 2019;39(2):98−103.
21. Duff SV, Aaron DH, Gogola GR, Valero-Cuevas FJ. Innovative evaluation of dexterity in pediatrics. *J Hand Ther.* 2015; 28(2):144−149.
22. Tissue CM, Velleman PF, Stegink-Jansen CW, Aaron DH, Winthrop BG, Gogola GR. Validity and reliability of the functional dexterity test in children. *J Hand Ther.* 2017; 30(4):500−506.
23. Tremblay J, Curatolo S, Leblanc M, et al. Establishing normative data for the functional dexterity test in typically developing children aged 3−5 years. *J Hand Ther.* 2019; 32(1):93−102.
24. Poole JL, Burtner PA, Torres TA, et al. Norm scores of the box and block test for children age 3−10 years. *J Hand Ther.* 2005;18(3):348−351.
25. Jongbloed-Pereboom M, Nijhuis-van der Sanden MW, Steenbergen B. Norm scores of the box and block test for children age 3−10 years. *Am J Occup Ther.* 2013;67: 312−318.
26. Gardner RA, Broman M. The Purdue pegboard: normative data on 1334 school children. *J Child Adolesc Psychopharmacol.* 1979;8(3):156−162.
27. Wilson BC, Wilson JJ, Iacoviello JM, Risucci D. Purdue Pegboard performance of normal preschool children. *J Clin Exp Neuropsychol.* 1982;4(1):19−26.
28. Reedman SE, Beagley S, Sakzewski L, Boyd RN. The Jebsen Taylor test of hand function: a pilot test re-rest reliability study in typically developing children. *Phys Occup Ther Pediatr.* 2016;36(3):292−304.
29. Walsh JM, Chee N. Replantation. In: Saunders RJ, Astifidis RP, Burke SL, Higgins JP, McClinton MA, eds. *Hand and Upper Extremity Rehabilitation: A Practical Guide.* 4th ed. St. Louis: Elsevier; 2016:431−439.
30. Koczan BJ, Ware LC. Digital amputation and ray resection. In: Saunders RJ, Astifidis RP, Burke SL, Higgins JP, McClinton MA, eds. *Hand and Upper Extremity Rehabilitation: A Practical Guide.* 4th ed. St. Louis: Elsevier; 2016: 441−446.
31. Berman B, Flores F. Comparison of a silicone gel-filled cushion and silicone gel sheeting for the treatment of hypertrophic or keloid scars. *Dermatol Surg.* 1999;25(6): 484−486.
32. Pettengill KM. Therapist's management of the complex injury. In: Skirven TM, Osterman AL, Fedorczyk JM, Amadio PC, eds. *Rehabilitation of the Hand and Upper Extremity.* 6th ed. Philadelphia: Elsevier; 2011:1238−1251.
33. Miller LK, Jerosch-Herold C, Shepstone L. Effectiveness of edema management techniques for subacute hand edema: a systematic review. *J Hand Ther.* 2017;30(4):432−446.
34. Villeco JP. Edema: a silent but important factor. *J Hand Ther.* 2012;25(2):153−162.
35. Granhaug KB. Splinting the upper extremity of a child. In: Henderson A, Pehoski C, eds. *Hand Function in the Child: Foundations for Remediation.* 2nd ed. St. Louis: Mosby; 2006:403−427.

36. Timms J, Carus C. Mirror therapy for the alleviation of phantom limb pain following amputation: a literature review. *Int J Ther Rehabil.* 2015;22(3):135–145.

37. Nilsen DM, DiRusso T. Using mirror therapy in the home environment: a case report. *Am J Occup Ther.* 2014;68(3): e84–e89.

38. Ramachandran VS, Altschuler EL. The use of visual feedback, in particular mirror visual feedback, in restoring brain function. *Brain.* 2009;132(7):1693–1710.

39. James MA, Bagley AM, Brasington K, Lutz C, McConnell S, Molitor F. Impact of prostheses on function and quality of life for children with unilateral congenital below-the-elbow deficiency. *J Bone Joint Surg Am.* 2006;88(11): 2356–2365.

40. Cannon NM. Amputation. In: Cannon NM, ed. *Diagnosis and Treatment Manual for Physicians and Therapists: Upper Extremity Rehabilitation.* Indianapolis: The Hand Rehabilitation Center of Indiana PC; 2001:1.

41. Cannon NM. Replantation. In: Cannon NM, ed. *Diagnosis and Treatment Manual for Physicians and Therapists: Upper Extremity Rehabilitation.* Indianapolis: The Hand Rehabilitation Center of Indiana PC; 2001:1.

42. Silverman PM, Willette-Green V, Petrilli J. Early protective motion in digital revascularization and replantation. *J Hand Ther.* 1989;2(2):84–101.

FURTHER READING

1. Griffet J. Amputation and prosthesis fitting in paediatric patients. *Orthop Traumatol Surg Res.* 2016;102:S161–S175.

2. Valencia J, Leyva F, Gomez-Bajo GJ. Pediatric hand trauma. *Clin Orthop Relat Res.* 2005;(432):77–86.

CHAPTER 23

Pediatric Hand Burn Therapy Chapter

CAROLYN M. LEVIS, MD, MSC, FRCSC • DANIEL WALTHO, MD, (RESIDENT) •
REBECCA NEIDUSKI, PHD, OTR/L, CHT

INTRODUCTION

Burn injuries are common in the pediatric population, representing the fourth leading cause of emergency department visits in the western world. Burns affecting the hand present a significant challenge to the surgeon and therapist.[1] Furthermore, pediatric hand burns require their own unique approach to management and benefit from a multidisciplinary team of surgeons, hand therapists, child life specialists, and other pediatric support staff. These injuries can significantly compromise hand function and growth and therefore necessitate timely and appropriate management to ensure optimal outcomes and quality of life. The challenges of managing hand burns in both children and adults have led to strong recommendations for definitive management at a dedicated burn center whenever possible.[2]

Although burn injuries may result from electricity, chemicals, or radiation, thermal injuries represent most hand burns in children. Most pediatric burns are accidental; however, a high index of suspicion toward nonaccidental injuries should be exercised in this population. In young children, scald injuries tend to be the most frequently observed. Contact burns are another common injury in this age group typically affecting the palmar surface of the hand; whereas, friction injuries have emerged as a common injury to the dorsum of the hand and are almost always due to treadmill belts. Flame burns become more prevalent with increasing age.[3]

Depending on the type and extent of burn injury to the hand, appropriate surgical and postoperative management is critical to optimize hand function. This chapter will review the pertinent anatomy, classifications, surgical management, and rehabilitation relevant to pediatric hand burns.

ANATOMY

The skin comprises epidermis and dermis. The dermis contains important structures of the skin, including the base of hair follicles, sebaceous and sweat glands, capillaries, and nerve endings. The dermis can be further divided into papillary and reticular layers, the latter of which contains many of the aforementioned structures (Fig. 23.1). The palm has hairless, glabrous skin with a relatively thicker dermis. The greatest dermal thickness in the body is found in the volar fingertips.

The anatomic differences between the pediatric and adult hands have clinical implications. First, the layers of skin are thinner in children, resulting in greater vulnerability to thermal exposure and making full-thickness injury more likely. Children, however, have more adipose tissue underlying the skin, which protects deeper structures such as tendons, nerves, and vessels. The excess adipose tissue also lends itself to both the excision of eschar and harvesting of full-thickness grafts. Prolonged

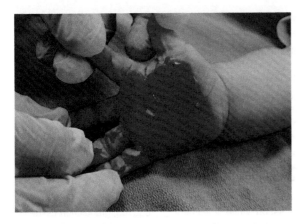

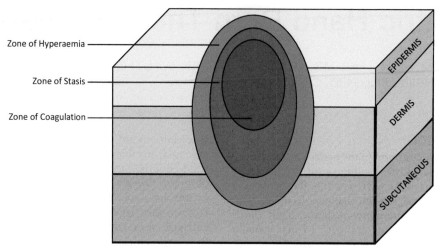

Zone of Hyperaemia

Zone of Stasis

Zone of Coagulation

EPIDERMIS

DERMIS

SUBCUTANEOUS

FIG. 23.1 Jackson's burn model.

exposure to the burn source and in friction burns, such as when a child's hand is in contact with a moving tread-mill, can cause extensive injuries to tendons, nerves, and vessels deep to skin and adipose layers.

Another critical difference between adult and pediatric hand burns pertains to the consequences on the growth of the hand. More severe burns and those affecting very young children will have a greater negative impact on the growth of the hand. This is related to the potential for scar contractures of skin and joints that restrict growth.

CLASSIFICATION

This classification of burns is based on the depth of skin exposure (Table 23.1).

Specific classifications of hand-related burns in children have also been proposed to guide therapy. Burns causing *flexion* contractures at the proximal interphalangeal (PIP) joints of the fingers and the thumb may be classified according to Stern et al. (Table 23.2).[5] Moreover, burns causing *hyperextension* contractures of the metacarpophalangeal (MCP) joints may be classified according to Graham et al. (Table 23.3).[6]

TABLE 23.1
Classification of Burns based on Depth of Involved Skin.

Burn Classification		Depth	Clinical Features	Healing
Superficial		Epidermis	Mild-to-moderate pain; intact sensation; erythematous skin	Nonscarring healing within 7 days
Partial thickness	Superficial	Papillary dermis	Significant tenderness; sensation usually intact; blistering, pink, blanchable skin	Nonscarring healing within 2−3 weeks
Partial thickness	Deep	Reticular dermis	Dull to no tenderness; sensation reduced; mottled skin with slow capillary refill	Scarring usually occurs; healing within 2−3 weeks
Full thickness		Through dermis into subcutaneous tissue	No tenderness; loss of sensation; white or leathery skin; severe edema	Excision and coverage required; granulation tissue forms within 3−7 days
Complete		Muscle, fascia, or bone	Systemic toxic reaction; sepsis; no edema	Excision and coverage required; granulation tissue forms within 3−7 days

Cowan AC, Stegink-Jansen CW. Rehabilitation of hand burn injuries: current updates. Injury. 2013;44(3):391−396.

TABLE 23.2 Classification: PIP Joint Flexion Contractures.	
Type I	Involves scar alone; full passive PIP extension with maximum MCP joint flexion
Type II	Articular structures involved; reduced passive PIP extension with maximum MCP joint flexion
Type III	Fixed flexion deformity; no passive PIP extension with maximum MCP joint flexion; joint arthrodesed/irregular

Stern PJ, Neale HW, Graham TJ, Warden GD. Classification and treatment of postburn proximal interphalangeal joint flexion contractures in children. J Hand Surg Am. May 1987;12(3):450—457.

TABLE 23.3 Classification: MCP Joint Hyperextension Contractures.	
Type I	Greater than 30 degrees of metacarpophalangeal flexion with the wrist fully extended
Type II	Less than 30 degrees of metacarpophalangeal flexion with the wrist maximally extended
Type III	Metacarpophalangeal joint fixed in greater than 30 degrees of metacarpophalangeal hyperextension

Graham T, Stern P, True M. Classification and treatment of postburn metacarpophalangeal joint extension contractures in children. J Hand Surg Am 1990;15:450—456.

APPROACH TO TREATMENT

Robson et al.[7] outlines core principles for improving outcomes in hand burn injuries. These principles include prevention of burn propagation to deeper structures, prompt wound closure/grafting, preservation of range of motion both at the level of the hand and the remainder of the extremity, prevention and control of infection (to mitigate extension of nonviable tissue), and early retraining. Robson advocates for a multidisciplinary team consisting of physician, nurse, occupational therapist, physical therapist, vocational rehabilitation counselor, and social worker.[7]

Clinically significant burns should be initially managed according to the advanced burn life support[8] and advanced trauma life support[9] when associated with concomitant trauma protocols. Specific management of pediatric hand burns should be implemented once the patient is medically stable.

Preoperative Evaluation

A focused history should be obtained including timing, type, and duration of burn injury as well as other concomitant injuries to the hand(s). Nonaccidental injuries, either neglect or abuse, should be promptly identified and reported to the appropriate child protection services. Incidence of nonaccidental burns has reportedly been as high as 25%.[10] In addition to the history of presenting injury, certain burn patterns identified during examination may lead to a higher likelihood of neglect or abuse. Burns to certain anatomic sites should raise the suspicion of abuse, such as burns to perineum, ankles, plantar aspect of the feet, wrists, and palmar aspect of the hand. Burns with a clean line of demarcation in a glove and/or stocking pattern, or symmetric burns should raise the suspicion for nonaccidental injury.

The burn depth can be assessed using the aforementioned classification system (Table 23.1). Extent can be determined based on percentage of total body surface area (TBSA) using a Lund and Browder Chart (Fig. 23.2); however, a detailed description of dorsal and palmar involvement of digits and joints should be documented. Careful assessment is essential to rule out any circumferential burns or other signs of vascular compromise that will require immediate intervention. Appropriate physical examination may require initial debridement that is usually performed under conscious sedation in the emergency department, burn treatment room or the operating room.

Treatment

Depending on the characteristics of the injury, there are a number of possible treatment options for the pediatric hand burn. Initially, burns should be managed with cooling, irrigation, and elevation. Excessive and prolonged cooling particularly in greater TBSA burns must be avoided to prevent hypothermia particularly in the pediatric population. Superficial partial-thickness burns will heal within 2—3 weeks and should be treated with appropriate dressings. Deep partial-thickness and full-thickness burns will require surgical debridement; however, it can be temporized with an antibiotic topical ointment or cream. Although it is common practice to change hand dressings frequently, the current trend is to reduce the frequency of dressing changes in children to minimize pain and anxiety

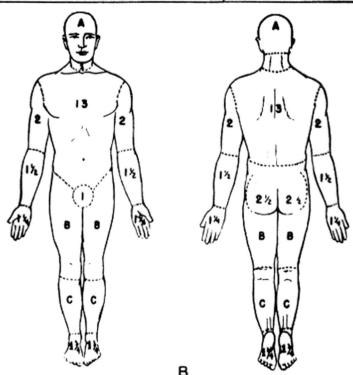

B

FIG. 23.2 Lund and Browder Chart.

associated with dressing changes as well as the need for resource-intense, conscious sedation. Dressings should be applied sparingly to encourage early mobilization, as bulky dressings often impair range of motion and affect design and fit of splints.

MANAGEMENT OF VASCULAR COMPROMISE

Consequences of certain burn injuries and resuscitation efforts can lead to acute compartment syndrome in one or more fascial compartments of the hand and forearm.

Compartment syndrome occurs when the tissue pressure within a compartment is greater than the perfusion pressure (~ 30 mmHg), resulting in ischemic changes and ultimately tissue necrosis of muscles and nerves. This outcome can significantly impair hand function and even viability. Expedient diagnosis is therefore essential and is usually made clinically including direct tissue pressure monitoring though this is an invasive technique that may require conscious sedation. Occasionally, adjunctive investigations (elevated Creatine Kinase (CK) and myoglobin) may be used to support the diagnosis. One should have a high index of suspicion for compartment syndrome in electrical, significant thermal burns and those associated with other injuries such as fractures. Compartment syndrome, when diagnosed, requires urgent surgical management with decompression of all affected muscle compartments.

Circumferential full-thickness burns of the hand and forearm may lead to an *extrinsic* compartment syndrome and will demand prompt *escharotomy* if distal perfusion is in jeopardy of compromise. Areas distal to a circumferential, full-thickness burn may appear vascularly intact on initial assessment, however, may become compromised over time particularly as fluid resuscitation progresses. The recommended locations for escharotomies are demonstrated in Fig. 23.3. Dorsal escharotomies are located over the second and fourth metacarpals. Radial and ulnar escharotomies are placed over the thenar and hypothenar eminences, respectively, at the border of glaborous—nonglaborous skin. Digital escharotomies are made at the glaborous—nonglaborous junction, ulnarly on the thumb and radially on other digits. Proximally, forearm escharotomies are carried out along the radial and ulnar aspects, with the ulnar incision being performed anterior to the medial epicondyle of the humerus so as to avoid the ulnar nerve. These incisions can be extended distally to the thenar and hypothenar incision in the hand.

In certain cases, thermal damage or fluid resuscitation may lead to an intrinsic compartment syndrome. If escharotomy has not sufficiently decompressed the hand, or in the absence of a circumferential burn, an urgent fasciotomy may be indicated if the intercompartmental pressure is determined to be high. Incisions in the hand are the same as in an escharotomy with the addition of a carpal tunnel release. Forearm incisions are made on the dorsal and volar aspect as illustrated in Fig. 23.4, with the volar incision being extended to include the decompression of the carpal tunnel. A successful fasciotomy should decompress the involved compartments and neurovascular structures, resulting in clinical resolution of any signs/symptoms.

SURGICAL DEBRIDEMENT AND COVERAGE

Indications for surgical debridement are dependent on the viability of skin and underlying tissue. According to Jackson's burn model (Fig. 23.1), the zone of coagulation represents nonviable tissue in the central area of a burn and is typically debrided in the initial procedure. The zone of hyperemia represents inflammatory tissue on the periphery of a burn and will likely remain viable, thus obviating the need for debridement. However, the zone of stasis represents an area of uncertainty between the two aforementioned zones, wherein time, fluid resuscitation, and other factors will determine the viability of involved tissue. Therefore, full-thickness burns should be excised promptly as early as day 1–3; however, decisions to debride surrounding tissue should be delayed for approximately 48 hours to allow nonviable tissue to declare itself as to its depth of burn.

Excision of a burn can be done in a fascial or tangential fashion. Fascial excision involves removing all cutaneous and subcutaneous tissue to the level of the muscle fascia. Tangential excision involves sequential removal of tissue in graduated depths until healthy bleeding tissue is reached. Fascial excision limits the amount of intraoperative blood loss, whereas tangential excision preserves maximal tissue, the latter of which is

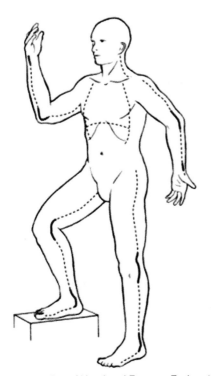

FIG. 23.3 Location of Hand and Forearm Escharotomies.

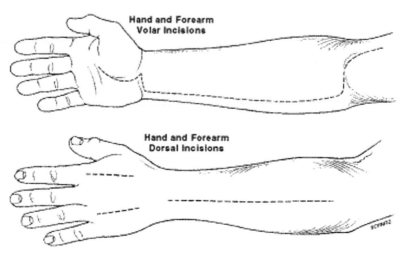

FIG. 23.4 Location of Forearm and Hand Fasciotomies.

desired in the upper extremity. Tangential debridement of tissue in the pediatric hand and forearm should be performed under tourniquet control to minimize blood loss and to allow for optimal hemostasis. The tourniquet is released following debridement to visualize healthy bleeding tissue for subsequent coverage.

Decisions for coverage of a hand burn following surgical debridement depend on location and extent of injury. Skin grafts can provide adequate and definitive coverage for most hand burns. For the dorsum of the hand and digits, split-thickness skin grafts (STSG) can be used. Donor sites for STSG include, but are not limited to, the thigh, back, lateral abdominal wall, and scalp. With the small surface area of the hand, meshing of the skin graft should be avoided to ensure optimal cosmesis and to limit contracture. The amount of wound contracture that is covered with a skin graft depends upon the amount of dermis included, with less dermis resulting in greater wound contracture. Therefore, for the palm of the hand and digits, a thicker STSG or full-thickness skin graft (FTSG) should be used. Common donor sites for FTSGs to be used in hand burns include supraclavicular, antecubital, groin, and abdomen. These donor sites can typically be closed primarily in cases of upper extremity coverage, or a local flap may be indicated. Skin graft take occurs in 5–7 days and therefore, recipient site dressings should be maintained for at least 7 days to ensure that graft is adequately protected throughout these stages.

In severe cases of very deep burns that involve bone, tendon, or muscle, a more involved debridement is needed to allow for coverage. These injuries will require coverage with a soft tissue flap. Options include local,

regional, distant, or free flaps. If the injury is too extensive for functional coverage, amputation may be required. One of the major considerations in the care of children with hand burns, is the need for frequent and long-term follow-up to assess the relationship between scars and growth. Burn scars may not result in contractures in the acute and subacute phase, however it is very possible that with growth, scar and joint contractures can develop and therefore surgery and even multiple revisions may be required until the growth phase is complete. These revisions may include scar lengthening in the form of z-plasties, skin grafts or even fasciocutaneous flaps. Subsequent surgeries would then require the involvement of a therapist for appropriate care.

Postoperative Immobilization and Splinting

Immobilization of the involved hand joints is critical to skin graft take/flap healing in the pediatric population. Patients should be immobilized with a splint, cast, or placement of Kirschner wires for a period of 1–2 weeks. The hand should be immobilized to optimize the graft take and prevent contractures with 20 degrees of extension at the wrist, 30 degrees of MCP flexion, and interphalangeal joints maintained in full extension. The Kirschner wires are removed once the grafts have healed at 1–2 weeks. Range of motion and hand therapy can then be initiated.

Splinting is an extremely important adjunct for palmar hand burns to prevent flexion contractures that can lead to irreversible growth disturbances and the need for complex reconstruction when the child is older or as an adult. Prevention of flexion contractures presents a particular challenge in the pediatric palmar hand burn, due to compliance. Ideally, fiberglass or thermoplastic materials are used to splint the joints in extension as they are lighter than plaster. A number of different splint types can be used to achieve this position, including a dorsal/volar sandwich, dorsal pan, palmar conforming, slot-through, and volar slab. Certain variations on these splints have been described to address difficulties incompliance for injuries to digits 2–5. Some hyperextension has been met with success in pediatric populations less than 4 years old. Additionally, incorporating a pressure garment directly into the splint has resulted in better patient compliance.[11,12]

POSTOPERATIVE REHABILITATION

Outcomes following pediatric burns are heavily influenced by postoperative rehabilitation that involves active and passive range of motion, fabrication of orthoses, and issuance of compression garments and/or silicone inserts. Assessment of range of motion, scar, and participation in activities of daily living are essential throughout the rehabilitative process. Ideally, the child should be followed by a hand therapist experienced in burn management.

Following 2–3 weeks of postoperative immobilization, progressive hand therapy is initiated. It is imperative to identify the patient's active and passive range of motion for each joint to establish a baseline, carefully noting joints and web spaces susceptible to contractures during the healing process. Incidence of contractures has been correlated with burn size and depth, immobilization, pain, edema, and adherence to orthosis and exercise regimens.[13] Contracture tendencies at each joint of the upper extremity are as follows: typically aligned with burns in or near the anatomic "spaces" that allow a wide range of motion, such as the axilla, cubital fossa, and first webspace. The glenohumeral joint has a tendency to contract toward adduction, with scar tissue building in the anterior and posterior axillary spaces limiting upward mobility toward flexion and abduction (Fig. 23.5). The elbow has a tendency to contract toward flexion, decreasing the ability to produce full extension and impacting the child's ability to reach forward (Fig. 23.6). The wrist can contract toward flexion or extension based on burn location (Fig. 23.7). Wrist mobility is directly related to grasp and release; a flexion contracture will severely limit a child's strong and agile use of the fingers and thumb.

Dorsal hand burns tend to be more common when hands are used to cover the face or body in response to trauma. Dorsal skin is notably thinner and more pliable, with minimal subcutaneous tissue to protect

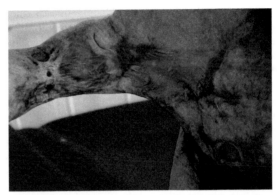

FIG. 23.5 Contracture of the axilla limiting full abduction.

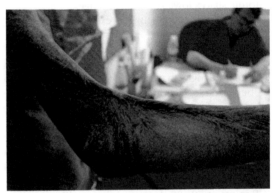

FIG. 23.6 Contracture bands at the elbow limiting full extension.

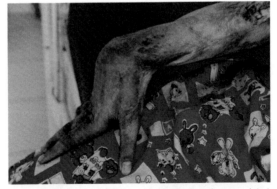

FIG. 23.7 Contracture bands traversing from wrist to thenar eminence.

the extensor mechanism.[14] An intrinsic minus, or claw hand, can result with MCP joints contracting toward extension and interphalangeal (IP) joints toward flexion. Boutonniere and mallet deformities can result from central slip and terminal tendon necrosis, respectively. Both volar and dorsal hand burns can draw the first webspace toward adduction, severely limiting functional grasp and release. Web spaces between fingers typically contract toward adduction.

The likelihood of contractures following burns in and around anatomical spaces of the upper extremity necessitates both careful range of motion measurements in the clinic and consistent range of motion programs at home. Progression toward full range of motion following skin grafts is pursued both consistently and cautiously, with attention to wound edges to minimize disruption. Children and family members should be educated on surface anatomy, tendency for contractures, and low load active and passive range of motion exercises that will gently, yet effectively, move joints and anatomic spaces toward their end range.

Orthoses are used between exercises and during sleep to create optimal joint positioning during the healing process. Creating an abduction or "airplane" orthosis for the glenohumeral joint requires careful planning and rigid materials (Fig. 23.8). A beach ball can be used during orthosis breaks throughout the day as a comfortable, albeit not as effective alternative (Fig. 23.9). Elbow extension orthoses are relatively simple to construct, however, may be difficult to adhere with as they significantly limit wrist and hand function (Fig. 23.10). Intrinsic plus positioning of the wrist and hand, with the wrist at 20–30 degrees of extension, MCP joints at 70–90 degrees of flexion, IP joints fully extended, and thumb maximally, palmarly abducted, is recommended for hand burns.[14]

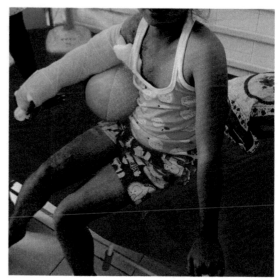
FIG. 23.9 Use of a beach ball as a comfortable break from the airplane orthosis.

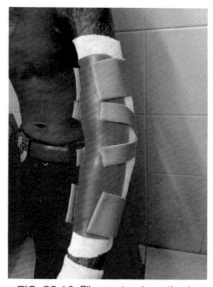
FIG. 23.10 Elbow extension orthosis.

It is important to recognize that hard plastic, custom orthoses can effectively position joints but are limited in their ability to intimately fit within anatomic spaces. Compression garments, also called as pressure therapy, are prescribed for 23 hours per day of wearing to maintain anatomical spaces and to help organize and control scar tissue. These garments are continued for 6 months to a year after injury.[14] These garments should provide a pressure gradient of 24 mm Hg to overcome capillary

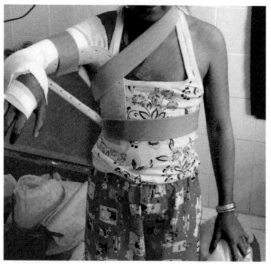
FIG. 23.8 An airplane orthosis to maintain abduction of the glenohumeral joint.

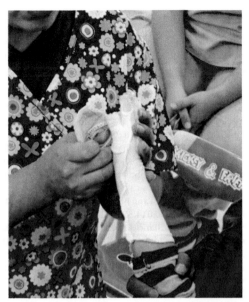

FIG. 23.11 Custom-made compression garment for the wrist and hand.

pressure. Compression garments can be custom-made in rehabilitation units by garment fitters (Fig. 23.11); they can also be ordered based on measurements taken in the clinic. Sudhakar and Le Blanc[15] offered an interesting and alternative design where an orthosis is incorporated directly into a custom fit compression garment. This design was intended to afford ease of donning and doffing along with increased adherence to the wearing schedule.

Once burn wounds have healed, silicone gel and inserts can be used in conjunction with or in lieu of compression garments to simultaneously provide compression and soften scar tissue. Silicone is perceived to have moisturizing properties and decrease the tension of scar tissue. Massage with lotions or oils is also effective to increase moisture and soften scars through gentle pressure and friction. It is important to teach caregivers how to monitor any maceration and/or irritation that could occur.

OUTCOMES MEASUREMENT

Outcome measures can be used throughout the rehabilitative process to assess multiple aspects of recovery, from appearance to functional use. A scar assessment, such as the Vancouver Scar Scale or Burn Scar Index,[16] can be used to document hypertrophy and change in scar appearance. This tool is completed by the therapist, and the final score is calculated by totaling subscores in categories of scar vascularity, pigmentation, pliability, and height. Thirteen points are possible on this tool with a higher score indicating a more hypertrophic and potentially contracted scar. This tool has been used extensively in burn research and noted to have moderate-to-high interrater reliability as well as construct and divergent validity.

In addition to scar assessment, it is vital to consider how burns impact a child's ability to use their arm and hand to complete everyday tasks and participate in meaningful activities. A comprehensive review of outcome measures is offered in Chapter 4 of this text. When used alongside body structure and function measures such as range of motion, grip strength, and pinch strength, outcome measures provide a holistic view of the impact of a burn injury on a child's function.

The final aspect to consider is the psychological impact of the burn on the patient and their caregivers, potentially due to the traumatic incident or a resultant, altered appearance. A recent systematic review by Bakker et al.[17] noted that while children are likely to demonstrate anxiety, stress, and behavioral responses to burn injuries in the months immediately following, long-term impairments in self-esteem or body image were not prevalent in the patients studied. In comparison, parents were described as having posttraumatic stress, depression, and guilt in the short term as well as persistent psychological problems. These outcomes were correlated with severity of burns; more severe burns led to higher incidences of long-term psychological responses in both parents and children. Acknowledgment of the impact of trauma on the coping mechanisms of the child and caregivers is a vital aspect of the rehabilitative process, especially in the months immediately following a burn injury.

CONCLUSION

Management of the physical and psychological aspects of pediatric upper extremity burns requires a multidisciplinary approach. Familiarity with burn anatomy, classification, surgical management, and rehabilitative approaches enables therapists to effectively treat these difficult and traumatic injuries and help children return to full function and quality of life.

REFERENCES

1. Svientek S, Levine J. Pediatric burns of the hand. *Plast Surg Nurs.* 2015;35(2):80–81.
2. Rotondo MF, Cribari C, Smith RS, American College of Surgeons Committee on Trauma. *Resources for Optimal*

Care of the Injured Patient. Chicago: American College of Surgeons; 2014:6.

3. Norbury WB, Herndon DN. Management of acute pediatric hand burns. *Hand Clin.* May 2017;33(2):237−242.

4. Cowan AC, Steginik-Jansen CW. Rehabilitation of hand burn injuries: current updates. *Injury.* March 2013;44(3): 391−396.

5. Stern PJ, Neale HW, Graham TJ, Warden GD. Classification and treatment of postburn proximal interphalangeal joint flexion contractures in children. *J Hand Surg Am.* May 1987;12(3):450−457.

6. Graham T, Stern P, True M. Classification and treatment of postburn metacarpophalangeal joint extension contractures in children. *J Hand Surg Am.* 1990;15:450−456.

7. Robson MC, Smith Jr DJ, VanderZee AJ, et al. Making the burned hand functional. *Clin Plast Surg.* 1992;19(3): 663−671.

8. American Burn Association. *Advanced Burn Life Support Providers Manual.* 2005 (Chicago, IL).

9. ATLS Subcommittee; American College of Surgeons' Committee on Trauma; International ATLS working group. Advanced trauma life support (ATLS®): the ninth edition. *J Trauma Acute Care Surg.* May 2013;74(5): 1363−1366.

10. Bousema S, Stas HG, van de Merwe MH, Oen IM, Baartmans MG, van Baar ME, Dutch Burn Repository group, Maasstad Hospital Rotterdam. Epidemiology and screening of intentional burns in children in a Dutch burn centre. *Burns.* September 2016;42(6):1287−1294.

11. Schwanholt C, Daugherty MB, Gaboury T, Warden GD. Splinting the pediatric Palmar burn. *J Burn Care Rehabil.* 1992 Jul-Aug;13(4):460−464.

12. Sudhakar G, Le Blanc M. Alternate splint for flexion contracture in children with burns. *J Hand Ther.* 2011 Jul-Sep;24(3):277−279. https://doi.org/10.1016/j.jht.2010.10.008. Epub 2010 Dec 24.

13. Schneider JC, Holavanahalli R, Helm P, O'Neil C, Goldstein R, Kowalske K. Contractures in burn injury part II: investigating joints of the hand. *J Burn Care Res.* 2008;29:606−613.

14. Fufa DT, Chang S-S, Yang J-Y. Postburn contractures of the hand. *J Hand Surg.* 2014;39(9):1869−1876.

15. Sudhakar G, Le Blanc M. Alternate splint for flexion contracture in children with burns. *J Hand Ther.* 2011; 24(3):277−279.

16. Baryza MJ, Baryza GA. The vancouver scar scale: an administration tool and its interrater reliability. *J Burn Care Rehabil.* 1995;16(5):535−538.

17. Bakker A, Maertens KJP, Van Son MJM, Van Loey NEE. Psychological consequences of pediatric burns from a child and family perspective: a review of the empirical literature. *Clin Psychol Rev.* 2013;33:361−371.

CHAPTER 24

Pediatric Sports Injuries: Little League Elbow, Osteochondritis Dissecans of the Elbow, Gymnast Wrist

HETA PARIKH, OTR/L, MPH • ALEXANDRIA L. CASE, BSE • DANIELLE A. HOGARTH, BS • JOSHUA M. ABZUG, MD

INTRODUCTION

Pediatric sports are a cornerstone of childhood in the United States. According to a 2008 report compiled by the Women's Sports Foundation, approximately 69% of girls and 75% of boys participate in organized team sports.[1] The increased intensity, pressure, and expectations of these young competitive athletes lead to an increased risk of musculoskeletal injury.[2,3] Approximately two million children each year seek medical intervention due to repetitive stress injuries pertaining to sports-related activities.[4] An even higher incidence is likely present, as sport injuries in which the player continues to "play through pain" are not represented in the aforementioned number.[2] The most common sports-related pediatric overuse injuries include inflammatory conditions, fractures, sprains, strains, and contusions.[5,6]

Key intrinsic factors impacting injury to the growing child include open growth plates, muscle imbalance, and incoordination due to growth.[6] The need for high intensity and frequency of training to master one sport-specific skill increases the probability of an overuse injury. Young athletes are intensifying training, playing on multiple teams, and playing all year round, thereby not allowing their bone, muscle, and tendons time to recover from the repetitive stress of the season.[2,3] Adolescents are particularly at risk for injury due to the imbalance of ossifying bone. The porous ossifying bone is highly susceptible to fracture as it lengthens during a growth spurt.[6,7] A wide variety of sports-related trauma, both acute and chronic, can develop in the upper extremity including fractures, tendonitis/tendonopathies, apophysitis, epiphysitis, growth plate damage, and tendon

rupture.[5] Three common overuse sports injuries affecting the child's upper extremity discussed in this chapter include little league elbow, osteochondritis dissecans (OCD), and gymnast wrist.

Anatomical Overview

Pediatric bone is most vulnerable to injury about the physes (growth plates), which contribute to longitudinal bone growth. Biomechanically, open growth plates are the weakest points within the pediatric musculoskeletal system, and therefore they are more prone to injury than fully ossified bone.[6–8] The surrounding ligaments are 2–3 times stronger than the physis and are therefore less susceptible to injury in the skeletally immature patient.[9] The ossifying bones are the first areas impacted by repetitive compressive and tensile forces in gymnastics and high frequency throwing sports in young athletes.

The physis, situated between the metaphysis and epiphysis, consists of germinal cells responsible for increasing bone length.[7,10] The physis is further separated into three chondrocyte zones: reserve/resting, proliferative, and hypertrophic. The reserve/resting zone, which is adjacent to the epiphysis, is known to have irregular chondrocytes, low rates of proliferation, and cartilage for bone growth, putting this zone at the greatest risk of a growth arrest injury (Fig. 24.1). As the chondrocytes multiply, they become stacked and organized in the proliferative zone, where actual bone growth takes place. The cells then travel from the proliferative zone to the hypertrophic zone where they mature, degenerate, and begin calcification. The hypertrophic zone is considered the weakest zone and is at greatest

Pediatric Hand Therapy. https://doi.org/10.1016/B978-0-323-53091-0.00024-5

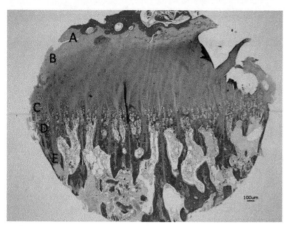

FIG. 24.1 Histological photograph identifying the normal human physis anatomy: **(A)** Epiphyseal bone, **(B)** resting/reserve zone, **(C)** proliferative zone **(D)** hypertrophic zone, and **(E)** metaphyseal bone. (Courtesy of Motomi Entomo-Iwamoto, DDS, PhD.)

risk for fracture. Overuse injuries at the hypertrophic zone can potentially lead to physeal widening, calcification, fracture, and premature closure of the physis.[9]

An apophysis is the region of the bone where tendon attaches to the ossifying cartilaginous area. The tension of the tendon attachment on the apophysis can adversely affect the formation of the bone via prolonged, high velocity loading. Inadequate healing of ossifying bone can influence the player's future success in their sport of choice.[8,11] Pediatric sports-related injuries are greatly impacted by the frequency, velocity, and direction of forces to bone, tendon, and ligaments.

LITTLE LEAGUE ELBOW

Little league elbow, an injury observed in youth athletes, can also be called as medial epicondyle apophysitis. A traction and shearing force injury occurs due to the valgus stress placed on the medial elbow during overhead-throwing activities. Radiographs may reveal a widening of the physis at the medial epicondyle apophysis or a frank medial epicondyle fracture.[12] This overuse injury is most commonly diagnosed between the ages of 9 and 12 years, before closure of the medial epicondyle apophysis.[3,13] Athletes at risk for medial elbow pain include pitchers, catchers who throw the ball back to the pitcher following every pitch, quarterbacks, and tennis players. Reportedly, 70% of baseball players from ages 7 to 19 years have elbow pain at some point during sport participation, including 28% of young pitchers.[8,14]

Anatomy and Classification

The elbow consists of the ulnohumeral joint, radiocapitellar joint, and proximal radioulnar joint. Congruency of the elbow joint allows for extension, flexion, and axial rotation of the forearm. The ligaments of the elbow consist of the medial collateral ligament (also known as the ulnar collateral ligament or UCL), the pronator/flexor mass, and the lateral collateral ligament (also known as the radial collateral ligament or RCL), all of which contribute to elbow stability. Although the pronator/flexor mass primarily protects against valgus torque, the lateral collateral ligament complex stabilizes the radial head from posterior subluxation, in addition to protecting against varus stress. Three bundles form the medial collateral ligament: the anterior, posterior, and transverse bundles. The anterior bundle serves as the primary stabilizer against valgus and internal rotary forces, while the posterior bundle is a secondary stabilizer at 120 degrees of elbow flexion. Both of these bundles attach directly to the medial epicondyle. The transverse bundle does not contribute to stability of the elbow.[15]

Six physes about the elbow ossify between 1 and 17 years old, with high variability regarding the exact timing of physeal closure depending on the individual. Use of the mnemonic, CRITOE (capitellum, radial head, internal/medial epicondyle, trochlea, olecranon, external/lateral epicondyle) starting at 1 year old and continuing in 2-year increments, is helpful in remembering the ossification sequence about the elbow (Fig. 24.2). Ossifying physes at the elbow in the preadolescent athlete contribute to the risk of injury at the elbow.[9,13] The medial epicondyle begins ossification around 6 years old, but does not fuse to the humerus until 14–17 years old, forming a vulnerable area susceptible to valgus forces, predominantly in overhead-throwing athletes. The valgus distraction (displacement or force away from the midline of the body/stress on the medial aspect of elbow) on the medial epicondyle apophysis can lead to little league elbow.[13,16,17]

Clinical Assessment

Patients with medial epicondyle apophysitis (little league elbow) present with insidious and gradual onset of medial elbow pain. The patient may report arm fatigue, particularly during the stride/early cocking and cocking stages of throwing motion (Fig. 24.3). Complaints of point tenderness at the medial epicondyle, edema, and decreased throwing velocity and strength are common. Range of motion about the elbow is typically unaffected; however, a contracture greater than 15 degrees, ecchymosis, catching or a "popping" sound when throwing, is indicative of an avulsion fracture.

Furthermore, as throwing involves the entire upper extremity, it is important to note that excessive external rotation of the shoulder, with concomitant decreased internal rotation of the shoulder, a condition known as glenohumeral rotation deficit (GIRD) can lead to increased valgus stress being placed on the medial aspect of the elbow. It is always important to obtain a detailed history of pitch counts and pitch types, as these injuries are often a result of repetitive high valgus forces.[13,16,17]

The diagnosis of medial epicondyle apophysitis is largely based on the clinical examination given the variability of radiographic findings.[8] However, obtaining radiographs of the contralateral side can assist in observing if there is apophysis widening or a fracture present.[12] (Fig. 24.4). A widening of the medial epicondyle physis is indicative of early injury, and if play is continued, progression to a UCL tear or medial epicondyle avulsion fracture is possible.[18] The older athlete may also have

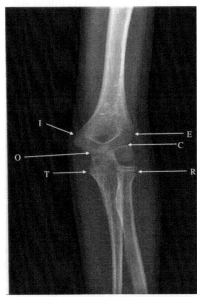

FIG. 24.2 Radiograph of a 7-year-old male with labeled ossification centers about the elbow: (C) capitellum, (R) radial head, (I) internal/medial epicondyle, (T) trochlea, (O) olecranon, and (E) external/lateral epicondyle. (Courtesy of Joshua M. Abzug, MD.)

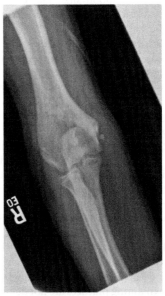

FIG. 24.4 Plain radiograph (AP view) of a 13-year-old baseball pitcher with little league elbow. Note the physeal widening of the medial epicondyle epiphysis. (Courtesy of Joshua M. Abzug, MD.)

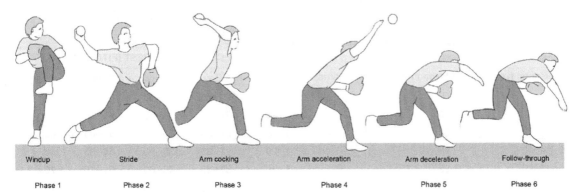

Windup	Stride	Arm cocking	Arm acceleration	Arm deceleration	Follow-through
Phase 1	Phase 2	Phase 3	Phase 4	Phase 5	Phase 6

FIG. 24.3 Stages of throwing in baseball. (Adapted from Pinkowsky G, Hennrikus W. The throwing athlete. In: Abzug JM, Kozin SH, Zlotolow DA, editors. *The Pediatric Upper Extremity*. New York: Springer; 2015: 1635–1666.)

ulnar nerve irritation or even instability of the nerve during throwing. A study by Wei et al. showed that magnetic resonance imaging (MRI) does not commonly provide findings beyond the information obtained from a thorough history, physical examination, and plain radiographs and is therefore not necessary for true cases of medial epicondyle apophysitis.[19]

Prevention

Rest is of utmost importance in the prevention of medial epicondyle apophysitis. Pitchers are not the only athletes at risk for medial epicondyle apophysitis; catchers, volleyball players, tennis players, and football quarterbacks are also vulnerable to the valgus stresses of the overhead thrower. Such athletes should play a maximum of 8 months out of the year to allow their bodies time to rest and prevent long-term damage. Avoidance of participation in more than one game per day, playing on multiple teams, pitching and catching in the same game, and pitching for more than three consecutive days are also measures that should be taken to prevent injury. Young athletes should not play through pain.[20] Both the Major League Baseball Association and the Little League Association support the need for young players to rest their throwing arm between games. As a preventative measure, the USA Baseball organization with collaboration from the American Sports Medicine Institute has set forth pitching guidelines and recommendations via the Pitch Smart Program (Table 24.1). However, the amount and types of pitches thrown during practices are not defined or taken into account in these counts. On a positive note, the minimum age for the types of pitches has begun to be considered in their recommendations.

The importance of resting between games and making sure every young athlete has an off-season from overhead-throwing sports, at least 3 months (4 months preferred), is integral to preventing overuse injuries. Pitching more than 100 pitches in a year can significantly increase the risk for injury.[21] Lyman et al. reported that pitchers who threw 600–800 pitches in one season were 234% more likely to sustain an elbow injury.[22] The combination of fatigue and overuse greatly impact biomechanical form when throwing. When tired, young athletes are less likely to maintain optimal stance amplifying potential valgus elbow injury.[23]

Additionally, overall conditioning of the core, pelvis, and shoulder girdle are essential in preventing elbow injuries in overhead-throwing athletes. The biomechanical form of the shoulder girdle should be evaluated to minimize stress on the shoulder and elbow.[10] Proper pitching mechanics from trunk to hand and conditioning addressed in childhood can limit overuse injuries as the athlete ages.[20]

Yukutake et al. formulated a risk evaluation tool consisting of six questions to identify risk factors for sustaining throwing injuries.[24] The authors found the most significant indicators to be pain in the extremity during the preseason and the participation of 7 days of independent training.[24] (Appendix 1). Education is a critical component in the prevention of these injuries. Providing simple surveys, such as those composed by Yukatake et al., can bring awareness of risk factors to players, their families, and the coaching staff.[24] Instruction on the importance of listening to one's body and resting after experiencing pain is another necessary part of prevention, particularly in the ever-increasing competitive sporting world that often promotes a

TABLE 24.1
Recommended Pitch Count for Little League Baseball Suggested by USA Baseball With Collaboration From the American Sports Medicine Institute.

Age Range (years)	Maximum Pitches per Game	RECOMMENDED REST (PITCHES)				
		0 Days	1 Day	2 Days	3 Days	4 Days
7–8	50	1–20	21–35	36–50	N/A	N/A
9–10	75	1–20	21–35	36–50	51–65	66+
11–12	85	1–20	21–35	36–50	51–65	66+
13–14	95	1–20	21–35	36–50	51–65	66+
15–16	95	1–30	31–45	46–60	61–75	76+
17–18	105	1–30	31–45	46–60	61–75	76+
19–22	120	1–30	31–45	46–60	61–75	76+

Adapted from Pitch Smart USA Baseball. Guidelines for Youth and Adolescent; 2018. https://www.mlb.com/pitch-smart/pitching-guidelines.

"play through the pain" mentality.[20] General pitching guidelines do not include pitches thrown in practices and types of pitches; however, the hazards of throwing breaking pitches (ex. curveball, slider, or slurve) in young athletes are a source of continued debate (Table 24.2). The technique involves greater finger involvement and wrist movement causing the ball to spin and change trajectory.[13] In general, it is considered risky and ill-advised practice for any athlete under 14 years old to throw breaking pitches due to their decreased neuromuscular control and limited biomechanical form.[13,14,25,26] Additional factors associated with prevention of injury include physical condition, nutrition, hydration, and environment. These previously mentioned factors influence the overall health and endurance of the young athlete and should not be overlooked.[20]

Conservative Treatment

In the absence of a medial epicondyle fracture, conservative treatment of medial epicondyle apophysitis consists of 4–6 weeks of complete rest from all sports-related activities, supplemented with icing and antiinflammatory medication. Practitioners may also recommend a long-arm orthosis if compliance is in question or the patient is in substantial pain. If the radiographs demonstrate a widening of the apophysis and/or an avulsion fracture with less than 5 mm of displacement, the patient should be placed in a long arm cast or orthosis at 90 degrees of flexion with the forearm in neutral rotation for 4 weeks[13] (Fig. 24.5). A course of occupational or physical therapy is subsequently recommended to gradually rehabilitate and strengthen the affected extremity. A progressive therapy program that starts with joint mobility and range of

motion (ROM), followed by the initiation of biomechanical patterns needed for throwing and ending with increasing stress to facilitate tissue adaption for throwing is recommended to fully rehabilitate the upper extremity.[27] Return to throwing within a structured sport is not recommended for at least 3 months.[3] The patient's throwing mechanics and technique must be evaluated and modified as necessary during this time period.

Progressive medial epicondyle apophysitis may also lead to a partial or complete tear of the UCL, particularly in the preadolescent and adolescent populations. The conservative management of a UCL tear depends on the severity of the tear: a 1–2 week immobilization period in a hinged elbow brace may be recommended with ice and antiinflammatory medications in partial tears. Early protected motion can be introduced to limit elbow stiffness and muscle atrophy, which consists of a hinged elbow brace limiting valgus force and elbow extension/flexion motion in a pain-free arc of movement, typically 10–100 degrees. The brace facilitates realigning the tears in the collagen fibers, as the ligament begins to heal. Additionally, performing isometric exercises to the shoulder, elbow, and wrist will also assist in limiting atrophy while the affected extremity is immobilized. During the initial 2 weeks postinjury, passive shoulder external rotation should be avoided due to the valgus force it can produce on the elbow. The nonpainful arc of motion is progressed by 5–10 degrees per week in both elbow extension and flexion, with return of full motion by week 4, including forearm rotation. At approximately week 5, static and dynamic stability exercises are introduced. Advancing to isotonic exercises for the upper extremity by weeks 6–7 and advanced strengthening such as the Thrower's Ten exercises (Appendix 2) (Appendix 3) and plyometrics are included in the rehabilitation.[10] Following the completion of the throwing program, stability, and isotonic exercises without return of symptoms, the athlete may start an interval sport program completely pain-free and then may return to competitive sports. Such interval sport programs consist of evaluation of sport-specific drills with the use of a plyometric ball.[11] Return of symptoms and pain need to be monitored, particularly with increased throwing distances or frequencies throughout therapy.[10]

Although most patients with little league elbow can be treated conservatively with success, if medial elbow pain persists or worsens there is an increased likelihood of progression to a medial epicondyle avulsion fracture or complete tear of the UCL requiring surgical intervention.

Operative Intervention

Displaced medial epicondyle avulsion fractures in overhead-throwing athletes are best treated surgically

---

TABLE 24.2

Ages for Which Pitches Should be Learned Based on Order of Growth Plate Closure in Elbow.

Pitch Type	Age at which Pitch Should Be Introduced
Fastball	8
Change-up	10
Curveball	14
Knuckleball	15
Slider	16
Splitter	16
Screwball	17

Adapted from Lyman S, Fleisig GS, Andrews JR, Osinski ED. Effect of pitch type, pitch count, and pitching mechanics on risk of elbow and shoulder pain in youth baseball pitchers. *Am J Sports Med.* 2002; 30(4):463–8.

(A) **(B)**

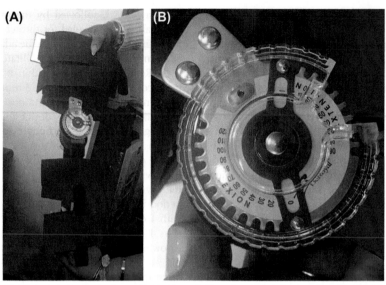

FIG. 24.5 (A) Clinical photograph of a pediatric hinged elbow brace in full extension. (B) Note the adjustable range of motion dial that can be modified as therapy progresses. (Courtesy of Joshua M. Abzug, MD.)

with open reduction and internal fixation. Early active range of motion (AROM) is begun at 2–3 weeks postoperatively. For cases with an associated UCL tear, reconstruction via the Tommy-John procedure or repair via the docking procedure, may be performed warranting a specific, regimented rehabilitation protocol. The general guidelines and timeline for rehabilitation following UCL surgery utilizing either an autograft or the docking surgical technique can be seen in Appendices 4 or 5, respectively.

Rehabilitation

At the initiation of therapy, general conditioning and postural control should be assessed. In addition, it is fundamental to evaluate scapular and shoulder function, as it directly impacts the forces on the elbow.[21,28] The therapist should use the nonthrowing side for comparison, given that the throwing scapula often postures anteriorly tilted, protracted, and depressed.[29] Kyphotic posture can mask a weak serratus anterior by orienting the scapula in a protracted position. The serratus anterior is weak if the thoracic spine is extended and the scapula wings while in a quadruped position.[23] Frequently, overhead-throwing athletes will display decreased internal rotation and horizontal adduction, described as GIRD, with an associated excessive amount of external rotation. In such instances, the use of the sleeper stretch for prevention of posterior capsule tightness is important to include as part of a comprehensive home exercise program. Evaluation of the glenohumeral

joint is necessary to assess for muscle imbalances contributing to an anterior positioning of the humeral head, even after scapular realignment is addressed.[28] Examining the position of the humeral head and palpation of the rotator cuff muscles, in addition to manual muscle testing of the shoulder, assist the practitioner in deducing the cause of protracted positioning. The pulling of the humeral head anteriorly can be attributed to pectoralis tightness, limited thoracic extension, lower trapezius weakness, posterior capsule tightness, and forward head posture.[23,30] In throwing, scapular control by the upper trapezius, serratus anterior, and lower trapezius ensure that the scapula is tilted posteriorly, is elevated, and is upwardly rotated to achieve a successful throw. As such, sequential firing, scapular kinematics, stability, and control of the proximal muscles should be addressed through neuromuscular reeducation and isometric exercises for the shoulder and scapula in the early stages of therapy, before progressing to therapy for the elbow.[23,25,31,32] The therapist should also assess synergistic core activation of all the abdominal muscles: rectus abdominus, transverse abdominis, obliques, and lower abdominals including the pelvic floor. Ensuring that the patient is utilizing diaphragmatic breathing as opposed to accessory breathing, which can lead to shortening of the periscapular muscles, particularly in the pediatric patient, is necessary.[23]

Concurrently, the initial phase of rehabilitation should focus on decreasing inflammation and elbow ROM in a pain-free arc. Edema management can be addressed with cryotherapy and compression. AROM is initiated in a pain-free arc, progressing to active assistive range of motion (AAROM) if a flexion contracture is present before immobilization, until full ROM is obtained. If possible, obtaining elbow extension measurements preseason and/or preinjury is helpful in planning rehabilitation goals, as the preinjury elbow motion may lack 3–5 degrees of full extension and is more likely to develop flexion contractures. Tightness in the joint capsule, formation of scar tissue in the brachialis and adhesions in the anterior capsule limit the full extension of the elbow and bilateral measurements can differ by as much as 5–6 degrees.[33] In addition to AAROM, grade I and II mobilizations may assist in improving ROM. Specifically, when end range of elbow extension is difficult to obtain, humeroulnar posterior glide oscillations and low-load long duration stretch can be helpful. The intensity of mobilizations and stretching is dependent on the healing of the tissues and the report of pain during limited motion. If there is pain before application of resistance, gentle and graded stretching supports the healing structures in the safest manner.[10]

The second phase of rehabilitation should include isometric elbow strengthening along with continued strengthening of the shoulder and scapula. Rotator cuff muscle strengthening against gravity and the use of exercise bands is added. Isotonic elbow strengthening is included when full AROM is achieved.[10] It is best to begin with concentric and progress to eccentric elbow extension/flexion, wrist extension/flexion, and forearm supination/protonation. Beginning proprioceptive training to limit muscle fatigue may also be initiated in this phase.[34] Graded closed chained exercises are also added to dynamically strengthen the upper extremity stabilizers and core.[30]

The third phase of rehabilitation consists of further dynamic strengthening of the core and upper extremities. Increased strengthening of eccentric elbow flexion is an important focus, as eccentric control limits abutment of the olecranon in the fossa during deceleration and the biceps acts as a stabilizer during follow-through of a throw.[35] Dynamic closed chained exercises, plyometrics, and a throwing program should be completed during this phase of rehabilitation (Video 1). Throughout this process, it is important to keep in mind skeletal maturity, workload limits, and the biomechanics of throwing. The amount of torque at the shoulder and elbow during an overhead throw increases between the ages of 12 and 15, thereby increasing the importance of biomechanical control while throwing to limit the risk of injury, as the skeletal system achieves maturity.[21] A comprehensive list of

dynamic exercises that are commonly incorporated into rehabilitation protocols for athletes recovering from little league elbow can be found in Appendix 6.

Various throwing programs have been created to promote full preinjury recovery given the biomechanical demands unique to each throwing phase. Early and late cocking stages apply significant valgus overload and distraction to the medial elbow.[17] The position of the pelvis, trunk, and ipsilateral one-foot balance during the windup stage impacts the arm speed during acceleration. Peak elbow valgus torque is present just before the acceleration, right before maximum shoulder external rotation.[25] Observation and feedback are necessary to provide the patient with optimal pitching technique as they return to throwing. The "Thrower's Ten program" and the "Advanced Thrower's Ten Program" are two common throwing programs for youth athletes to follow, both in-season and for out of season training.[30] (Appendix 2) (Appendix 3). In addition, the University of Delaware and the Mayo Clinic created training programs, the Interval Throw Program, which provides throwing limits based on distance and intensity for little league players based on age.[36] (Appendixes 7–9). Following the completion of a throwing program without return of pain or symptoms, the athlete is advised to complete an interval sports program as it is much more comprehensive and focuses on the use of the extremity and its demands relevant to different sports.[10]

OSTEOCHONDRITIS DISSECANS

OCD was first described in 1874 by Paget and has continued to plague the medical profession with its unclear etiology and debated methods of treatment.[37] OCD is an osteochondral injury that can lead to the development of loose bodies within a joint. In the upper extremity, it is most commonly observed in the capitellum of the elbow, but can also be seen about the elbow in the trochlea, radial head, and olecranon.[12,38] Multiple etiological factors are considered to be responsible for an OCD lesion including repetitive compressive forces, inflammation, genetics, vascular abnormalities, and environmental factors.[39] Baseball players and gymnasts are at increased risk of developing OCD about the elbow due to the repetitive nature of upper extremity movements in these overhead and weight-bearing sports, respectively.[37,39] For example, in baseball, the greatest valgus compressive force is applied at the lateral elbow during deceleration when the ball leaves the hand.[17] This compressive force adds to the mitigating factors of the ossifying centers between the radial head and humeral capitellum. A valgus torque is also present during the arm-cocked position during ball release with elbow extension causing impingement of the posterior elbow.[20] The highest incidences of OCD of the elbow have been observed in adolescent athletes, ages 11−17.[40,41] Young athletes participating in overhead throwing sports are at risk of developing OCD of the elbow with high frequency and intensity of throws.

Anatomy and Classification

OCD of the elbow is commonly observed on the distal anterolateral aspect of the humerus due to the poorly vascularized capitellum.[12] OCD of the capitellum affects the subchondral bone as well as the overlying cartilage of the central or lateral aspect of the capitellum. OCD is differentiated from Panner's disease, which is an osteochondrosis of the entire capitellum and occurs in younger patients, 5−10 years old. Panner's disease does not present with loose bodies.[38]

Initially when an OCD occurs, the capitellum will demonstrate some subchondral flattening or sclerotic bone with disturbance of the articular cartilage. As the disease progresses, limited blood supply to the area causes the bone and cartilage to separate and form a loose body, which can impact motion, cause pain and lead to a popping/catching sensation with elbow motion.

Clinical Assessment

Patients with OCD classically report pain on the lateral or central aspect of the elbow and may remark about a "catching or popping" due to a loose body. Less than 20% of patients present with edema over the affected region.[37,40] Radiocapitellar tenderness to palpation may be present, along with decreased elbow extension or crepitus. The active radiocapitellar compression test, in which the examiner places the patient's elbow in full extension and the patient actively pronates and supinates the forearm, can be used to illicit lateral elbow pain in a patient with an OCD. A positive test result reveals either an OCD or medial ulnar collateral ligament weakness and indicates the need for further work-up, typically with advanced imaging such as an MRI.[40]

Given the limited symptomatic presentation before fragmentation, radiographic imaging is a crucial component of the diagnostic work-up. Radiographs positive for an OCD will demonstrate subchondral flattening, sclerotic bone, and/or radiolucency during the early stages (Fig. 24.6). If plain radiographs do not demonstrate an abnormality, an MRI can be obtained to further evaluate for an OCD lesion (Fig. 24.7). In the context of the diagnostic evaluation, assessing the

stability of the OCD lesion is imperative, as instability may impact the decision for surgical intervention.

Prevention

As a result of the multifactorial etiology of OCD of the capitellum, preventive strategies are limited. Due to a possible genetic link, if the patient has a family history of OCD, it may be recommended that they limit the amount of time participating in an overhead-throwing sport or upper extremity weight-bearing sport, such as gymnastics.[42] In general, a pediatric athlete is unaware of the development of the OCD until there are obvious signs of pain or difficulty with ROM. Once a lesion on the subchondral bone of the elbow is identified, compliance to activity modification of limiting axial load on the radiocapitellar joint and rest is imperative. Early detection of an OCD and immediate activity modification with cessation of the sport and rest have been observed to induce spontaneous healing.[39] However, the importance of continued monitoring of the subchondral bone in the wake of recovery is recommended to safeguard against OCD reoccurrence.

Conservative Treatment

The optimal method of nonoperative treatment of OCD of the capitellum is debated and varies across current literature. Current treatments include termination of the aggravating sport, casting, utilizing a hinged elbow brace, and rest.[16,37,40] Management is dependent on the stability of the lesion, the cartilage integrity, and the condition of the capitellar physis. Stable lesions can be treated with a hinged elbow brace, activity modification, and rest and typically demonstrate improvement of symptoms within 3−12 weeks.[39] Additional indications for conservative management include an open capitellar physis, less than a 20-degree limitation in elbow extension/flexion, and/or a primarily intact capitellum on radiographs without fragmentation or instability.[40] Current literature supports nonoperative management for stable OCD lesions, particularly in the young athlete.[40,43,44]

Patients should be followed with radiographs in 6−8 week increments to ensure consistency between radiograph improvements and verbalized pain symptoms. Despite reports of improvements in pain, radiographs may not always reflect the same improvements in the radiolucency about the lesion. Therefore, initiation of exercises and activities needs to be carefully weighed with images and patient reports, because increased radiocapitellar stress can cause regression in an unprepared elbow.[16,40] As radiographs demonstrate recalcification and the patient reports anecdotal

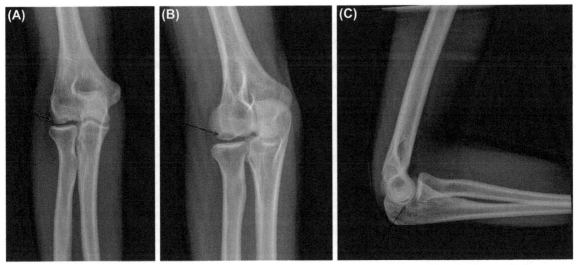

FIG. 24.6 Radiographs of an elbow OCD in a 13-year-old female volleyball player. Note the lucency in the capitellum: **(A)** AP view, **(B)** oblique view, and **(C)** lateral view. (Courtesy of Joshua M. Abzug, MD.)

improvements, gentle ROM is initiated in occupational or physical therapy. Although patients may be anxious to return to their sport, the patient and family should be counseled to avoid overhead and extended elbow activity to allow the articular surface of the capitellum to fully heal.[16] In the case of failed conservative treatment, surgical intervention may be required.

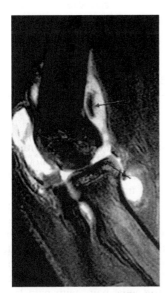

FIG. 24.7 Sagittal slice of an elbow MRI with an OCD lesion of the capitellum (bottom arrow) and a corresponding loose body in the joint space (top arrow). (Courtesy of Joshua M. Abzug, MD.)

Operative Intervention

Once operative intervention is determined to be necessary, the specific procedure performed will be dictated by the location and size of the OCD lesion, as well as the presence/absence of a stable cartilage cap or loose bodies. For example, lateral uncontained lesions may be preferably treated with an osteochondral autograft transfer (OATS) procedure, while contained lesions located centrally on the capitellum may be optimally treated with microfracture.

When loose bodies are present, arthroscopic removal or fragment fixation may be attempted. When unstable OCD lesions are observed, in situ fixation may be the ideal intervention. This can be performed using bone pins, Kirschner wires, absorbable pins, Herbert screw fixation, or other implants, such as darts, designed specifically to stabilize OCD lesions.

When full excision of the OCD lesion is not necessary, the surgeon may elect to proceed with a microfracture procedure. Following the removal of any fraying cartilage, a microfracture pick is used to place a number of small holes in the subchondral bone to stimulate bleeding and an inflammatory response with the goal of new cartilage formation. Cartilage restoration using osteochondral autograft transfer (OATS), is indicated for large, unstable lesions, and those covering most the articular surface. These procedures involve the harvesting of bone and intact articular cartilage, typically from the knee in an area with less weight-bearing. The osteochondral plugs are then grafted at the site of the OCD lesion.

Rehabilitation

Depending on the surgical procedure performed, the severity of the injury, and complications, postoperative care will vary. Control of pain and edema are in the forefront of rehabilitation and patients are reminded to avoid aggravating activities, such as prematurely returning to sports and radiocapitellar stress by avoiding full elbow extension on the affected upper extremity. General guidelines for rehabilitation following arthroscopic debridement, microfracture (Table 24.3), and alternative operative procedures warrant 3—5 months for full return to sport (Table 24.4).

GYMNAST WRIST

Gymnastics is a physically and psychologically demanding sport, with widespread popularity increasing with every Olympics.[45] Muscle memory,

TABLE 24.3
General Rehabilitation Protocol Following Microfracture or Arthroscopic Debridement of OCD of the Capitellum.

Weeks Post-Op	Focus of Rehab
Week 1	• Transition from postoperative dressing to hinged elbow brace and initiate gentle active range of motion under the guidance of an occupational or physical therapist • Edema management • Scar management
Week 4	• Following physician clearance, initiate active assistive range of motion if full range of motion not achieved
Week 6	• Following physician clearance, initiate passive range of motion if full range of motion is not achieved
Weeks 8–12	• Wean from hinged brace when no pain or complications with motion • Begin light strengthening when no pain and full range of motion is achieved
Weeks 10–12	• Dynamic stability and strengthening to entire affected upper extremity • Throwing program
Months 3–4	• Full return to sport

TABLE 24.4
General Rehabilitation Protocol Following Alternative Operative Procedures Such as OATS for OCD of the Capitellum.

Weeks Post-Op	Focus of Rehab
Week 1	• Transition from postoperative dressing to hinged elbow brace and initiate gentle active range of motion under the guidance of an occupational or physical therapist • Edema management • Scar management
Week 4	• Following physician clearance, continue active range of motion if full range of motion not achieved. • Consider NMES for neuromuscular retraining
Week 6	• Following physician clearance, initiate active assistive range of motion if full range of motion not achieved
Weeks 8–12	• Following physician clearance, initiate passive range of motion if full range of motion not achieved • Wean from hinged elbow brace when no pain or complications with motion • Begin light strengthening when no pain and full range of motion is achieved
Weeks 12–14	• Dynamic stability and strengthening to entire affected upper extremity • Throwing program
Months 4–5	• Full return to sport

strength, stability, balance, and neuromuscular control are needed for completion of meticulous routines. During the 10—15-year career of a professional/competitive gymnast, 50 h of training per week during the peak of competition years is common.[46–48] Chronic wrist pain is prevalent at all levels of gymnastics; however, the skeletally immature wrist is at greater risk for bony injury due to the developing growth plates, whereas soft tissue injuries are more prevalent in postpubescent athletes.[49,50] Specifically, 50% of beginning to midlevel gymnasts report wrist pain, with pain lasting at least 6 months in 45% of those participants.[51] Correspondingly, up to 79% of gymnasts report wrist pain at the collegiate level.[50–52] A variety of injuries contribute to wrist pain in gymnasts. Specifically, the frequent weight-bearing at the wrist level can develop into a positive ulnar variance, which is seen in 40%–80% of professional gymnasts.[53,54] The wrist's primary role of optimizing strength and dexterity in the forearm and digits for fine motor control is transformed into a weight-bearing joint in gymnastics.[46,51] Changing the function of a joint changes the biomechanics of the wrist over time.

During training, the upper extremities are tasked with managing frequent, high-velocity loading and traction forces at the wrist.[16,54,55] A back handspring or pommel horse routine can generate forces up to 16 times the gymnast's body weight at the level of the wrist.[56,57] One common cause of wrist pain is a physeal injury to the distal radius physis, frequently referred to as gymnast wrist. Another common name for this injury is distal radius epiphysitis.[46] Distal radius epiphysitis is an overuse injury caused by axial loading on the hyperextended wrist with open growth plates. The frequent rotational and traction force causes a stress reaction between the distal radius physis and epiphysis.[3,58] This can lead to premature closure of the distal radius physis which contributes to positive ulnar variance and ultimately, growth arrest and degenerative arthritis[46,53,59–63] (Fig. 24.8).

Elite gymnasts typically start training around 3–6 years old.[64] Frequency and intensity of training increases with age; however, the bones within the upper extremity continue to develop and ossify up to 17 years old for females and 19 years old for males.[65] Female gymnasts tend to injure their wrist more than males, while male gymnasts tend to injure their shoulders more, most likely due to their participation in the rings and pommel horse events.

Gymnasts report most pain in the dorsum of the wrist, describing the most symptoms during weight-bearing with the wrist extended.[50,51,58] Kox et al. found that the peak incidence of wrist pain in young gymnasts was between the ages of 9 and 14 years.[66] Although specific research is limited in the impact of weight-bearing on carpal development, the correlation between the increase of wrist pain and the development of the carpus warrants further investigation. As a gymnast ages, axial forces at the wrist increase due to greater body mass, practice time, and training intensity associated with higher levels of gymnastics.

Repetitive forces negatively impact the open physes.[49,59,67] DiFori et al. reported that hyperextended wrist weight-bearing in gymnasts increases positive ulnar variance as compared to same age peers.[49] Repetitive microtrauma advances to abnormal endochondral ossification, which can progress to distal radial physeal growth arrest and subsequent positive ulnar variance, due to rotational and traction forces compromising the blood supply.[3,50] Positive ulnar variance may lead to ulnar impaction syndrome,[68] TFCC injury,[69] and/or osteomalacia of the ulnar carpal bones.[70,71] Reportedly, 50% of midlevel gymnasts describe having wrist pain.[50,72]

As the young athlete ages, the open growth plates are at most risk for injury. In 1998, Gabel divided the progression of stress about the distal radius physis into three stages.[46] Stage I is diagnosed with a clinical assessment and patient interview, as there are no notable changes in the radiographs. Stage II reflects both clinical (pain) and radiographic findings (changes at the distal radial physis are evident). Stage III consists of notable clinical findings, radiographic changes to the distal radial physis, and the presence of positive ulnar variance. Often, this late stage (stage III) in elite gymnasts is present without symptoms of pain as the change in the radius, ulna, and carpus alignment is chronic and has become normalized.[46] It is also likely in stage III that ulnar variance has impacted other aspects of the wrist including ligament complexes, such as the TFCC, and/or carpal bones (Fig. 24.9).

Additional repetitive overuse conditions observed in upper extremity weight-bearing athletes include dorsal impingement, scaphoid impaction syndrome, and extensor retinaculum impingement. The end result of

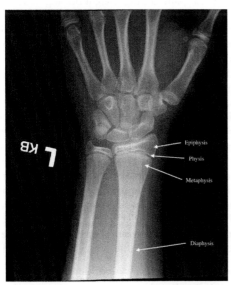

Epiphysis

Physis

Metaphysis

Diaphysis

FIG. 24.8 Radiograph (PA view) of a 13-year-old female with open growth plate anatomy. (Courtesy of Joshua M. Abzug, MD.)

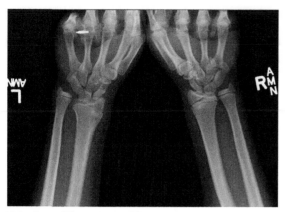

FIG. 24.9 Bilateral wrist PA radiograph of an 11-year-old female gymnast with left ulnar impaction syndrome, characteristic of stage III gymnast wrist. (Courtesy of Joshua M. Abzug, MD.)

all of these conditions is dorsal wrist pain that is caused by wrist hyperextension; however, each of these diagnoses and their treatments differ.

Primary dorsal impingement is described as tenderness about the dorsal radius and carpal rims during active and passive extension. The frequent impaction forces may cause dorsal capsulitis or synovitis leading to thickening of the capsule. Eventual osteophyte formation along the dorsal radius, scaphoid, and/or lunate is possible. When diagnosed early, immobilization, rest, antiinflammatories, and corticosteroid injections have successfully resolved symptoms. If symptoms persist, debridement via wrist arthroscopy and posterior interosseous nerve excision may be warranted.[46,64]

Scaphoid impaction syndrome, described by Linscheid and Dobyns, is when the dorsal rim of the scaphoid and dorsal lip of the radius are pushed together during hyperextension and is most commonly seen in floor routines, pressure from the weight bar in weight lifters, or with too many push-ups.[73] Clinically, the patient reports tenderness along the dorsoradial aspect of the wrist over the dorsal rim of the scaphoid and pain with wrist flexion and ulnar deviation. Immobilization, rest, and avoidance of forced wrist hyperextension are the initial conservative treatments, with corticosteroid injections considered at times.[73] Surgical intervention involves a cheilectomy of the dorsal rim of the scaphoid and/or dorsal lip of the radius. Following 2 weeks of cast immobilization and gradual reintroduction of ROM, the patient may return to activities as tolerated.[64,73]

Extensor retinaculum impingement, a relatively newer diagnosis, occurs when the extensor retinaculum pathologically thickens causing impingement and subsequent pain in the dorsum of the wrist during repetitive extension. Clinically, patients will complain of pain and present with swelling along the distal border of the extensor retinaculum. To confirm this diagnosis, a positive provocative test is warranted to elicit reproducible pain during resisted digital extension while the wrist is maintained in the end range of extension. If there are suspicions of this diagnosis, obtaining an MRI is recommended, as radiographs are not always sensitive for this diagnosis. Conservative treatment consisting of rest, ice, and antiinflammatories should be attempted before providing a corticosteroid injection. With failed conservative management, surgical treatment including a tenosynovectomy of the extensor tendons and resection of the extensor retinaculum will alleviate symptoms. Postoperatively, the patient is immobilized in a short-arm cast for 1 month, followed by AROM and progression toward wrist and forearm strengthening according to progress and pain.[74,75]

Gymnasts are more likely to develop dorsal wrist pain due to the high frequency and intensity of load bearing on their extended wrists during various gymnastic events.[74] Dorsal impingement, scaphoid impaction syndrome, and extensor retinaculum impingement are differential diagnoses not as recognizable as distal radius epiphysitis; however, they fall under the umbrella of gymnast wrist injuries and one should be aware of the various presentations.

Clinical Assessment

Patients with distal radius epiphysitis will complain of dorsal wrist pain during weight-bearing that lessens with rest. Point tenderness at the distal radial physis is present along with pain with axial loads to the wrist in extension. The push-off test is used to reproduce symptoms by weight-bearing on a tabletop. The patient may also have swelling, decreased ROM, and/or decreased grip strength in advanced cases.[46,66] Radiographs may reveal a widened, sclerotic, and/or calcifying distal radial physis.[54,67] In addition, the use of MRI may provide additional information, depending on the severity of the injury (Fig. 24.10). Differential diagnoses of wrist pain in gymnasts can be due to several other issues including triangular fibrocartilage complex tears/sprains, scapholunate or lunotriquetral ligament tears, scaphoid impaction syndrome, dorsal impingement, and/or carpal instability.[58,64,76] These differential diagnoses can be due to progressive, chronic gymnast wrist or they may be present concurrently with earlier stages of gymnast wrist.

Prevention

Factors impacting the risk of gymnast wrist include limited training techniques, improper use of equipment (such as soft mats), previous injury, growth spurts, and

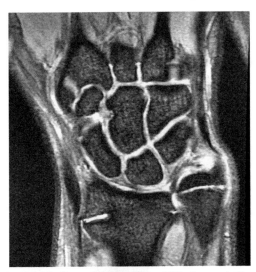

FIG. 24.10 Coronal slice of an MRI demonstrating a partially closed distal radial growth plate and open distal ulnar growth plate resulting in positive ulnar variance. (Courtesy of Joshua M. Abzug, MD.)

persistent pain.[72,77] During initiation of training, the gymnast's proper technique and how equipment is safely used should be stressed. For example, the use of soft mats leads to increased wrist hyperextension causing more stress on the wrist and therefore firm mats are recommended. Evaluation of the trunk, shoulder complex, elbow and wrist for stability, alignment, strength, and flexibility should be constant. With training, closed chained exercises provide insight into how the wrist is absorbing tensile forces. During closed chained kinetic exercises, the extremity is in contact with a fixed immobile surface, such as weight-bearing with the hand down on a vault. When completing beam routines, the elbows are locked and the wrists are absorbing rotational forces during maneuvers. Lack of strength and control in core muscles and the shoulder contribute to negative forces being applied to the distal upper extremity.[72,78]

Alignment and form need to be continuously assessed and critiqued, not only with increased complexity, but also with growth. Often growth causes imbalances between muscles and bone, and time is needed for the gymnast to adapt to changes in their limbs and body.[50] For example, increased ulnar deviation in the wrist during weight-bearing increases the risk of radial impaction, particularly after repetitive and high velocity drills such as the vault.[56,72,78]

A video or photograph of the gymnast completing floor routines, pommel horse, or beam work can be particularly useful in assessing upper extremity positioning. Use of wrist supports thatprevent end range hyperextension, such as tiger paws or taping, may assist in alignment and limiting the traction force on the epiphysis.[55] Research supporting the use of supports is limited; however, anecdotal evidence is positive from gymnasts. Coaches and trainers need to advocate proper form from the very beginning when introducing new routines. Regular conditioning, strengthening, proprioception training, and stability exercises outside of actual gymnastic techniques are key to preventing injury.[77] Throughout all levels of gymnastics, athletes should be educated on the importance of obtaining medical attention for persistent pain, especially in the upper extremity. Persistent pain should not be ignored and evaluation by a medical professional may limit the progression of an injury.

Conservative Treatment

Stage I distal radius epiphysitis is treated with a course of ice, rest, and antiinflammatory medications. Medical management is individualized depending on other diagnostic findings, and may include immobilization, therapy, and/or corticosteroid injections. Rest and avoidance of aggravating activities is recommended for at least 4 weeks, with return to sport only after the patient has no pain or point tenderness. In stage II, immobilization of the wrist for 4–6 weeks is prescribed with rest from activity (Fig. 24.11). If compliance with a removable orthosis is doubted, casting should be considered. Following clinical improvement, it is important to follow-up with physical or occupational therapy to receive a comprehensive evaluation and treatment to manage wrist rehabilitation.[3,46] The patient should not return to gymnastics until the radiographs have normalized. Stage III intervention is dependent on the severity of symptoms and clinical presentation. Immobilization with casting for 6–8 weeks can be considered; however, at this late stage surgical intervention is often necessary. Although not typically recommended in prepubescent athletes, some physicians consider corticosteroid injections for pain management in the skeletally mature gymnast[79,80] Follow-through with a comprehensive occupational or physical therapy rehabilitation program is essential following immobilization or rest. In instances where pain persists and extensive injury to the wrist is not improved through conservative management, surgery options are considered.

Operative Intervention

In cases where a physeal bar is identified about the distal radius, a physeal bar resection and interposition grafting

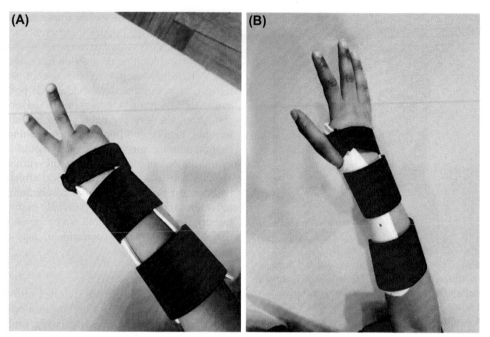

FIG. 24.11 Clinical photographs of a volar wrist splint commonly utilized for gymnast wrist immobilization: **(A)** dorsal view and **(B)** radial view. (Courtesy of Heta Parikh, OTR/L.)

or completion epiphysiodesis (completion of the growth arrest) may be warranted to prevent ulnar abutment syndrome from occurring or worsening. A physeal bar resection removes the bony formation within the physis to allow for continued growth along the remaining active physis. Local fat is typically interposed to fill the void created by the removed bony bar. These procedures can be complicated by damaged physis surrounding the physeal bar thatcan complicate healing. As such, these procedures are only recommended in young children who have substantial growth remaining.

Patients with a history of ulnar impaction syndrome are best treated with an ulnar shortening osteotomy. This procedure involves the removal of a wedge of bone within the ulna, to decrease the ulnar variance, thus eliminating the impaction of the ulna into the lunate or triquetrum. The osteotomy is performed as distal as possible to minimize the risk of nonunion. Placement of the plate volarly is common practice to minimize the risk of irritation from the hardware. The adjustment of alignment at the wrist can normalize wrist mechanics and may also alleviate pain associated with TFCC tears (Fig. 24.12).

TFCC tears can cause substantial wrist pain as well. Arthroscopic debridement or repair can improve wrist function and minimize pain, although these procedures are sometimes more successful when combined with an ulnar shortening osteotomy.

Rehabilitation

Rehabilitation of the young wrist is separated into three main phases. The first phase focuses on proximal and core evaluation ensuring neuromuscular control and mobility of the trunk, abdomen, scapula, and shoulder. Periscapular mobility, stability, and strength provide balance to the distal extremity under axial load.[80] Joint mobilizations and manual therapy techniques are initiated to focus on mobilization of the proximal extremity to enable pain-free distal extremity ROM. Introduction of isometric strengthening and stabilizing exercises are included with open kinetic chain activities without pain. Phase II of the rehabilitation consists of progression of dynamic isometric exercises and introduction of isotonic exercises by strengthening of the entire extremity. Periscapular and shoulder musculature are strengthened via rotator cuff exercises and use of exercise bands, weights, or resistive machines. Closed kinetic chain activities are practiced with particular focus paid to alignment, control, and proximal activation without pain. Pain-free, partial weight-bearing can then be trialed bilaterally (Fig. 24.13) (Video 2),

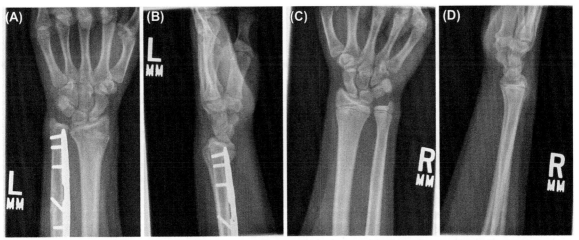

FIG. 24.12 Radiographs following a left ulnar shortening osteotomy and bilateral distal ulnar epiphysiodesis to correct left ulnar impaction syndrome and bilateral distal radial physeal arrest, respectively: **(A)** PA view of left wrist, **(B)** lateral view of left wrist, **(C)** PA view of right wrist, and **(D)** lateral view of right wrist. (Courtesy of Joshua M. Abzug, MD.)

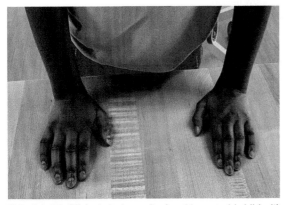

FIG. 24.13 Clinical photograph of an 11-year-old child with bilateral hand placement for upper extremity weight-bearing assessments. Note the ulnar deviation of the wrists most likely due to the misalignment of the hands not directly in line with the shoulders. Continued wrist misalignment can cause further dorsal impaction and complications related to gymnast wrist. (Courtesy of Heta Parikh, OTR/L, MPH.)

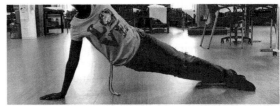

FIG. 24.14 Clinical photograph of an 11-year-old child demonstrating unilateral wrist weight-bearing via T-pose. (Courtesy of Heta Parikh, OTR/L, MPH.)

and on the isolated affected extremity (Fig. 24.14). During phase III, further strengthening and challenging of dynamic exercises are continued and progressed. Similar to various throwing programs for little league elbow, phase III focuses on more routine-specific activities such as handstands, progressing to backbends in an attempt to address movement patterns. Dynamic

closed chained exercises such as planks on a Bosu Ball and open chained sequences such as floor routines without breaks should be reinstituted to challenge neuromuscular control, strength, and proprioceptive feedback.[72] (Video 3). The patient is encouraged to practice skills in the clinic and then reinitiate routines on gymnastic equipment. During the return to sport, correct form is critical, and a gradual return should be timed on pain-free reintegration into typical routines.[72]

Rehabilitation stages following surgery is dependent on the surgery completed; however, it is similar to conservative management, following the initial postsurgical care period. Initially, orthosis fabrication, scar care, and edema management is addressed, followed by specific physician-related therapy orders. AROM, assessment of correct form, neuromuscular activation of movement patterns, proximal stability, and strength without pain in nonweight-bearing planes is commenced in phases I and II. More challenging and dynamic exercises related to gymnastics are resumed in the final phase.

CONCLUSION

In conclusion, the phenomena of the year-round athlete is a contemporary condition in which the young competitor is perpetually stressed. Increasing intensity, frequency, and participation in sports limit the recovery and rest needed for the still developing body. The child athlete undergoes repetitive compressive, tensile, and axial forces impacting the skeletal system's joints and physes. The difference in children and adults is not only size, but an immature musculoskeletal system consisting of open growth plates, which are the weakest location of the developing skeleton. Physes are susceptible to overuse and repetitive motions created when a sport is played continually without rest and recovery from stress. Three upper extremity diagnoses that are common in young athletes related to overuse include little league elbow, osteochondritis dissecans, and gymnast wrist. With over 30 million children participating in sports every year, the likelihood of increased prevalence is eminent.[81] The importance of proper diagnosis and treatment is irrefutable and permanently impacts the athlete's future. Appropriate and timely treatment is relevant to everyone, from tomorrow's weekend warrior to the next gold medal Olympian.

APPENDIX 2 Thrower's Ten Program to Be Done 1–2 Times a Day While in Season and 2–3 Times a Day During Off-season.
Exercise
Diagonal pattern D2 extension Diagonal pattern D2 flexion
External rotation at 0 degrees abduction Internal rotation at 0 degrees abduction
Shoulder abduction to 90 degrees
Scaption, external rotation ("full can")
Side-lying external rotation
Prone horizontal abduction Prone horizontal abduction (full external rotation, 100 degrees abduction) Prone rowing Prone rowing into external rotation
Press-ups
Push-ups
Elbow flexion Elbow extension
Wrist extension Wrist flexion
Wrist supination Wrist pronation

Data from Wilk KE, Arrigo CA, Hooks TR, Andrews JR. Rehabilitation of the overhead throwing athlete: there is more to it than just external rotation/internal rotation strengthening. *Pharm Manag PM R*. 2016;8(3 suppl):S78–S90.

APPENDICES

APPENDIX 1 Evaluation Tool Utilized for Determining Risk Factors of Throwing Injuries.
Questions
1. Have you experienced shoulder or elbow pain while throwing in the preceding 12 months?
2. Have you ever experienced a shoulder or elbow injury requiring medical treatment?
3. Do you participate in team training >4 days per week?
4. Do you participate in self-training 7 days per week?
5. Are you in the starting lineup?
6. Does your pitching arm often feel fatigued while playing baseball?

Data from Yukutake T, Kuwata M, Yamada M, Aoyama T. A preseason checklist for predicting elbow injury in little league baseball players. *Orthop J Sports Med*. 2015;3(1):2325967114566788.

APPENDIX 3
Advanced Thrower's Ten Program to Be Done
1–2 Times a Day While in Season and 2–3 Times a Day During Off-season.

Exercise

External rotation at 0 degrees abduction while seated on a stability ball
Internal rotation at 0 degrees abduction while seated on a stability ball

External rotation at 0 degrees abduction with sustained hold while seated on a stability ball
Internal rotation at 0 degrees abduction with sustained hold while seated on a stability ball

Shoulder abduction to 90 degrees with sustained hold while seated on a stability ball

Scaption, external rotation ("full can") with sustained hold on while seated on a stability ball

Side-lying external rotation

Prone horizontal abduction with sustained hold on a stability ball
Prone horizontal abduction (full external rotation, 100 degrees abduction) with sustained hold on a stability ball
Prone row on a stability ball
Prone row into external rotation with sustained hold on a stability ball

Seated scapular retraction into external rotation on a stability ball
Seated low trap on a stability ball

Seated neuromuscular control on a stability ball

Tilt-board push-ups

Elbow flexion on a stability ball
Elbow extension on a stability ball

Wrist extension
Wrist flexion

Wrist supination
Wrist pronation

Data from Wilk KE, Arrigo CA, Hooks TR, Andrews JR. Rehabilitation of the overhead throwing athlete: there is more to it than just external rotation/internal rotation strengthening. *Pharm Manag PM R*. 2016;8(3 suppl):S78–S90.

APPENDIX 4
Postoperative Guidelines Following a UCL Reconstruction with Autogenous Graft.

Time Postoperative	Therapy Type	Instructions
0 days	Splinting	• Long arm orthosis—elbow at 90 degrees of flexion, forearm neutral
2 weeks	Splinting	• Hinged elbow brace allowing extension/flexion of 30/100 degrees of motion
	Range of motion	• Begin gentle active range of motion (AROM) and active assisted range of motion (AAROM) at elbow (within confines of brace) and wrist • Full digital AROM/AAROM • Scapular AROM
3 weeks	Splinting	• Hinged elbow brace allowing extension/flexion of 10/110 degrees of motion
	Range of motion	• Continue AROM/AAROM to elbow/wrist within brace ROM limits • Isometric shoulder internal rotation, abduction, wrist extension/flexion, elbow flexion

Continued

APPENDIX 4
Postoperative Guidelines Following a UCL Reconstruction with Autogenous Graft.—cont'd

Time Postoperative	Therapy Type	Instructions
4 weeks	Splinting	• Hinged elbow brace allowing extension/flexion of 10/120 degrees of motion
	Range of motion	• Begin gentle in session PROM to elbow within ROM limits if needed
		• Initiate light resistance isotonics to shoulder (IR/ER, abduction, flexion), elbow, forearm and wrist protecting medial aspect of elbow during all shoulder exercises
5 weeks	Splinting	• Hinged elbow brace allowing extension/flexion of 5/130 degrees of motion
	Range of motion	• Continue AROM/AAROM to elbow/wrist within ROM limits
		• Continue gentle and controlled PROM to elbow within ROM limits if needed
6 weeks	Splinting	• Hinged elbow brace allowing extension/flexion of 0/130 degrees of motion
	Range of motion	• Continue AROM/AAROM to elbow/wrist within ROM limits
		• Continue gentle and controlled PROM to elbow within ROM limits if needed
		• Introduce elbow positions allowing some valgus forces during ROM and stretching
6–8 weeks	Splinting	• Begin to wean from brace
	Range of motion	• Thrower's Ten exercises (see Appendices 2 and 3)
	Modified sport involvement	• No running/throwing
10 weeks	Range of motion	• Obtain and maintain full elbow ROM
	Strength	• Increase strength and endurance—provided no pain with exercises
		• Initiate plyometrics
		• Begin eccentric/concentric elbow flexion exercises
	Modified sport involvement	• Still no running/throwing
13 weeks	Strength	• Rotator cuff and scapular strengthening and conditioning should be maximized
		• Stabilization exercises for elbow and shoulder with arm at side to protect medial aspect of elbow
		• Add two-handed plyometrics
		• Shoulder, core, and lower extremity strengthening
	Modified sport involvement	• Throwing education and throwing mechanics more advanced
16 weeks	Strength	• Rotator cuff and scapular strengthening and conditioning should be maximized
		• Stabilization exercises for elbow and shoulder with arm at side to protect medial aspect of elbow
		• Add two-handed plyometrics
		• Shoulder, core, and lower extremity strengthening
	Modified sport involvement	• Throwing education and throwing mechanics more advanced
		• Gradual running and jumping can be added

APPENDIX 4
Postoperative Guidelines Following a UCL Reconstruction with Autogenous Graft.—cont'd

Time Postoperative	Therapy Type	Instructions
20 weeks	Modified sport involvement	• Interval throwing program (longer distance and increased frequency) • Dynamic stability and closed chained exercises • Interval sport program
9 months	Return to sport	• Full, unrestricted return to competitive sport

Adapted from Ellenbecker TS, Wilk KE, Altchek DW, Andrews JR. Current concepts in rehabilitation following ulnar collateral ligament reconstruction. *Sports Health*. 2009;1(4):301–13.

APPENDIX 5
Postoperative Therapy Guidelines Following a UCL Repair with Docking Procedure.

Time Postoperative	Therapy Type	Instructions
0 days	Splinting	• Long arm orthosis—elbow at 90 degrees offlexion, forearm neutral
1–4 week	Splinting Range of motion Strength Other modalities	• Removal of splint and replace with a hinged elbow brace • Begin gentle range of motion (AROM) allowing extension/flexion of 30/90 degrees of motion in brace • Wrist active range of motion • Scapula isometrics • Gripping exercises • Cryotherapy • Home exercise program
4–6 weeks	Splinting Range of motion Strength	• Hinged elbow brace • Gentle range of motion allowing extension/flexion of 15/115 degrees of motion in brace • Manual scapula stabilization exercises with proximal resistance • Isometric wrist flexion/extension exercises • Isometric deltoid exercises • Isometric elbow flexion/extension exercises
6–12 weeks	Splinting Range of motion Strength	• Removal of hinged elbow brace • Continue elbow AROM • Isotonic scapular, shoulder, elbow, forearm, and wrist exercises • Neuromuscular and proprioception facilitation • Slowly incorporate eccentric training, when strength is adequate
12–16 weeks	Range of motion Strength	• Full upper extremity AROM • Internal/external rotation 90/90 position • Trunk and lower extremity strength • Plyometric program
4–9 months	Strength Return to sport	• Continue strength program • Begin interval throwing programs, 4 months • Begin hitting program, 5 months
1 year	Return to sport	• Full return to activity

Adapted from Ellenbecker TS, Wilk KE, Altchek DW, Andrews JR. Current concepts in rehabilitation following ulnar collateral ligament reconstruction. *Sports Health*. 2009;1(4):301–13.

Appendix 6. Series of clinical videos demonstrating dynamic strength exercises commonly incorporated into Little League elbow rehabilitation.

Supplementary Materials for Appendix 6

Supplementary data related to Appendix 6 can be found online at https://doi.org/10.1016/B978-0-323-53091-0.00024-5.

APPENDIX 7		
Interval Throwing Program for Skeletally Immature (8–12 years old) Baseball Players.		
	Short Toss—12 s Rest Between Throws, 6–8 min Rest Between Sets	**Long Toss—12 s Rest Between Throws, 6–8 min Rest Between Sets**
Phase I	15 throws at 20′ 15 throws at 20′ 20 throws at 20′ Intensity to tolerance	10 min rest between short and long toss 65% target distance 25 throws Intensity to tolerance
Phase II	15 throws at 30′ 15 throws at 30′ 20 throws at 30′ Intensity to tolerance	10 min rest between short and long toss 70% target distance 25 throws Intensity to tolerance
Phase III	15 throws at 40′ 15 throws at 40′ 20 throws at 40′ Intensity to tolerance	10 min rest between short and long toss 75% target distance 25 throws Intensity to tolerance
Phase IV	15 throws at 46′ (mound) 20 throws at 46′ (mound) 20 throws at 46′ (mound) Intensity up to half speed	10 min rest between short and long toss 80% target distance 25 throws Intensity to tolerance
Phase V	15 throws at 46′ (mound) 20 throws at 46′ (mound) 20 throws at 46′ (mound) Intensity up to three-quarter speed	10 min rest between short and long toss 85% target distance 25 throws Intensity to tolerance
Phase VI	20 throws at 46′ (mound) 20 throws at 46′ (mound) 20 throws at 46′ (mound) Full speed	10 min rest between short and long toss 90% target distance 25 throws Intensity to tolerance
Phase VII	20 throws at 46′ (mound) 20 throws at 46′ (mound) 25 throws at 46′ (mound) Full speed Breaking ball 3:1	10 min rest between short and long toss 95% target distance 25 throws Intensity to tolerance
Phase VIII	20 throws at 46′ (mound) 20 throws at 46′ (mound) 25 throws at 46′ (mound) Full speed Breaking ball 3:1	10 min rest between short and long toss 100% target distance 25 throws Intensity to tolerance
Phase IX	Simulated game	

Adapted from Axe MJ, Snyder-Mackler L, Konin JG, Strube MJ. Development of a distance-based interval throwing program for little league-aged athletes. *Am J Sports Med*. 1996;24(5):594–602.

APPENDIX 8
Interval Throwing Program for Skeletally Immature (13–14 years old) Baseball Players.

PHASE I—RETURN TO THROWING

Step 1	15 throws at 30′ 15 throws at 30′ 15 throws at 30′	20 long tosses to 60′
Step 2	15 throws at 45′ 15 throws at 45′ 15 throws at 45′	20 long tosses to 75′
Step 3	15 throws at 60′ 15 throws at 60′ 15 throws at 60′ Fastballs: From level ground following crow hop	20 long tosses to 90′

PHASE II—RETURN TO PITCHING

Step 4	20 Fastballs (50%) 16 fastballs (50%) 16 fastballs (50%)	25 long tosses to 105′
Step 5	20 fastballs (50%) 20 fastballs (50%) 20 fastballs (50%)	25 long tosses to 120′
Step 6	20 fastballs (50%) 20 fastballs (50%) 16 fastballs (50%)	25 long tosses to 120′

PHASE III—INTENSIFIED PITCHING

Step 7	20 fastballs (50%) 20 fastballs (75%) 20 fastballs (75%)	25 long tosses to 160′
Step 8	20 fastballs (75%) 21 fastballs (50%) 21 fastballs (75%) 20 fastballs (50%)	25 long tosses to 160′
Step 9	25 fastballs (75%) 24 fastballs (50%) 24 fastballs (75%) 25 fastballs (50%)	25 long tosses to 160′
Step 10	25 fastballs (75%) 25 fastballs (75%) 25 fastballs (75%) 25 fastballs (75%)	25 long tosses to 160′
Step 11	Active rest 20 throws at 60′ (75%) 15 throws at 80′ (75%)	Warm-up toss to 120′
Step 12	20 throws at 60′ (75%) 15 throws at 80′ (75%) 20 fast balls (100%) 20 fast balls (75%) 6 off-speed pitches (75%) 20 fastballs (100%)	20 long tosses to 160 ft

Continued

Step 13	20 fastballs (75%) 6 off-speed pitches (75%) 20 fastballs (75%) 4 throws to 1st (75%) 15 fastballs (100%) 10 off-speed pitches (100%) 20 fastballs (100%) 5 off-speed pitches (75%) 20 fastballs (75%) 4 throws to 1st (75%)	25 long tosses to 160′ 25 long tosses to 160′
Step 14	20 fastballs (100%) Throws to 1st (100%) 15 fastballs (100%) 10 off-speed pitches (100%) 20 fastballs (100%) 5 throws to 1st (75%)	25 long tosses to 160′
Step 15	Batting practice 100–110 pitches Bunts and comebacks	
Step 16	Simulated game	

Adapted from Axe MJ, Snyder-Mackler L, Konin JG, Strube MJ. Development of a distance-based interval throwing program for little league-aged athletes. *Am J Sports Med*. 1996;24(5):594–602.

APPENDIX 9
Interval Throwing Program for Skeletally Mature (High School, College, and Professional Level) Baseball Players.

PHASE I—RETURN TO THROWING

Step 1	15 throws at 30′ 15 throws at 30′ 15 throws at 30′	20 long tosses to 60′
Step 2	15 throws at 45′ 15 throws at 45′ 15 throws at 45′	20 long tosses to 75′
Step 3	15 throws at 60′ 15 throws at 60′ 15 throws at 60′	20 long tosses to 90′
Step 4	15 throws at 75′ 15 throws at 75′ 15 throws at 75′	20 long tosses to 105′
Step 5	15 throws at 90′ 20 throws at 90′ 15 throws at 90′	20 long tosses to 120′
Step 6	20 throws at 105′ 20 throws at 105′ 15 throws at 105′	20 long tosses to 120′
Step 7	20 throws at 120′ 20 throws at 120′ 20 throws at 120′	20 long tosses to 120′ Throws at effort level given

PHASE II—RETURN TO PITCHING

Step 8	15 throws at 60.5′ (75%) 20 throws at 60.5′ (75%) 20 throws at 60.5′ (75%) 15 throws at 60.5′ (75%)
Step 9	20 throws at 60.5′ (75%) 20 throws at 60.5′ (75%) 20 throws at 60.5′ (75%) 20 throws at 60.5′ (75%)
Step 10	20 fastballs (50%) 20 fastballs (50%) 20 fastballs (50%) 20 fastballs (50%) 25 throws at 60.5′ (75%)
Step 11	20 fastballs (50%) 20 fastballs (75%) 20 fastballs (50%) 15 fastballs (75%) 25 throws at 60.5′ (75%)
Step 12	25 fastballs (50%) 20 fastballs (75%) 20 fastballs (75%) 20 fastballs (75%) 20 fastballs (75%)

PHASE III—INTENSIFIED PITCHING

Step 13	25 fastballs (75%) 20 fastballs (100%) 10 fastballs (75%) 15 fastballs (100%) 25 fastballs (75%)
Step 14	Active rest 20 throws at 80′ 20 throws at 80′ 20 throws at 80′ 20 throws at 80′
Step 15	20 fastballs (75%) 20 fastballs (100%) 5 off-speed pitches 15 fastballs (100%) 5 off-speed pitches 20 fastballs (100%) 5 off-speed pitches Field blunts and comebacks
Step 16	20 fastballs (100%) 15 fastballs (100%) 5 off-speed pitches 5 pickoff throws to 1st 20 fastballs (100%) 5 off-speed pitches 20 fastballs (100%) 5 off-speed pitches

Continued

Step 17	15 fastballs (100%) 5 off-speed pitches 15 fastballs (100%) 3 pickoff throws to 1st 20 fastballs (100%) 5 off-speed pitches 15 fastballs (100%) 3 pickoff throws to 2nd 15 fastballs (100%) 5 off-speed pitches
Step 18	Active rest 20 throws at 80′ 20 throws at 80′ 20 throws at 80′ 20 throws at 80′
Step 19	20 fastballs (100%) 5 off-speed pitches 20 fastballs (100%) 3 pickoff throws to 1st 20 fastballs (100%) 3 pickoff throws to 2nd 15 fastballs (100%) 5 off-speed pitches 15 fastballs (100%) 5 off-speed pitches
Step 20	Batting practice 110–120 pitches Field bunts and comebacks
Step 21	Simulated games

Adapted from Axe MJ, Snyder-Mackler L, Konin JG, Strube MJ. Development of a distance-based interval throwing program for little league-aged athletes. *Am J Sports Med.* 1996;24(5):594–602.

SUPPLEMENTARY MATERIALS

Supplementary data related to this article can be found online at https://doi.org/10.1016/B978-0-323-53091-0.00024-5.

REFERENCES

1. Myer GD, Jayanthi N, DiFiori JP, et al. Sports specialization, part II: alternative solutions to early sport specialization in youth athletes. *Sports Health.* 2016;8(1):65–73.
2. Luke A, Lazaro RM, Bergeron MF, et al. Sports-related injuries in youth athletes: is overscheduling a risk factor? *Clin J Sport Med.* 2011;21(4):307–314.
3. Hoang QB, Mortazavi M. Pediatric overuse injuries in sports. *Adv Pediatr.* 2012;59(1):359–383.
4. Stracciolini A, Casciano R, Friedman HL, Meehan 3rd WP, Micheli LJ. A closer look at overuse injuries in the pediatric athlete. *Clin J Sport Med.* 2015;25(1):30–35.
5. Caine D, Caine C, Maffulli N. Incidence and distribution of pediatric sport-related injuries. *Clin J Sport Med.* 2006;16(6):500–513.
6. Davis KW. Imaging pediatric sports injuries: upper extremity. *Radiol Clin N Am.* 2010;48(6):1199–1211.
7. Maffuli N, Baxter-Jones AD. Common skeletal injuries in young athletes. *Sports Med.* 1995;19(2):137–149.
8. Migliaccio D, Wang NE. Common pediatric upper extremity overuse injuries. *Pediatr Em Med Rep.* 2017;22(1):1–13.
9. Paz DA, Chang GH, Yetto Jr JM, Dwek JR, Chung CB. Upper extremity overuse injuries in pediatric athletes: clinical presentation, imaging findings, and treatment. *Clin Imag.* 2015;39(6):954–964.

10. Wilk KE, Macrina LC, Cain EL, Dugas JR, Andrews JR. Rehabilitation of the overhead athlete's elbow. *Sports Health.* 2012;4(5):404−414.

11. Reinold MM, Wilk KE, Reed J, Crenshaw K, Andrews JR. Interval sport programs: guidelines for baseball, tennis, and golf. *J Orthop Sports Phys Ther.* 2002;32(6):293−298.

12. Zellner B, May MM. Elbow injuries in the young athlete-an orthopedic perspective. *Pediatr Radiol.* 2013;43(suppl 1): S129−S134.

13. Elder KE. Little league elbow. *Athl Train Sports Health Care.* 2010;2(3):100−102.

14. Lyman S, Fleisig GS, Andrews JR, Osinski ED. Effect of pitch type, pitch count, and pitching mechanics on risk of elbow and shoulder pain in youth baseball pitchers. *Am J Sports Med.* 2002;30(4):463−468.

15. Kijowski R, Tuite M, Sanford M. Magnetic resonance imaging of the elbow. part I: normal anatomy, imaging technique, and osseous abnormalities. *Skeletal Radiol.* 2004; 33(12):685−697.

16. Ellington MD, Edmonds EW. Pediatric elbow and wrist pathology related to sports participation. *Orthop Clin N Am.* 2016;47(4):743−748.

17. Burton-Cahn MS. Elbow injuries in the youth athlete. *Pediatr Ann.* 2012;41(7):292−295.

18. Benjamin HJ, Briner Jr WW. Little league elbow. *Clin J Sports Med.* 2005;15(1):37−40.

19. Wei AS, Khana S, Limpisvasti O, Crues J, Podesta L, Yocum LA. Clinical and magnetic resonance imaging findings associated with little league elbow. *J Pediatr Orthop.* 2010;30(7):715−719.

20. Fleisig GS, Andrews JR. Prevention of elbow injuries in youth baseball pitchers. *Sports Health.* 2012;4(5):419−424.

21. Fleisig GS, Andrews JR, Cutter GR, et al. Risk of serious injury for young baseball pitchers. *Am J Sports Med.* 2011;39(2):253−257.

22. Lyman S, Fleisig GS, Waterbor JW, et al. Longitudinal study of elbow and shoulder pain in youth baseball pitchers. *Med Sci Sports Exerc.* 2001;33(11):1803−1810.

23. Leahy I, Schorpion M, Ganley T. Common medial elbow injuries in the adolescent athlete. *J Hand Ther.* 2015; 28(2):201−210.

24. Yukutake T, Kuwata M, Yamada M, Aoyama T. A preseason checklist for predicting elbow injury in little league baseball players. *Orthop J Sports Med.* 2015;3(1), 2325967114566788.

25. Fleisig GS, Barrentine SW, Zheng N, Escamilla RF, Andrews JR. Kinematic and kinetic comparison of baseball pitching among various levels of development. *J Biomech.* 1999;32(12):1371−1375.

26. Osbahr DC, Chalmers PN, Frank JS, Williams 3rd RJ, Widmann RF, Green DW. Acute, avulsion fractures of the medial epicondyle while throwing in youth baseball players: a variant of little league elbow. *J Shoulder Elbow Surg.* 2010;19(7):951−957.

27. Mueller MJ, Maluf KS. Tissue adaptation to physical stress: a proposed "physical stress theory" to guide physical therapist practice, education, and research. *Phys Ther.* 2002; 82(4):383−403.

28. Reinold MM, Escamilla RF, Wilk KE. Current concepts in the scientific and clinical rationale behind exercises for glenohumeral and scapulothoracic musculature. *J Orthop Sports Phys Ther.* 2009;39(2):105−117.

29. Nakamizo H, Nakamura Y, Nobuhara K, Yamamoto T. Loss of glenohumeral internal rotation in little league pitchers: a biomechanical study. *J Shoulder Elbow Surg.* 2008;17(5):795−801.

30. Wilk KE, Arrigo CA, Hooks TR, Andrews JR. Rehabilitation of the overhead throwing athlete: there is more to it than just external rotation/internal rotation strengthening. *Pharm Manag PM R.* 2016;8(3 suppl): S78−S90.

31. Kibler WB, Sciascia A. Kinetic chain contributions to elbow function and dysfunction in sports. *Clin Sports Med.* 2004; 23(4):545−552.

32. Wiesner SL. Rehabilitation of elbow injuries in sports. *Pharm Manag PM R.* 1994;5(1):81−113.

33. Wright RW, Steger-May K, Wasserlauf BL, O'Neal ME, Weinberg BW, Paletta GA. Elbow range of motion in professional baseball pitchers. *Am J Sports Med.* 2006;34(2): 190−193.

34. Voight ML, Hardin JA, Blackburn TA, Tippett S, Canner GC. The effect of muscle fatigue on and the relationship of arm dominance to shoulder proprioception. *J Orthop Sports Phys Ther.* 1996;23(6):348−352.

35. Fleisig GS, Escamilla RF. Biomechanics of the elbow in the throwing athlete. *Op Tech Sports Med.* 1996;4(2): 62−68.

36. Axe MJ, Snyder-Mackler L, Konin JG, Strube MJ. Development of a distance-based interval throwing program for little league-aged athletes. *Am J Sports Med.* 1996;24(5): 594−602.

37. Edmonds EW, Polousky J. A review of knowledge in osteochondritis dissecans: 123 years of minimal evolution from König to the ROCK study group. *Clin Orthop Relat Res.* 2013;471(4):1118−1126.

38. Lam KY, Siow HM. Conservative treatment for juvenile osteochondritis dissecans of the talus. *J Orthop Surg.* 2012;20(2):176−180.

39. Takahara M, Shundo M, Kondo M, Suzuki K, Nambu T, Ogino T. Early detection of osteochondritis dissecans of the capitellum in young baseball players. Report of three cases. *J Bone Joint Surg Am.* 1998;80(6):892−897.

40. Giuseffi SA, Field LD. Osteochondritis dissecans of the elbow. *Oper Tech Sports Med.* 2014;22(2):148−155.

41. Bradley JP, Petrie RS. Osteochondritis dissecans of the humeral capitellum. Diagnosis and treatment. *Clin Sport Med.* 2001;20(3):565−590.

42. Richie LB, Sytsma MJ. Matching osteochondritis dissecans lesions in identical twin brothers. *Orthopedics.* 2013;36(9): e1213−e1216.

43. Mihara K, Tsutsui H, Nishinaka N, Yamaguchi K. Nonoperative treatment for osteochondristis dissecans of the capitellum. *Am J Sports Med.* 2009;37(2):298−304.

44. Matsuura T, Kashiwaguchi S, Iwase T, Takeda Y, Yasui N. Conservative treatment for osteochondrosis of the humeral capitellum. *Am J Sports Med.* 2008;36(5):868−872.

45. Atiković A, Kalinski SD, Čuk I. Age trends in artistic gymnastic across world championships and the Olympic games from 2003 to 2016. *Sci Gymnastics J.* 2017;9(3):251–263.

46. Gabel GT. Gymnastic wrist injuries. *Clin Sports Med.* 1998;17(3):611–621.

47. Buckner SB, Bacon NT, Bishop PA. Recovery in level 7-10 Women's USA artistic gymnastics. *Int J Exerc Sci.* 2017;10(5):734–742.

48. The Associated Press. *Gymnastics Walks Fine Line between Training and Overtraining;* 2016. https://www.usatoday.com/story/sports/olympics/2016/07/10/gymnastics-walks-fine-line-between-training-and-overtraining/86920938/.

49. DiFiori JP, Caine DJ, Malina RM. Wrist pain, distal radial physeal injury, and ulnar variance in the young gymnast. *Am J Sports Med.* 2006;34:840–849.

50. Mandelbaum BR, Bartolozzi AR, Davis CA, Teurlings L, Bragonier B. Wrist pain syndrome in the gymnast. Pathogenetic, diagnostic, and therapeutic considerations. *Am J Sports Med.* 1989;17(3):305–317.

51. DiFiori JP, Puffer JC, Aish B, Dorey F. Wrist pain, distal radial physeal injury and ulnar variance in young gymnasts: does a relationship exist? *Am J Sports Med.* 2002;30(6):879–885.

52. DiFiori JP, Puffer JC, Mandelbaum BR. Mar S. Factors associated with wrist pain in the young gymnast. *Am J Sports Med.* 1996;24(1):9–14.

53. Aubergé T, Zenny JC, Duvallet A, Godefroy D, Horreard P, Chevrot A. Bone maturation and osteoarticular lesions in top level sportsmen. apropos of 105 cases. *J Radiol.* 1984;65(8–9):555–561.

54. Roy S, Caine D, Singer KM. Stress changes of the distal radial epiphysis in young gymnasts. A report of twenty-one cases and a review of the literature. *Am J Sports Med.* 1985;13(5):301–308.

55. Wolf MR, Avery D, Wolf JM. Upper extremity injuries in gymnasts. *Hand Clin.* 2017;33(1):187–197.

56. Markolf KL, Shapiro MS, Mandelbaum BR, Teurlings L. Wrist loading patterns during pommel horse exercises. *J Biomech.* 1990;23(10):1001–1011.

57. Koh TJ, Grabiner MD, Weiker GG. Technique and ground reaction forces in the back handspring. *Am J Sports Med.* 1992;20(1):61–66.

58. Cornwall R. The painful wrist in the pediatric athlete. *J Pediatr Orthop.* 2010;30(Suppl 2):S13–S16.

59. De Smet L, Claessens A, Lefevre J, Beunen G. Gymnast wrist: an epidemiologic survey of ulnar variance and stress changes of the radial physis in elite female gymnasts. *Am J Sports Med.* 1994;22(6):846–850.

60. Kozin SH, Abzug JM. Wrist Injuries in the immature athlete. *Oper Tech Sports Med.* 2016;24:148–154.

61. Benjamin HJ, Engel SC, Chudzik D. Wrist pain in gymnasts: a review of common overuse wrist pathology in the gymnastics athlete. *Curr Sports Med Rep.* 2017;16(5):322–329.

62. Mehlman CT, Araghi A, Roy DR. Hyphenates history – the Hueter-Volkmann law. *Am J Ortho (Belle Mead NJ).* 1997;26(11):798–800.

63. Abzug JM, Little K, Kozin SH. Physeal arrest of the distal radius. *J Am Acad Orthop Surg.* 2014;22(6):381–389.

64. Webb BG, Rettig LA. Gymnastic wrist injuries. *Curr Sports Med Rep.* 2008;7(5):289–295.

65. Gilsanz V, Ratib O. Indicators of skeletal maturity in children and adolescents. In: Gilsanz V, Ratib O, eds. *Hand Bone Age: A Digital Atlas of Skeletal Maturity.* Berlin (Heidelberg, Germany): Springer; 2005:9–17.

66. Kox LS, Kuijer PP, Kerkhoffs GM, Maas M, Frings-Dresen MH. Prevalence, incidence and risk factors for overuse injuries of the wrist in young athletes: a systematic review. *Br J Sports Med.* 2015;49(18):1189–1196.

67. Carter SR, Aldridge MJ, Fitzgerald R, Davies AM. Stress changes of the wrist in adolescent gymnasts. *Br J Radiol.* 1988;61:109–112.

68. Iwasaki N, Ishikawa J, Kato H, Minami M, Minami A. Factors affecting results of ulnar shortening for ulnar impaction syndrome. *Clin Orthop Relat Res.* 2007;465:215–219.

69. Nakamura R, Horii E, Imaeda T, Nakao E, Kato H, Watanabe K. The ulnocarpal stress test in the diagnosis of ulnar-sided wrist pain. *J Hand Surg Br.* 1997;22(6):719–723.

70. Nishiwaki M, Nakamura T, Nagura T, Toyama Y, Ikegami H. Ulnar-shortening effect on distal radioulnar joint pressure: a biomechanical study. *J Hand Surg Am.* 2008;33(2):198–205.

71. Altman E. The ulnar side of the wrist: clinically relevant anatomy and biomechanics. *J Hand Ther.* 2016;29(2):111–122.

72. Boucher B, Smith-Young B. Examination and physical therapy management of a young gymnast with bilateral wrist pain: a case report. *Phys Ther Sport.* 2017;27:38–49.

73. Linscheid RL, Dobyns JH. Athletic injuries of the wrist. *Clin Orthop Rel Res.* 1985;198:141–151.

74. VanHeest AE, Luger NM, House JH, Vener M. Extensor retinaculum impingement in the athlete: a new diagnosis. *Am J Sports Med.* 2007;35(12):2126–2130.

75. Wilson SM, Dubert T, Rozenblat M. Extensor tendon impingement in a gymnast. *J Hand Surg Br.* 2006;31B(1):66–67.

76. Pengel KB. Common overuse injuries in the young athlete. *Pediatr Ann.* 2014;43(12):e297–308.

77. Colston MA. Core stability, part 2: the core-extremity link. *Int J Athl Ther Train.* 2012;17(2):10–15.

78. Vaseghi B, Jaberzadeh S, Kalantari KK, Naimi SS. The impact of load and base of support on electromyographic onset in the shoulder muscle during push-up exercises. *J Bodyw Mov Ther.* 2013;17(2):192–199.

79. Fufa DT, Goldfarb CA. Sports injuries of the wrist. *Curr Rev Musculoskelet Med.* 2013;6(1):35–40.

80. Kalantari KK, Ardestani SB. The effect of base of support stability on shoulder muscle activity during closed kinematic chain exercises. *J Bodyw Mov Ther.* 2014;18(2):233–238.

81. Adirim TA, Cheng TL. Overview of injuries in the young athlete. *Sports Med.* 2003;33(1):75–81.

82. Ellenbecker TS, Wilk KE, Altchek DW, Andrews JR. Current concepts in rehabilitation following ulnar collateral ligament reconstruction. *Sports Health.* 2009;1(4):301–313.

83. Pitch Smart USA Baseball. *Guidelines for Youth and Adolescent;* 2018. https://www.mlb.com/pitch-smart/pitching-guidelines.

FURTHER READING

1. Little League. *Regular Season Pitching Rules;* 2019. https://www.littleleague.org/playing-rules/pitch-count/.

2. Marshall KW, Marshall DL, Busch MT, Williams JP. Osteochondral lesions of the humeral trochlea in the young athlete. *Skeletal Radiol.* 2009;38(5):479–491.

3. American Medical Society for Sports Medicine. *TFCC Injections;* 2019. https://www.sportsmedtoday.com/tfcc-injections-va-173.htm.

CHAPTER 25

Pediatric Hand Therapy—Sports Shoulder: Throwing Athletes

RYAN KROCHAK, MD • ELLIOT GREENBERG, PT, DPT, PHD •
DANIEL W. SAFFORD, PT, DPT • THEODORE J. GANLEY, MD

INTRODUCTION/PERTINENT ANATOMY

As youth sports participation continues to increase, there has been a corresponding increase in the amount of injuries seen, especially shoulder injuries in overhead athletes.[1] Traumatic injuries such as fractures are common across the spectrum of competitive sports. Overuse injuries, however, tend to predominate in the pediatric throwing athlete and comprise approximately 60% of all sports injuries in children and adolescents.[2]

Baseball and throwing in particular has been the focus of extensive research with regards to shoulder injuries. The incidence of shoulder pain and symptoms ranges from 32% to 35% within a season of youth baseball and the incidence of injury for pitchers has been shown to be 37.4% versus only 15.3% for position players.[3,4]

Throwing places a significant amount of stress on the shoulder and overhead athletes require a delicate balance between shoulder mobility and stability to meet the functional demands of their sport. During pitching, peak angular velocities of the humerus have been recorded up to 7550 degrees/second, the generation of internal rotation torques have been reported as high as 67–92 Nm, and it has been demonstrated that a compressive force of up to 1090 N is produced on the shoulder.[5-7]

Although youth athletes may present with many of the same complaints as more mature athletes, differences in anatomy and throwing technique often leads to age-specific injuries. Injuries in youth throwing athletes are typically caused by repeated stress and cumulative trauma to the developing physis of the proximal humerus as well as adaptive changes in the soft tissue stabilizers of the glenohumeral joint.

In pediatric athletes, the proximal humerus growth plate typically remains open until 14–16 years old in girls and 16–18 years old in boys.[8] Open physeal plates, increased joint laxity, and underdeveloped musculature about the shoulder are three unique aspects of the developing skeleton that lead to inherent susceptibility for injuries in the pediatric overhead athlete.[9]

Similarly, in adults, the rotator cuff muscles, long head of the biceps, and scapular stabilizers contribute dynamic stability to the shoulder joint, while the capsule and ligaments of the glenohumeral joint provide static stability to the shoulder. The static stabilizers function primarily at the extremes of motion and different portions of the capsule tighten depending on the position of the athletes arm.

The anterosuperior capsule, superior glenohumeral ligament, and other rotator interval structures function to limit inferior and posterior translation of the humeral head with the arm adducted. The middle glenohumeral ligament functions to limit anterior–posterior translation in the midrange of abduction and external rotation (∼45 degrees). The inferior glenohumeral ligament functions to limit anterior–posterior translation in the abducted (90 degrees) and maximally externally rotated arm. The posterior capsule does not have any direct posterior ligamentous reinforcement but is important in limiting posterior translation in the adducted, internally rotated, and forward-flexed arm.[10]

LITTLE LEAGUE SHOULDER
Background/Epidemiology

Little league shoulder (LLS) is an overuse injury of the shoulder (specifically the physis) in youth athletes that presents as pain and is accompanied by radiographic evidence of widening of the proximal humeral physis. In 1953, Dotter first described it in a case report in the Guthrie Clinical Bulletin.[11] Since then, it has been described by numerous authors and referred to as osteochondrosis of the proximal humeral epiphysis, proximal humeral epiphysiolysis, or as a rotational stress fracture of the proximal humeral epiphyseal plate.[12–14]

Pediatric overuse injuries are most common in children between 11 and 16 years old with LLS presenting most commonly at age 13–14 years in boys.[13,15] Although most commonly seen in male baseball pitchers, LLS can also occur in females, catchers, baseball position players, and other overhead athletes such as tennis players, quarterbacks, and cricket players.[15]

The inherent susceptibility of the developing shoulder plays a predominant role in the development of LLS. Additionally, poor throwing technique or mechanics also increases susceptibility. Other risk factors include the quantity and frequency of pitches thrown, the pitch type, muscular imbalance, and glenohumeral internal rotation deficits (GIRD).[16,17] In a study by Heyworth et al., almost one-third of patients with LLS had GIRD on physical exam and the odds of recurrence in this subgroup were 3.6 times greater than in those without GIRD.[15]

As the incidence of LLS is increasing, it is important for practitioners to be aware of this condition when considering the spectrum of disorders that affect the pediatric shoulder. Additionally, educating players, parents, trainers, and coaches on risk factors along with the symptoms, such as shoulder fatigue, pain, and decreased velocity, may help identify LLS earlier and lead to prompt and appropriate treatment.[3,18]

Mechanism/Pathophysiology

LLS is the result of repetitive microtrauma to the physis of the proximal humerus. Skeletally immature athletes tend to develop stress reactions of the proximal humeral physis, as the physis is the weak point in the upper arm compared with the surrounding bony, muscle/tendinous, and ligamentous structures.[13] Additionally, epiphyseal growth cartilage is more susceptible to injury by repetitive microtrauma than is adult cartilage and the growth plate is also especially weak during periods of rapid bone growth, such as puberty.[19]

Within the physis, the zone of hypertrophy tends to be the affected area due to its vertically oriented columns of cells and collagen fibers with little structural matrix, thus making it the weakest portion of the growth plate and most susceptible to injury.[13,17]

Two major types of loading have been implicated in the pathogenesis of proximal humeral epiphysiolysis. The first and most important is rotational stress or torque applied to the physis during throwing, which can result in repetitive trauma, possibly causing a fatigue fracture or a local inflammatory reaction to the growth plate.[20] The second is a distraction force on the physis at the time of ball release. In response to this distraction force, the rotator cuff muscles contract to create a proximally directed force on the humeral head to keep the glenohumeral joint intact.[21]

A biomechanical study of youth baseball pitchers by Sabick et al. showed that shear stresses on the physis arising from high torque during throwing were approximately 18 Nm or equivalent to 400% of the shear force that growth plate cartilage can normally tolerate and large enough to cause deformation of the weak proximal humeral epiphyseal cartilage.[21] Therefore, proximal humeral epiphysiolysis or LLS is the pathological response to these stresses over time and results in clinical symptoms.

Presentation/Clinical Evaluation

Patients typically present with diffuse shoulder pain during throwing that is often worse in the late cocking or deceleration phases. Rest usually relieves the pain but some patients may progress to having pain with activities of daily living or even at rest. Initially, patients may also complain of a decrease in velocity or control while throwing.

On examination, there is often a focal tenderness or pain over the anterolateral shoulder at the level of the proximal humerus physis. There may be swelling, weakness, atrophy, and loss of motion in the involved shoulder; however, these are all uncommon and nonspecific findings in LLS.[13] Shoulder motion, flexibility, and strength should be examined along with evaluating for scapular dysfunction and assessing other components of the kinetic chain. Additionally, clinical evaluation and provocative testing to exclude other potential causes of shoulder pain in the throwing athlete should also be assessed as clinical suspicion warrants.

Imaging

X-rays of the symptomatic shoulder should be obtained and will classically show physeal widening and possibly some increased sclerosis, demineralization, metaphyseal calcification, or fragmentation adjacent to the physis (Fig. 25.1).[15] These findings tend to be most identifiable in the anterolateral region of the physis, so an external rotation view of the shoulder may be helpful in addition to an AP view. Contralateral shoulder X-rays are also recommended for comparison to help confirm the diagnosis.

Advanced imaging, such as an MRI, will show edema around the physis but it is typically not necessary and

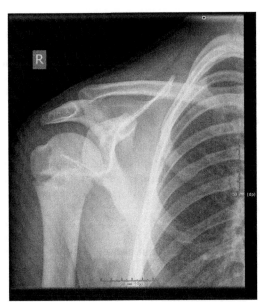

FIG. 25.1 Right shoulder X-ray showing widening of the proximal humeral physis as seen in little league shoulder.

reserved for patients with refractory cases or those with instability, where it may be used to rule out other pathology, such as a labral tear.

Treatment

Different from adult throwing injuries that often require surgery, conservative treatment of LLS is highly effective. Please see the rehabilitation section later for a detailed discussion of physical therapy treatment.

SHOULDER INSTABILITY

Background/Epidemiology

Anterior shoulder instability is a common problem in pediatric athletes that most often results from a traumatic episode and is more commonly seen in contact and collision sports rather than in overhead athletes. The throwing athlete more commonly may present with anterior microinstability or multidirectional instability.

The overhead athlete is presented with a unique paradox in which there is a fine line between ideal excess laxity to allow for full range of motion (ROM) while throwing and instability leading to subluxation of the humeral head.[22] Microinstability is subtle, atraumatic asymmetry of glenohumeral translation in the overhead athlete that may lead to impingement findings and pain secondary to this laxity. Multidirectional instability (MDI) is defined by atraumatic glenohumeral instability in at least two planes, arising from weakness of the joint capsule and surrounding rotator cuff muscles.[23]

It is estimated that 4%–13% of the pediatric population exhibits some degree of joint hypermobility, although this incidence may be even higher in youth overhead athletes due to overuse and adaptive changes.[24] Although not all athletes with hypermobility suffer from shoulder instability, some throwers experience recurrent subluxations that gradually stress and lengthen their capsule and ligamentous structures, leading to symptomatic microinstability or multidirectional instability.

Mechanisms/Pathophysiology

Although traumatic anterior shoulder macroinstability is typically caused by an anterior directed force on the arm while the shoulder is in abduction and external rotation, microinstability and multidirectional instability are not typically caused by a single traumatic event. Their underlying mechanism is either microtrauma from overuse or due to generalized ligamentous laxity that may be associated with a connective tissue disorder such as Ehlers–Danlos syndrome. However, it is important to note that children frequently display greater shoulder laxity compared with adults due to an increased proportion of type III collagen in their ligaments.[25]

Anterior microinstability can develop from repetitive throwing, as external rotation during the overhead motion places tremendous stress on the anterior capsule and ligamentous structures leading to ligamentous laxity overtime. Initially, the periscapular and rotator cuff muscles can compensate but these dynamic stabilizers fatigue with repetitive activity and anterior translation ensues with subsequent development of instability.[26]

Although the exact pathogenesis of symptomatic multidirectional instability is still unclear, it can be postulated that inherent laxity and instability in the youth shoulder may predispose these patients to symptomatic chronic instability when combined with the repetitive overhead stress of throwing. Affected athletes typically possess underlying laxity that is exacerbated by repetitive traumatic insults, resulting in the inability to maintain dynamic stability.[26]

Both MDI and microinstability can lead to secondary impingement syndrome, a condition in which it is difficult for the humeral head to stay centered in the glenoid fossa while the arm is in motion, due to ligamentous laxity and weakness in the rotator cuff muscles.[27]

Presentation/Clinical Evaluation

In overhead athletes with microinstability or MDI, symptom onset is usually gradual, atraumatic, and may correlate with an increase in training. Patients are usually most symptomatic during late arm cocking and early acceleration phases, when the arm is in maximal external rotation.[27] Their chief complaint is often pain more than instability but they may have a subjective feeling of laxity with overhead activities or complaints of popping or catching. MDI patients may also experience concomitant recurrent transient episodes of numbness, tingling, and weakness in the affected extremity, while microinstability patients often have findings of rotator cuff inflammation and impingement secondary to underlying recurrent microinstability.[8]

Examination of the shoulder should reveal instability in two or more planes to be defined as multidirectional instability, while in patients with microinstability more subtle asymmetries of glenohumeral translation between the affected and unaffected side may be present.

Both shoulders should be evaluated and any signs of scapular dysfunction should be noted. Some specific tests to be performed include the following:

- The Sulcus Sign—Visible indentation is created between the acromion and the lateral deltoid/humeral head when inferior traction is pulled on the arm
- Apprehension Testing—With the patient supine, the examiner flexes the patient's elbow to 90 degrees and abducts the patient's shoulder to 90 degrees, maintaining neutral rotation. The examiner then slowly applies an external rotation force to the arm to 90 degrees while carefully monitoring the patient. Patient apprehension from this maneuver is considered a positive test
- Relocation Test—This test is administered as a second part to a positive Apprehension test. With the arm still in 90 degrees of abduction and external rotation, the examiner applies a posteriorly directed force to the shoulder. If the patient's apprehension is reduced, the Relocation test is considered to be positive
- Anterior and Posterior Load and Shift tests—With patient seated or supine, the examiner stabilizes the scapula, axially loads the humerus, and applies anterior/posterior translation forces. This should then be compared to the contralateral side. The test is positive when there is greater than 50% movement of the humeral head or increased translation compared to the contralateral side.

Testing for generalized ligamentous laxity should also be performed using the Beighton nine-point scoring system for hypermobility. This involves testing the patient's ability to touch their palms to the floor while bending at the waist, testing for hyperextension of the knees, elbows, and MCP joints, and testing for the ability to abduct the thumb to the ipsilateral forearm.[28]

Imaging

Although X-rays and MRI are often ordered, imaging usually will not demonstrate significant abnormalities, underscoring the importance of the history and physical exam.

As with LLS, AP radiographs should be taken in both internal and external rotation, but additional axillary and scapular Y views can also be helpful to rule out proximal humeral physeal fractures and other bony pathology.[22]

MRI, specifically MR arthrogram with the addition of intraarticular contrast, may provide a more diagnostic image of the shoulder with instability; however, routine use of an MRI for instability secondary to overuse is not needed unless the clinician suspects associated damage.[29] Notable findings may include a patulous and expanded joint capsule and an increased rotator interval.[30,31] Additionally, labral tears and/or other intraarticular pathology can be ruled out.

Treatment

Nonoperative

See the rehabilitation section of this chapter later.

Operative

Most cases of instability in the pediatric throwing athlete can be successfully treated nonoperatively with activity modification and an inclusive physical therapy program. If the patient continues to be symptomatic after a 6-month trial of nonoperative management, surgical intervention for stabilization is an option.[29]

Traditionally, stabilization was accomplished via an open technique and performing an inferior capsular shift to minimize capsular redundancy.[32] Despite the elimination of instability and good return of functionality, return to play at preoperative levels was only found in 69% of patients.[33] However, as arthroscopic surgery and techniques have improved over time, most are now occurring arthroscopically.[1] In contrast to open surgery, arthroscopic capsulorrhaphy allows improved access to all portions of the joint, allows the surgeon to address anterior, inferior, and posterior disease at the same time, and minimizes postoperative external rotation loss, which is critical in the overhead athlete.[34] Newer arthroscopic suture anchor techniques also allow the surgeon to tighten the capsule and attach it to the glenoid rim.

The results of arthroscopic treatment have been encouraging for those subset of patient's that have failed nonoperative treatment, with recurrence rates reported between 2% and 12% and with improved patient satisfaction and return to sport compared with traditional open techniques.[35,36] In a study by Baker et al. that assessed 2–5-year clinical outcomes, most patients had good to excellent pain scores, 91% of patients had full or near full ROM, 98% had normal or near normal strength, and 86% of patients were able to return to sports.[37]

However, it is important to note that in adolescents with connective tissue disorders, such as Ehlers–Danlos syndrome, results are not as optimistic, with return to play at 64% and only 47% reporting no further episodes of instability at 8-year follow-up.[38]

Post-Op Rehab

Rehabilitation after surgery is outlined in detail later within the rehabilitation section of this chapter.

SLAP TEARS
Background/Epidemiology

Superior labral anterior–posterior (SLAP) lesions are another pathology seen in overhead athletes, although much less common in younger patients. A study of 490 baseball players ranging from 13 to 22 years old revealed that players' ages 13–15 had only a 5.2% incidence of SLAP injury, which is significantly lower than high school and college aged throwers.[39] In contrast to younger athletes, mature throwers more often develop disorders of the superior glenoid labrum, as once the proximal humeral physis closes, the static and dynamic stabilizers of the shoulder are more likely to be injured.

Other risk factors that can predispose the adolescent athlete for the development of a superior labral injury include alterations in shoulder and scapular motion. Although it is controversial whether an incidental finding of GIRD is a measure of injury risk, studies have shown that throwers with GIRD of at least 18 degrees had a 1.9× higher risk of a shoulder injury including SLAP tears.[40]

SLAP tears were originally classified by Snyder in 1990 and although others, such as Maffet, have expanded his classification, the original Snyder classification remains the most widely recognized and describes four major variants.[41]

Type I lesions involve labral fraying with localized degeneration. The superior labral and biceps anchor attachments remain intact.

Type II lesions involve detachment of the superior labrum/biceps anchor complex from the glenoid. They have abnormal mobility and are the most common and clinically significant SLAP tear in overhead athletes.

Type III lesions involve a bucket handle tear of the superior labrum with an intact biceps tendon anchor (biceps separates from bucket handle tear).

Type IV lesions also involve a bucket handle tear of the labrum but have extension of the tear into the biceps tendon. This often creates a split appearance of the biceps tendon with a portion attached to bucket handle tear and a portion remaining attached to the glenoid.

Mechanisms/Pathophysiology

A variety of injury mechanisms have been proposed for SLAP tears including forceful traction loads to the arm, direct compression loads to the arm, and repetitive overhead throwing activities.

The strength of the superior labrum–biceps complex has been examined in multiple studies simulating overhead throwing and these studies have shown that the stability of the biceps anchor and pattern of injury is dependent on shoulder position. SLAP tears are most frequently shown to occur in the late cocking position with one cadaver study showing that the biceps anchor demonstrated 20% less strength in the late cocking phase than in the early deceleration phase.[42] Another study examining simulated loads on the biceps because of throwing showed that strain in the superior labrum was significantly increased in the late cocking phase.[43]

Several factors predispose the overhead athlete to SLAP tears. This includes increased external rotation of the shoulder, which creates a dynamic "peel back" of the biceps anchor during the late cocking phase, resulting in a torsional force at the posterior superior aspect of the glenoid labrum. The labrum and biceps displace medially ("peel back") over the glenoid rim with each throw and this leads to attritional tears. Additionally, in patients with GIRD, there is increased stress on the labrum from altered glenohumeral kinematics. The posterior capsular contracture seen in GIRD leads to abnormal posterosuperior positioning of the humeral head on the glenoid during arm rotation and creates shear forces across the posterosuperior labrum that can lead to the development of an SLAP tear.[44–46]

Presentation/Clinical Evaluation

Throwers with an SLAP tear typically present with an insidious onset of shoulder pain, most often during the late cocking phase, and this may be associated with a decrease in velocity or "dead arm."[47] Patients may complain of a dull aching sensation within the joint, a catching feeling when throwing, and/or difficulty sleeping because of shoulder discomfort. However, the pattern and location of pain are often nonspecific. The pain may localize deep within the shoulder or radiate to the anterior or posterior aspects of the shoulder, mimicking symptoms from biceps pathology, anterior and posterior labral tears, or acromioclavicular joint disease. Typically, the symptoms are worse not only with throwing and overhead motion but with heavy lifting and pushing.[48]

The clinical diagnosis of SLAP tears on physical examination is often difficult, as patients with SLAP tears frequently have coexistent pathology and examination tests to detect SLAP tears lack sensitivity and specificity. Additionally, studies of provocative testing have mainly been performed in the adult population, and further studies are needed to appreciate their utility in the youth athlete. Two of the most commonly used maneuvers for evaluating patients with suspected SLAP tears include the O'Brien's active compression test and the dynamic labral shear test.

The active compression test (O'Brien) is performed by forward flexing the affected arm to 90 degrees. The arm is then adducted 10–15 degrees across the body and then pronated, so the thumb is pointing down. The examiner applies downward force to the wrist while the patient resists. The patient then supinates the forearm so the palm is up and the examiner once again applies force to the wrist while the patient resists. A positive test for SLAP tear is when there is pain "deep" in the glenohumeral joint while the forearm is pronated but not when the forearm is supinated.

The dynamic labral shear test was developed by Dr. O'Driscoll and reproduces the shearing mechanism that can cause SLAP tears. It is performed by standing behind the patient, holding the wrist of the patient with one hand and applying an anteriorly directed force on the proximal humerus near the joint line with the other hand. The patient's arm is then elevated in the plane of the body from the side to maximal abduction. The test is considered positive when the patient reports pain or the examiner feels a click in the patient's posterior shoulder between 90 degrees and 120 degrees of elevation.

Imaging

Diagnostic imaging is often helpful in confirming an SLAP lesion in a youth athlete who continues to experience symptoms after nonoperative treatment.

Radiographic evaluation includes standard views of the shoulder to identify any other potential sources of shoulder pain while an MRI is the preferred imaging modality for patients with suspected SLAP tears (Fig. 25.2). An MRI is also helpful in identifying other abnormalities that frequently coexist in the shoulder.

Distinguishing SLAP tears from normal variable anatomy of the anterosuperior labrum can be difficult, and the sensitivity and specificity have been reported to range from 84% to 98% and 63% to 91%, respectively.[48] The accuracy of MRI may be improved with the addition of contrast into the joint, with one study showing that MR arthrograms have a sensitivity of 90%.[49]

Findings suggestive of an SLAP tear on MRI include high signal intensity and intraarticular contrast extension under the superior labrum/biceps root on coronal images and anteroposterior extension of high signal intensity at the superior labrum on axial imaging.

Treatment
Nonoperative

Nonoperative treatment for SLAP tears is discussed in detail later within the rehabilitation section of this chapter.

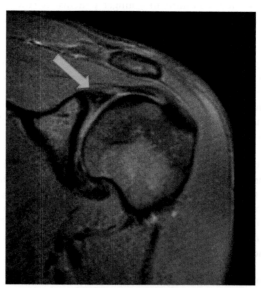

FIG. 25.2 Left shoulder T2-weighted coronal MRI image showing increased signal within the superior labrum characteristic of a SLAP tear.

Operative

When a period of rest and physical therapy does not resolve symptoms, surgery may be indicated. However, indications for surgery are variable and dependent on multiple factors, as surgery does not always reliably restore overhead athletes to their preinjury level of function. In one study of 40 overhead athletes following type II SLAP repair, 90% of patients had good to excellent results but only 75% returned to their preinjury sport level.[50] In another study, return to play was 73% for all athletes but only 63% for overhead athletes.[51] Athletes with SLAP tears who are able to perform at a high level are generally allowed to finish a competitive season, while early intervention is considered in athletes with evidence of concurrent suprascapular nerve compression secondary to a paralabral cyst.

Surgical treatment of SLAP lesions is performed arthroscopically. During surgery the superior labrum is examined for erythema and probed for signs of detachment and abnormal mobility to decide if repair is indicated. Type I lesions are treated with debridement when they are significantly frayed but such lesions do not necessarily require treatment. Unstable type II lesions should be repaired when the history and exam are consistent with an SLAP tear in young athletic patients. In contrast type II degenerative tears associated with other shoulder lesions in older less active patients do not require repair. Type III lesions are treated with resection of the unstable labral fragment and repair of the middle glenohumeral ligament (MGHL) if the ligament is attached to the torn fragment. Type IV lesions are generally treated with labral repair and biceps repair. Depending on the extent of trauma to the biceps tendon, biceps debridement, repair, tenodesis, or tenotomy may be required.

Surgical repair involves freeing up the tear, debridement of the articular cartilage above the face of the glenoid to create a bleeding bony bed for healing, and placement of suture anchor fixation. Although biomechanical studies have presented conflicting data regarding the ideal suture anchor configuration for SLAP repairs, it is important to note that the biceps anchor has some normal physiologic motion and over constraint during repair may contribute to postoperative stiffness.[48]

Additionally, normal anatomic variations of the anterosuperior labrum are important to distinguish from pathologic conditions, as errant repair can result in a significant loss of external rotation. The three main normal variations include a sublabral foramen (3.3% patients), a sublabral foramen with a cord-like MGHL (8.6% patients), and an absent anterosuperior labrum with a cord-like MGHL, also known as a Buford complex (1.5% patients).[52]

Post-Op Rehab

Rehabilitation after surgery is outlined in detail later within the rehabilitation section of this chapter.

REHABILITATION OVERVIEW

The key to successful rehabilitation of the youth throwing athlete lies in the therapists' ability to understand the unique physical features associated with these athletes, while being able to identify and address the underlying pathological features that may have predisposed this athlete to injury. Modifiable risk factors for injury can be broadly classified as external or internal factors. External factors are those that occur because of the environment in which the athlete plays and include things such as playing volume and pitch counts. Internal risk factors are those specific to the player and include things such as soft tissue abnormalities or muscle strength. The key principle that must be acknowledged during the examination and treatment of the throwing athlete is that the throwing motion is a highly coordinated, fast moving task that involves the entire body. Although shoulder pain may be the primary complaint of the athlete, to facilitate optimal recovery, a detailed examination, inclusive of the entire kinetic chain, is necessary. This section of the chapter will first focus on the principles of examination necessary to identify both external and internal factors that may contribute to the development of injury. Foundational principles of rehabilitation that are common across all throwing injuries will then be presented, with specific modifications necessary for specific injury types highlighted. Finally, return to sports considerations, including outcomes testing and pitching evaluation will be discussed.

Examination

History and evaluation of external risk factors

The therapy examination of the pediatric throwing athlete should begin with a thorough history, seeking insight into important details of the injury characteristics, including the level of irritability and predisposing factors for injury. Exposure-related variables, such as playing baseball more than 8 months each year, high overall volume of pitches thrown per game or per season, inadequate rest between pitching outings, and pitching with arm fatigue are well-established risk factors for injury among youth baseball players.[53-57] Therefore, a thorough review of the athletes baseball-specific activities is required. In addition to these volume dependent factors, the examiner should identify the type of pitches the athlete typically throws, as research has identified children who throw breaking pitches (i.e., curveball or sliders) are more likely to develop arm pain.[58] This information is essential for parent and patient education during the reintroduction of sports activities during the late phase of rehabilitation, and also helpful during counseling regarding reducing the risk of future injuries upon discharge. The examiner will find that the pediatric or adolescent patient will typically forget or gloss over details that may be important for clinical decision-making. As a result, we recommend the examiner use very specific questioning, with age appropriate terminology, while also enlisting the assistance of the parent or guardian, to obtain a complete history. In addition to baseball-specific questions, the examiner should ascertain the athlete's overall sports participation and external training activities, as these may contribute to overall workloads and the development of injury.[59]

Posture

Generally, the physical examination of the youth athlete's shoulder should begin with a detailed postural examination. In particular, the examiner should note resting scapular position, degree of thoracic kyphosis, and general muscular bulk or appearance. Although the exact correlation of scapular position or dysfunction with shoulder injury is unclear, abnormal scapular motion (termed scapular dyskinesis) has been associated with decreased shoulder mobility, increased likelihood of shoulder pathology, and impaired muscle activation and therefore should be addressed as part of an inclusive rehabilitation program.[60,61] Normal scapular motion consists of smooth and symmetrical scapular upward rotation, posterior tilting, and external rotation during active elevation of the shoulders.[61] The presence of scapular dyskinesis can be determined by observing the patient from behind, while the patient actively elevates and lowers both arms first in the frontal, and then in the sagittal plane. The scapulae should be observed, judging for any abnormal degree of motion or altered pattern of mobility. Several visual observation methods of determining scapular dyskinesis have been described and shown to be reliable in distinguishing normal from abnormal motion.[62–64] Medial scapular border prominence (i.e., scapular winging) and loss of smooth motion during eccentric lowering are common abnormalities observed within the youth thrower. If scapular dyskinesis is present, any correlation to complaints of pain should be noted and the surrounding anatomic structures should be evaluated further, to determine the factors that may be causing dysfunction. This should include an assessment of thoracic spine mobility and flexibility of the pectoralis

minor. Pectoralis minor length can be assessed by obtaining a linear measurement from the treatment table to the posterior aspect of the acromion while the patient is lying supine or by measuring the distance while the patient is standing with their back against a wall.[60,61] Normal measurement distances have been described; however, these may be highly population dependent and thus comparison can be made to the contralateral side to determine relative tightness. In addition, isolated muscle performance testing of scapular stabilizing muscles should be performed, which will be covered in detail later in this chapter.

Shoulder range of motion

Before performing a specific examination of shoulder mobility, the patient should be screened for generalized ligamentous laxity using the Beighton scoring system outlined earlier, as generalized ligamentous laxity may lead to higher than normal ROM.[65]

Accurate assessment and treatment of shoulder ROM deficits is a key concept in the treatment of the youth throwing athlete. Throwing athletes exhibit a pattern of increased glenohumeral external rotation (ER) and limited glenohumeral internal rotation (IR) in their dominant shoulder.[60,66–68] Often the increase in ER is balanced by a concurrent loss of IR, such that the total arc of motion is the normal, just shifted toward an external rotation bias. Thus, upon examination, the typical healthy throwing athlete will demonstrate a greater degree of shoulder ER (external rotation gain), a lower degree of shoulder IR (GIRD), and a symmetrical amount of total shoulder rotational motion (ER + IR) between the dominant and nondominant sides.

Although most studies outlining this ROM profile were performed within adult baseball players,[69] recent evidence demonstrates this asymmetrical shoulder rotation profile can be found in children as young as 8 years old and should be considered normal for this population.[70,71] Deviations in shoulder motion, specifically GIRD >20 degrees,[60] total arc of motion deficits of >5 degrees,[72] flexion deficits of >5 degrees,[73] and horizontal adduction deficits of >15 degrees,[74] have all been identified as risk factors for injury among throwing athletes and should be assessed and addressed as part of a comprehensive treatment plan.

When assessing shoulder motion, it is important to stabilize the scapula, as unwanted accessory motion from the scapulothoracic joint may impact the accuracy true glenohumeral joint motion.[75] The authors recommend stabilizing the scapular and assessing shoulder motion using standardized techniques as outlined in Fig. 25.3.

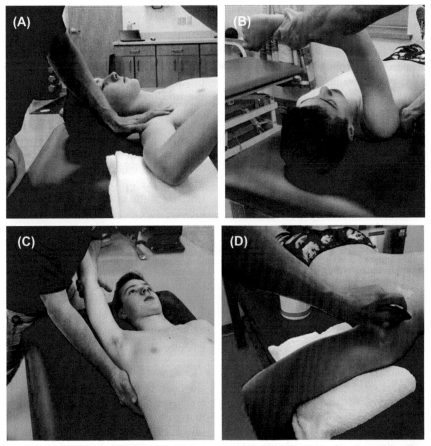

FIG. 25.3 **(A)** To accurately assess internal rotation range of motion, a posterior force should be placed at the coracoid process to keep the scapula from anteriorly tilting. **(B)** Cross-body adduction stretch with the scapula blocked. **(C)** Flexion stretching with the scapula blocked. **(D)** Instrument-assisted soft tissue mobilization to the posterior shoulder.

Motor performance

As the shoulder girdle is arguably the least structurally stable joint in the body, the importance of assessing motor or muscular performance cannot be overstated. Various aspects of motor performance, including strength (more accurately described as force production), endurance, and control are crucial for the throwing athlete, and thus require specific evaluation during rehabilitation.

Force production

Manual muscle testing (MMT) may be utilized initially to screen the patient for large strength deficits; however, it should be noted that MMT may lack the sensitivity required to identify strength deficits within this population, particularly within the rotator cuff musculature.[76] Although isokinetic dynamometry is the gold standard,[77] handheld dynamometry (HHD) is an accurate and more clinically feasible alternative.[78,79] Primary testing should consist of glenohumeral internal and external rotation at neutral elevation and 90 degrees of abduction. A ratio of at least 66% for ER to IR glenohumeral force production has been proposed as ideal and may be associated with reduced injury rates.[77,79–82] Although the formal MMT for shoulder flexion and abduction is performed at end range,[83] testing elevation at 90 degrees in the plane of the scapula, otherwise known as the "full can" position, is a better and more functional position. Testing of scapular musculature should not be overlooked, as diminished stability at the scapulothoracic joint has been associated with increased injury risk.[84,85] Prone horizontal abduction testing at 90 degrees biases the middle trapezius, while the position at 120 degrees biases the lower trapezius. By placing the testing force at the distal radius, greater functional information of the kinetic chain can be garnered, but isolation of the trapezius musculature is better achieved with resistance at the spine of the scapula. Isolated testing of the serratus anterior may also be of particular value if scapular dyskinesis is observed.

Endurance

Adolescents tend to have less muscular endurance,[86] and upper extremity fatigue has been associated with pain and injury in baseball players,[3,18] making identification and treatment of muscular endurance deficits an important aspect of rehabilitation. Multiple endurance testing protocols exist for the upper extremity including isokinetics and repeated motions.[87–89] The authors recommend use of the prone Y fatigue test, as decreased performance has been associated with injury,[88] and seems to be most appropriate for throwers. These tests are likely not appropriate at the initial evaluation, but may be utilized later in the course of care for return to sport decision-making, or in the patient that complains of symptoms that seem to be associated with fatigue.

Control

Proprioceptive impairments have been identified in individuals with shoulder or upper extremity pain,[90,91] and such impairments may increase the risk of injury or reinjury.[92,93] Proprioceptive abilities may be reliably measured with isokinetic equipment, a laser pointer, or inclinometer.[94] Yet, there is mixed evidence as to whether isolated proprioceptive training compared to more conventional treatment leads to improved outcomes.[95–97] As such, specific examination of upper extremity proprioception and isolation of it as an outcome is likely unnecessary as long as it is addressed within the treatment plan.

Kinetic chain

The kinetic chain is the interaction of individual parts of the whole athlete to best produce a desired action. In throwing, the kinetic chain functions to transfer force from the ground to the ball, and optimal transfer of energy has been associated with injury prevention and improved performance.[84,85] The examination of the throwing athlete must also include assessment of the spine, core, and lower extremities. Examination of every aspect of these regions is unreasonable, so key measurements and movement screens have been highlighted.

Spinal rotation should be measured grossly and if deficits are found, thoracic rotation should be examined more closely. Deficits in hip ROM have been associated

with groin and throwing arm injuries in baseball players,[98,99] and sufficient hip ROM has been proposed as necessary for optimal throwing mechanics.[100] Similarly, at least 20 degrees of weight-bearing ankle dorsiflexion is necessary for proper wind-up mechanics, to provide sufficient propulsion from the ground into the driveline of a pitch, and also for allowance of deceleration on the lead leg at the end of the throwing motion.[101] Lower extremity motor performance and balance control can be quickly screened with a single leg squat or lateral step down test.

The core musculature plays an important role in throwing, as it provides the link for the transference of force from the lower extremities to the upper extremities. A number of specific examination measures, such as timed planks, have been described in the literature.[102–105] However one criticism of these tests is that they capture isometric endurance, which may not simulate the sport-specific action in baseball, in which motion is fast, dynamic, and often plyometric in nature. Nevertheless, we recommend use of these tests to gauge the athlete's baseline level of physical ability and develop interventions to address identified deficits.

Treatment Considerations

The components of a successful rehabilitation program are driven by the details of the examination findings of that particular patient. There are many common elements of rehabilitation across the various thrower-specific conditions discussed in this chapter, and thus we will present treatment principles for many of these common elements here. At the conclusion of this section, we will present aspects of rehabilitation that are specific to the pathology or surgical procedure that was performed.

In general the rehabilitation program should be structured to respect the individual athlete's pathoanatomical diagnosis (e.g., SLAP tear), identified impairments, and level of tissue irritability.[106] The level of irritability relates to the tolerance for stress within the affected tissue and helps guide the clinician to select the appropriate level of intensity for therapeutic intervention. For example, after injury, the athlete may be experiencing high levels of pain and diminished shoulder motion. The treatment program at this time will emphasize patient education in activity modification, modalities to improve pain, and manual therapy to reduce pain and restore mobility. As the patient's level of irritability decreases, the physical stress associated with rehabilitation exercises should be increased accordingly to more specifically target deficits in strength, motion, neuromuscular control, and other impairments identified during the evaluation that are contributing to dysfunction or impairing performance. Any modifications to rehabilitation based upon pathoanatomy or surgical restrictions will be layered over top of these general principles of rehabilitation progression.

When compared to their adult counterparts, one of the unique features of the youth athlete that makes rehabilitation challenging, but fun, is the necessity for more individual supervision during rehabilitation exercises. The youth athlete will require increased attention to ensure proper form and utilization of intended muscle groups, as substitution patterns are very common and sometimes difficult to identify. Use of visual feedback via mirror or video recording, along with tactile and verbal cuing, will be necessary to achieve optimal performance of exercises. Adherence to the prescribed home exercise program is also sometimes difficult. Typically, adherence can be improved by keeping the volume of exercises at home low, incorporating 4—6 exercises, which can be accomplished in 15 minutes or less. Additionally, variation of home exercise prescription is helpful to keep the program fresh, limiting boredom and keeping the athlete engaged. Parental supervision and involvement can be extremely helpful in improving compliance, while also assisting with monitoring for proper form while performing exercises outside of the clinic.

Posture and scapular dyskinesis

Treatment directed toward improving postural abnormalities and scapular dyskinesis can usually begin during the early phases of rehabilitation. Pectoralis minor tightness can be treated with unilateral corner stretch or manual stretching techniques, in which the scapula is brought into a position of retraction and posterior tilting.[107] Manual stretching techniques may be improved by having the patient lie on a foam roller placed longitudinally along the spine. Manual therapy techniques to improve thoracic spine mobility may also be incorporated to improve posture and have also been shown to improve scapular muscle activity and strength.[61] Various types of posterior to anterior mobilization or manipulation techniques have been described in sitting, supine, or prone. The therapist should determine the best technique for each patient based upon several factors including irritability of symptoms, body positions that may exacerbate patient symptoms, and body morphology. A thorough explanation of the intended mobilization procedure should be explained to both the parent and patient before engaging in this aspect of treatment, to obtain consent

and optimize the effects of treatment. Appropriate screening for contraindications should be performed before initiating treatment. Although thoracic manipulation is safe, its use within growing children should be considered a precaution,[108] and thus should be monitored carefully. In addition, the authors do not recommend utilizing manipulation techniques on children with hypermobility or significant ligamentous laxity.

Scapular strengthening exercises should also be incorporated here to improve scapular positioning and control during motion. Early exercises, such as shoulder external rotation with a stable scapula or serratus punches, can be initiated during periods of high irritability. As the patient's irritability level decreases, exercises should be advanced to include those that target the middle and lower trapezius, such as prone I's, T's, and Y's. Advanced exercises, such as closed chain serratus push-ups and dynamic stabilization in an open or closed chain, with more focus on endurance-based exercise prescription, should be incorporated in the late phases of rehabilitation (Fig. 25.4).

Shoulder range of motion

Due to the relationship of limited shoulder mobility to upper extremity injury in throwing athletes, addressing any identified deficits in motion is a critical component of rehabilitation within this population. Pathological GIRD or loss of IR motion can be the result of increased humeral retrotorsion,[70,71] decreased flexibility within the posterior capsular/ligamentous structures,[109] or decreased flexibility of the posterior rotator cuff.[110] Thus, to adequately treat IR deficit within the throwing athlete, all of these factors should be considered. Clinical techniques for quantifying humeral retrotorsion, using either palpation[111] or musculoskeletal ultrasound,[112] have been described, but may not be appropriate for widespread clinical adoption at this time. Although there is evidence indicating the posterior capsule may become thickened because of throwing, it is currently unknown whether this thickening results in impaired capsular mobility, leading to glenohumeral IR motion loss.[60,109] McClure et al. demonstrated that cross-body adduction stretching, targeting the posterior rotator cuff, results in greater improvements in shoulder IR motion than the "sleeper" stretch, which is intended to preferentially stretch the posterior capsule.[113] More recently, Bailey et al.[110] demonstrated that changes in rotator cuff stiffness, not glenohumeral joint mobility or humeral torsion, were most likely associated with the internal rotation deficits observed in a group of adolescent baseball players. Taken together, the

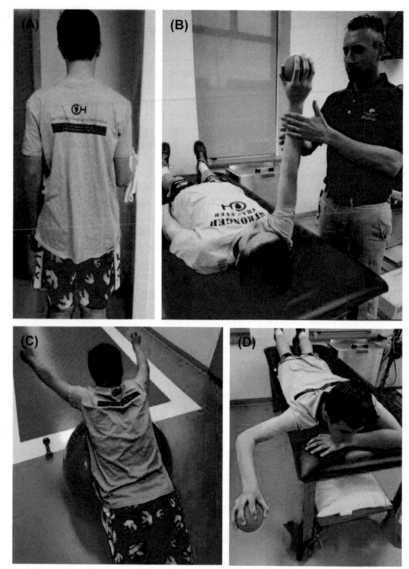

FIG. 25.4 **(A)** Isometric GH ER/IR performed at neutral elevation against a wall. **(B)** Manual rhythmic stabilizations performed at the "balance point"—90–100 degrees of flexion with 10 degrees of horizontal abduction in supine. **(C)** Prone Y's on a physioball, emphasizing scapular and core control simultaneously. **(D)** Prone "drop and catch" with a weighted ball at 90/90 to improve eccentric control and endurance.

evidence indicates that effective treatment for shoulder IR loss should focus on muscle/tendon techniques, such as cross-body adduction stretching, modified sleeper stretching, and manual stretching to the posterior rotator cuff (Fig. 25.3). In addition, recent evidence has demonstrated the use of instrument-assisted soft tissue mobilization (IASTM) to the posterior shoulder can improve shoulder horizontal adduction and internal rotation motion in baseball players (Fig. 25.3).[114] It is the authors' experience that IASTM techniques are usually well tolerated within the adolescent population, but may not be as useful in younger athletes. Any deficits in shoulder flexion mobility can be addressed using manual stretching while blocking the scapula (Fig. 25.3) and patient-centered stretches targeting the latissimus dorsi or teres major complex.

Shoulder motor performance interventions

Motor performance impairments should also be addressed based on stage of irritability[106] and safe level of tissue physical stress. Although well-designed phased progressions have been presented,[115,116] dosage should exist on a continuum in parallel to patient irritability and will likely ebb and flow in the natural course of the rehabilitative process. Those experiencing high irritability should be prescribed active-assisted ROM and low-intensity isometrics in low elevation and midrange positions with gradually increasing volume. Rhythmic stabilizations should also be incorporated for early neuromuscular control integration. These can be performed in the plane of the scapula with the elbow flexed to 90 degrees or in the balance point position of 90–100 degrees of flexion and 10 degrees of horizontal abduction inducing glenohumeral compression (Fig. 25.4).[117] Even in patients with high irritability, scapular control and strengthening exercises can be initiated against manual resistance or in an open chain fashion.

Isotonic resistance training should be added once irritability decreases. These should be initiated with higher volume and low intensity in positions of increasing elevation and rotation, emphasizing the scapular stabilizers and external rotators. The Thrower's Ten exercise program[81] is an excellent resource for a well-rounded shoulder girdle motor performance regimen. Prone Y's and resisted ER/IR at increasing elevations should be prioritized (Fig. 25.4). Rhythmic stabilization training may be progressed by addition of weighted balls or resistance bands in open chain or via perturbation in closed chain positions. These interventions should be progressed to unilateral performance and include altered surfaces to integrate core and kinetic chain training.

As the patient reaches low irritability, intensity of strength training should be increased, muscular endurance should be specifically addressed, plyometrics should be introduced, and integration of dynamic core control should occur. Circles on a wall with weighted balls, isometric contractions, or "burn-out" sets can all be used to promote muscular endurance. Wilk et al.[115] have suggested performing an isometric hold on one side during an isotonic movement contralaterally to capture multiple aspects of muscular training simultaneously. During this phase, it is important to emphasize eccentric training within the posterior shoulder musculature, as these groups are responsible for arm deceleration after ball release during pitching. Once the athlete has established a base of foundational strength, plyometric training can begin. Open chain plyometrics should begin two-handed,[115] and progress to unilateral, which can be performed with a rebounder. We recommend beginning with approximately 30–40 repetitions of plyometric activity for skeletally immature throwers, with slow progression and careful monitoring for symptoms. Prone "drop and catch" exercises in Y, T, or 90/90 positions are excellent to emphasize eccentric control and posterior shoulder endurance (Fig. 25.4). "Reverse throwing" is an excellent activity to target arm deceleration and tends to be a fun activity for kids. Closed kinetic chain stability exercises, such as unstable quadruped reaching, arm walks on a physioball, and moving planks can be instituted, and may be particularly useful for individuals with issues related to instability.

Additional kinetic chain considerations

Even in stages of higher irritability, aerobic and lower extremity strengthening interventions should be applied to maintain fitness, address kinetic chain impairments, and provide analgesic and antiinflammatory effects.[118–121] Stationary cycling, leg press, and knee extension machines can be used to begin lower extremity training with minimal upper extremity stress. As shoulder stability is established, band-resisted hip abduction/walks and single leg squats (Fig. 25.5)—which have demonstrated high gluteal activation[122,123]—along with heel raises, and static balance exercises may be incorporated. Patients should return to running and light agility exercises as symptoms diminish and after physician clearance.

Injury-Specific Treatment Considerations
Little League Shoulder

The initial treatment of LLS consists of a period of relative rest in which the player will refrain from any throwing or other irritating activities. Therapy is typically initiated during this period with the treatment directed toward specific examination findings, while respecting the level of symptom irritability. As the underlying pathology in LLS is related to high amounts of stress being transferred across the proximal humeral physis, all factors that may contribute to this increase in stress should be evaluated and addressed as necessary. These will include external risk factors (e.g., throwing volume and rest days) and internal or player-specific risk factors, such as shoulder motion, posture, strength, and other considerations covered in the previous examination section. Postural deficits and pathological loss of shoulder flexion, internal rotation, and horizontal adduction are commonly encountered in those with LLS and should be addressed accordingly. Commonly,

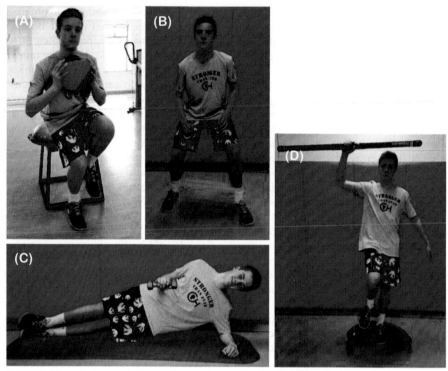

FIG. 25.5 **(A)** Singe leg squat; both a test and an exercise for the kinetic chain. **(B)** Anterolateral "monster" bandwalks. **(C)** Side plank with resisted GH ER combines core and rotator cuff strengthening. **(D)** Single leg stance on foam while oscillating a bodyblade at 90/90 integrates core control with plyometric and endurance training of the shoulder musculature in a functional and sport-specific position.

pain involved with LLS resolves relatively quickly and the therapist should progress the patient through the spectrum of more advanced strengthening and neuromuscular control activities. A progressive return to throwing program can begin once the patient has met the necessary clinical milestones for progression, typically 3–4 months after injury. To reduce the potential for reinjury, these patients and parents should be heavily counseled on overuse injury risk factors, pitch count/type limitations, and recommendations for 3–4 months of rest per year from overhead sports activity, before discharge.

Gross and Microinstability

Although patients with instability-related diagnoses will predominantly be treated with similar concepts as mentioned earlier, some nuances should be considered. Severity and chronicity of the instability will guide the initial treatment. A patient experiencing a recent traumatic dislocation will likely require a short period of sling immobilization, more low-level isometric activities, and a slower overall rehabilitation progression, whereas an individual with chronic subluxation may be able to progress to more challenging rehabilitation

exercises earlier. The predominant focus of rehabilitation with these individuals should be optimizing muscular strength, motor control, and endurance to achieve active control of the shoulder with daily and sport-related activities. Therapist-controlled rhythmic stabilization in nonprovocative positions and low-level CKC stability exercises may be safely initiated early on, during periods of high irritability. Rehabilitation progression should then focus on neuromuscular re-education and dynamic stability training, moving from less provocative to more provocative positions (e.g., arm at side to overhead activity) and finally focusing on sport-specific movements (e.g., rhythmic stabilization in cocking position of throwing).

Specific progression of postoperative care following capsulorraphy or other surgical stabilization procedures will be dictated by surgeon protocol (*Appendix*). However, generally speaking submaximal isometrics can usually be instituted in the first 1–2 weeks postoperatively if the patient's pain is well controlled and the exercises can be performed relatively pain free. Rehabilitation progression should proceed according to the principles outlined earlier, while making specific modifications based upon procedure-related precautions or surgical protocol. Traditionally, some slight restriction in external rotation may be considered advantageous after capsular repair; however, for the throwing population, in particular pitchers, a loss of external rotation motion may impair performance and increase the risk of subsequent shoulder or elbow injury. Thus, the therapist must cautiously progress ROM exercises to restore optimal shoulder mobility; however, aggressive stretching beyond 90 degrees should not begin until at least 12 weeks postoperatively.[124]

SLAP tear
Nonoperative treatment of patients with a SLAP tear can progress according to the basic principles outlined throughout this chapter. As symptom presentation may vary considerably within these athletes, specific attention should be paid to individual provocative positions. Early emphasis on active rest, refraining from activities or positions that cause pain, is important to move the patient toward lower irritability levels. Detailed assessment and treatment of localized strength, ROM, or scapular dyskinesis should be performed, while employing factors related to kinetic chain abnormalities, is important for an inclusive rehabilitation program (Appendix). After the resolution of pain and the patient has achieved satisfactory performance criteria, an interval throwing program can be initiated (see full discussion later). The patient should be monitored closely and if symptoms return or the patient is unable to achieve satisfactory performance during throwing, the patient may need to be referred back to the physician for surgical consultation.

Similar to the previous discussion for capsulorraphy, the postoperative rehabilitation will vary depending upon the extent of injury and surgical procedure performed. However, the overriding principle that will apply to all SLAP rehabilitation programs is protection of the healing tissue. ROM will be slowly progressed after an initial period of immobilization and comprehensive rehabilitation activities will progress in a graded fashion. During the later phases of rehabilitation, the therapist should be mindful of the "peel-back mechanism" discussed earlier and the role of the long head of the biceps brachii during deceleration following ball release. Following ball release, rapid elbow extension is slowed by the eccentric activity of the biceps brachii, transferring stress to the long head's attachment to the superior labrum and site of surgical repair.[85] Additional time, and a more gradual progression for eccentric training and high velocity throwing, may be necessary to allow safe tissue adaptation to occur.

Interval Sport Program and Return to Play: Clearance and Application
As the patient progresses to the later stages of care, a gradual return to sport—beginning with an interval sport program and ending with full return to play—is strongly recommended. Criteria-based decisions, guided by "soreness rules,"[125–127] should be emphasized for clearance to initiate and progress through these stages (Table 25.1).[76,81,82,115,116,128] Physician

TABLE 25.1 *Predominantly Used in Older Adolescents **Recommended[125] ***.	
Criteria to Initiate Interval Throwing Program	**Criteria for Return to Play**
• Near to full sport-specific ROM	• Full sport-specific ROM
• >80% force production compared to contralateral uninjured upper extremity—measured via HHD	• >90%–95% force production compared to contralateral uninjured upper extremity—measured via HHD
• Minimal to no pain with current activities/interventions	• Successful completion of interval throwing program
	• >90% endurance and functional testing compared to contralateral uninjured upper extremity or norms*
	• >90% self-reported outcome measure**

SORENESS RULES*
- If no soreness, advance one step every throwing day.
- If sore during warm-up but soreness is gone within the first 15 throws, repeat the previous workout. If shoulder becomes sore during this workout, stop and take 2 days off. Upon return to throwing, drop down one step.
- If sore more than 1 hour after throwing, or the next day, take 1 day off and repeat the most recent throwing program workout.
- If sore during warm-up and soreness continues through the first 15 throws, stop throwing and take 2 days off. Upon return to throwing, drop down one step.

clearance may be required as well, particularly for the postoperative population.

An interval throwing program is a graded progression of throwing activity designed to provide a safe return to play by slowly increasing the stress transferred to the shoulder through manipulation of variables such as volume, intensity, type of throw, and recovery time. Although multiple interval throwing programs exist,[125,128] the authors recommend the one developed by Axe et al.[125] as it provides progressions stratified for the age of the patient. If the upper extremity in question is the nondominant arm, then the same criteria should be met for clearance; however, throwing programs may not be necessary. Batting has related but specific physical requirements as compared to throwing, so a batting interval program[76] should be similarly applied. Arguably, the athlete returning to full play should demonstrate proper throwing mechanics that can be identified using slow-motion video analysis (outlined later).

Functional testing procedures, such as the closed kinetic chain upper extremity stability test (CKCUEST), upper quarter Y-balance test, or single-arm shot put, may be valuable, as they assess multiple aspects of performance. Although normative and reliability values[102,129–132] for some of these tests have been reported, they are generally not well studied within the pediatric population. However, these values along with endurance testing might be appropriate for consideration when assessing older adolescent patients, or as a marker for comparison considering typical muscular development trends in the pediatric population.

Throwing Evaluation

Pitching is a complex and highly coordinated motion. Abnormalities in the pitching motion may contribute to the development of injury; although a highly detailed discussion of pitching biomechanics may be outside the scope of this chapter, the general clinician treating the youth thrower should be capable of performing a basic throwing evaluation to determine if further referral for improving pitching mechanics is warranted. Fleisig

et al. have shown that youth pitchers are capable of replicating the throwing mechanics demonstrated by professional pitchers, and thus, established that achieving sound pitching mechanics can be accomplished at an early age, and should be a focus for injury prevention early in an athlete's pitching career.[133] The proliferation of slow-motion digital technology and improved camera functionality in handheld devices (phones, tablets, etc.) now allows the clinician to more easily perform throwing analysis within the clinic. Several authors have shown that clinic-based 2D motion analysis can be accurate and clinically meaningful. To perform a 2D pitching analysis, the clinician will need to obtain two views of the pitcher: a frontal view (as if standing at home plate) and a lateral view (as if standing at first base for left-handed, third base for right-handed pitchers). The video is replayed in slow motion and the clinician can focus on body position or sequencing at specific points within the pitching motion, to identify common flaws that may predispose the player to injury. The reader is referred to DeFroda et al.[134] for a comprehensive summary of pitching abnormalities and 2D pitching analysis. If any of these common errors are noted, the clinician can attempt to resolve them through additional intervention strategies (e.g., additional hip stretching) or can refer the patient to a pitching coach, with specific instructions to work on the identified deficits.

SUMMARY

As youth sports participation continues to increase, there has been a corresponding increase in the amount of injuries seen, especially overuse injuries of the shoulder. Although youth athletes may present with many of the same complaints as more mature athletes, differences in anatomy often lead to age-specific injuries. This chapter covers the presentation, diagnosis, and treatment of several pediatric throwing injuries including LLS, shoulder instability, and SLAP lesions. Additionally, risk factors, throwing evaluation, interval throwing programs, and return to play are discussed.

APPENDIX

UNIVERSITY OF PENNSYLVANIA HEALTH SYSTEM
SHOULDER AND ELBOW SERVICE

REHABILITATION GUIDELINES FOLLOWING ANTERIOR CAPSULORRHAPHY

Phase I: 0–4 weeks:
Goals:
1. Patient independent with precautions and home exercise program before discharge from hospital (typical inpatient hospital stay = 1 day).
2. Permit capsular healing.
3. Control pain and inflammation.
4. Range of motion exercises will be initiated depending on surgeon's preference.

POD # 1:
1. Educate patient on precautions.
2. Pendulum exercises (25 times in each direction)—depending on surgeon
3. Elbow AROM, hand squeeze exercises
4. Ice (instruct patient on use of ice at home)

Phase II: 4–6 weeks:
Goals:
1. Decreased pain and inflammation
2. Normal arthrokinematics of glenohumeral and scapulothoracic joint
3. Improve strength
Treatment:
1. Continue with above treatment
2. Add phase I stretching (forward elevation and external rotation in POS)
   -Limit ER to 45 degrees
3. Manual resistance for glenohumeral and scapulothoracic stabilization
4. Add phase I strengthening
5. Add shoulder shrugs and scapular retraction
6. Bodyblade in nonprovocative positions

Phase III: 6–12 weeks:
Goals:
1. Increase strength of rotator cuff and deltoid
2. Increase strength of scapular muscles
3. Increase total arm strength (biceps, triceps, forearms, etc.)
4. Initiate strengthening in provocative positions
Treatment:
1. Continue with that mentioned earlier (decrease frequency of stretching exercises)
2. Add phase II stretching (extension, IR, cross-body adduction)
3. Add phase II strengthening (abduction, forward elevation, ER @ 45 ⤙ in POS)
4. Variable resistance and/or free weight resistance
5. Bodyblade in functional positions
6. Plyoball progression (begin with chest pass)

Phase IV: 12–16 weeks:
Goals:
1. Initiate return to sport or occupational activity[a]
Treatment:
1. Bodyblade in overhead positions
2. Plyoball throwing
3. Work/sport-specific activities[a]

---

[a] Applies to athlete or laborer. 1/2007, BGU MJK.

⊕H The Children's Hospital
of Philadelphia®

Theodore Ganley, MD Lawrence Wells, MD J. Todd Lawrence, MD, PhD

Postoperative Rehabilitation Protocol Following Arthroscopic.
   SLAP Debridement.

This protocol guides a progressive return to full activity beginning **at 6 months** if all other criteria are achieved. If the criteria are met sooner, the patient must restrict his/her activity level until the **end of the sixth postoperative month. If patient has a concomitant injury/repair (such as a rotator cuff repair) treatment will vary. Please consult with surgeon.**

Weeks 0–6:
Goals:
1. Permit capsule-ligamentous-labral healing
2. Minimize effects of immobilization
3. Decrease pain and inflammation
4. Patient education
5. Discontinue brace use **after 6 weeks**

Treatment:
- **No formal physical therapy**
- Home exercise program of pendulums, elbow and wrist ROM, gripping exercises, and ice as needed
- Elbow PROM (no biceps activation)

Weeks 7–12:
Goals:
1. Normalize arthrokinematics of glenohumeral and scapulothoracic joints
2. Full shoulder ROM by week 10
3. Increase total arm/scapular strength
4. Initiate strength and proprioceptive training
5. Decrease pain and inflammation

Treatment
Weeks 7–9:
- Address shoulder ROM (ER at 90 degrees to 90 degrees; FE to 180 degrees)
- Shoulder strength (IR/ER/extension/abduction/forward elevation) with bands/weights (begin with nonprovocative positions)

- Begin biceps AROM
- Thrower's Ten
- PNF D2 manual resistance
- Nonprovocative neuromuscular and proprioceptive activities (i.e., bodyblade, rhythmic stabilization)
- Scapular stabilization
- Prone rows
- Supine ½ foam roll pectoralis stretch arms at side

Weeks 10–12:
- Continue strength/ROM as mentioned earlier
- **Initiate double-arm open chain plyometrics (begin with chest pass)**
- **Initiate ER/IR strengthening at 90 degrees abduction**
- **Initiate full weight-bearing activity/closed kinetic chain at week 10**
- Incorporate lower extremity/core stability into program

Weeks 13–20.
Goals:
1. Full AROM and PROM
2. Improve muscular strength and endurance
3. Initiation of functional activities

Treatment:
Weeks 13–16:
- Continue strength/ROM as mentioned earlier
- **Initiate single-arm open chain plyometrics**
- Functional and overhead strengthening

Weeks 16–20:
- Continue as mentioned earlier
- **Initiate interval throwing program (for most injuries, expect return to throwing by 3–6 months; throwing at full velocity is typically delayed until 6 months)**
- Initiate sport-specific drills

Weeks 21–26.
Goals:
1. Enhance muscular strength and endurance
2. Maximize neuromuscular control
3. Maintain shoulder ROM

Treatment:

- Continue strengthening program
- Continue neuromuscular control drills
- Continue plyometric drills
- Continue interval throwing program with progression to position-specific throwing program

6—9 months.
Goals:

1. Gradual return to full unrestricted sport activities
2. Maintain ROM, stability, and neuromuscular control
3. Achieve maximal strength and endurance

Criteria to Discharge for Return to Full Sport Activities

- *Normal arthrokinematics of GH and ST joint*
- *Satisfactory clinical exam*
- *Strength testing >90% contralateral side*
- *Subjective scoring (Penn Shoulder Score >90 points) (DASH<15)*
- *Completion of both interval and position-specific throwing program*

This protocol is designed to be administered by a licensed physical therapist and/or certified athletic trainer. Please do not hesitate to contact our office should you have any questions concerning the rehabilitation process.
Protocol adapted from Wilk et al., JOSPT, 2005.

Sports medicine and performance center at the Children's Hospital of Philadelphia

Specialty Care Center in King of Prussia
550 South Goddard Blvd.
King of Prussia, PA 19046
267—425—9105

Specialty Care Center in Chalfont
500 W Butler Pike
Chalfont, PA 18914
215—590—6930

Department of physical therapySports Medicine
Children's Seashore House—2nd Floor
34th and Civic center Boulevard
Philadelphia, PA 19104
215—590—5819

Specialty care at Virtua

Health and Wellness center, 2nd Floor
200 Bowman Dr. Suite D-260

Voorhees, NJ 08043
866—486—3225 (x37524)

REFERENCES

1. Moyer JE, Brey JM. Shoulder injuries in pediatric athletes. *Orthop Clin N Am.* 2016;47(4):749—762.
2. Stracciolini A, Casciano R, Friedman HL, Meehan 3rd WP, Micheli LJ. A closer look at overuse injuries in the pediatric athlete. *Clin J Sport Med.* 2015;25(1):30—35.
3. Lyman S, Fleisig GS, Waterbor JW, et al. Longitudinal study of elbow and shoulder pain in youth baseball pitchers. *Med Sci Sport Exerc.* 2001;33(11):1803—1810.
4. Shanley E, Rauh MJ, Michener LA, Ellenbecker TS. Incidence of injuries in high school softball and baseball players. *J Athl Train.* 2011;46(6):648—654.
5. Dillman CJ, Fleisig GS, Andrews JR. Biomechanics of pitching with emphasis upon shoulder kinematics. *J Orthop Sport Phys Ther.* 1993;18(2):402—408.
6. Fleisig GS, Andrews JR, Dillman CJ, Escamilla RF. Kinetics of baseball pitching with implications about injury mechanisms. *Am J Sports Med.* 1995;23(2):233—239.
7. Fleisig GS, Barrentine SW, Escamilla RF, Andrews JR. Biomechanics of overhand throwing with implications for injuries. *Sport Med.* 1996;21(6):421—437.
8. Wasserlauf BL, Paletta Jr GA. Shoulder disorders in the skeletally immature throwing athlete. *Orthop Clin N Am.* 2003;34(3):427—437.
9. Ireland ML, Hutchinson MR. Upper extremity injuries in young athletes. *Clin Sports Med.* 1995;14(3):533—569.
10. Cole BWJ. Anatomy, biomechanics, and pathophysiology of glenohumeral instability. In: Iannotti JGW, ed. *Disorders of the Shoulder: Diagnosis and Management.* New York: Lippincott Williams & Wilkins; 1999:207—232.
11. Dotter WE. Little leaguer's shoulder: a fracture of the proximal epiphysial cartilage of the humerus due to baseball pitching. *Guthrie Clin Bull.* 1953;23(1):68—72.
12. Adams JE. Little league shoulder: osteochondrosis of the proximal humeral epiphysis in boy baseball pitchers. *Calif Med.* 1966;105(1):22—25.
13. Carson Jr WG, Gasser SI. Little Leaguer's shoulder. A report of 23 cases. *Am J Sports Med.* 1998;26(4):575—580.
14. Tullos HS, Fain RH. Little league shoulder: rotational stress fracture of proximal epiphysis. *J Sport Med.* 1974; 2(3):152—153.
15. Heyworth BE, Kramer DE, Martin DJ, Micheli LJ, Kocher MS, Bae DS. Trends in the presentation, management, and outcomes of little league shoulder. *Am J Sports Med.* 2016;44(6):1431—1438.
16. Kocher MS, Waters PM, Micheli LJ. Upper extremity injuries in the paediatric athlete. *Sport Med.* 2000;30(2): 117—135.
17. Osbahr DC, Kim HJ, Dugas JR. Little league shoulder. *Curr Opin Pediatr.* 2010;22(1):35—40.
18. Olsen 2nd SJ, Fleisig GS, Dun S, Loftice J, Andrews JR. Risk factors for shoulder and elbow injuries in adolescent baseball pitchers. *Am J Sports Med.* 2006;34(6):905—912.

19. Bright RW, Burstein AH, Elmore SM. Epiphyseal-plate cartilage. A biomechanical and histological analysis of failure modes. *J Bone Joint Surg Am.* 1974;56(4):688–703.

20. Tibone JE. Shoulder problems of adolescents. How they differ from those of adults. *Clin Sports Med.* 1983;2(2):423–427.

21. Sabick MB, Kim YK, Torry MR, Keirns MA, Hawkins RJ. Biomechanics of the shoulder in youth baseball pitchers: implications for the development of proximal humeral epiphysiolysis and humeral retrotorsion. *Am J Sports Med.* 2005;33(11):1716–1722.

22. Tisano BK, Estes AR. Overuse injuries of the pediatric and adolescent throwing athlete. *Med Sci Sport Exerc.* 2016;48(10):1898–1905.

23. Taylor DC, Krasinski KL. Adolescent shoulder injuries: consensus and controversies. *J Bone Joint Surg Am.* 2009;91(2):462–473.

24. Smucny M, Kolmodin J, Saluan P. Shoulder and elbow injuries in the adolescent athlete. *Sport Med Arthrosc Rev.* 2016;24(4):188–194.

25. Walton J, Paxinos A, Tzannes A, Callanan M, Hayes K, Murrell GA. The unstable shoulder in the adolescent athlete. *Am J Sports Med.* 2002;30(5):758–767.

26. Chen FS, Diaz VA, Loebenberg M, Rosen JE. Shoulder and elbow injuries in the skeletally immature athlete. *J Am Acad Orthop Surg.* 2005;13(3):172–185.

27. Zaremski JL, Krabak BJ. Shoulder injuries in the skeletally immature baseball pitcher and recommendations for the prevention of injury. *PM & R.* 2012;4(7):509–516.

28. Schenk TJ, Brems JJ. Multidirectional instability of the shoulder: pathophysiology, diagnosis, and management. *J Am Acad Orthop Surg.* 1998;6(1):65–72.

29. Milewski MD, Nissen CW. Pediatric and adolescent shoulder instability. *Clin Sports Med.* 2013;32(4):761–779.

30. Dewing CB, McCormick F, Bell SJ, et al. An analysis of capsular area in patients with anterior, posterior, and multidirectional shoulder instability. *Am J Sports Med.* 2008;36(3):515–522.

31. Kim KC, Rhee KJ, Shin HD, Kim YM. Estimating the dimensions of the rotator interval with use of magnetic resonance arthrography. *J Bone Joint Surg Am.* 2007;89(11):2450–2455.

32. Neer 2nd CS, Foster CR. Inferior capsular shift for involuntary inferior and multidirectional instability of the shoulder. A preliminary report. *J Bone Joint Surg Am.* 1980;62(6):897–908.

33. Pollock RG, Owens JM, Flatow EL, Bigliani LU. Operative results of the inferior capsular shift procedure for multidirectional instability of the shoulder. *J Bone Joint Surg Am.* 2000;82-A(7):919–928.

34. Wiley WB, Goradia VK, Pearson SE. Arthroscopic capsular plication-shift. *Arthroscopy.* 2005;21(1):119–121.

35. Gaskill TR, Taylor DC, Millett PJ. Management of multidirectional instability of the shoulder. *J Am Acad Orthop Surg.* 2011;19(12):758–767.

36. Yeargan 3rd SA, Briggs KK, Horan MP, Black AK, Hawkins RJ. Determinants of patient satisfaction following surgery for multidirectional instability. *Orthopedics.* 2008;31(7):647.

37. Baker 3rd CL, Mascarenhas R, Kline AJ, Chhabra A, Pombo MW, Bradley JP. Arthroscopic treatment of multidirectional shoulder instability in athletes: a retrospective analysis of 2- to 5-year clinical outcomes. *Am J Sports Med.* 2009;37(9):1712–1720.

38. Vavken P, Tepolt FA, Kocher MS. Open inferior capsular shift for multidirectional shoulder instability in adolescents with generalized ligamentous hyperlaxity or Ehlers-Danlos syndrome. *J Shoulder Elb Surg.* 2016;25(6):907–912.

39. Han KJ, Kim YK, Lim SK, Park JY, Oh KS. The effect of physical characteristics and field position on the shoulder and elbow injuries of 490 baseball players: confirmation of diagnosis by magnetic resonance imaging. *Clin J Sport Med.* 2009;19(4):271–276.

40. Wilk KE, Macrina LC, Fleisig GS, et al. Correlation of glenohumeral internal rotation deficit and total rotational motion to shoulder injuries in professional baseball pitchers. *Am J Sports Med.* 2011;39(2):329–335.

41. Snyder SJ, Karzel RP, Pizzo WD, Ferkel RD, Friedman MJ. Arthroscopy classics. SLAP lesions of the shoulder. *Arthroscopy.* 2010;26(8):1117.

42. Kuhn JE, Lindholm SR, Huston LJ, Soslowsky LJ, Blasier RB. Failure of the biceps superior labral complex: a cadaveric biomechanical investigation comparing the late cocking and early deceleration positions of throwing. *Arthroscopy.* 2003;19(4):373–379.

43. Pradhan RL, Itoi E, Hatakeyama Y, Urayama M, Sato K. Superior labral strain during the throwing motion. A cadaveric study. *Am J Sports Med.* 2001;29(4):488–492.

44. Burkhart SS, Morgan CD, Kibler WB. The disabled throwing shoulder: spectrum of pathology. Part II: evaluation and treatment of SLAP lesions in throwers. *Arthroscopy.* 2003;19(5):531–539.

45. Burkhart SS, Morgan CD, Kibler WB. The disabled throwing shoulder: spectrum of pathology Part I: pathoanatomy and biomechanics. *Arthroscopy.* 2003;19(4):404–420.

46. Grossman MG, Tibone JE, McGarry MH, Schneider DJ, Veneziani S, Lee TQ. A cadaveric model of the throwing shoulder: a possible etiology of superior labrum anterior-to-posterior lesions. *J Bone Joint Surg Am.* 2005;87(4):824–831.

47. Braun S, Kokmeyer D, Millett PJ. Shoulder injuries in the throwing athlete. *J Bone Joint Surg Am.* 2009;91(4):966–978.

48. Keener JD, Brophy RH. Superior labral tears of the shoulder: pathogenesis, evaluation, and treatment. *J Am Acad Orthop Surg.* 2009;17(10):627–637.

49. Amin MF, Youssef AO. The diagnostic value of magnetic resonance arthrography of the shoulder in detection and grading of SLAP lesions: comparison with arthroscopic findings. *Eur J Radiol.* 2012;81(9):2343–2347.

50. Ide J, Maeda S, Takagi K. Sports activity after arthroscopic superior labral repair using suture anchors in overhead-throwing athletes. *Am J Sports Med.* 2005;33(4):507–514.

51. Sayde WM, Cohen SB, Ciccotti MG, Dodson CC. Return to play after Type II superior labral anterior-posterior lesion repairs in athletes: a systematic review. *Clin Orthop Relat Res.* 2012;470(6):1595−1600.

52. Rao AG, Kim TK, Chronopoulos E, McFarland EG. Anatomical variants in the anterosuperior aspect of the glenoid labrum: a statistical analysis of seventy-three cases. *J Bone Joint Surg Am.* 2003;85-A(4):653−659.

53. Fleisig GS, Andrews JR. Prevention of elbow injuries in youth baseball pitchers. *Sport Health.* 2012;4(5):419−424.

54. Fleisig GS, Weber A, Hassell N, Andrews JR. Prevention of elbow injuries in youth baseball pitchers. *Curr Sports Med Rep.* 2009;8(5):250−254.

55. Ray TR. Youth baseball injuries: recognition, treatment, and prevention. *Curr Sports Med Rep.* 2010;9(5):294−298.

56. Fleisig GS, Andrews JR, Cutter GR, et al. Risk of serious injury for young baseball pitchers: a 10-year prospective study. *Am J Sports Med.* 2011;39(2):253−257.

57. Petty DH, Andrews JR, Fleisig GS, Cain EL. Ulnar collateral ligament reconstruction in high school baseball players: clinical results and injury risk factors. *Am J Sports Med.* 2004;32(5):1158−1164.

58. Lyman S, Fleisig GS, Andrews JR, Osinski ED. Effect of pitch type, pitch count, and pitching mechanics on risk of elbow and shoulder pain in youth baseball pitchers. *Am J Sports Med.* 2002;30(4):463−468.

59. Windt J, Gabbett TJ. How do training and competition workloads relate to injury? The workload-injury aetiology model. *Br J Sports Med.* 2017;51(5):428−435.

60. Kibler WB, Kuhn JE, Wilk K, et al. The disabled throwing shoulder: spectrum of pathology-10-year update. *Arthroscopy.* 2013;29(1):141−161 e26.

61. McClure P, Greenberg E, Kareha S. Evaluation and management of scapular dysfunction. *Sport Med Arthrosc Rev.* 2012;20(1):39−48.

62. Kibler WB, Uhl TL, Maddux JW, Brooks PV, Zeller B, McMullen J. Qualitative clinical evaluation of scapular dysfunction: a reliability study. *J Shoulder Elb Surg.* 2002;11(6):550−556.

63. McClure P, Tate AR, Kareha S, Irwin D, Zlupko E. A clinical method for identifying scapular dyskinesis, part 1: reliability. *J Athl Train.* 2009;44(2):160−164.

64. Uhl TL, Kibler WB, Gecewich B, Tripp BL. Evaluation of clinical assessment methods for scapular dyskinesis. *Arthroscopy.* 2009;25(11):1240−1248.

65. Boyle KL, Witt P, Riegger-Krugh C. Intrarater and interrater reliability of the Beighton and horan joint mobility index. *J Athl Train.* 2003;38(4):281−285.

66. Crockett HC, Gross LB, Wilk KE, et al. Osseous adaptation and range of motion at the glenohumeral joint in professional baseball pitchers. *Am J Sports Med.* 2002;30(1):20−26.

67. Bigliani LU, Codd TP, Connor PM, Levine WN, Littlefield MA, Hershon SJ. Shoulder motion and laxity in the professional baseball player. *Am J Sports Med.* 1997;25(5):609−613.

68. Ellenbecker TS, Roetert EP, Bailie DS, Davies GJ, Brown SW. Glenohumeral joint total rotation range of motion in elite tennis players and baseball pitchers. *Med Sci Sport Exerc.* 2002;34(12):2052−2056.

69. Greenberg EM, Fernandez-Fernandez A, Lawrence JT, McClure P. The development of humeral retrotorsion and its relationship to throwing sports. *Sport Health.* 2015;7(6):489−496.

70. Greenberg EM, Lawrence JT, Fernandez-Fernandez A, McClure P. Humeral retrotorsion and glenohumeral motion in youth baseball players compared with age-matched nonthrowing athletes. *Am J Sports Med.* 2017;45(2):454−461.

71. Hibberd EE, Oyama S, Myers JB. Increase in humeral retrotorsion accounts for age-related increase in glenohumeral internal rotation deficit in youth and adolescent baseball players. *Am J Sports Med.* 2014.

72. Wilk KE, Meister K, Andrews JR. Current concepts in the rehabilitation of the overhead throwing athlete. *Am J Sports Med.* 2002;30(1):136−151.

73. Wilk KE, Macrina LC, Fleisig GS, et al. Deficits in glenohumeral passive range of motion increase risk of elbow injury in professional baseball pitchers: a prospective study. *Am J Sports Med.* 2014;42(9):2075−2081.

74. Shanley E, Kissenberth MJ, Thigpen CA, et al. Preseason shoulder range of motion screening as a predictor of injury among youth and adolescent baseball pitchers. *J Shoulder Elb Surg.* 2015;24(7):1005−1013.

75. Wilk KE, Reinold MM, Macrina LC, et al. Glenohumeral internal rotation measurements differ depending on stabilization techniques. *Sport Health.* 2009;1(2):131−136.

76. Monti R. Return to hitting: an interval hitting progression and overview of hitting mechanics following injury. *Int J Sports Phys Ther.* 2015;10(7):1059−1073.

77. Ellenbecker TS, Davies GJ. The application of isokinetics in testing and rehabilitation of the shoulder complex. *J Athl Train.* 2000;35(3):338−350.

78. Riemann BL, Davies GJ, Ludwig L, Gardenhour H. Hand-held dynamometer testing of the internal and external rotator musculature based on selected positions to establish normative data and unilateral ratios. *J Shoulder Elb Surg.* 2010;19(8):1175−1183.

79. Byram IR, Bushnell BD, Dugger K, Charron K, Harrell Jr FE, Noonan TJ. Preseason shoulder strength measurements in professional baseball pitchers: identifying players at risk for injury. *Am J Sports Med.* 2010;38(7):1375−1382.

80. Ivey Jr FM, Calhoun JH, Rusche K, Bierschenk J. Isokinetic testing of shoulder strength: normal values. *Arch Phys Med Rehabil.* 1985;66(6):384−386.

81. Wilk KE, Obma P, Simpson CD, Cain EL, Dugas JR, Andrews JR. Shoulder injuries in the overhead athlete. *J Orthop Sport Phys Ther.* 2009;39(2):38−54.

82. Shanley E, Thigpen C. Throwing injuries in the adolescent athlete. *Int J Sports Phys Ther.* 2013;8(5):630−640.

83. Hislop HJAD, Brown M. *Daniels and Worthingham's Muscle Testing.* 9th ed. St. Louis, Missouri: Elsevier; 2014.

84. Chu SK, Jayabalan P, Kibler WB, Press J. The kinetic chain revisited: new concepts on throwing mechanics and injury. *PM & R*. 2016;8(3 Suppl):S69–S77.

85. Seroyer ST, Nho SJ, Bach BR, Bush-Joseph CA, Nicholson GP, Romeo AA. The kinetic chain in overhand pitching: its potential role for performance enhancement and injury prevention. *Sports Health*. 2010;2(2):135–146.

86. Huang T-F, Wei S-H, Jung-Chi C, Hsu M-J, Chang H-Y. Isokinetic evaluation of shoulder internal and external rotators concentric strength and endurance in baseball players: variations from pre-pubescence to adulthood. *Isokinet Exerc Sci*. 2005;13(4):237–241.

87. Moore SD, Uhl TL, Kibler WB. Improvements in shoulder endurance following a baseball-specific strengthening program in high school baseball players. *Sports Health*. 2013;5(3):233–238.

88. Pontillo M, Spinelli BA, Sennett BJ. Prediction of in-season shoulder injury from preseason testing in division I collegiate football players. *Sports Health*. 2014;6(6):497–503.

89. Roy JS, Ma B, Macdermid JC, Woodhouse LJ. Shoulder muscle endurance: the development of a standardized and reliable protocol. *Sports Med Arthrosc, Rehabil Ther Technol*. 2011;3(1):1.

90. Anderson VB, Wee E. Impaired joint proprioception at higher shoulder elevations in chronic rotator cuff pathology. *Arch Phys Med Rehabil*. 2011;92(7):1146–1151.

91. Fyhr C, Gustavsson L, Wassinger C, Sole G. The effects of shoulder injury on kinaesthesia: a systematic review and meta-analysis. *Man Ther*. 2015;20(1):28–37.

92. Tripp BL, Yochem EM, Uhl TL. Functional fatigue and upper extremity sensorimotor system acuity in baseball athletes. *J Athl Train*. 2007;42(1):90–98.

93. Laudner KG, Meister K, Kajiyama S, Noel B. The relationship between anterior glenohumeral laxity and proprioception in collegiate baseball players. *Clin J Sport Med*. 2012;22(6):478–482.

94. Vafadar AK, Cote JN, Archambault PS. Interrater and intrarater reliability and validity of 3 measurement methods for shoulder-position sense. *J Sport Rehabil*. 2016. Technical Report 19:2014-0309.

95. Dilek B, Gulbahar S, Gundogdu M, et al. Efficacy of proprioceptive exercises in patients with subacromial impingement syndrome: a single-blinded randomized controlled study. *Am J Phys Med Rehab*. 2016;95(3):169–182.

96. Marzetti E, Rabini A, Piccinini G, et al. Neurocognitive therapeutic exercise improves pain and function in patients with shoulder impingement syndrome: a single-blind randomized controlled clinical trial. *Eur J Phys Rehabil Med*. 2014;50(3):255–264.

97. Martins LV, Marziale MH. Assessment of proprioceptive exercises in the treatment of rotator cuff disorders in nursing professionals: a randomized controlled clinical trial. *Rev Brasileira Fisioterapia*. 2012;16(6):502–509.

98. Saito M, Kenmoku T, Kameyama K, et al. Relationship between tightness of the hip joint and elbow pain in adolescent baseball players. *Orthopaedic J Sports Med*. 2014;2(5), 2325967114532424.

99. Li X, Ma R, Zhou H, et al. Evaluation of hip internal and external rotation range of motion as an injury risk factor for hip, abdominal and groin injuries in professional baseball players. *Orthop Rev*. 2015;7(4):6142.

100. Holt T, Oliver GD. Hip and upper extremity kinematics in youth baseball pitchers. *J Sport Sci*. 2016;34(9):856–861.

101. Kageyama M, Sugiyama T, Kanehisa H, Maeda A. Difference between adolescent and collegiate baseball pitchers in the kinematics and kinetics of the lower limbs and trunk during pitching motion. *J Sport Sci Med*. 2015;14(2):246–255.

102. Westrick RB, Miller JM, Carow SD, Gerber JP. Exploration of the y-balance test for assessment of upper quarter closed kinetic chain performance. *Int J Sports Phys Ther*. 2012;7(2):139–147.

103. Tong TK, Wu S, Nie J. Sport-specific endurance plank test for evaluation of global core muscle function. *Phys Ther Sport*. 2014;15(1):58–63.

104. Allen BA, Hannon JC, Burns RD, Williams SM. Effect of a core conditioning intervention on tests of trunk muscular endurance in school-aged children. *J Strength Cond Res*. 2014;28(7):2063–2070.

105. Strand SL, Hjelm J, Shoepe TC, Fajardo MA. Norms for an isometric muscle endurance test. *J Hum Kinet*. 2014;40:93–102.

106. McClure PW, Michener LA. Staged approach for rehabilitation classification: shoulder disorders (STAR-Shoulder). *Phys Ther*. 2015;95(5):791–800.

107. Borstad JD, Ludewig PM. Comparison of three stretches for the pectoralis minor muscle. *J Shoulder Elb Surg*. 2006;15(3):324–330.

108. Puentedura EJ, O'Grady WH. Safety of thrust joint manipulation in the thoracic spine: a systematic review. *J Man Manip Ther*. 2015;23(3):154–161.

109. Thomas SJ, Swanik CB, Higginson JS, et al. A bilateral comparison of posterior capsule thickness and its correlation with glenohumeral range of motion and scapular upward rotation in collegiate baseball players. *J Shoulder Elb Surg*. 2011;20(5):708–716.

110. Bailey LB, Shanley E, Hawkins R, et al. Mechanisms of shoulder range of motion deficits in asymptomatic baseball players. *Am J Sports Med*. 2015;43(11):2783–2793.

111. Feuerherd R, Sutherlin MA, Hart JM, Saliba SA. Reliability of and the relationship between ultrasound measurement and three clinical assessments of humeral torsion. *Int J Sports Phys Ther*. 2014;9(7):938–947.

112. Bailey LB, Beattie PF, Shanley E, Seitz AL, Thigpen CA. Current rehabilitation applications for shoulder ultrasound imaging. *J Orthop Sport Phys Ther*. 2015:1–44.

113. McClure P, Balaicuis J, Heiland D, Broersma ME, Thorndike CK, Wood A. A randomized controlled comparison of stretching procedures for posterior shoulder tightness. *J Orthop Sport Phys Ther*. 2007;37(3):108–114.

114. Laudner K, Compton BD, McLoda TA, Walters CM. Acute effects of instrument assisted soft tissue mobilization for improving posterior shoulder range of motion in collegiate baseball players. *Int J Sports Phys Ther*. 2014;9(1):1−7.

115. Wilk KE, Arrigo CA, Hooks TR, Andrews JR. Rehabilitation of the overhead throwing athlete: there is more to it than just external rotation/internal rotation strengthening. *PM & R*. 2016;8(3 Suppl):S78−S90.

116. Wilk KE, Macrina LC, Cain EL, Dugas JR, Andrews JR. Rehabilitation of the overhead athlete's elbow. *Sports Health*. 2012;4(5):404−414.

117. Ellenbecker TS, Elmore E, Bailie DS. Descriptive report of shoulder range of motion and rotational strength 6 and 12 weeks following rotator cuff repair using a mini-open deltoid splitting technique. *J Orthop Sport Phys Ther*. 2006;36(5):326−335.

118. Hoffman MD, Shepanski MA, Mackenzie SP, Clifford PS. Experimentally induced pain perception is acutely reduced by aerobic exercise in people with chronic low back pain. *J Rehabil Res Dev*. 2005;42(2):183−190.

119. Hoffman MD, Shepanski MA, Ruble SB, Valic Z, Buckwalter JB, Clifford PS. Intensity and duration threshold for aerobic exercise-induced analgesia to pressure pain. *Arch Phys Med Rehabil*. 2004;85(7):1183−1187.

120. Koltyn KF, Brellenthin AG, Cook DB, Sehgal N, Hillard C. Mechanisms of exercise-induced hypoalgesia. *J Pain*. 2014;15(12):1294−1304.

121. Petersen AM, Pedersen BK. The anti-inflammatory effect of exercise. *J Appl Physiol*. 2005;98(4):1154−1162.

122. Distefano LJ, Blackburn JT, Marshall SW, Padua DA. Gluteal muscle activation during common therapeutic exercises. *J Orthop Sport Phys Ther*. 2009;39(7):532−540.

123. Macadam P, Cronin J, Contreras B. An examination of the gluteal muscle activity associated with dynamic hip abduction and hip external rotation exercise: a systematic review. *Int J Sports Phys Ther*. 2015;10(5):573−591.

124. Wilk KE, Macrina LC. Nonoperative and postoperative rehabilitation for glenohumeral instability. *Clin Sports Med*. 2013;32(4):865−914.

125. Axe M, Hurd W, Snyder-Mackler L. Data-based interval throwing programs for baseball players. *Sports health*. 2009;1(2):145−153.

126. Arundale A, Silvers H, Logerstedt D, Rojas J, Snyder-Mackler L. An interval kicking progression for return to soccer following lower extremity injury. *Int J Sports Phys Ther*. 2015;10(1):114−127.

127. Adams D, Logerstedt DS, Hunter-Giordano A, Axe MJ, Snyder-Mackler L. Current concepts for anterior cruciate ligament reconstruction: a criterion-based rehabilitation progression. *J Orthop Sport Phys Ther*. 2012;42(7):601−614.

128. Reinold MM, Wilk KE, Reed J, Crenshaw K, Andrews JR. Interval sport programs: guidelines for baseball, tennis, and golf. *J Orthop Sport Phys Ther*. 2002;32(6):293−298.

129. Tucci HT, Martins J, Sposito Gde C, Camarini PM, de Oliveira AS. Closed Kinetic Chain Upper Extremity Stability test (CKCUES test): a reliability study in persons with and without shoulder impingement syndrome. *BMC Musculoskeletal Disorders*. 2014;15:1.

130. Sciascia A, Uhl T. Reliability of strength and performance testing measures and their ability to differentiate persons with and without shoulder symptoms. *Int J Sports Phys Ther*. 2015;10(5):655−666.

131. Negrete RJ, Hanney WJ, Kolber MJ, et al. Reliability, minimal detectable change, and normative values for tests of upper extremity function and power. *J Strength Cond Res*. 2010;24(12):3318−3325.

132. Pontillo MSB, Horneff JG. Profile of upper extremity rotator cuff strength and function in division 1 collegiate athletes. *J Orthop Sport Phys Ther*. 2011;41(1):A45.

133. Fleisig GS, Barrentine SW, Zheng N, Escamilla RF, Andrews JR. Kinematic and kinetic comparison of baseball pitching among various levels of development. *J Biomech*. 1999;32(12):1371−1375.

134. DeFroda SF, Thigpen CA, Kriz PK. Two-dimensional video analysis of youth and adolescent pitching biomechanics: a tool for the common athlete. *Curr Sports Med Rep*. 2016;15(5):350−358.

Index

Note: Page numbers followed by "t" indicate tables and "f" indicate figures.

Printed and bound by CPI Group (UK) Ltd, Croydon, CR0 4YY

03/10/2024

01040300-0012